Understanding Crisis in Critical Care

NOTICE

Medicine is an ever-changing science. As new research and clinical experience broaden our knowledge, changes in treatment and drug therapy are required. The author and the publisher of this work have checked with sources believed to be reliable in their efforts to provide information that is complete and generally in accord with the standards accepted at the time of publication. However, in view of the possibility of human error or changes in medical sciences, neither the author nor the publisher nor any other party who has been involved in the preparation or publication of this work warrants that the information contained herein is in every respect accurate or complete, and they disclaim all responsibility for any errors or omissions or for the results obtained from use of the information contained in this work. Readers are encouraged to confirm the information contained herein with other sources. For example and in particular, readers are advised to check the product information sheet included in the package of each drug they plan to administer to be certain that the information contained in this work is accurate and that changes have not been made in the recommended dose or in the contraindications for administration. This recommendation is of particular importance in connection with new or infrequently used drugs.

Understanding Crisis in Critical Care

Ronaldo C. Go, MD
Assistant Professor of Medicine
Hackensack Meridian School of Medicine
Nutley, New Jersey
Department of Critical Care
Hackensack University Medical Center
Hackensack, New Jersey

New York   Chicago   San Francisco   Athens   London   Madrid
Mexico City   New Delhi   Milan   Singapore   Sydney   Toronto

Understanding Crisis in Critical Care

1 2 3 4 5 6 7 8 9 LCR 26 25 24 23 22 21

ISBN 978-1-264-25871-0
MHID 1-264-25871-2

This book was set in Times NR MT Std by MPS Limited.
The editors were Jason Malley and Kim J. Davis.
The production supervisor was Richard Ruzycka.
Project management was provided by Poonam Bisht, MPS Limited.
The cover designer was W2 Design.

Library of Congress Cataloging-in-Publication Data

Names: Go, Ronaldo Collo, editor.
Title: Understanding crisis in critical care/[edited by] Ronaldo C. Go.
Description: New York : McGraw Hill Education, [2022] | Includes
    bibliographical references and index. | Summary: "This book explores the
    new standard of critical care from the perspective of physicians during
    the heart of the initial U.S. COVID-19 crisis"— Provided by publisher.
Identifiers: LCCN 2021017769 (print) | LCCN 2021017770 (ebook) | ISBN
    9781264258710 (paperback) | ISBN 9781264258727 (ebook)
Subjects: MESH: Critical Care—methods | Communicable Disease
    Control—methods | Pandemics—prevention & control | Critical Illness |
    Emergencies
Classification: LCC RC86.7 (print) | LCC RC86.7 (ebook) | NLM WX 218 |
    DDC 616.02/8—dc23
LC record available at https://lccn.loc.gov/2021017769
LC ebook record available at https://lccn.loc.gov/2021017770

McGraw Hill books are available at special quantity discounts to use
as premiums and sales promotions, or for use in corporate training
programs. To contact a representative, please visit the Contact Us
pages at www.mhprofessional.com.

Contents

Contributors...*xi*
Preface...*xxi*
Dedication..*xxiii*

SECTION I: RESOURCES

Chapter 1
Accommodating the Crisis Surge 3
Ronaldo C. Go and Keith M. Rose

Chapter 2
Nursing 23
Caroline Castro, Jacqueline Siatti, and Katerina Korunovski

Chapter 3
Inflammation and Reperfusion 35
Ronaldo C. Go

Chapter 4
Repurposing Therapies for COVID-19 42
Ronaldo C. Go

Chapter 5
Personal Protective Equipment 71
Avalon Mertens and Ronaldo C. Go

Chapter 6
Thrombosis and Transfusions 90
Alina Dulu, Padmastuti Akella, Mustapha Serhan, and Stephen M. Pastores

Chapter 7
Shock 121
Sung Hong and Karan Omidvari

Chapter 8
Analgesia, Sedation, and Mechanical Ventilation 162
Ronaldo C. Go, Ruchi Jain, Jason Steinfeld, and Bisma Alam

Chapter 9
Endocrinologic Issues During Crisis. 195
Shruti Pandiri, Anne Marie Van Hoven, and Colette M. Knight

Chapter 10
Strategies in Acute Respiratory Distress Syndrome 206
Anjan Devaraj and Michael McBrine

Chapter 11
Acute Kidney Injury and Renal Replacement Therapy. . . 228
Renu D. Muttana

Chapter 12
Transplantation 245
Ella Illuzzi and John Oropello

Chapter 13
Extracorporeal Membrane Oxygenation
Use During Crisis in Critical Care. 257
Samantha K. Brenner

Chapter 14
Post Critical Care in the Geriatric Population 300
Laurie G. Jacobs and Robert A. Zorowitz

Chapter 15
Psychiatric Issues. 321
Francis Aguilar

Chapter 16
Children's Mental Health Issues in Critical Care 338
Aurora Tompar Tiu

Chapter 17
Treating Critically Ill Pediatric Patients 350
Reut Kassif Lerner, Oshri Zaulan, and Itai M. Pessach

Chapter 18
Coping Strategies 370
Aurora Tompar Tiu and Anna C. Go

SECTION II: CRISES IN PANDEMICS

Chapter 19
SARS and MERS 381
Jerry Jomi and Taaran Ballachanda

Chapter 20
COVID-19 402
Danit Arad, Anuja Pradhan, and Zhiyong Peng

Chapter 21
Influenza 434
Steven J. Sperber

Chapter 22
Plague 462
Robert Lee

Chapter 23
Tularemia 473
Han Nguyen

Chapter 24
Ebola and Marburg Virus 478
Armand Gottlieb

Chapter 25
Dengue, Yellow Fever, Chikungunya, Lassa Fever, and Crimean-Congo Hemorrhagic Fever 495
Lopa Maharaja

Chapter 26
Nipah, Hendra, and Rift Valley Fever Viruses 512
Jodi Galaydick

Chapter 27
Pediatrics in Pandemics 526
Katharine N. Clouser, Saranga Agarwal, and Karen Eigen

SECTION III: CRISES IN WAR AND NATURAL DISASTERS

Chapter 28
Bioterrorism 553
Ronaldo C. Go

Chapter 29
Chemical Warfare 578
Abdulrahman Elabor, Nikhita Gadi, Marianne Minock,
Andre Sotelo, and Ronaldo C. Go

Chapter 30
Natural Disasters, Evacuation, and Critical
Care in Austere Conditions 597
Ronaldo C. Go

Chapter 31
Traumatic Brain Injury 604
Ari M. Wachsman

Chapter 32
Thoracic Trauma 626
Avi Benov and Aran N. Gilead

Chapter 33
Abdominal Trauma 645
Jasmin Neal and Matthew Giangola

Chapter 34

Orthopedic Trauma **660**
Adam Gitlin

Chapter 35

Burns **674**
Kailash Kapadia, Haripriya Ayyala, Michael Marano, and Edward S. Lee

Chapter 36

Inhalation Injuries **695**
Bar Cohen, Shaul Gelikas, and Avi Benov

Chapter 37

Immersion, Submersion, and Crush Injuries **704**
Aminat Ibikunle, Anna C. Go, Christina Hajicharalambous, and Chinwe Ogedegbe

Index *711*

Contributors

Saranga Agarwal, MBBS, DCH, MD
Assistant Professor
Department of Pediatrics
Pediatric Critical Care Unit
Joseph M. Sanzari Children's Hospital
Hackensack Meridian School of Medicine
Hackensack, New Jersey
27. Pediatrics in Pandemics

Francis Aguilar, MD
Associate Program Director
Department of Psychiatry and Behavioral Health
Cooper University Hospital
Clinical Instructor
Cooper Medical School of Rowan University
Physician Informaticist
Cooper Medical Informatics and Care Delivery Innovation
Camden, New Jersey
15. Psychiatric Issues

Padmastuti Akella, MD
Critical Care Medicine Fellow
Department of Anesthesiology and Critical Care Medicine
Memorial Sloan Kettering Cancer Center
New York, New York
6. Thrombosis and Transfusions

Bisma Alam, MD
Assistant Professor of Medicine
Hackensack Meridian School of Medicine
Nutley, New Jersey
Department of Critical Care at Hackensack University Medical Center
Hackensack, New Jersey
8. Analgesia, Sedation, and Mechanical Ventilation

Danit Arad, MD, FACP
Assistant Professor of Medicine
Hackensack Meridian School of Medicine
Chief, Division of Hospital Medicine
Hackensack University Medical Center
Hackensack, New Jersey
20. COVID-19

Haripriya Ayyala, MD
Division of Plastic and Reconstructive Surgery
Rutgers New Jersey Medical School
Newark, New Jersey
35. Burns

Taaran Ballachanda, MD
Department of Critical Care
Hackensack University Medical Center
Hackensack, New Jersey
19. SARS and MERS

Avi Benov, MD, MHA
Head, Trauma and Combat Medicine Branch
Israel Defense Force – Medical Corps
32. Thoracic Trauma
36. Inhalation Injuries

Samantha K. Brenner, MD, MPH
Core Assistant Professor of Internal Medicine
Hackensack Meridian School of Medicine
Nutley, New Jersey
13. Extracorporeal Membrane Oxygenation Use During Crisis in Critical Care

Caroline Castro, DNP, FNP-C, BSN, RN
Hackensack University Medical Center
Hackensack, New Jersey
2. Nursing Issues

Katharine N. Clouser, MD
Assistant Professor of Pediatrics
Hackensack Meridian School of Medicine
Nutley, New Jersey
Department of Pediatrics
Hackensack University Medical Center
Hackensack, New Jersey
27. Pediatrics in Pandemics

Bar Cohen, MD
The Trauma and Combat Medicine Branch
Surgeon General's Headquarters
Israel Defense Forces
Ramat Gan, Israel
36. Inhalation Injuries

Anjan Devaraj, MD
Fellow
Division of Pulmonary, Critical Care and Sleep Medicine
Tufts Medical Center
Boston, Massachusetts
10. Strategies in Acute Respiratory Distress Syndrome

Alina Dulu, MD
Associate Professor of Medicine in Clinical Anesthesiology
Weill Cornell Medical College
Associate Attending Physician, Critical Care Medicine
Department of Anesthesiology and Critical Care Medicine
Memorial Sloan Kettering Cancer Center
New York, New York
6. Thrombosis and Transfusions

Karen Eigen, MD
Department of Pediatrics
Hackensack University Medical Center
Hackensack, New Jersey
27. Pediatrics in Pandemics

Abdulrahman Elabor, MD
Fellow, Department of Critical Care
Rutgers New Jersey Medical School
Newark, New Jersey
29. Chemical Warfare

Nikhita Gadi, MD
Resident, Department of Internal Medicine
Hackensack University Medical Center
Hackensack, New Jersey
29. Chemical Warfare

Jodi Galaydick, MD, MPH
Garnet Health Medical Center
Middletown, New York
26. Nipah, Hendra, and Rift Valley Fever Viruses

Shaul Gelikas, MD, MBA
The Trauma and Combat Medicine Branch
Surgeon General's Headquarters
Israel Defense Forces
Ramat Gan, Israel
36. Inhalation Injuries

Matthew Giangola, MD
Assistant Professor of Surgery
Associate Program Director
Hofstra-Northwell Department of Surgery
Long Island Jewish Medical Center
New Hyde, New York
33. Abdominal Trauma

Aran N. Gilead, MD
Department of Thoracic Surgery
Rambam Health Care Campus
Haifa, Israel
32. Thoracic Trauma

Adam Gitlin, MD
Assistant Professor, Department of Orthopedic Surgery and Rehabilitation
University of Florida College of Medicine – Jacksonville
Jacksonville, Florida
34. Orthopedic Trauma

Anna C. Go, MD
UV-Gullas College of Medicine
Cebu, Philippines
18. Coping Strategies
37. Immersion, Submersion, and Crush Injuries

Ronaldo C. Go, MD
Assistant Professor of Medicine
Hackensack Meridian School of Medicine
Nutley, New Jersey
Department of Critical Care
Hackensack University Medical Center
Hackensack, New Jersey
1. Accommodating the Surge
3. Inflammation and Reperfusion
4. Repurposing Therapies for COVID-19
5. Shortages and Solutions to Personal Protective Equipment
8. Analgesia, Sedation, and Mechanical Ventilation
28. Bioterrorism
29. Chemical Warfare
30. Natural Disasters, Evacuation, and Critical Care in Austere Conditions

Armand Gottlieb, MD
Division of Pulmonary, Critical Care, and Sleep Medicine
Tufts Medical Center
Boston, Massachusetts
24. Ebola and Marburg Virus

Christina Hajicharalambous, DO, MS, MSEd
Residency Program Director
Department of Emergency Medicine
Hackensack University Medical Center
Hackensack, New Jersey
37. Immersion, Submersion, and Crush Injuries

Sung Hong, MD
Resident, Department of Internal Medicine
Hackensack University Medical Center
Hackensack, New Jersey
7. Shock

Aminat Ibikunle, MD
PGY3 Emergency Medicine Resident
Department of Emergency Medicine
Hackensack University Medical Center
Hackensack, New Jersey
37. Immersion, Submersion, and Crush Injuries

Ella Illuzzi, MSN, ANP-BC
Head ANP, Transplant ICU
Institute for Critical Care Medicine
Mount Sinai Hospital, New York, NY
Adjunct Clinical Professor
New York University
New York, New York
12. Transplantation

Laurie G. Jacobs, MD, FACP, AGSF
Professor and Chair
Department of Internal Medicine
Hackensack Meridian School of Medicine
Hackensack University Medical Center
Hackensack, New Jersey
14. Post Critical Care in the Geriatric Population

Ruchi Jain, PharmD
Department of Pharmacy
Hackensack University Medical Center
Hackensack, New Jersey
8. Analgesia, Sedation, and Mechanical Ventilation

Jerry Jomi, MD
Division of Pulmonary, Critical Care and Sleep Medicine
Rutgers University Hospital
Newark, New Jersey
19. SARS and MERS

Kailash Kapadia, MD
Division of Plastic and Reconstructive Surgery
Rutgers New Jersey Medical School
Newark, New Jersey
35. Burns

Colette M. Knight, MD
Department of Endocrinology
Hackensack University Medical Center
Hackensack, New Jersey
9. Endocrinologic Issues During Crisis

Katerina Korunovski, BSN, RN, CCRN
Hackensack University Medical Center
Hackensack, New Jersey
2. Nursing Issues

Edward S. Lee, MD
Division of Plastic and Reconstructive Surgery
Rutgers New Jersey Medical School
Newark, New Jersey
35. Burns

Robert Lee, MD
Division of Pulmonary, Critical Care and Sleep Medicine
Hackensack University Medical Center
Hackensack, New Jersey
22. Plague

Reut Kassif Lerner, MD
Department of Pediatric Intensive Care
The Edmond & Lily Safra Children's Hospital Sheba Medical Center
Ramat Gan, Israel
Sackler School of Medicine
Tel Aviv University, Tel Aviv, Israel
17. Treating Critically Ill Pediatric Patients

Lopa Maharaja, MD
Division of Infectious Diseases
Hackensack University Medical Center
Hackensack, New Jersey
25. Dengue, Yellow Fever, Chikungunya, Lassa Fever, and Crimean-Congo Hemorrhagic Fever

Michael Marano, MD
Saint Barnabas Medical Center-The Burn Center
RWJ Barnabas Health
Livingston, New Jersey
35. Burns

Michael McBrine, MD
Program Director
Pulmonary and Critical Care Fellowship
Tufts Medical Center
Boston, Massachusetts
10. Strategies in Acute Respiratory Distress Syndrome

Avalon Mertens, DO
Fellow
Division of Pulmonary, Critical Care and Sleep Medicine
Rutgers New Jersey Medical School
Newark, New Jersey
5. Shortages and Solutions to Personal Protective Equipment

Marianne Minock, MSN, APN-C
Department of Critical Care,
Hackensack University Medical Center,
Hackensack, New Jersey
29. Chemical Warfare

Renu D. Muttana, MD
Attending Physician
Jacobi Medical Center
Bronx, New York
11. Acute Kidney Injury and Renal Replacement Therapy

Jasmin Neal, MD
Resident
Hofstra-Northwell Department of Surgery
Hempstead, New York
33. Abdominal Trauma

Han Nguyen, MD
Division of Infectious Diseases
Hackensack University Medical Center
Hackensack, New Jersey
23. Tularemia

Chinwe Ogedegbe, MD, MPH
Department of Emergency Medicine
Hackensack University Medical Center
Hackensack, New Jersey
37. Immersion, Submersion, and Crush Injuries

Karan Omidvari, MD
Associate Professor of Medicine
Hackensack Meridian School of Medicine
Nutley, New Jersey
7. Shock

John Oropello, MD
Director, Transplant ICU
Institute for Critical Care Medicine
Mount Sinai Hospital,
Professor of Surgery and Medicine
Department of Surgery
Mount Sinai School of Medicine
New York, New York
12. Transplantation

Shruti Pandiri, MD
Department of Endocrinology
Hackensack University Medical Center
Hackensack, New Jersey
9. Endocrinologic Issues During Crisis

Stephen M. Pastores, MD
Professor of Medicine and Anesthesiology
Weill Cornell Medical College
Program Director, Critical Care Medicine
Department of Anesthesiology and Critical Care Medicine
Memorial Sloan Kettering Cancer Center
New York, New York
6. Thrombosis and Transfusions

Zhiyong Peng, MD
Professor and Chair of Critical Care Medicine
Zhongnan Hospital of Wuhan University
Wuhan, Hubei, China
20. COVID-19

Itai M. Pessach, MD, PhD, MPH, MHA
Director
The Edmond and Lily Safra Children's Hospital
Sheba Medical Center, Tel-Hashomer
Assistant Professor of Pediatrics
Sackler Faculty of Medicine
Tel-Aviv University
Tel-Aviv, Israel
17. Treating Critically Ill Pediatric Patients

Anuja Pradhan, MD
Assistant Professor of Medicine
Hackensack Meridian School of Medicine
Hackensack University Medical Center
Division of Pulmonary & Critical Care Medicine
Division of Infectious Disease
Hackensack, New Jersey
20. COVID-19

Keith M. Rose, MD
Associate Professor of Medicine
Hackensack Meridian School of Medicine
Nutley, New Jersey
Chair, Department of Critical Care
Hackensack University Medical Center
Hackensack, New Jersey
1. Accommodating the Surge

Mustapha Serhan, MD
Critical Care Medicine Fellow
Department of Anesthesiology and Critical Care Medicine
Memorial Sloan Kettering Cancer Center
New York, New York
6. Thrombosis and Transfusions

Jacqueline Siatti, BSN, RN, CCRN
Hackensack University Medical Center
Hackensack, New Jersey
2. Nursing Issues

Andre Sotelo, MD
Assistant Professor of Medicine
Hackensack Meridian School of Medicine
Hackensack, New Jersey
29. Chemical Warfare

Steven J. Sperber, MD, FACP, FIDSA
Associate Professor of Medicine
Hackensack Meridian School of Medicine
Chief, Division of Infectious Diseases
Hackensack University Medical Center
Hackensack, New Jersey
21. Influenza

Jason Steinfeld, BHA, RRT
Clinical Specialist
Northeast Region
8. Analgesia, Sedation, and Mechanical Ventilation

Aurora Tompar Tiu, MD
Voluntary Child/Adolescent Psychiatrist
Department of Psychiatry
Montefiore Medical Center
Bronx, New York
16. Children's Mental Health Issues in Critical Care
18. Coping Strategies

Anne Marie Van Hoven, MD
Department of Endocrinology
Hackensack University Medical Center
Hackensack, New Jersey
9. Endocrinologic Issues During Crisis

Ari M. Wachsman, MD
Assistant Professor of Neurology and Neurosurgery
Case Western Reserve School of Medicine
Director, Neurocritical Care Unit
MetroHealth Medical Center
Cleveland, Ohio
31. Traumatic Brain Injury

Oshri Zaulan, MD, MHA
Department of Critical Care Medicine
Division of Cardiac Critical Care and Cardiology
The Labatt Family Heart Centre
The Hospital for Sick Children
Toronto, Ontario, Canada
17. Treating Critically Ill Pediatric Patients

Robert A. Zorowitz, MD, MBA, FACP, AGSF, CMD
Regional Vice President, Health Affairs
Northeast
Humana Inc.
New York, New York
14. Post Critical Care in the Geriatric Population

Preface

Understanding Crisis in Critical Care is a narrative on accommodating an overwhelming surge of critically ill patients from pandemics, natural disasters, or war, while ensuring the safety of the healthcare staff. During crisis, the standard of critical care is dictated by the available resources. Triage models are used to provide treatment based on the best level of evidence for the available resources. Various stakeholders continuously reassess the supply with the patient load. Drugs are repurposed to meet the time of need. Healthcare providers go beyond their specialty to provide care for any patient.

Inspired by coronavirus disease 2019, the narrative is driven by this pandemic. The initial approach for any crisis is similar. However, each cause of crisis can have unique challenges.

I hope this book provides insight into the present and any future crises.

Ronaldo C. Go, MD
Assistant Professor of Medicine
Hackensack Meridian School of Medicine
and
Department of Critical Care
Hackensack University Medical Center
Hackensack, New Jersey

Dedicated to:

Pater Noster

Qui es in coelis

Jesu, Joseph, Anthony, Jude, Pio, Mary, Michael, Gerard, Bernadette, Faustina

Evangeline, Benjamin, Anna, Jean, Gabriela, Rafeala, Juan, Esther, Aida

Collo, Go, Truyol, Bediones, and Rodriguez families

Cresencia, Leah, Jose

Norma, Robert

Sam, June, Rosie

Natalio, Brigida

Maring, Saring

Our patients

Deo confidimus

SECTION I
Resources

ACCOMMODATING THE CRISIS SURGE 1

Ronaldo C. Go, MD and Keith M. Rose, MD

▍INTRODUCTION

A health care crisis is triggered by a natural disaster, an infectious disease, or acts of war. The surge can occur over a short period or linger for a prolonged period of time. It can also evolve, with ever-changing treatment guidelines. With inadequate planning, transition from resource rich to resource poor conditions can occur.

The recent health crisis is coronavirus disease 2019 (COVID-19). According to the World Health Organization (WHO), there are 155,506,494 cases and 3,247,228 deaths worldwide.[1] As of May 6, 2021, there were 32,356,034 cases with 576,238 deaths in the United States.[2] The New York City (NYC) region was an epicenter for COVID-19 during the initial surge from March to June 2020. One expected the volume at a local hospital to double every three to five days.[3] Hackensack University Medical Center (HUMC) is a 771 bed hospital in northern New Jersey just outside of New York City, and had one of the largest inpatient COVID-19 cases in one hospital.

We would like to describe our protocol to accommodate the first COVID-19 surge from March to June 2020 by the conversion of 47 intensive care unit (ICU) beds to 190 ICU beds, and our plan to return to normal operations. We performed daily surveillance for new peer reviewed literature and guidance from the Centers for Disease Control and Prevention (CDC), WHO, American College of Chest Physicians (ACCP), and Society of Critical Care Medicine (SCCM).[1–7] We consolidated their recommendations and adjusted for our hospital, resources, and patient needs. The strategies included tier-based staffing models, mechanical ventilator allocation, adjustments for medication shortages, cleaning and reusing of personal protective equipment (PPE), as well as designated teams for vascular access, intubations, prone positioning, and updating of families, counseling for health care workers, and decontamination of COVID-19 designated floors once the COVID-19 census decreased.

▌DAILY COVID-19 MEETINGS

This was a multidisciplinary assessment of the current number of patients, opening and conversion of various units, available PPE, mechanical ventilation, medical supplies, and new treatment options. A follow-up meeting in the afternoon re-assessed and identified any adjustments to the action plan.

To accommodate the surge in patients, coordination and input from various stakeholders were essential. The clinical teams include medicine, emergency medicine, surgery, critical care (physicians, nursing, and respiratory), as well as the departments of Engineering, Biomedical Engineering, Plant Operations, Environmental Services, Information Technology, Capacity management/Bed Board, and Hospital Leadership/ Administration.[4]

▌IDENTIFICATION OF PATIENTS

Maximizing the containment to reduce community impact is key. Patients under investigation (PUI) are rapidly identified through their history, physical examination, and laboratory values. They are isolated in the emergency department (ED) and triaged to the appropriate ward or unit according to the lab results.

▌COHORT

We geographically cohorted COVID-19 patients to minimize health care personnel exposure and conserve supplies.[8] As the COVID-19 patient population grew, future COVID-19 wards were identified in weekly meetings. Generally, we planned and reviewed the next two areas for conversion daily for both ICU and medical wards.

Creating Additional ICU Space

We normally function with 47 ICU beds. During the COVID-19 crisis, we increased our capacity to 170 ICU beds by creating additional intensive care units (10 additional units, 12 in total) with the immediate ability to extend to 190. We favored single room occupancy, but if not possible, two beds were placed in one room at least two meters apart. We incrementally converted medical and surgical floors into ICUs. When one ICU was nearing capacity, we ensured we had plans for the next two unit conversions. Each new ICU space was adapted to create negative pressure rooms compliant with CDC guidelines. Floors were chosen for ICU conversion primarily based on their ability to be converted to negative pressure rooms, but also with considerations for geographic location and physical layout. Floors that had rooms with large windowed doors were favored as this greatly improved patient visibility. If needed, doors were adapted to have windows. As doors must be kept closed, this higher visibility proved paramount in recognizing emergent situations.

Floors that had their own isolated air handlers were most easily converted to negative pressure rooms. When unable to be converted to negative pressure rooms using the ventilation system, rooms were individually modified using high efficiency particulate air (HEPA) filter air scrubbers (Figure 1-1) and vented outside. HEPA filters can remove airborne particles as low as 0.3 um.[9] Minimum efficiency reporting values (MERVs) report the filter's efficiency to capture particles.[9] A MERV rating of 1–4 can capture particle size 3–10 um with efficiency < 20% whereas a MERV rating of 16 can capture particle size 0.3–0.1 um with ≥ 75% efficiency.[9] Since the particle size of SARS-CoV-2 was < 5 um,

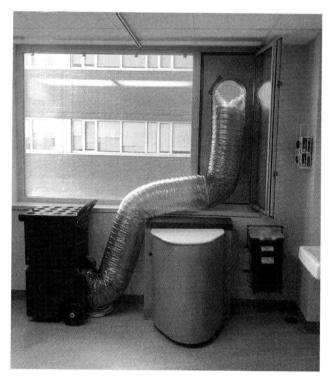

Figure 1-1 • Room is modified using HEPA filter air scrubbers with ventilation to outside.

this method allows 6–12 changes per hour and pressure and airflow direction was from the corridor to the room and then exhausted outside through the room's modified windows.[10] Rooms were then regularly spot-checked using smoke tests to ensure negative pressure was maintained.

Creating Additional Medical Space

In addition to ICU space, the hospital also needed to expand the capacity of medical beds, quickly growing from a 770 bed facility to one with 954 beds. Further plans were made to expand to 1,100 beds. Canceling all elective procedures and surgeries, and facilitating appropriate medical discharges helped alleviate the non-COVID-19 volume of patients and allowed for expansion into these existing wards. When these spaces were exhausted, non-conventional space was utilized. We converted a large seating area of the cafeteria (9,500 square feet) to a 76 bed COVID-19 medical ward. This entire area was made negative pressure as opposed the individual rooms, necessitating the continuous use of N95 masks by all medical staff in this area.

Additional non-ICU growth capacity was continually pre-identified and further unconventional spaces were considered. Plans were made for several areas to host exterior tents to accommodate these patients. Although not yet needed, we have a formalized plan to externalize nearly the entire ED to a tented space, leaving the traditional ED space to be used as both critical care rooms (with negative pressure) and medical ward rooms. One section of the ED had rooms that were already capable of maintaining negative pressure, making an easy conversion to ICU space.

PERSONAL PROTECTIVE EQUIPMENT

PPE is designed to protect the health care provider from any contact with chemical or biologic hazards.[6–21] As per CDC, optimization of the supply of PPE follows a sequential order from conventional capacity, contingency capacity, and crisis capacity.[12] In crisis capacity, all elective and non-urgent procedures are canceled. N95 respirators and face masks are used beyond the manufacturer's shelf-life, approved under standards from other countries, or reused.[12] Isolation gowns' use are extended, or cloth isolation gowns are reused.[12] Eye protection devices and gloves are used beyond their shelf life.[12]

There are four levels, and with COVID-19, a modified Level A is advocated (Table 1-1). The current evidence suggested airborne risk. We

Table 1-1 LEVELS OF PPE[7]	
Level	Description
A	• Highest level of respiratory, skin, eye, and mucous membrane protection needed • Positive pressure, self contained breathing apparatus (SCBA), or positive pressure supplied with air respirator with SCBA • Chemical suit • Inner and outer chemical resistant gloves • Chemical resistant boots
B	• Highest level of respiratory, but lesser level for skin and eye • Positive pressure, self contained breathing apparatus (SCBA), or positive pressure supplied with air respirator with SCBA • Chemical resistant clothing • Inner and outer chemical resistant gloves • Chemical resistant boots
C	• Airborne substance is known, and skin and eye exposure unlikely • Full face or half mask, air purifying respirator • Chemical resistant clothing • Inner and outer chemical resistant gloves • Chemical resistant boots
D	• Work uniform

practiced donning and doffing of PPE as suggested by the CDC.[2] To conserve our resources, we limited the number of health care personnel entering the room. When available, we had dedicated staff monitoring that the PPE was worn properly prior to entering the room. Fit tested National Institute of Occupational Safety and Health (NIOSH) N95 masks were reused if a surgical mask was worn on top of it. Face shields can be reused if they are cleaned with germicidal wipes and air dried. Hand washing is key, even while wearing gloves. Shortages of PPE made these conservation efforts paramount. Powered air-purifying respirators (PAPRs) were alternatives, particularly for those who are intubating patients (Figure 1-2).

Due to shortages, methods of PPE decontamination such as hydrogen peroxide vaporization, UV treatment, moist heat, and dry heat were explored. The method must demonstrate a $\geq 6 \log_{10}$ reduction of bacterial spores and $< 3 \log_{10}$ reduction in viral infectivity. In our institution, we used UV light to sterilize N95. The number of times a N95 can be reused is limited to fit, filtration performance, contamination and soiling,

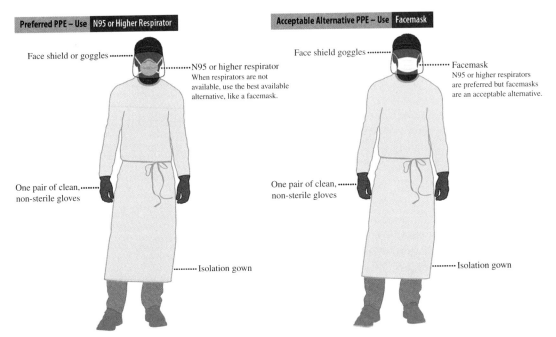

Figure 1-2 • Preferred PPE and alternative PPE as per CDC.[13] (Used with permission from Centers for Disease Control and Prevention. https://www.cdc.gov/coronavirus/2019-ncov/downloads/A_FS_HCP_COVID19_PPE.pdf.)

and damage. The masks were placed in a personally labeled brown bag and collected for cleaning twice daily. These masks were taken for UV light treatment and returned to the drop off site by the next shift. We limited this process to three sessions due to data suggesting that frequent use of UV light can degrade the N95 mask fibers (Figure 1-3).[14,15]

Face shields were reused by being cleaned with germicidal disposable wipes. They were then air dried for 2 minutes. Later, we had shortages of disposable wipes, so bags of towels or wipes soaked in bleach or germicidal fluid in plastic bags were distributed daily throughout the units.

COMMAND CENTER

The command center helped ensure every unit had enough supplies to care for the rapidly surging population of patients. They coordinated with purchasing and distribution departments to continually update the clinical teams and provide support where needed.

TELEMEDICINE

Telemedicine helped attenuate transmission of SARS-CoV-2 between health care professionals and patients while providing patient care.[22]

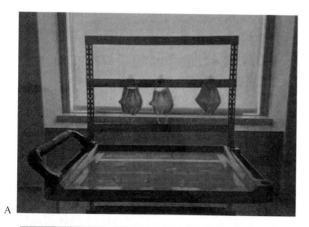

A

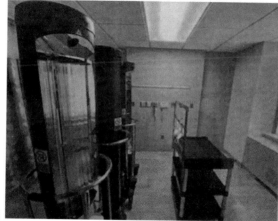

B

Figure 1-3 • A. N95 masks hung for UV cleaning. **B.** Position of UV lights and N95 masks.

There are three modalities: (1) synchronous, which is real-time telephone or live audio interaction via smartphone or computer; (2) asynchronous, where previously recorded images and/or messages are interpreted or responded later; and (3) remote patient monitoring.[22] For the most part, we used synchronous and asynchronous modalities to help with our outpatient clinics.

BLOOD WORK AND IMAGING STUDIES

Ancillary services were also stressed with the increased volume of patients and tests. We made attempts to limit routine blood work including arterial blood gases (ABGs) to once a day. However, if clinically necessary they were performed as needed. Labs were generally drawn by the bedside nurse in the morning. Similarly, we made efforts to avoid unnecessary radiographic imaging.

▌ PHARMACY

As the COVID-19 surge peaked, we had several medication shortages. Drug shortages can cause consequences such as medication errors with drug omission, dispensing, or administration, and alternative treatment may be less effective or have higher adverse events.[23] The pharmacy team designed evidence-based treatment guidelines and algorithms with treatment alternatives and drug demand analysis, and implemented medication sparing strategies.[23]

For sedation, we initially preferred fentanyl and propofol as per SCCM guidelines.[24] Benzodiazepines were avoided, but with sedation shortages and patients requiring heavier sedation, midazolam infusions were used. Hydromorphone infusions were also used with fentanyl shortages. This led to midazolam shortages, prompting us to use ketamine infusions.[25,26] Prior to this, ketamine had been used only for procedural sedation and had not been for longer term use in critically ill patients. We worked closely with our clinical pharmacists to continually strategize what would be the next substitute in case of other anticipated medication shortages.

For COVID-19 specific treatment, direct access including compassionate use medications were re-evaluated on a weekly basis. We were involved in clinical trials. There were multiple ongoing studies, and the process was streamlined. Physicians would place an order in the electronic medical record (EMR) for clinical trial referral, and the cases were then reviewed by a research team to determine which studies the patient would be eligible for. This information was then relayed back to the primary team.

Our COVID-19 treatment algorithm was continually evolving based on data as it became available. Treatment options included hydroxychloroquine, Azithromycin, tocilizumab, remdesivir, convalescent plasma, and corticosteroids. Corticosteroids were used to mitigate the inflammatory response in the late phase of the illness. They were generally given for 5–7 days consistent with recommendations from Surviving Sepsis Campaign regarding Acute Respiratory Distress Syndrome (ARDS).[27,28] This was later modified from methylprednisolone to dexamethasone 6 mg IV/PO daily for up to 10 days for patients requiring oxygen supplementation.[29]

Certain treatment guidelines were modified to preserve PPE and decrease health care provider and patient contact. One example is treatment modifications for diabetic ketoacidosis (DKA). Although we advocated for continuous insulin drip and glucose checks every hour, we were aware of alternatives such as: (1) SC lispro 0.15 units/kg and glucose checks every 2 hours and once glucose < 250 mg/dL, interval increased to every 4 hours and (2) glargine 0.25 units/kg within 12 hours of initiation of IV insulin.[30–37] Another is the preference for enoxaparin therapeutic dose instead of heparin drip to treat acute coronary syndrome and pulmonary embolism (PE).

▌TIERED-BASED STAFFING FOR PHYSICIANS

Most of the ICUs can accommodate 26 patients. We modified SCCM's Tiered Staffing Strategy for the pandemic.[38] We favored having a full time faculty intensivist to cover 13 beds, and recruited other non-intensivist physicians to cover the other 13 beds. This allowed one intensivist in each unit to troubleshoot for all 26 patients. We had cardiologists, surgeons, pediatric intensivists, and hospitalists working alongside our critical care physicians. We also staffed each unit with non-critical care fellows, medical residents, or Advanced Practice Provider (APP) to assist in the care of these patients.

▌TIERED-BASED STAFFING FOR NURSES

Nurse staffing proved to be the most difficult task. Creating a tiered model, intensive care unit nurses served as mentors and worked alongside step-down and medical-surgical nurses in converted COVID-19 critical care units. We also made use of traveler nurses to help staff the newly transformed medical wards and ICUs. Having one or two experienced critical care nurses on a critical care floor with non-ICU nurses proved effective, and this leadership by experienced critical care nurses proved invaluable.

It is particularly important on the day a new ICU is opened to have extra critical care nurses on duty. These shifts tend to have multiple new patients arriving on a unit in succession, often with high intensity needs.

ICU nursing staffing ratios were stretched from traditional 2:1 to 3:1 or even 4:1 when needed. Helpers were recruited to assist in the care of these patients to ensure the nurse could deliver specialized nursing care to all the patients.

Nursing Adjustments

To minimize health care personnel exposure without compromising patient care, extension tubing (MRI tubing is long without the side ports) was used to administer continuous infusions. By doing this, the pumps could be kept outside of the rooms. Minor adjustments in drip rates could then be made more efficiently without using PPE. This also allowed quick administration of certain meds without requiring the extra time to put on the proper PPE. Care was taken to protect these long stretches of tubing and minimize direct contact with the floor. Medications that require frequent monitoring such as insulin drips were avoided but sometimes needed. Store bought baby monitors (audio and video) were used to help monitor the patients as the doors to the rooms were necessarily closed.

RESPIRATORY FAILURE

The goal was to improve oxygenation while preventing aerosolization. If patients on nasal cannula required higher levels of oxygenation supplementation, we favored non-rebreather masks to minimize aerosol generation. High flow nasal cannula was also employed, though patients were advised to wear a surgical mask over the high flow nasal cannula to help minimize potential aerosols. Non-invasive ventilation using traditional BiPAP masks was generally avoided, though we were aware some centers were using this modality with a closed mask and a filter on the expiratory limb of the device. Despite this, we still had significant concerns with this approach given significant mask leak potential and concerns that patients often remove the masks themselves, increasing the potential to generate aerosols. We did not have access to helmet Continuous Positive Airway Pressure (CPAP) devices at the time of this pandemic, though there is interest in using this modality in this disease.

Similarly, we avoided use of nebulized medications. Bronchodilators were mainly given via meter dose inhalers (MDI) with or without ventilators. MDI with spacer is preferred, allowing the patient to take slow deep breaths and improve medication delivery.[5] If nebulizers were used with a ventilator circuit, a one way valve was placed to mitigate this aerosolization risk. To facilitate mobilization of secretions in non-intubated patients, flutter valves were occasionally used.

Some ventilators have a detachable interphase, which could be placed outside the ICU room. Although we did not utilize this technology, this could allow vent changes more readily without going into the room.

Intubation

Pre-oxygenation was delivered via non-rebreather or high flow nasal cannula (HFNC). Both modalities were often used together for the most severely hypoxemic patients. We favored rapid sequence intubation (RSI) via video laryngoscopy, performed by the most experienced operator on hand, which was typically an anesthesiologist.[39] Bag valve mask (BVM) was minimized or avoided if possible due to further concerns of aerosolization. If needed, BVM was performed using an attached filter.

We formed intubation teams led by an Anesthesiologist to assist with the large number of intubations. However, if an unplanned extubation or sudden clinical decompensation occurred, the intensivist at the bedside would typically perform the intubation given the urgency of the situation.

Intubation boxes made of clear plastic were purchased and kept on each floor to help protect the operator during the procedure. These tended to be somewhat bulky but were successfully used. Alternative, more portable options are also available.

Mechanical Ventilation

This was advocated for COVID-19 patients with rapid clinical decline or worsening PaO_2. We invoked a strategy of watchful waiting and accepting significant hypoxemia while using high flow nasal O_2 and 100% non-rebreather masks, often simultaneously in severe cases. Despite tolerating the relative hypoxemia, intubation was often inevitable. All patients were initiated on ARDSnet protocol with a low tidal volume strategy.[40] We used moderate PEEP in these patients to achieve oxygenation. Treatment threshold goals include: Plateau pressure < 30 cm H_2O, pH > 7.20 with permissive hypercapnia, and tidal volume 6–8 ml/kg per IBW.[40] Each ventilator had a HEPA filter or pleated hydrophobic filter in the expiratory ports. Heat and moisture exchanger should be used instead of heated humidifier.

Due to limitations in availability of mechanical ventilators, we applied a six-tiered approach to ventilator allocation.[41] Tier 1 referred to conventional critical care ventilators; Tier 2 included transport ventilators or BiPAP V60s with modified circuits (these non-invasive ventilation devices can be converted to pressure control ventilators); Tier 3 were disaster and disposable ventilators; Tier 4 were anesthesia machines; Tier 5 was considered having two patients on one ventilator; Tier 6 referred to rationing of equipment. We were able to manage with Tier 1 and Tier 2 ventilators but were prepared to go higher. We were able to purchase additional Tier 1 ventilators as we began ramping up our response. We recommended increasing ventilator capacity as much as feasible in anticipation of a local epidemic/surge in COVID-19 cases.

A plan for resource allocation was necessary in the event the supply of ventilators or other life sustaining equipment became limited. We worked closely with our bioethics department and formulated a plan to deal with this possible contingency. In turn, legal implications were also considered. Co-venting (two patients sharing one ventilator) was considered, but ultimately felt to be a last resort that would only be considered before the bioethical dilemma of choosing which patient would not be able to get a ventilator. It was important, though, to consider this option, and establish a proof of concept to better understand all the challenges that may arise from it. Other authors have suggested using prognostic scores such as Sequential Organ Failure Assessment (SOFA) or reassess every seven days to determine who would benefit the most from mechanical ventilation.[42]

Prone Position

Due to the results of the PROSEVA trial,[43] we advocated for the early prone position in moderate to severe ARDS (PaO_2/FiO_2 ratio < 200). Most of our patients responded exceedingly well to prone positioning with significant improvement in oxygenation. We continued prone positioning (16 hours prone) daily for most patients until there was significant improvement in their oxygenation with most patients, requiring it for at least five days. This was discontinued when the patient was able to be maintained with a FiO_2 of 50% and PEEP of 10 if they did not develop significant worsening of hypoxemia while supine. The decision, however, was ultimately at the discretion of the primary team.

To facilitate this workload, we created a dedicated "prone team" that rounded on all on COVID-19 ICUs daily. The team kept a patient list and schedule and were reachable on a direct phone line to discuss new cases, changes in schedules, or any concerns. After discussion with the primary team and nursing, patients were placed in prone position for a maximum of 16 hours per day, and then placed supine for eight hours. The dramatic improvement in oxygenation while in prone position for most patients was found to often immediately reverse while returning to the supine position. We created a specialized COVID-19 ARDS protocol to accommodate this effect. FiO_2 adjustments were made while both prone and supine; however, PEEP adjustments were only made while supine. FiO_2 was also typically increased by 10%–20% just before supinating in anticipation of the changes. This prevented the vast majority of decompensations while returning to the supine position.

Because of these dramatic improvements in oxygenation with prone positioning of intubated COVID-19 patients, select patients that were not intubated were asked to self-prone. This was done for four-hour intervals and also encouraged while sleeping. An "awake prone" protocol was created to help guide nursing and staff on both critical care units and medical wards.

IV Access and Continuous Blood Pressure Monitoring

We found early central venous catheter and arterial catheter placement helpful in the majority of our mechanically ventilated patients, particularly in candidates for prone positioning. Axillary arterial catheters were favored due to ease of placement and less problems with positional alterations. A line team was created consisting predominantly of surgeons and surgery residents. They were available 24 hours a day to place these catheters and also change them when necessary.

NUTRITION

We continued enteral nutrition with continuous tube feeds; however, the pumps for tube feeds soon were also in short supply. Bolus feeds were initiated in these cases. We maintained our goal nutritional targets whether prone or supine. Feeds were only held one hour before transitions between prone and supine positions. Although there has been no general consensus on bolus feeds versus continuous feeds, and trophic feeds versus full feeds, we attempted to fully meet our patients' nutritional goals.[44-48]

FAMILY COMMUNICATION

Due to restrictions on visitors, communication was primarily done by phone, which was considerably time consuming. To help manage these demands, we developed a dedicated team of medical staff that would make daily calls and give updates to the families of our patients. The communication team was made up primarily of staff physicians who volunteered as well as some medical students. Goals of care, treatment, and consent discussions, however, were always performed by the primary medical team. There were numerous requests by families to use FaceTime so they could actually see their loved ones. We were able to accommodate this, but needed to ensure Health Insurance Portability and Accountability Act (HIPAA) compliance.

GOALS OF CARE

This is discussed in the emergency department and prior to invasive mechanical ventilation. However, during a pandemic, with limited resources, the typical standard approach does not necessarily apply. This is referred to as crisis standard of care (CSOC), to allocate resources. Do not attempt resuscitation (DNAR) is similar to do not resuscitate (DNR) except no formal consent from patient or surrogate is required. This was deemed important to prevent doing CPR with significant exposure to the staff in cases that would not benefit from CPR. The conditions that needed to be met to enact this directive were (1) the patient will likely re-arrest within 24 hours; (2) a second physician not involved in the care of the patient concurs; (3) patient or surrogate notified; (4) documentation in chart; (5) involvement of bioethics; and (6) can be revoked if patient improves.

CODE CARTS AND CARDIAC ARREST

Due to limited supply, and concerns over contaminating a full code cart, COVID-19 CODE bags were made. Contents include 5 epinephrine 1 mg/10 mL, 1 calcium chloride 1 g/10 mL, 2 sodium bicarbonate, and 2 amiodarone 150 mg/3 mL. Code trays will not enter the room. Full code trays are available outside of the room if additional medications are needed. Prior to resuscitation, a full length transparent plastic cover can be placed on top of the patient to help protect from contamination of the staff.

CONSENTS

Verbal consents are obtained from the patient if they are competent via hospital phone or by health care proxy or surrogate.

NON-COVID-19 CRITICALLY ILL PATIENTS

Due to staffing constraints, patients who were admitted for non-COVID-19 related causes were initially assessed by the medical ICU team, but were then managed by the surgical intensive care unit (SICU) intensivists. The medical team was available to follow these patients if any issues arose. Patients who were considered as patients under investigation (PUI) or "rule-out COVID" remained in the ED until the results of the PCR test were available. Prior to the availability of rapidly available testing, a specific PUI unit was created. This unit had negative pressure single rooms and served as a staging area prior to admission to COVID or non-COVID units. If a PUI required ICU level care, they could be admitted to a single occupancy, negative pressure room in one of the COVID ICUs.

POST-COVID-19

Starting at the end of April, the numbers of new COVID-19 admissions have been decreasing, and non-COVID–related admissions are increasing. Less urgent surgeries are being performed and more routine radiographic imaging services have resumed. COVID-19 floors are being converted back to non-COVID-19 floors in a controlled, stepwise fashion. To maintain a buffer, we ensure that we have 12 available COVID ICU beds available prior to closing a unit. When the threshold gets close, the selected unit begins to not take new admissions. Once the threshold is achieved, the remaining patients on that unit can be moved to other COVID-19 ICUs.

Discontinuation of Precautions and Patient Discharge

Discontinuation of precautions should depend on severity of illness and onset of symptoms.[49] Precautions can be removed upon resolution of symptoms and fever without anti-pyretics and two negative FDA approved SARS-CoV-2 RNA assay, $\geq$ 24 hours apart.[49] However, discontinuation of precautions is not a prerequisite from hospital discharge. As per CDC guidelines, patients who have mild to moderate illness can be discharged if $\geq$ 10 days have passed from the initiation of symptoms, $\geq$ 24 hours since last fever without any anti-pyretics, and symptoms improved.[49] Patients who have severe to critical illness or are immunocompromised can be discharged if $\geq$ 10–20 days since initiation of symptoms, $\geq$ 24 hours from last fever without any anti-pyretics, symptoms improved, and consultation with infectious disease physicians.[49]

Severity of Illness	Description
Mild	Fever, cough, sore throat, malaise, headache, muscle pain without shortness of breath or abnormal chest radiograph
Moderate	Respiratory symptoms, oxygen saturation (SpO_2) $\geq$ 94%, and abnormal radiograph
Severe	Respiratory rate > 30 breaths per minute, SpO_2 < 94% on room air or 3% decrease from baseline, arterial partial pressure of oxygen to fraction of inspired oxygen (PaO_2/FiO_2) < 300 mm Hg or lung infiltrates > 50%
Critical	Respiratory failure, septic shock, and/or multi-organ dysfunction

If there is lack of available SARS-CoV-2 PCR and concern for prolonged viral shedding below the limit of detection, we would considering using WHO's recommendations: for symptomatic patients, 10 days from onset of symptoms plus > 3 additional days without symptoms and fever.[50]

Decontamination

We needed to create a new non-COVID ICU as the traditional ICU was fully occupied by COVID-19 cases with many patients on extracorporeal membrane oxygenation (ECMO) that are difficult to move and require specialized care. We chose to convert one of the COVID-19 ICUs that was being closed as it was already fitted with proper monitoring stations, etc. Considerations for this non-COVID-19 ICU weighed heavily on the unit having its own air handler, allowing us to better protect that environment from any possible contamination. We preferred to create entire COVID-19 and non-COVID-19 floors within the hospital.

Once a unit was emptied of patients, a conversion team was set in place. This team consists of a team leader, nursing manager, and bed flow coordinator, environmental services, bed assignment, and staffing. Initially, the floor undergoes a walkthrough for terminal cleaning, which lasts between 6 and 8 hours. Linen was removed, papers discarded, and cabinets and drawers are opened. Supplies that could not be cleaned were boxed, labeled, and stored for a minimum of 14 days. This was followed by a second walkthrough. Then electrostatic fogging with an Environmental Protection Agency (EPA) approved disinfectant was sprayed. UV light was utilized in the patient rooms. Rooms were left untouched for 2–3 days. Then there was a second unit cleaning with floor stripping and waxing. The HVAC system filters were changed and air ducts were all cleaned and decontaminated. Prior to reopening, multiple surface and air sample testing were performed to ensure environmental cleaning was effective. Decontamination took approximately six days.

Continuous Screening

All the new admissions to the hospital were now considered PUIs for COVID-19 until viral testing was negative. Employees and visitors were screened near the entrances with body temperature scanners and were still mandated to wear face masks.

Counseling

The COVID-19 experience has left some health care providers with emotional scars. Counseling was made continually available. We had psychiatrists and psychologists as well as a chaplain lead open sessions for staff members to participate in as well as made available for individual counseling. Staff were reminded often that this service is available 24 hours a day and 7 days a week.

▌CONCLUSION

The pre-pandemic standard of care is modified to crisis standard of care. An incremental strategy in staffing, mechanical ventilation, and ICU rooms and proactive multidisciplinary updates on COVID-19 helped us manage this pandemic and approach unforeseen issues. The same approach helped us de-escalate COVID-19 to non-COVID-19 critical care floors and staffing. As de-escalation occurs, we continue to perform COVID-19 surveillance with the current patient population and staff in anticipation for a second peak.

▌REFERENCES

1. Coronavirus Disease (COVID-19) Pandemic. who.int. https://www.who.int/emergencies/diseases/novel-coronavirus-2019. Updated May 6, 2021. Accessed May 7, 2021.
2. Cases of Coronavirus Disease (COVID-19). cdc.gov. https://www.cdc.gov/coronavirus/2019-ncov/cases-updates/cases-in-us.html. Updated May 6, 2021. Accessed May 7, 2021.
3. Sanche S, Lin YT, Xu C, Romero-Severson E, Hengartner N, Ke R. High contagiousness and rapid spread of severe acute respiratory syndrome coronavirus 2. *Emerg Infect Dis*. 2020;26(7):1470-1477.
4. Sandrock CE. Care of the critically ill and injured during pandemics and disasters: Groundbreaking results from the Task Force on Mass Critical Care. *CHEST*. 2014;881-883.
5. Halpern NA, Kaplan LJ, Rausen M, Yang JJ. Configuring ICUs in the COVID-19 era. https://www.sccm.org/COVID19RapidResources/Resources/Configuring-ICUs-in-the-COVID-19-Era-A-Collection. Updated June 15, 2020. Accessed October 29, 2020.
6. Guidance for US Healthcare Facilities about Coronavirus (COVID-19). cdc.gov. https://www.cdc.gov/coronavirus/2019-ncov/hcp/us-healthcare-facilities.html. Updated July 12, 2020. Accessed October 31, 2020.
7. Country and Technical Guidance – Coronavirus Disease (COVID-19). https://www.who.int/emergencies/diseases/novel-coronavirus-2019/technical-guidance. Accessed October 31, 2020.
8. Chopra V, Toner E, Waldhorn R, et al. How should U.S. hospitals prepare for coronavirus disease 2019 (COVID-19). *Ann Intern Med*. 2020;172(9):621-622.
9. What Is a HEPA Filter? epa.gov. https://www.epa.gov/indoor-air-quality-iaq/what-hepa-filter-1. Updated April 3, 2019. Accessed October 21, 2020.

10. Rosenbaum R, Benyo J, O'Connor R, et al. Use of a portable forced air system to convert existing hospital space into a mass casualty isolation area. *Ann Emerg Med*. 2004;44:628-634.

11. Chemical Hazards Emergency Medical Management. chemm.nlm.nih.gov. https://chemm.nlm.nih.gov/ppe.htm. Updated September 14, 2020. Accessed October 21, 2020.

12. Summary for Healthcare Facilities: Strategies for Optimizing the Supply of PPE during Shortages. cdc.gov. https://www.cdc.gov/coronavirus/2019-ncov/hcp/ppe-strategy/strategies-optimize-ppe-shortages.html. Updated July 16, 2020. Accessed October 21, 2020.

13. Use Personal Protective Equipment (PPE) When Caring for Patients with Confirmed or Suspected COVID-19. cdc.gov. https://www.cdc.gov/coronavirus/2019-ncov/downloads/A_FS_HCP_COVID19_PPE.pdf. Accessed October 21, 2020.

14. Lindsley WG, Martin SB, Twelis RE et al. Effects of ultraviolet germicidal irradiation (UVGI) on N95 respirator filtration performance and structural integrity. *J Occup Environ Hyg*. 2015;12:509-517.

15. Mills D, Harnish DA, Lawrence C, Sandoval-Powers M, Heimbuch BK. Ultraviolet germicidal irradiation of influenza-contaminated N95. *Am J Infect Control*. 2018;46:e49-e55.

16. Cheng VCC, Wong SC, Kwan GSW, Hui WT, Yuen KY. Disinfection of N95 respirators by ionized hydrogen peroxide in pandemic coronavirus disease (COVID-19) due to SARS-CoV-2. *J Hosp Infect*. 2020;105(2):358-359.

17. Heilingloh CS, Aufdehorst UW, Schipper L, et al. Susceptibility of SARS-CoV-2 to UV irradiation. *Am J Infect Control*. 2020;48:1273-1275.

18. Daeschler S, Manson N, Joachim K, et al. Effect of moist heat reprocessing of N95 respirators on SARS-CoV-2 inactivation and respirator function. *CMAJ*. 2020;192:E1189-97.

19. Anderegg L, Meisenhelder C, Ngooi CO, et al. A scalable method of applying heat and humidity for decontamination of N95 respirators during the COVID-19 crisis. *PLoS One*. 2020;15(7):e0234851.

20. Oh C, Araud E, Puthussery JV, et al. Dry heat as a decontamination method for N95 respirator reuse. *Environ Sci Technol Lett*. 2020;7:677-682.

21. Guide to Local Production: WHO – Recommended Handrub Formulations. who.int. https://www.who.int/gpsc/5may/Guide_to_Local_Production.pdf?ua=1. Accessed October 18, 2020.

22. Using Telehealth to Expand Access to Essential Health Services during the COVID-19 Pandemic. cdc.gov. https://www.cdc.gov/coronavirus/2019-ncov/hcp/telehealth.html. Updated June 10, 2020. Accessed October 31, 2020.

23. Baldrelin HA, Atallah B. Global drug shortages due to COVID-19: Impact on patient care and mitigation strategies. *Res Social Adm Pharm*. 2021;17(1):1946-1949.

24. Devlin J, Skrobik Y, Gelinas C, et al. Clinical practice guidelines for the prevention and management of pain, agitation/sedation, delirium, immobility, and sleep disruption in adult patients in the ICU. *Crit Care Med*. 2018;46(9):e825-e873.

25. Umunna BP, Tekwani K, Barounis D, Kettaneh N, Kulsted E. Ketamine for continuous sedation of mechanically ventilated patients. *J Emerg Trauma Shock*. 2015;8(1):11-15.

26. Groetzinger LM, Rivosecchi RM, Bain W, et al. Ketamine infusion for adjunct sedation in mechanically ventilated adults. *Pharmacotherapy*. 2018;38(2): 181-188.

27. Meduri GU, Siemieniuk RAC, Seyler SJ. Prolonged low dose methylprednisolone treatment is highly effective in reducing duration for mechanical ventilation and mortality in ARDS. *J Intensive Care*. 2018;6(53):1-7.

28. Alhazzani W, Moller MH, Arabi YM, et al. Surviving Sepsis Campaign: Guidelines on the management of critically ill adults with coronavirus disease 2019. United States Resource Availability for COVID-19. Society of Critical Care Medicine. https://sccm.org/Blog/March-2020/United-States-Resource-Availability-for-COVID-19. Accessed April 10, 2020.

29. Recovery Collaborative Group, et al. Dexamethasone in hospitalized patients with COVID-19 – Preliminary report. *N Engl J Med*. 2021;384(8):693-704.

30. Priyambada L, Wolsfdorf JI, Brink SJ, et al. ISPAD Clinical Practice Consensus Guideline: Diabetic ketoacidosis in the time of COVID-19 and resource-limited settings – role of subcutaneous insulin. *Pediatr Diabetes*. 2020;1-9.

31. Palermo NE, Sadhu AR, McDonnell ME. Diabetic ketoacidosis in COVID-19: Unique concerns and consideration. *J Clin Endocrinol Metab*. 2020;105:2819-2829.

32. Hsia E, Seggelke S, Gibbs J, et al. Subcutaneous administration of glargine to diabetic patients receiving insulin infusion prevents rebound hyperglycemia. *J Clin Endocrinol Metab*. 2012;97(9):3132-3137.

33. Della Manna T, Steinmetz L, Campos PR, et al. Subcutaneous use of a fast-acting insulin analog: An alternative treatment for pediatric patients with diabetic ketoacidosis. *Diabetes Care*. 2005;28(8):1856-1861.

34. Ersoz HO, Ukinc K, Kose M, et al. Subcutaneous lispro and intravenous regular insulin treatments are equally effective and safe for the treatment of mild and moderate diabetic ketoacidosis in adult patients. *Int J Clin Pract*. 2006;60(4): 429-433.

35. Karoli R, Fatima J, Salman T, Sandhu S, Shankar R. Managing diabetic keto-acidosis in non-intensive care unit setting: role of insulin analogs. *Indian J Pharmacol*. 2011;43(4):398-401.

36. Umpierrez GE, Cuervo R, Karabell A, Latif K, Freire AX, Kitabchi AE. Treatment of diabetic ketoacidosis with subcutaneous insulin aspart. *Diabetes Care*. 2004;27(8):1873-1878.

37. Umpierrez GE, Latif K, Stoever J, et al. Efficacy of subcutaneous insulin lispro versus continuous intravenous regular insulin for the treatment of patients with diabetic ketoacidosis. *Am J Med*. 2004;117(5):291-296.

38. United States Resource Availability for COVID-19. sccm.org. https://sccm.org/Blog/March-2020/United-States-Resource-Availability-for-COVID-19. Updated March 13, 2020. Accessed March 13, 2020.

39. Benger JR. Rethinking rapid sequence induction of anaesthesia in critically ill adults. *Lancet Respir Med*. 2019;7(12):997-999.

40. ARDS Clinical Network Mechanical Ventilation Protocol Summary. ardsnet.org. http://www.ardsnet.org/files/ventilator_protocol_2008-07.pdf. Accessed April 18, 2020.

41. Goh KJ, Wong J, Tien JCC, et al. Preparing your intensive care unit for the COVID-19 pandemic: Practical considerations and strategies. *Crit Care*. 2020; 24(215):1-12.

42. Ehmann MR, Zink EK, Levin AB, et al. Operational recommendations for scare resource allocation in a public health crisis. *CHEST*. September 2020. https://doi.org/10.1016/j.chest.2020.09.246. Accessed October 1, 2020.

43. Guerin C, Reignier J Richard JC, et al. Prone position in severe acute respiratory distress syndrome. *N Engl J Med*. 2013;368:2159-2168.

44. Reignier J, Thenoz-Jost N, Fiancette M, et al. Early enteral nutrition in mechanically ventilated patients in the prone position. *Crit Care Med*. 2004;32:94-9.

45. Linn DD, Beckett RB, Foellinger K. Administration of enteral nutrition to adult patients in the prone position. *Intensive Crit Care Nurs*. 2015;31:38-43.

46. Reignier J, Dimet J, Martin-Lefevre L, et al. Before and after study of a standardized ICU protocol for early enteral feeding in patients turned in the prone position. *Clin Nutr*. 2010;29:210-216.

47. De la Fuente IS, de la Fuente JS, Estelles MDQ, et al. Enteral nutrition in patients receiving mechanical ventilation in prone position. *JPEN J Parenter Enteral Nutri*. 2016;250-255.

48. McClave SA, Taylor BE, Martindale RG, et al. Guidelines for the provision and assessment of nutrition support therapy in the adult critically ill patient: Society of Critical Care Medicine (SCCM) and American Society for Parenteral and Enteral Nutrition (ASPEN). *J Parenter Enteral Nutr*. 2016;40:159-211.

49. Discharging COVID-19 Patients. cdc.gov. https://www.cdc.gov/coronavirus/2019-ncov/hcp/disposition-hospitalized-patients.html#definitions. Updated August 10, 2020. Accessed October 31, 2020.

50. Criteria for Releasing COVID-19 Patients from Isolation. who.int. https://www.who.int/news-room/commentaries/detail/criteria-for-releasing-covid-19-patients-from-isolation. Updated May 27, 2020. Accessed October 31, 2020.

NURSING 2

Caroline Castro, DNP, FNP-C, BSN, RN, Jacqueline Siatti, BSN, RN, CCRN, and Katerina Korunovski, BSN, RN, CCRN

▌ INTRODUCTION

The COVID-19 healthcare crisis caused significant strain on health care professionals such as nurses. Protocols were implemented to guide with staffing, medication administration, providing nutrition, and moving patients from supine to prone position while ensuring the safety of the nurses.

Nurse Staffing

In a survey performed by the American Association of Critical Care Nurses (AACN), out of 164 ICU nurses, 39% had less than two years of experience and 73% had less than five.[1] The recent COVID-19 pandemic forced a crisis of standard of care where health care resources, including nursing staff, were limited. This forced many non-ICU nurses to assume care for ICU level patients.[1]

The SCCM published a tier-based model taken by the University of Pittsburg Medial Center for surge staffing of critical care physicians and nursing under crisis.[2] For every 24 mechanically ventilated patients, the unit should be staffed with 4 ICU nurses and 12 non-ICU nurses.[3] Each nurse must be familiar with the unit including where intubation boxes, intubation medications, and code blue carts are located. Because hospitals under crisis may stop or slow surgeries, the operating room (OR) and post-anesthesia care unit (PACU) staff become available to incorporate into the model. Nurses who may not have ICU experience but are familiar with devices such as ventilators used in ORs are beneficial in assisting in the care of the ICU patient under crisis.[3] Other hospitals recruited nurses with prior critical care experience to return to critical care units during pandemic-related surge capacity.[4] The SCCM also suggests incorporating intermediate care, telemetry, or stepdown nurses into the team-based care approach similar to SCCM's model.[4] For nurses returning to the bedside after six months or more away, a surge plan orientation, skills lab, shift with a preceptor, and e-module training should be offered.[5-7] Validation in essential nursing skills such as assessment, medication administration, documentation, and dressing changes is recommended. Furthermore, it is recommended that these nurses assist with patient assignments but not take their own full patient load.[5]

Nurse Safety

According to the AACN, nurses spend an average of 33% of their shift at the bedside contributing to both health and safety concerns and fatigue.[1] Nurses who had became infected followed hospital protocol and quarantined with location and duration depending on severity of symptoms.[8,9] Nurses were under significant psychological pressure at the bedsides of critically ill and dying patients of a poorly understood disease.[8] Based on research from previous pandemics such as SARS, MERS-CoV, Ebola, and H1N1, nurses suffered from anxiety, depression, physical and mental fatigue, insomnia, and post-traumatic stress after being in close contact with patients with these diseases. With the Ebola pandemic, 45% of caregivers sought psychological counseling and 29% felt lonely. Depression was present in 38.5% of nurses during the SARS pandemic while 37% experienced insomnia and 33% had post-traumatic stress.[8] The First Affiliated Hospital of Henan University of Science and Technology conducted research based on qualitative analyses of 20 nurses involved in treating patients with COVID-19 to determine the psychological impact of the pandemic.[8] Through face to face and telephone interviews, they found that all 20 nurses had significant negative emotions when they first began caring for COVID-19 patients and that their workload increased 1.5–2 times normal. Furthermore, they all said their fear increased as they entered negative pressure rooms and all were concerned about the well-being of their own families. Nurses also reported physical fatigue such as headaches, chest tightness, ear pain, sweating, and body pain from the uncomfortable protective gear that was worn for hours.[8] It is recommended that early psychological intervention and support systems be established to aid nurses and health care workers in a crisis situation. Confidence in safety, availability of supplies, and adequate training also had a positive effect on mental health of nurses.[8] Coping mechanisms such as mediation, music, and emotional venting along with cohesive teamwork and support assist nurses' mental health during these times.

The CDC set forth specific guidelines for health care providers, which varied drastically from the guidelines for the general public, to optimize available staff. Health care providers with confirmed or suspected mild to moderate COVID-19 were able to return to work after 24 hours of last fever without fever-reducing agents, 10 days since symptoms first appeared, or when symptoms improved.[9]

"Prone Position" Team

Prone position improved oxygenation and mortality in acute respiratory distress syndrome (ARDS) and was used during the COVID-19 pandemic for patients with a $PaO_2/FiO_2 < 150$ for 12 to 16 hours a day but preferably 16 hours.[10–16] It was not advised for patients with facial or pelvic fractures, burns or open wounds on ventral surfaces, spinal instability, increased intracranial pressure, or life threatening arrythmias. According to the ACCN, without the use of assistive devices such as the RotoProne, four to five staff members are required.[13] Sometimes, two nurses and one respiratory therapist are the only ones available. These dedicated "prone position" teams would round in each unit and discuss with the medical team which patients needed to be placed in prone position. Nursing preparation includes gathering sufficient staff, assessing mental status, turning off tube feeding one hour prior, applying skin protection to areas of pressure, mouth and eye care, hemodynamic status, assessing endotracheal tubes (ETT) position and securement method, capnography monitoring, positioning of central and arterial lines, tubes, and drains to prevent kinking and pulling, and preoxygenation.[13] Two nurses are on each side of the bed and a respiratory therapist at the head of the bed.[13] The patient is then flipped to prone position (Figure 2-1).

While the patient is in the prone position, the ICU nurse is responsible for monitoring the patient's tolerance and response through frequent vital sign monitoring, respiratory effort and compliance with the ventilator, and blood gas interpretation. Furthermore, the nurse is expected to reposition the patient's head hourly, frequently assess skin, provide

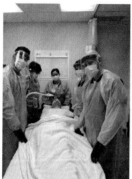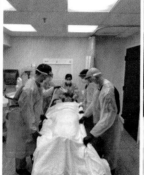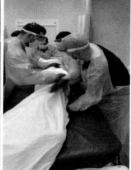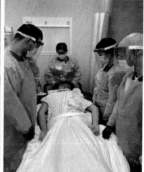

Figure 2-1 • Prone position team.

oral care and airway suctioning, provide eye care, manage tube feeding, and continue all other monitoring and care responsibilities of the ICU patient.[13] The COVID-19 pandemic put constraints on the nurse's ability to perform many of these responsibilities and prioritized simply getting the patient safely in the prone position to optimize oxygenation.

Prone position complications include unplanned removal of central catheter, unplanned extubation, pressure sores, and ventilator-associated pneumonia.[10] A systemic review and meta-analysis of prone position for ARDS showed no difference in the incident of these events in prone versus supine position except for an increased risk of endotracheal tube obstruction and pressure sores in the prone position.[10] In a retrospective analysis of prone position complications in 170 patients, 58% of patients survived, 14% developed pressure sores, and only 0.4% experienced removal of a respiratory device and no removal of central line catheters when five trained and skilled health care professionals were involved in the manual proning of the patient following a dedicated protocol.[17] In further support of minimizing complications, the AACN recommends using an interdisciplinary team approach including providers, clinical nurses, respiratory care providers, physical therapists, and wound ostomy continence nurses.[18]

Medication Administration

The Institute of Medicine (IOM) has noted the various barriers and challenges that can present for nurses to successfully complete this task, which led to the development of the medication administration rights. In addition, regulations have been set forth by the IOM and other accrediting agencies such as The Joint Commission (TJC) to guide nurses to prevent medication errors.[19] Overall, this can be considered the most complex and time-consuming nursing task throughout a typical shift. During any large-scale disaster or emergency such as a global pandemic or other crises, additional safety challenges can arise for nursing staff when administering medications. The bundling of medication administration with other nursing tasks, such as phlebotomy or nutrition, is recommended.[20] Similarly, it is encouraged that long extension tubing be utilized to allow all infusion pumps outside of the patient's room.

Many institutions developed a procedural change to remove all intravenous (IV) medication poles and pumps outside of the patients' rooms and into anterooms and hallways during the COVID-19 pandemic (Figure 2-2). This practice change approved by the Food and Drug Administration (FDA) intended to limit delays of initiating and titrating life sustaining medications by donning Personal Protective Equipment (PPE) less frequently.[21,22] This additionally allowed nurses to avoid entering patient rooms when not necessary, consequently reducing staff

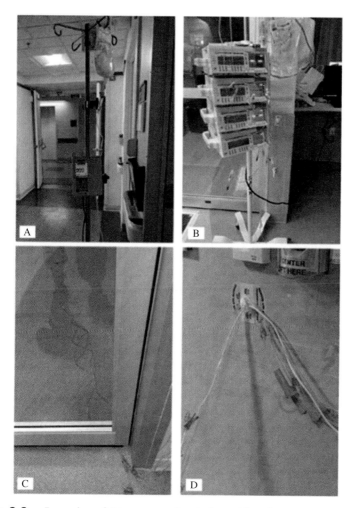

Figure 2-2 • Examples of IV pumps relocated outside of patient rooms during COVID-19. (Reproduced with permission of American Association of Critical-Care Nurses from Blake JWC, Giuliano KK. Flow accuracy of IV smart pumps outside of patient rooms during COVID-19. *AACN Adv Crit Care*. 2020;31(4):357–363; permission conveyed through Copyright Clearance Center, Inc.)

exposure. The change conserved PPE and allowed nursing staff to quickly change medication bags and to respond to alarms promptly. An example of the set up from the AACN can be seen in Figure 2-2.[22] Nursing responsibilities included ensuring that IV lines were not kinked and that infusion pump accuracy was met despite differing rates and resistance from numerous tubing sizes and lengths.[21] It is of concern that medication volume be considered when administering medications via this new tactic. Additionally, when numerous medications are being continuously infused, it is a nursing responsibility to ensure that all medications are compatible.[22] Nurses must be educated and vigilant of potential safety implications associated with this practice change. Relocating IV pumps is ideal for circumstances of crisis, limited resources, and time. The Institute for Safe Medicine Practices noted that this practice allows nurses to barcode medications, but not patients directly at the bedside for each administration.[23]

Medication use should be limited to treat the acute disease to reduce medication burden and delay medication shortage, and less frequent doses and monitoring should be advocated.[24,25]

Documentation

During a critical crisis or disaster, documentation requirements are changed while optimized for the clinician and patient's best interests.[26] In 2008, the American Nurses Association released a report to help guide nurses and professionals who may come across an extreme emergency. This report recommends that institutional policies are developed during such circumstances to guide standards of care for nursing staff.[27] Many institutions then rely on the executive orders set forth by the state government, the department of health (DOH), and Center of Medicaid Services (CMS) for guidance and recommendations to be made for documentation requirements. Additionally, the CMS and TJC issue waivers when emergency operations plans are in place to assist with documentation requirements. Ultimately, the organization in which the nurse is practicing determines the final policy.[28]

The CMS waived all nursing care plans and education requirements to allow more time throughout a shift to be dedicated to direct patient care.[28] This varies from normal standards as many institutions require a nursing physical exam to be completed and documented once a shift or typically every twelve hours in addition to an individualized nursing care plan for each patient.

In correspondence with the crisis guidelines put forth by the American Nurses Association, institutions can further develop documentation guidelines to guide nurses.[29] For example, many institutions emphasize that nurses should only chart by exception during these difficult times, which is also not prohibited by TJC.[20,30] However, there is vital documentation that cannot be eliminated at any time. This includes but is not limited to restraints, medication administration, and blood transfusions, for example, as dictated by New York state developed by recommendations set forth in a New York executive order.[31] This policy, "Streamlining Documentation during State of Emergency," emphasizes that pertinent clinical findings should always be documented by the nurse. Pertinent clinical findings and changes are at the forefront of documentation during this time. All documentation relevant to a patient's skin, IV lines, drains, or airway is to be charted by exception only. Other states heavily impacted by the pandemic developed similar policies. Additionally, some institutions used nursing staff to alleviate documentation burdens. For example, non-ICU nursing staff can assist critical care nurses by documenting vital signs or telemetry cardiac strips (USE JAX'S). Overall, nurses maintain the same professional standards of care while balancing documentation throughout a shift with guidelines set forth by institutions and governing bodies.

Nutrition

In the ICU, nutrition is key to optimal medical management and recovery. It is recommended that oral nutritional support is encouraged each time a staff member has an encounter with a patient who is capable of oral hydration. This model, the "every contact counts" model, can significantly improve nutrition and hydration status.[32] Food intake is significantly reduced due to both the patient's condition and the environment in which they reside during their hospital stay.[33] The patient's symptoms, such as dyspnea and weakness, as well as lack of staff support can contribute to developing malnourishment. Nurses can advocate for patients who are not intubated, yet not obtaining nutrition via oral feeding due to weakness and deteriorating conditions. These patients should receive enteral nutrition when able.

Patients with mechanical ventilation secondary to respiratory failure require enteral nutritional support. Numerous recommendations encourage nasogastric tubes despite frequent prone positioning for this population.[32] It is important for feedings to be stopped by nursing staff an hour before assuming the prone position or returning to supine or semi fowler's position. Feeds should always be given through an enteral pump if accessible, and rates should not exceed 60–85 ml/hour.[32] Remember that there may be a lack of feeding pumps during a critical time. In this circumstance, nurses can deliver gravity or bolus feeds. Whenever available, pumps should first be used with ventilated patients. The nurse, with communication from a registered dietician specialist, can advocate for patients to be started on nutrition within 36–48 hours of hospitalization or 12 hours after intubation.[33] If patients are hemodynamically stable and can be fed via the gastrointestinal tract, enteral nutrition should be encouraged.[34] The feeding schedule should be coordinated with the nurse's entrance into the patient room to minimize exposure. It is not encouraged to monitor gastric residual volumes, due to increased infection risk, yet to assess for intolerance or vomiting.[33] Standard safety checks with nasogastric and orogastric tube feedings must continue even during unprecedented times. Overall, nurses play a significant role in optimizing nutrition care of critically ill COVID-19 patients.

Decubitus Ulcers

Typically, due to the severe acuity of the patient population, ICUs have a high incidence of pressure ulcer development in mechanically ventilated patients, particularly in ARDS.[35,36] Pressure ulcers are defined as partial to full thickness tissue injury to the skin or muscle, usually over bony prominences due to pressure and shear, or from medical devices.[37] Prophylactic dressings can be placed on the patient by nursing staff to prevent skin injury on high risk regions. Moreover, a negative fluid balance is preferred in ARDS patients, which can further alter their skin integrity.[37] Proper skin hygiene, eliminating body fluids on the skin, and moisturizing the skin prevents maceration and minimizes friction.[37] Urine and fecal containment devices are frequently adopted for patients who are prone to help reduce moisture-associated skin damage.[38] Nurses have a significant role in reducing pressure injuries by thorough assessments and numerous interventions.

Less frequent contact with the patients during this time made it more of a challenge to prevent and manage pressure injuries. To overcome this obstacle, strategically placing foam protective dressings on pressure points (face, thorax, knees, toes, breast region, iliac crest) benefits prevention of pressure injury development.[38]

Mucosal pressure injuries to the lips and tongue were often found in prone positioned patients.[37] ETT are secured with twill to help with prone/supine position changes, but often cause circumferential injury to the head, neck, and cheeks. Placing a silicone pressure-reducing strip or gauze protective dressing can be used as prophylaxis to skin breakdown.[36] It is recommended to perform head position changes two or three times during the 16-hour prone position, and ETT position changes between each prone session.[36] Pillows are placed underneath the chest, pelvic area, and shins to alleviate excessive pressure on the neck, genitals, and toes, respectively. Pink foam pillows in a semilunar shape can be placed under the patient's head to help cradle the head with an outlet for the ETT.[36] Prior to the pandemic, incidence of pressure ulcers in prone positioning was 56%.[37]

Rapid Response Team

Rapid response teams (RRT) consist of an advanced practice nurse or physician, two ICU nurses, and an anesthesiologist to perform intubations.[39] Anesthesiologists have specialized training in airway management, which helps minimize intubation attempts, reducing COVID-19 exposure.[40] Studies have shown limited success with in-hospital cardiac arrest (IHCA), with only about 25% of patients surviving to hospital discharge.[39] A recent study regarding COVID-19 patients and IHCA was conducted between 31 patients with a median age of 69. Seventy-one percent were males, 55% had cardiovascular disease, and 42% were African American.[41] The median resuscitation time was 14 minutes with 100% mortality rate.[41] The severity of this illness and the outcomes of IHCA only conclude that cardiopulmonary resuscitation is ineffective in this patient population. Likelihood of success is further decreased due to less experienced code team members during times of staffing shortages and the time delays of donning PPE.[39]

Patient Monitoring

As the pandemic surge progresses, rooms are modified to accommodate more patients.[42-44] Some rooms may make it difficult for nursing staff to hear patients, bed alarms, telemetry alarms, and ventilators alarming. Virtual critical care nurses may help support less experienced nurses or remote monitoring via smartphone apps that can visualize vital signs.[45] There are even smartphone apps for monitoring and adjusting mechanical ventilators remotely. One-way baby monitors are enhancing nurses' interaction with patients, preserving PPE, and allowing nurses to frequently check on their patients through closed doors.[46]

▌ REFERENCES

1. Arneson SL, Tucker SJ, Mercier M, Singh J. Answering the call: Impact of tele-ICU nurses during the COVID-19 pandemic. *Crit Care Nurse*. 2020;40(4):25-31.
2. Harris GH, Baldisseri MR, Reynolds BR, Orsino AS, Sackrowitz R, Bishop JM. Design for implementation of a system-level ICU pandemic surge staffing plan. *Crit Care Explor*. 2020;2(6):e0136.
3. Halpern NA, Tan KS. United States resource availability for COVID-19. SCCM. org. https://sccm.org/getattachment/Blog/March-2020/United-States-Resource-Availability-for-COVID-19/United-States-Resource-Availability-for-COVID-19.pdf?lang=en-US. Published May 12, 2020. Accessed September 1, 2020.
4. Martland AM, Huffines M, Henry K. Surge priority planning COVID-19: Critical care staffing and nursing considerations. Resources - American College of Chest Physicians. http://www.chestnet.org/Guidelines-and-Resources/Resources/Surge-Priority-Planning-COVID-19-Critical-Care-Staffing-and-Nursing-Considerations. Accessed September 1, 2020.

5. Miller J. Professional development nurses respond to the COVID-19 crisis. aacn. org. https://www.aacn.org/blog/professional-development-nurses-respond-to-the-covid-19-crisis. Published March 26, 2020. Accessed September 18, 2020.

6. Surge Capacity-Education and Training for a Qualified Workforce. Archive. https://archive.ahrq.gov/news/ulp/btbriefs/btbrief7.htm. Accessed September 18, 2020.

7. Ragazzoni L, Barco A, Echeverri L, et al. Just-in-time training in a tertiary referral hospital during the COVID-19 pandemic in Italy. *Acad Med.* 2021;96(3): 336-339.

8. Sun N, Wei L, Shi S, et al. A qualitative study on the psychological experience of caregivers of COVID-19 patients. *American Journal of Infection Control.* https://www.ncbi.nlm.nih.gov/pmc/articles/PMC7141468/pdf/main.pdf. Accessed September 19, 2020.

9. Return-to-Work Criteria for Healthcare Workers. cdc.gov. https://www.cdc. gov/coronavirus/2019-ncov/hcp/return-to-work.html. Accessed September 18, 2020.

10. Munshi L, Del Sorbo L, Adhikari NKJ, et al. Prone position for acute respiratory distress syndrome. A systematic review and meta-analysis. *Ann Am Thorac Soc.* 2017;14(Supplement_4):S280-S288.

11. Mitchell DA, Seckel MA. Acute respiratory distress syndrome and prone positioning. AACN Advanced Critical Care. https://aacnjournals.org/aacnacconline/article/29/4/415/2281/Acute-Respiratory-Distress-Syndrome-and-Prone. Published December 15, 2018. Accessed September 18, 2020.

12. Lindahl SGE. Using the prone position could help to combat the development of fast hypoxia in some patients with COVID-19. *Acta Paediatr.* 2020;109(8):1539-1544.

13. Vollman K, Dickinson S, Powers J. Pronation therapy. AACN.org. https://www. aacn.org/docs/Photos/Procedure-19-pzjnnuht.pdf. Accessed September 17, 2020.

14. Guerin C, Reignier J, Richard JC. et al. Prone positioning in severe acute respiratory distress syndrome. *NEJM.* 2013;368:2159-2168.

15. Clinical Management of COVID-19. who.int. https://www.who.int/publications/i/item/clinical-management-of-covid-19. Published May 27, 2020. Accessed September 18, 2020.

16. Matsos S. Prone Team: Johns Hopkins Medicine. Prone Team | Johns Hopkins Medicine. https://www.hopkinsmedicine.org/coronavirus/articles/prone-team. html. Published May 6, 2020. Accessed September 18, 2020.

17. Lucchini A. Prone position in acute respiratory distress syndrome: Dimensions of critical care nursing. LWW. https://journals.lww.com/dccnjournal/Fulltext/2020/01000/Prone_Position_in_Acute_Respiratory_Distress.6.aspx. Accessed September 18, 2020.

18. Mitchell DA, Seckel MA. Acute respiratory distress syndrome and prone positioning. AACN Advanced Critical Care. https://aacnjournals.org/aacnacconline/article/29/4/415/2281/Acute-Respiratory-Distress-Syndrome-and-Prone. Published December 15, 2018. Accessed September 18, 2020.

19. Jennings BM, Sandelowski, M. Mark B. The nurse's medication day. *Qual Health Res.* 2011;21(10):1441-1451.

20. Farmer BM, Cole JB, Olives TD, et al. ACMT position statement: Medication administration and safety during the response to COVID-19 pandemic. *J Med Toxicol*. 2020;1-3.

21. Shah AG, Taduran C, Friedman S, et al. Relocating IV pumps for critically ill isolated coronavirus disease 2019 patients from bedside to outside the patient room. *Crit Care Explor*. 2020;2(8):e0168.

22. Blake JWC, Giuliano KK. Flow accuracy of IV smart pumps outside of patient rooms during COVID-19. *AACN Adv Crit Care*. 2020;e1-e7.

23. Institute for Safe Medication Practices: Special Edition Medication Safety Alert! 2020. https://ismp.org/acute-care/special-edition-medication-safety-alert-april-3-2020/covid-19. Accessed August 22, 2020.

24. Altevogt BM, Stroud C, Hanson SL, Hanfling D, Gostin LO, eds. *Guidance for Establishing Crisis Standards of Care for Use in Disaster Situations: A Letter Report*. Institute of Medicine. The National Academies Press; 2009.

25. Brandt N, Steinman MA. Optimizing medication management during the COVID-19 pandemic: An implementation guide for post-acute and long-term care. *J Am Geriatr Soc*. 2020;68(7):1362-1365.

26. Principles for Nursing Documentation. 2010. American Nurse's Association. https://www.nursingworld.org/~4af4f2/globalassets/docs/ana/ethics/principles-of-nursing-documentation.pdf.

27. *Adapting Standards of Care under Extreme Conditions: Guidance for Professionals during Disasters, Pandemics, and Other Extreme Emergencies*. Prepared for the American Nurses Association by the Center for Health Policy, Columbia University School of Nursing. American Nurses Association, Silver Spring, MD; 2008.

28. Campbell R. Documentation challenges under an emergency operations plan. The Joint commission. 2020. https://www.jointcommission.org/resources/news-and-multimedia/blogs/on-infection-prevention-control/2020/04/24/documentation-challenges-when-operating-under-an-emergency-operations-plan/.

29. Crisis Standard of Care COVID-19 Pandemic. American Nurses Association. https://www.nursingworld.org/~496044/globalassets/practiceandpolicy/work-environment/health--safety/coronavirus/crisis-standards-of-care.pdf.

30. COVID-19 Emergency Declaration Blanket Waivers for Healthcare Providers. cms.gov. https://www.cms.gov/files/document/summary-covid-19-emergency-declaration-waivers.pdf. Published April 8, 2021.

31. Nursing Streamlining Documentation during COVID-19 State of Emergency. Executive Order by Governor Cuomo. https://www.aonl.org/system/files/media/file/2020/04/EXAMPLE%201%20Nursing%20Streamlining%20Documentation%20During%20COVID-19%20State%20of%20Emergency.pdf.

32. Anderson L. Providing nutritional support for the patient with COVID-19. *Br J Nurs*. 2020;29(8):458-459.

33. Thibault R, Seguin P, Tamion F, Pichard C, Singer P. Nutrition of the COVID-19 patient in the intensive care unit (ICU): A practical guidance. *Crit Care*. 2020;24(1):447.

34. Handu D, Moloney L, Rozga M, Cheng F. Malnutrition care during the COVID-19 pandemic: Considerations for registered dietitian nutritionists evidence analysis center. *J Acad Nutr Diet*. 2020. [Online ahead of print]

35. Worsley PR, Spratt F, Bader DL. COVID-19: Challenging tissue viability in both patients and clinicians. *J Tissue Viability*. 2020;29(3):153-154.

36. Perrillat A, Foletti JM, Lacagne AS, Guyot L, Graillon N. Facial pressure ulcers in COVID-19 patients undergoing prone positioning: How to prevent an underestimated epidemic? *J Stomatol Oral Maxillofac Surg*. 2020;S2468-7855(20)30154-3.

37. Moore Z, Patton D, Avsar P, et al. Prevention of pressure ulcers among individuals cared for in the prone position: Lessons for the COVID-19 emergency. *J Wound Care*. 2020;29(6):312-320.

38. Davis CR, Beeson T. Mitigating pressure injury challenges when placing patients in a prone position: A view from here. *J Wound Ostomy Continence Nurs*. 2020; 47(4):326-327.

39. Kramer DB, Lo B, Dickert NW. CPR in the COVID-19 Era - An ethical framework. *N Engl J Med*. 2020;383(2):e6.

40. Sullivan EH, Gibson LE, Berra L, Chang MG, Bittner EA. In-hospital airway management of COVID-19 patients. *Crit Care*. 2020;24(1):292.

41. Sheth V, Chishti I, Rothman A, et al. Outcomes of in-hospital cardiac arrest in patients with COVID-19 in New York City. *Resuscitation*. 2020;155:3-5.

42. Panse S, Kanchi M, Chacko J, et al. Intensive care unit setup for COVID-19. *Journal of Cardiac Critical Care TSS*. 2020;4(1):5-11.

43. Phua J, Weng L, Ling L, et al. Intensive care management of coronavirus disease 2019 (COVID-19): Challenges and recommendations [published correction appears in Lancet Respir Med. 2020;8(5):e42]. *Lancet Respir Med*. 2020;8(5): 506-517.

44. Bambi S, Iozzo P, Lucchini A. New issues in nursing management during the COVID-19 pandemic in Italy. *Am J Crit Care*. 2020;29(4):e92-e93.

45. Naik BN, Gupta R, Singh A, Lal Soni S, Puri GD. Real-time smart patient monitoring and assessment amid COVID-19 pandemic: An alternative approach to remote monitoring. *J Med Syst*. 2020;44(131).

46. Baby Monitors Provide Innovative Angle to Treat COVID-19. Daily Dose. https://atriumhealth.org/dailydose/2020/05/06/baby-monitors-provide-innovative-angle-to-treat-covid19. Accessed September 21, 2020.

INFLAMMATION AND REPERFUSION 3

Ronaldo C. Go, MD

▌ INTRODUCTION

Inflammation, ischemia, and reperfusion are important mechanisms involved in pandemics and trauma.

▌ CYTOKINE STORM

Cytokine storm is an over-exaggerated inflammatory response with infectious and non-infectious causes.[1,2] The concept first appeared with graft versus host disease and then with cytomegalovirus, Epstein-bar virus associate hemophagocytic lymphohistiocytosis, group A streptococcus, influenza virus, variola virus, avian H5N1 influenza virus, and severe acute respiratory distress syndrome.[3-8] It has also been associated with use of muromonab-CD3 (OKTS), Coley's toxins, genetic diseases such as inappropriate inflammasome activation or idiopathic multicentric Castleman's disease, CAR T-cell therapy, hemophagocytic lymphohistiocytosis, and most recently SARS-CoV-2 infection.[2] There is no single definition of cytokine storm or cytokine release syndrome that is universally accepted.[2]

Cytokines

Cytokines are proteins with roles on intracellular signaling for communication[1] (Table 3-1 to 3-3). They are produced by cells of the innate immune system such as neutrophils, monocytes, and macrophages.[2] Neutrophils also produce extracellular traps and fibers that contribute to thrombi formation.[2] Macrophages' other roles include removal of senescent cells, antigen presentation, immune-regulation, and tissue repair.[2] NK cells have cytolytic roles.[2] The major types of cytokines include interferons, which regulate innate immunity with antiviral and anti-proliferative properties; interleukins, which may be pro-inflammatory or anti-inflammatory and growth of leukocytes; chemokines, which are generally pro-inflammatory

Table 3-1 ANTI-INFLAMMATORY CYTOKINES	
Cytokine	**Function**
IL-4	Decrease activate PI3K/Akt Pathway and decrease sensitivity of endothelial cells to complement mediated killing and apoptosis and upregulation of claudin-5 through JAK/STAT6 and FoXO1 activation decreases complement injury
IL-10	Mediates of vascular protection, Inhibit cytokine production by TH1 cells, monocytes, and neutrophil derived cytokines and attenuates ROS production and NAPDH oxidase activity
IL-13	Activate PI3K/Akt Pathway and decrease sensitivity of endothelial cells to complement mediated killing and apoptosis
IL-33	Induction of IL-4,IL-5, and IL-13 and suppresses IFN-y
Il-35	Generated by regulator T cells and B cells, produced by stimuli in endothelial cells, smooth muscle cells, and monocytes
IL-37	Suppresses IL-6, IL-1B, I-17, and IFN-y
TGF-β	Pleiotropic with anti-inflammatory and inflammatory properties and suppresses cytokine production and counters IL-1, IL-2, IL-6, and TNF

Source: Data from Fajgenbaum DC, June CH. Cytokine storm. *N Engl J Med*. 2020;383:2255-2273 and Ferrara JL, Abhyankar S, Gilliland DG. Cytokine storm of graft-versus-host disease: A critical effector role for interleukin-1. *Transplant Proc*. 1993;25:1216-1217.

for chemotaxis and leukocyte recruitment; colony-stimulating factors for hematopoietic progenitor cell proliferation and differentiation; and tumor necrosis factor, which activates cytotoxic T lymphocytes[1] The magnitude of chemokine and cytokine expression are related to pathogen-associated molecular patterns (PAMP).[1]

The adaptive immune system also can produce cytokines. Type 1 helper T cells regulate macrophages, Type 2 helper T cells help regulate eosinophils and basophils, Type 9 helper T cells help regulate mast cells, and Type 17 helper T cells help regulate neutrophils.[9] In cytokine storm, there is an exaggerated Type 1 helper T cell response.[2]

Pathogenesis

The cytokine response to eliminate a pathogen must be sufficient enough to eliminate triggers while avoiding collateral damage.[2] Cytokine storm

Table 3-2	PRO-INFLAMMATORY CYTOKINES
Cytokine	**Function**
IL-1	Pyrogenic and activates macrophages and T helper 17 cells
IL-2	Stimulate proliferation of Effector T cell and memory T cells
IL-6	Pleiotropic it has anti-inflammatory via classic signaling and pro-inflammatory via trans signaling that it binds to gp130 which activates Janus kinases and phosphorylation of tyrosine residues and activation of ras/raf/mitogen activated protein (MAP) kinase pathway Activates acute phase reactants
IL-9	Against helminths and activates mast cells
IL-12	Activates T helper 1 pathway and induction of interferon-γ
IL-17	Promotes neutrophils and against bacteria and fungus
IL-18	Activates T helper 1 pathway and synergistic with IL-12
interferon-γ	Activates macrophages
Tumor necrosis factor	Pyrogenic and increases vascular permeability
GM-CSF	Growth and differentiation for granulocyte and macrophage
VEGF	Promotes vascular growth

Source: Data from Fajgenbaum DC, June CH. Cytokine storm. *N Engl J Med.* 2020;383:2255-2273 and Ferrara JL, Abhyankar S, Gilliland DG. Cytokine storm of graft-versus-host disease: A critical effector role for interleukin-1. *Transplant Proc.* 1993;25:1216-1217.

occurs where there is a failure of negative feedback. It is also difficult to predict which patients will develop cytokine storm. It is dynamic, and the balance between pro- and anti-inflammatory markers may be dependent on inherent factors from the patient and the etiology of the cytokine storm.[1] The key cytokines in cytokine storm are Interferon-γ, interleukin-1, interleukin-6, TNF, and interleukin-18.[2] Therefore, they have been treatment targets.

Downstream signal transduction is regulated by Janus kinases (JAKs), signal transducer and activator of transcription 3 (STAT3), mammalian target of rapamycin (akt-mTOR), and mitogen-activated protein kinase-extracellular

Table 3-3 CHEMOKINES	
Chemokine	**Function**
CXCL9	Recruits macrophages, Th1 cells, NK cells, and dendritic cells
CXCL10	Recruits macrophages, Th1 cells, NK cells, and dendritic cells
CCL2	Recruits basophils, macrophages, Th2 cells, NK cells, and dendritic cells
CCL3	Recruits eosinophils, macrophages, Th1 cells, NK cells, and dendritic cells
CCL4	Recruits macrophages, Th1 cells, NK cells, and dendritic cells
CXCL13	Recruits B cells, CD4 T cells, and dendritic cells

Source: Data from Fajgenbaum DC, June CH. Cytokine storm. *N Engl J Med.* 2020;383:2255-2273 and Ferrara JL, Abhyankar S, Gilliland DG. Cytokine storm of graft-versus-host disease: A critical effector role for interleukin-1. *Transplant Proc.* 1993;25:1216-1217.

signal regulated kinase (MAPK-ERK) pathways.[2] Conformation changes with binding of IL-6 to IL-6R and to membrane-bound, ubiquitously expressed gp130-JAK-STAT3 results in systemic hyper-inflammation. This results in secretion of monocyte chemoattractant protein 1 (MCP-1), IL-8, more IL-6, vascular endothelial growth factor (VEGF), reduced E-cadherin expression.[2,10] TNF are inducers of NF-κB, which are pro-inflammatory. IL-18 and IL-1β are activated from inflammasome after detection of pathogens, and both are potent induces of IL-6 from macrophages.[2]

ISCHEMIC REPERFUSION INJURY

Ischemic reperfusion injury (IRI) occurs when blood flow is restored into a previously ischemic organ. It can cause a hyperinflammatory response, which can lead to multi-organ dysfunction. It is seen in circulatory shock, surgery such as post-transplantation, anoxic brain injury, and trauma.[1]

Pathophysiology

Ischemia

During ischemia, or when blood flow is less than required for normal function, anaerobic metabolism causes glycogen breakdown to produce adenosine triphosphate (ATP) and lactic acidosis.[11-16] The acidic pH causes a negative feedback loop to ATP production. ATP is broken down to adenosine diphosphate (ADP), adenosine monophosphate (AMP), and inosine monophosphate (IMP) and further into adenosine, inosine, hypoxanthine, and xanthine.[6] Lack of ATP ceases ATP dependent pumps such as Na^+/K^+ and Ca^{2+}.[16] As intracellular Na increases, it draws in water, resulting in cellular swelling.[16] K^+ and Ca^+ are released into the extracellular space. Ca^+ causes activation of cytosolic proteases such as calpain, which converts xanthine dehydrogenase into xanthine oxidase. Phospholipases degrade membrane lipids to increase circulating fatty acids.

Reperfusion

IRI involves activation of polymorphonuclear leukocytes, reactive oxygen species (ROS), cytokines, complement system, and eicosanoids or derivatives of arachidonic acid.[11–15] During reperfusion, the oxygen reacts with xanthine oxidase to convert hypoxanthine to xanthine and uric acid. Superoxide (O_2) is released and converted to hydroxyl radicals (OH-), and hydrogen peroxide (H_2O_2) is released, causing more oxidative stress.[17] As a consequence, there is peroxidation of lipid of cell membranes, followed by release of pro-inflammatory eicosanoids, cell permeability, and cell death. ROS activates endothelial cells, which leads to production of E-selection, vascular cell adhesion molecule-1 (VCAM-1), intercellular adhesion molecule-1 (ICAM-1), endothelial-leukocyte adhesion molecule (EMLM1 Am-1), plasminogen activator inhibotr-1 (PAi-1), tissue factor and IL-8, and increasing activity of NF-κB.[16] Other cytokines that are expressed during ischemia and reperfusion include TNF- α, IL-1, IL-6, and platelet activating factor.[16]

Eicosanoids help with the production of prostaglandins, thromboxanes, and leukotrienes.[16] Prostaglandin are short lived vasodilators, thromboxane A2 promote vasoconstriction and platelet aggregation, and leukotrienes are involved in the inflammatory cascade. Leukotrienes C4, D4, and E4 alter the cytoskeleton to increase vascular permeability and increase vasoconstriction. Leukotriene B4 leads to further neutrophil accumulation.[16,17]

There is a biphasic secretion of nitric oxide (NO), initially within 15 minutes of ischemia and a second surge after 3 hours of reperfusion. It can act as an antioxidant, but if combined with superoxide, it forms a peroxynitrite radical, a promoter of lipid peroxidation and cellular membrane disruption.[16]

Hypoxia, angiotensin II, noradrenaline, and growth factors stimulate production of endothelin from the vascular endothelium, which results in Ca^{2+} mediated vasoconstriction.[16,17]

The complement system can be activated by antibody-dependent classical, the alternative pathway, or mannose-binding lectin/mannose-binding lectin-associated serine protease pathways.[11] With the degradation of the cell membranes, including protective proteins such as decay-accelerating factor and membrane cofactor protein, complement activation occurs, leading the release to anaphylatoxins, complement factors 3a, 5a, and 5b-9.[11]

ENDOTHELIUM

The endothelium is a monolayer of endothelial cells which lines blood vessels and an integral battleground for inflammation and reperfusion injuries. Endothelial dysfunction is an imbalance between vasoconstriction and vasodilation.[18] There is an upregulation of cytokines and ROS and reduced NO production and anticoagulation properties.[18]

REFERENCES

1. Tisoncik JR, Korth MJ, Simmons CP, Farrar J, Martin TR, Katze MG. Into the eye of the cytokine storm. *Microbiol Mol Biol Rev.* 2012;76(1):16-32.
2. Fajgenbaum DC, June CH. Cytokine storm. *N Engl J Med.* 2020;383: 2255-2273.
3. Ferrara JL, Abhyankar S, Gilliland DG. Cytokine storm of graft-versus-host disease: A critical effector role for interleukin-1. *Transplant Proc.* 1993;25: 1216-1217.
4. Barry SM, Johnson MA, Janossy G. Cytopathology or immunopathology? The puzzle of cytomegalovirus pneumonitis revisited. *Bone Marrow Transplant.* 2000;26:591-597.
5. Imashuku S. Clinical features and treatment strategies of Epstein-Barr virus-associated hemophagocytic lymphohistiocytosis. *Crit Rev Oncol Hematol.* 2002;44:259-272.
6. Bisno AL, Brito MO, Collins CM. Molecular basis of group A streptococcal virulence. *Lancet Infect Dis.* 2003;3:191-200.
7. Yokota S. Influenza-associated encephalopathy—pathophysiology and disease mechanisms. *Nippon Rinsho.* 2003;61:1953-1958.
8. Jahrling PB, Hensley LE, Martinez MJ, et al. Exploring the potential of variola virus infection of cynomolgus macaques as a model for human smallpox. *Proc Natl Acad Sci U S A.* 2004;101:15196-15200.
9. Sallusto F. Heterogeneity of human CD4+ T cells against microbes. *Annu Rev Immunol.* 2016;34:317-334.
10. Kang S, Tanaka T, Narazaki M, Kishimoto T. Targeting interleukin-6 signaling in clinic. *Immunity.* 2019;50:1007-1023.

11. Arumugam TV, Shiels IA, Woodruff TM, Granger DN, Taylor SM. The role of the complement system in ischemia-reperfusion injury. *Shock*. 2004;21(5):401-409.

12. Carden DL, Granger DN. Pathophysiology of ischemia-reperfusion injury. *J Pathol*. 2000;190:255-266.

13. Rose S, Floyd RA, Eneff K, Buhren V, Massion W. Intestinal ischemia: Reperfusion-mediated increase in hydroxyl free radical formation as reported by salicylate hydroxylation. *Shock*. 1994;1:452-456.

14. Shames BD, Barton HH, Reznikov LL, et al. Ischemia alone is sufficient to induce TNF-alpha mRNA and peptide in the myocardium. *Shock*. 2002;17:114-119.

15. Riedemann NC, Ward PA. Complement in ischemia reperfusion injury. *Am J Pathol*. 2003;162:363-367.

16. Cowled P, Fitridge R. Pathophysiology of Reperfusion Injury. In: Fitridge R, Thompson M, eds. *Mechanisms of Vascular Disease: A Reference Book for Vascular Specialists* [Internet]. Adelaide (AU): University of Adelaide Press; 2011:18.

17. Wu MY, Yiang GT, Liao WT, et al. Current mechanistic concepts in ischemia and reperfusion injury. *Cell Physiol Biochem*. 2018;46(4):1650-1667.

18. Shao Y, Cheng Z, Li X, Chernaya V, Wang H, Yang X. Immunosuppressive/anti-inflammatory cytokines directly and indirectly inhibit endothelial dysfunction – A novel mechanism for maintaining vascular function. *J Hematol Oncol*. 2014;7:80.

4 REPURPOSING THERAPIES FOR COVID-19

Ronaldo C. Go, MD

▍ INTRODUCTION

New drug development is expensive, requires at least 10 years, and has a success rate of only 2.01%.[1] There are a large number of compounds to be tested and large number of randomized control trials with no clinical benefit or with toxicities.[2,3] There would also be a significant gap between the need and the availability of treatment. During the coronavirus disease 2019 (COVID-19) pandemic, drug repurposing was used to identify new indications of existing drugs.[4–6] It has been suggested that 75% of known drugs can be used for repurposing, re-profiling, re-tasking, or rescue.[6] Safety of these drugs have already been tested. Therefore, this technique is less expensive, and allows faster utilization via phase II and III clinical trials and compassionate use.

▍ METHODS TO IDENTIFY REPURPOSED DRUGS

The concept of repurposing is that a single drug can interact with multiple targets and the targets are associated with a number of biological processes.[5] In other words, one drug that targets one disease might target another through a shared protein-protein interaction network.[6] Due to the repository of medical knowledge in the form of gene expression, drug target interactions, protein networks, electronic medical records, clinical trials, and adverse event reports, computational methods are able to integrate and identify potential new drug mechanisms and indications.[5]

During COVID-19, there were computational-based repurposing approaches with network, structure, and artificial intelligence (AI).[7] Network approaches rely on clusters and propagation to find drug–disease, drug–drug, and drug–target relationships.[7] Therefore, medical knowledge graphs relations between diseases, drugs, and proteins and predicts new links.[2] The structural approach uses known or predicted 3D structure to see how chemicals bind to targets. AI uses linear and non-linear transformation in hierarchical way and biological sequencing.[7]

CHALLENGES OF REPURPOSED DRUGS

Considerations in new treatment targets for repurposed drugs include the heterogenous patient population with many genetic variations, drug mechanisms, stage of the disease, pharmacokinetics and pharmacodynamics, and disease course. Repurposed drugs also have additional challenges. Cellular or animal assays are not the same as the human environment, and repurposed drugs are not necessarily optimized for the new indication.[2] Expedited trials often have a small number of patients and lack clinical endpoints. The drug should target the particular severity of the disease; therefore, patients with milder forms of the disease might require analysis with greater sensitivity.[2]

REPURPOSED DRUGS FOR COVID-19 (MONOTHERAPY AND COMBINATION THERAPY)

Drugs that do not have retrospective or prospective studies in peer-reviewed journals as of March 1, 2021 are not included. Large randomized control trials currently in pre-print are included. These drugs are nitazoxanide, elbasvir, mefuparib, bevacizumab, melatonin, imatinib, darutinib, ibrutinib, dasutinib, cepharantine, camostat mesylate, fingolimod, pirfenidone, bamlanivimab, and auranofin.

Acalabrutinib

Acalabrutinib is a bruton tyrosine kinase (BTK) inhibitor that regulates macrophage signaling and activation.[8] It is suggested that in macrophages, toll-like receptors recognize RNA viruses such as SARS-CoV-2 and initiate BTK-dependent activation of NF-KB, which triggers inflammatory cytokines, chemokines, and phagocytosis.[9–14] BTK also activates NLRP3 inflammosome, which matures, and IL-1B.[9–15] An animal model suggested that BTK inhibition decreased inflammation and acute lung injury.[16] A small study (n = 19) were given off-label acalbrutinib.[8] The results showed 8/11 (72.7%) patients in the supplemental oxygen cohort had been discharged on room air, and 4/8 (50%) patients in the mechanical ventilation cohort had been successfully extubated, with 2/8 (25%) discharged on room air.[8]

Angiotensin-Converting Enzyme Inhibitor (ACEI) and Angiotensin Receptor Blocker (ARB)

Omission of a medication that might pose as a greater risk can be a form of "repurposed" treatment. It has been suggested that SARS-CoV-2 binds to the extracellular domain of transmembrane angiotensin-converting enzyme 2 (ACE2) to enter host cells, and ACEI and ARB upregulate ACE2 receptors.[17] A large cohort study (18,472) showed no associated between ACEI/ARB use and COVID-19 positive results (overlap propensity score – weighted odd's ratio 0.7 95% CI 0.81-1.15).[17] A single center study (n = 1178) showed that percentage of patients with hypertension on ACEI/ARB did not differ between severe and non-severe infections (32.9% versus 30.7% P = 0.65) nor did it differ between non-survivors and survivors (27.3% vs 33% P = 0.34).[18] Another study using Danish national administrative registries showed that ACEI/ARB use compared with other antihypertensive drugs was not significantly associated with higher incidence of COVID-19 (adjusted HR, 1.05 [95% CI, 0.80-1.36]).[19] A multi-center study (n = 13501) suggested that ACEI/ARB use was associated with marginal increase rate of positive SARS-CoV-2 compared to calcium channel blocker (CCB) use (aOR 1.17 95% CI 1-147) but not with non-users (aOR 1 95 CI 0.92-1.09).[20] Risk of ICU admission was 6.3% in ACEI/ARB versus 5.4% in CCB (RR 1.17 95% CI 0.64-2.16) while 30-day mortality was 12.3% in ACEI/ARB versus 13.9% in CCB RR 0.89, 95% CI 0.61-1.30).[20] Another prospective study (n = 19486) showed reduced risk of COVID-19 disease (adjusted HR 0.71 95% CI 0.67-0.74) but no increased risk of ICU care (aHR 0.89, 95% CI 0.75-1.06).[21] However, another study (15,504) suggested that ACEI/ARB lower the risk of 28-day all-cause mortality in patients with hypertension (adjusted HR, 0.32 [95% CI, 0.15–0.66]; P 0.002), hypertension combined with coronary artery disease (adjusted HR, 0.11 [95% CI, 0.04–0.31]; $P<0.001$), and coronary artery disease (adjusted HR, 0.38 [95% CI, 0.16–0.89]; P = 0.03).[22]

Arbidol

Arbidol is an antiviral that has established mechanisms against influenza A and B and hepatitis C but has been studied in Zika virus, respiratory synctial virus (RSV), adenovirus, parainfluenza, Ebola, and hepatitis B.[23,24] It blocks entry of virus into target cells.[30] A retrospective case series of 220 patients with mild COVID-19 suggested that fever resolution and clinical recovery was faster in males with arbidol 200 mg TID for 4–8 days.[24] A multicenter prospective study of 196 patients were treated with arbidol (200 mg, 3 times/d) + lopinavir / ritonavir (2 tablets, 1 time/12 h) as the triple combination antiviral treatment group and 41 patients were treated with lopinavir/ritonavir

(2 tablets, 1 time/12 h) as the dual combination antiviral treatment group. The time of virus nucleic acid turning negative in triple versus dual combination was (12.2 ± 4.7) and [(15.0 ± 5.0) days] respectively (t = 6.159, P<0.01).[25] The length of hospital stay between triple and dual therapy was [12 (9, 17) d] and [15 (10, 18) d] respectively (H = 2.073, P<0.05).[25]

Azithromycin

This antibiotic has immunodulating and antiviral properties. In vitro studies show that it influences intracellular mitogen-activated protein kinase (MAPK) through extracellular signal-regulated kinase ½ (ERK½) and NF-KB pathway downstream of ERK.[26–28] MAPK is involved in inflammatory cytokine production, cell proliferation, and mucin secretion.[26–28] In vitro studies also suggest antiviral properties in Zika virus, rhino virus, and Ebola.[29–32] There might be a synergistic role with osteltamivir for treatment with influenza A.[33] One study failed to show mortality benefit in Middle East respiratory syndrome (MERS).[34] The studies in COVID-19 have not been promising. One observational study failed to show clinical benefit in terms of lung function after 48 hours or length of hospital stay.[35] A small (n = 20) open label non-randomized clinical trial of 600 mg hydroxychloroquine and addition of azithromycin depending on clinical course suggested a synergistic benefit with viral clearance.[36] A larger observational study (n = 1438) failed to show significant differences in mortality for patients who received hydroxychloroquine and azithromycin HR 1.35 [95% CI 0.76-2.40)], hydroxychloroquine (HR 1.08 95% CI 0.63-1.85]), or azithromycin (UR 0.56 [95% CI 0.26-1.21]).[37] A randomized control trial of 447 patients randomized to azithromycin (500 mg PO daily) and standard of care that might have included hydrocloroquine (400 mg twice a day for 10 days) failed to show any statistical difference of primary endpoint of 15-day clinical status (OR 1.36 [95% CI 0.94-1.97] P = 0.11).[38] A multicenter, open label controlled trial of hospitalized COVID-19 patients (n = 667) randomized to hydroxychloroquine at 400 mg twice a day or hydroxychloroquine at 400 mg twice a day with azithromycin 500 mg daily for 7 days showed no difference with seven point ordinal scale at 15 days OR 1.21 [(95% CI 0.69-2.11) P = 1.00] or OR 0.99 [(95% CI 0.57-1.73 P = 1.00], respectively.[39]

Baricitinib

Baricitinib is a Janus kinase inhibitor (anti-JAK) used for rheumatoid arthritis. It is an anti-inflammatory and antiviral by reducing SARS-CoV-2 endocytosis through affinity for AP2-associated protein AAK1.[40,41]

A small case series (n = 12) showed improvement with fever (P = 0.0), SpO_2 (P = 0.0), PaO_2/FiO_2 (P = 0.017), CRP (P = 0.23), and Modified Early Warning Score (P = 0.016).[40] A double blind, randomized controlled trial (n = 1033) with remdesivir (< 10 days) and either baricitinib (< 14 days) or placebo showed that patients receiving non-invasive mechanical ventilation including high flow at enrollment had time to recovery 10 days with combination therapy compared to 18 days with control (rate ratio for recovery 1.51 95% CI 1.10-2.08).[42] Twenty-eight-day mortality was 5.1% in combination and 7.8% in the control group (hazard ratio for death 0.65 95% CI 0.39-1.09).[42]

Bacillus Calmette Guerin (BCG)

This vaccine was developed from live-attenuated *mycobacterium bovis* as a vaccine against tuberculosis (TB). It provides some immunity against some viruses, bacteria, and parasites as well as treatment from malignant tumors such as bladder cancer.[43] Studies have shown that BCG reduced infant mortality by 50%, which is from unrelated infectious agents.[43,44] BCG may reduce incidence of respiratory syncytial virus, influenza, and herpes.[44-53] It has been suggested that BCG induces trained immunity against SARS-CoV-2 since it induces a transcriptional, epigenetic, and metabolic reprograming of myeloid cells of BCG-vaccinated individuals.[43,50-54] Upon challenge with pathogen-associated molecular patterns (PAMPs) from SARS-CoV-2, the innate immune cells, such as monocytes and/or natural killer cells, have enhanced response.[43] One study suggested that 10% increase in BCG index was associated with a 10.4% reduction in COVID-19 mortality.[55] An ecological study from 173 countries also suggested reduced mortality with BCG vaccination.[56] A retrospective cohort showed a decrease incidence in sickness adjusted OR 0.58 (P<0.05) and lower incidence of extreme fatigue.[57] A multivariate analysis of 55 countries suggested a negative correlation with deaths per million from COVID-19 to the years of BCG administration.[58] The strongest negative correlation with BCG vaccination and deaths per million is seen in BCG vaccination 0–64 years or those within 15 years of vaccination.[59] A meta-analysis of 160 countries suggests that countries with < 70% BCG coverage reported 6.5 (95% CI −8.4 to −4.5) less COVID-19 infections per 10,000 as compared to countries with no coverage.[59] Those countries with > 70% coverage had 10.1 (95% CI −11.4 to −8.7) less COVID-19 infections per 10,000 population compared to countries with no coverage.[59] Another exploratory study suggested that countries with a BCG vaccination policy had 58% less mortality than those without IRR 0.42 (95% CI 0.18 – 0.95).[60]

Cyclosporine (CsA)

CsA is isolated from the fungus *Tolypocladium inflatum* and is currently being used to treat and prevent graft versus host disease in bone marrow transplantation; rejection in kidney, heart, and liver transplantation; and treatment for autoimmune diseases such as rheumatoid arthritis.[61] In vitro, it has been shown to inhibit SARS-CoV and MERS-CoV replication.[62,63] CsA binds to cyclophilin A (Cyp-A) and calcineurin, which prevents activation of NF-AT.[64–69] This prevents downstream signaling of T cell receptors.[64–69] In a retrospective study (n = 607), being treated with tocilizumab, glucocorticoids, lopinavir/ritonavir, hydroxychloroquine, or cyclosporine showed cyclosporine was associated with decreased mortality (0.24 [0.12-0.46] P<0001).[70]

Chloroquine and Hydrochloroquine (HCQ)

These are anti-malarial drugs that have been reported to have antiviral properties. They are weak bases and increase endosomal pH in host organelles, inhibiting autophagosome-lysosome fusion and inactivating enzymes required for viral replication, and affect the glycosylation of angiotension converting enzyme-2, which is required by SARS-CoV-2.[71–74] There are variable results from in vitro and animal studies for other viruses such as H5N1, Zika, Epstein-Barr, Ebola, and dengue.[75–82] It has been suggested that chloroquine inhibits SARS-CoV-2 in vitro.[83] A clinical trial of non-hospitalized probable or confirmed COVID-19 (n = 491) randomized to oral hydroxychloroquine (800 mg once followed by 600 mg every 6–8 hours and then 600 mg daily for 4 more days) or placebo did not show any change in 14-day symptom severity relative 12%; absolute −0.27 point [(95% CI −0.61 to −0.07) P = 0.117].[84] At 14 days, 24% of patients who received HCQ and 30% of patients who received placebo had on-going symptoms P = 0.21.[84] In an open label platform control trial of 1,561 patients randomized to HCQ group (loading dose of 800 mg followed by 400 every 12 hours for the next 9 days) and 3,155 patients who received usual care showed no difference for death within 28 days 27% versus 25% rate ratio 1.09 (95% CI 0.97-1.23 P = 0.15).[85] A randomized double blind placebo controlled trial on post exposure prophylaxis (n = 821) showed no difference between those that received HCQ (11.8%) versus placebo (14.3%) (−2.4 percentage points [95% CI − 7.0 to 2.2. P = 0.35]).[86]

Corticosteroids

Corticosteroids were considered for their anti-inflammatory properties although their prolongation of viral shedding in SARS and MERS and increased mortality in influenza prompted initial reservations.[87–89] The recovery study on dexamethasone (n = 2104), a randomized control trial of dexamethasone 6 mg PO for 10 days versus placebo, showed that 22.9% (n = 482) in dexamethasone arm and 25.7% (n = 1110) in usual care died within 28 days, CI 0.75 to 0.93; P<0.001.[90] Incidence of death was lower than the usual care group, particularly for those on invasive mechanical ventilation (29.3% vs 41.4%; rate ratio 0.63;95% CI 0.51 to 0.81) and those on oxygen (23.3% vs 26% rate ratio 0.82 95% CI 0.72 to 0.94).[90] A multicenter observational study (n = 173) showed that prolonged low dose methylprednisolone (80 mg IV followed by 80 mg/d in 240 ml normal saline at 10 ml/h for at least 8 days until $PaO_2:FiO_2 > 350$ or CRP < 20 mg/L, after which 16 mg PO or 20 mg IV twice a day until CRP < 20% of normal range or $PaO_2:FiO_2 > 400$) versus placebo had a HR 0.41; 95% CI 0.24-0.72, transfer to ICU 15 vs 27 (P = .07) and 14 vs 26 (P = .10).[91] In another study, early use of glucocorticoids (within 48 hours of admission) was not associated with mortality benefit, but those with a CRP > 20 mg/dL had reduced risk of mortality or mechanical ventilation (OR 0.23; 95% CI 0.08-0.70) while those with CRP < 10 mg/dL had increased risk of mortality or mechanical ventilation (OR 2.64; 95% CI 1.39-5.03).[92] An RCT of methylprednisolone 0.5 mg/kg BID for 5 days compared to placebo showed no 28-day mortality benefit except in patients > 60 years of age.[93]

Eculizumab

Eculizumab is a monoclonal antibody use to treat paroxysmal nocturnal hemoglobinuria (PNH), atypical hemolytic uremic syndrome (aHUS), generalized myasthenia gravis (MG), and neuromyeitis optica spectrum disorder (NMOSD).[94] It binds to terminal complement c5, preventing cleavage to C5a and C5b, and formation of C5b-9, which has lytic, pro-inflammatory, and prothrombotic properties.[94] Selective C5 blockade preserves upstream activity for micro-organism opsonization and prevention of immune disorders. Animal models on SARS-CoV, H5N1, MERS-CoV, and H7N9 suggest protective benefits.[95,96] A proof of concept study (n = 80) showed 15-day survival for eculizumab (900 mg IV on day 1, 7, 15, and 22) of 82.9% (95% CI: 70.4%–95.3%) versus 62.2% (48.1%–76.4%) without eculizumab (log-rank test, P = 0.04).[94–98] Another study (n = 4) showed a drop inflammatory markers and all recovered.[99] Another study (n = 3) showed improvement in inflammatory makers in critically ill COVID-19 patients recalcitrant to other therapies.[100] A controlled study (n = 10) of ruxolitinib (10 mg BID for 14 days) and eculizumab (900 mg IV per week for 3 weeks) showed improvement in respiratory symptoms, radiographic findings, and d-dimers.[101]

Famotidine

Famotidine is a histamine-2 receptor antagonist used for gastric acid production suppression.[102] In vitro, famotidine inhibits human immunodeficiency virus (HIV) replication.[103] Previously, computation methods identified famotidine as a drug that can inhibit 3-chyotrypsin-like protease (3CL^{pro}), which is essential for SARS-CoV-2 replication, but this has recently been discredited.[104–107] Another theory suggests that famotidine can interfere with SARS-CoV-2's pathologic histamine release and dysfunctional mast cell activation.[108–110] A propensity score matched cohort study suggested that the use of famotidine had a reduced risk of clinical deterioration, which lead to intubation or death (P<0.01).[102] Another propensity matched cohort (n = 878) showed the use of famotidine [20 mg/d (95.2% of patients) and 40 mg/day (4.8% of patients)] was associated with decreased risk of in-hospital mortality OR 0.37 (95% CI 0.16-0.86 P = 0.021) and combined death or intubation OR 0.47 (95% CI 0.23-0.96 P = 0.040).[111]

Favipiravir

Favipiravir is another RDRP inhibitor that was approved for novel influenza in China and Japan.[112] It has a broad spectrum activity against RNA viruses, and has been suggested for Ebola virus, Lassa virus, rabies, and severe fever with thrombocytopenia.[113–116] One retrospective study found that favipiravir had a lower case-fatality rate, 42% [31 out of 73] vs 57.8% [52 of 900] P = 0.053. The study did not show improved survival, although there was longer survival time in the favipiravir-treated group (P = 0.015).[117] The dose is 1.6 g twice a day on day 1 followed by 600 mg twice a day for 8–14 days or for mild to moderate COVID-19, 1.8 gram twice a day followed by 800 mg twice a day for 14 days. In a prospective study of 40 patients treated with a combination of favipiravir and oseltamivir versus 128 with oseltamivir, the combination group had a higher clinical improvement by day 14 [(62.5% versus 42.2%) P = 0.0247], although no significant differences in mortality outcomes.[118] An adaptive open labeled randomized phase II study on hospitalized moderate COVID-19 pneumonia of 60 patients were assigned to group 1 (avifavir 1600 mg followed by 600 mg BID for day 2-14), group 2 (avifavir 1800 mg BID followed by 800 mg IBD for day 2-14), and group 3, which is standard of care (SOC).[119] On day 5, viral clearance was found in 25/40 (62.5%) of avifavir versus 5/20 (30%) in SOC (P = 0.018) but by day 10, clearance was 37/40 (92.5%) and 16/20 (80%) in SOC (P = 0.155), 13/20 (65%) in group 1, 17/20 (85%) in group 2, and 17/20 (85%) in SOC were discharged by day 15.[119]

Heparin

It has been suggested that heparin has pleotropic effects such as an anti-coagulation due to its anti-thrombin III activity, anti-inflammatory effects due to effects on chemokines, growth factors, adhesion molecules, cyto-toxic peptides, and reducing release of IL-6 and IL-8, and is a haparan sulfate analogue, which is a protective layer of natural vascular barrier.[120] There are several dosing regimen. For enoxaparin or low molecular weight heparin, standard prophylactic dose is 40 mg daily or 30 mg daily if Creatine clearance is < 30 mL/min; intermediate dose is 0.5 mg/kg daily + 10% or 40 mg twice a day; and therapeutic dose of 1 mg/kg every 12 hours. For unfractionated heparin, standard prophylactic dose is 5,000 units twice or three times daily and intermediate dose if 7,500 units three times daily or 10,000 units two times daily. These may have to be adjusted for BMI>40 kg/m^2 or creatine clearance < 30 mL/min. RCT (n = 600) on intermediate dose enoxaparin (1 mg/kg daily) versus prophylactic dose (40 mg daily) did not result in significant difference in primary outcome of venous or arterial thrombosis, extracorporeal membrane oxygenation or 30 day mortality (OR 1.06 95% CI 0.76-1.48; P = 0.71).[121] A RCT In a large observational study (n = 3239) early therapeutic anticoagulation did not affect survival (HR 1.12 95% CI 0.92 to 1.35).[122] A RCT (n = 1074) comparing prophylactic versus therapeutic dose of heparin in critically ill patients requiring at least high flow nasal cannula showed no improved hospital survival (adjusted OR 0.88 95% credible interval 0.67-1.16).[123] Another RCT (n = 2219) of patients that were not critically ill, therapeutic anticoagulation showed increased organ support free days compared to prophylactic dose (adjused OR 1.29 95% credible interval 1.04-1.61).[124] The adjusted absolute increase in survival to discharge without organ support with therapeutic anticoagulation was 4.6% (95% credible interval 0.7 to 8.1).[124]

IL-6 Antagonists

Due to the IL-6 driven cytokine storm syndrome that follows the second week SARS-CoV-2 infection, much interest has been paid to IL-6 antagonists, Tocilizumab and Sarilumab. Toclizumab has been used for autoimmune disease such as rheumatoid arthritis, systemic sclerosis interstitial lung disease, and cytokine release syndrome. Sarilumab has been used in rheumatoid arthritis. A case series (n = 21) in Wuhan, China, suggested survival benefit with tocilizumab at 400 mg IV × 1.[125] A RCT (n = 243), where 45% were Hispanic and 80% of the patients were receiving < 6 liters on nasal cannula, showed no benefit in preventing intubation or death (HR 0.83 [95% CI 0.38 to 1.81; P = 0.64]) and for disease progression (HR 1.11 [95% CI 0.59 − 2.10; P = 0.73]).[126] A multi-center Italian RCT (n = 126) of patients with PaO_2/FiO_2 200–300 mm Hg randomized to tocilizumab (8 mg/kg to a maximum of 800 mg) followed by second dose 12 hours later compared to placebo showed clinical worsening of 17 patients (28.3%) in tocilizumab arm and 17 patients (27%) in placebo arm after 14 days.[127] Trial was stopped due to futility. Due to the higher mortality among minorities, another study on tocilizumab focused on non-Hispanic Blacks, Hispanics, and American Indians. EMPACTA (Evaluating Minority Patients with Acemtra) (n = 389) is an RCT comparing 8 mg/kg tocilizumab versus placebo.[128] It showed tocilizumab group received less mechanical ventilation or died by day 28 (12.0% [95% CI 8.5 to 1.9] vs 19.3% [95% CI 13.3-27.4]) (HR 0.56; 95% CI 0.33-0.7 P = 0.04).[128] The COVACTA study's primary outcome based on ordinal scale did not show improved 28 day mortality (19.7% in the tocilizumab group and 19.4% in the placebo group (95% CI −7.6 to 8.2; P = 0.94).[129] Median time to hospital discharge was 20 days in tocilizumab and 28 days in placebo (HR 1.35 95% CI 1.02-1.79).[129]

The post hoc analysis of patients not on mechanical ventilation at randomization showed only 29% (53 of 183) in tocilizumab arm versus 42.2% (38 of 90) in placebo arm experienced clinical failure (HR 0.614 [95% CI 0.40 to 0.94]).[129] A study comparing two IL-6 receptor antagonists on patients within 24 hours of organ support in the ICU and randomized to tocilizumab (n = 353) (8 mg/kg), sarilumab (n = 48) (400 mg) or standard care (n = 402) showed median organ support-free days of 10 for tocilizumab, 11 for sarilumab, and 0 for control, respectively.[130] Hospital mortality was 28% (98/350) for tocilizumab, 22.2% (10/45) for sarilumab, and 36% (142/397) for control.[130] 90-day surivival for pooled IL-6 antagonists (tocilizumab and sarliumab) compared to control group (HR 1.61 95% Credible interval 1.26-2.08).[130] Another open labeled RCT, Recovery, (n = 4116) compared tocilizumab (8mg/kg) and standard of care. Eighty-two percent received corticosteroids and 14% (n = 562) received invasive mechanical ventilation, 41% (n = 1686) non-invasive respiratory support, and 45% no respiratory support other than oxygen (n = 1868).[131] Twenty-nine percent (n = 596) from tocilizumab arm and 33% (n = 694) died within 28 days, RR 0.86 95% CI 0.77-0.96.[131] Patients also in tocilizumab arm were likely to be discharged from hospital alive within 28 days (54% vs 47% RR 1.22 95% CI 1.12-1.33 P<0.0001).[131] An adaptive, phase 2 (n = 457) and phase 3 (n = 1365) RCT on sarilumab showed that patients > 1 point improvement in clinical status (alive not receiving MV) at day 22 was 43.2% in sarilumab 400 mg and 25.5% in placebo (risk difference[RD] +7.5%; 95% CI -7.4 to 21.3 P = 0.3261).[132] Day 29 all cause mortality was 36.4% in sarilumab 400 mg versus 41.9%

placebo (RD −5.5% 95% CI −20.2 to −8.7).[132] Pooled post hoc analysis showed HR 0.76 (95% CI 0.51-1.13), improving to 0.49 (95% CI 0.25-0.94) with corticosteroids at baseline.[132]

Interferons (IFN)

This group of cytokines is produced as a response to viral infections and activates interferon stimulating genes (ISGs). These increase ACE2 but inhibit angiotensin II, which is believed to be lung protective.[133,134] They have variable response in SARS and MERS.[135–137] A randomized clinical trial (n = 92) showed that patients given interferon B-1a [44 ug/ml (2 million IU/ml)] subcutaneously (SQ) three times a week for 2 weeks showed lower 28-day mortality compared to placebo 19% versus 43.6% P = 0.015.[133] Another prospective study (n = 77) suggested that nebulized IFN-a2b (5 mU BID) reduced detectable SARS-CoV-2 and decreased inflammatory markers.[138] A small randomized control trial (n = 80) showed that patients given IFN B-1b (250 mcg SQ every other day for 2 weeks) compared to placebo had shorter time to clinical improvement and less ICU admission rates.[139] However, 28-day all cause mortality was 6.06% (IFN) and 18.18% (placebo) (P = 0.12).[139]

Lopinavir

Lopinavir is a human immunodeficiency virus (HIV) type I aspartate protease inhibitor which has in vitro activity against SARS-CoV, and MERS-CoV. Combined with ritonavir, which inhibits cytochrome P450, and prolonging lopinavir's plasma half-life, it has been suggested as potential treatment for COVID-19. An open labeled trial with 199 patients randomized to lopinavir-ritonavir (400 mg/100 mg PO twice a day for 14 days) or SOC found no difference in time to clinical improvement (hazard ratio 1.31; 95% CI 0.95-1.90) and 28 day mortality (19.2% versus 25%; difference −5.8 percentage points; 95% CI −17.3 to 5.7).[140] Another open label platform trial found that there was no difference in 28 day mortality between lopinavir-ritonavir compared to SOC (rate ratio 1.03 95% CI 0.91-1.17 P = 0.60).[141]

Ivermectin

Ivermectin is a macrocyclic lactone 22,23-dihydroavermectin B produced by the bacterium *Streptomyces avermitilis* and has been used to treat onchocerciasis, filariasis, strongyloidiasis, ascariasis, ectoparisites, pediculosis, and rosacea.[142] It has been found to be effective in multiple viruses through multiple mechanisms. It inhibits the NS3 helicase in yellow fever, dengue virus, and West Nile virus; inhibits nonstructural protein 5 (NS5), which is required for viral replication, in Zika virus and dengue virus; inhibits the transmission of the Hendra virus and Venezuelan equine encephalitis virus through IMP a1/B1; reduces viral production in chikungunya virus, semliki forest virus, and sindbis virus; prevents the nuclear transmission of viral ribonucleoprotein complexes; reduces the intracellular expression of PRSRRV N protein in porcine reproductive and respiratory syndrome virus (PRRSV); inhibits the entry of DNA polymerase accessory subunit UL42 into nucleus and reduces viral loads in pseudorabies virus; decreases porcine circovirus 2 viral loads due to its effect on nuclear localization signal (NLS)-mediated nuclear import pathway; and inhibits the IMP a/B medicated nuclear import in BK polyomavirus, bovine herpes virus 1, and SARS-COV-2.[143–170] A multivariate analysis of a retrospective chart review of 280 patients with COVID-19 showed that mortality was lower in the ivermectin group (200 ug/kg $\times$ 1 but can be repeated after 7 days) compared to no ivermectin (OR 0.27; 95% CI 0.22-0.99 P = 0.03).[171] In the propensity matched cohort of 190 patients, mortality was lower in the ivermectin group (13.3% vs 24.5%; OR, 0.47; 95% CI, 0.22-0.99; P<.05), an 11.2% (95% CI, 0.38%-22.1%) absolute risk reduction, with a number needed to treat of 8.9 (95% CI, 4.5-263).[171] A double blinded RCT (n = 476) of ivermectin 300 ug/kg of body weight per day for five days compared to placebo did not significantly improve the time to resolution of symptoms.[172]

Methylene Blue

Some have hypothesized that hypoxia in COVID-19 is related to methemoglobinemia, secondary to oxidation of hemoglobin's iron from ferrous to ferric form, giving the rationale of use of methylene blue (MB).[173] Administration of MB at 1 mg/kg with vitamin C 1,500 mg/kg and N-acetyl cysteine (1,500 mg/kg) in 5 patients increased the SPO_2 with delayed effect in improvement in inflammatory markers.[173] MB has been studied in conjunction with ultraviolet light (UV) to decreased infectivity of SARS-CoV, Crimean-Congo haemorrhagic fever virus (CCHFV), and NIPAH virus (NiV) in plasma and platelet transfusions, and another study shows inhibition of SARS-CoV-2 in vitro.[174,175]

Remdesivir

This RNA-dependent RNA polymerase (RDRP) inhibitor had in vitro effects against SARS-CoV-1, Middle East Respiratory Syndrome (MERS-CoV), and SARS-CoV-2.[176–180] A cohort study of hospitalized COVID-19 patients who received compassionate use of remdesivir, at 200 mg IV on day one followed by 100 mg IV on days 2–10 found that 36 out of 53 patients had clinical improvement.[181] An open labeled randomized phase 3 trial with 397 patients found no significant benefit between 5-day versus 10-day course.[182] A randomized, double blinded placebo controlled study of 1,062 patients showed that 15-day mortality for remdesivir was 6.7% compared to placebo, which was 11.9% and by day 29, 11.4% with remdesivir and 15.2% with placebo (hazard ratio 0.73; 95% CI (0.52-1.03).[183] The World Health Organization (WHO)'s solidarity study of 4 repurposed antiviral drugs (n = 11,330) advised against the use of remdesivir based on their study's interim results.[184] Death occurred in 301 out of 2743 pateints with remdesivir and 303 out of 2708 in control group (Rate Ratio[RR] 0.95; 95% CI 0.81-1.11 P = 0.50).[184] They also advised against hydroxychloroquine (RR 1.19 95% CI 0.89-1.59 P = 0.23), Lopinavir (RR 1 95% CI 0.79-1.25 P = 0.97) and interferon (RR 1.16 95% CI 0.96-1.39 P = 0.11).[184]

Ribavarin

Ribavarin is a guanosine analogue that interferes with RNA and DNA viral replication, and also interferes with RNA capping, which prevents RNA degradation.[185] It is part of the treatment for hepatitis C and RSV. It has been studied in Crimean Congo hemorrhagic fevers, Lassa fevers, Ebola, SARS-CoV-2, and MERS-CoV with no established clinical benefit.[185–187] It was one of first five drugs to have in vitro efficacy against strains of SARS-CoV-2.[186] An open label phase 2 trial of 127 patients with mild to moderate COVID-19 were randomized to two groups: group 1 (14 day of lopinavir 400 mg and ritonavir 100 mg every 12 hours, ribavirin 400 mg every 12 hours, and three doses of 8 million international units of interferon beta-1b on alternate days) versus group 2 [14 days of lopinavir 400 mg and ritonavir 100 mg every 12 hours (control)].[188] Patients in group 1 or treatment group had shorter median time to negative nasopharyngeal swab [7 days (IQR 5-11)] than control group [12 days IQR (8-15)] P = 0.0010.[188]

Ruxolitinib

Ruxolitnib is used for primary myelofibrosis, post polycythemia vera, and post-essential thrombocythemia myelofibrosis. It is a selective Janus kinase (JAK) 1 and 2 inhibitor and modest to marked selectively of tyrosine kinase (TYK)2 and JAK3, respectively.[189] Efficacy is related to anti-inflammatory effects to IL-1, IL6, IL-8, IL-12, TNF-a, IFN-y, VEGF, TGF-B, FGF, PDGF, GM-CSF, and G-CSF.[190] A small study (n = 14) showed that 12 out of 14 patients who had COVID-19 inflammatory score

(CIS) > 10 and were given ruxolitinib (7.5 mg BID and increased to 15 mg BID) had > 25% reduction of CIS by day 7, and 11 of these had sustained clinical improvement.[189] Another small study (n = 18) with COVID-19 ARDS (acute respiratory distress syndrome) patients were given ruxolitinib (20 mg BID for the first 48 hours and de-escalated to 10 mg BID and then 5 mg BID for 14 days). It suggested rapid clinical improvement in 16 patients after 2 days; 11 of these patients had full recovery with PO_2 > 98% with spontaneous breathing after 7 days; and 16 of these patients had complete recovery of lung function after day 14.[190]

Sofosbuvir

Sofosbuvir, an antiviral used to treat hepatitis C, became a candidate to fight COVID-19 via sequence analysis and docking models.[191] It targets the RDRP, and in vitro has activity against positive strand RNA viruses such as yellow fever, Zika, dengue, and chikungunya.[192–195] A multi-center, open labeled controlled trial on 66 moderate to severe COVID-19 patients randomized to sofosbuvir and daclatasvir (400 mg / 60 PO mg daily for 14 days) versus standard of care found that 14-day clinical recovery was achieved in 29/33 (88%) treatment arm versus 22/33 (67%) in control arm (P 0.076).[196] However, the treatment arm had a shorter duration of hospitalization (6 days vs 9 days), P = 0.029.[196]

Statins

Statins are used to treat hyperlipidemia but also have anti-inflammatory properties. They have been studied in influenza and Ebola.[197,198] One study (n = 156) suggested that patients on long-term statins for dyslipidemia had lower chance of ICU admission compared to patients not on statins [CoEff (risk difference) – 0.12 (−0.23 to 0.01); P = 0.028].[199] Another retrospective single center study showed that 30-day prior to admission use of statins was associated with reduced risk of severe COVID-19 (adjusted OR 0.29, 95% CI 0.11-0.71 P<0.01) and faster time to recovery among those without severe disease (adjusted HR for recovery 2.69 95% CI 1.36 to 5.33 P<0.01).[200] A retrospective study (n = 13,981) where 1,219 patients received statin compared to no statin was found to have 28-day all-cause mortality of 5.2% and 9.5%, respectively (adjusted hazard ratio 0.58).[201] Another study (n = 4252) showed that statin use was associated with reduced mortality in patients with diabetes mellitus (HR 0.88 95% CI 0.84-0.92 P<0.01).[202] A meta-analysis of nine studies (n = 3449) showed that statins did not improve severity outcomes [OR 1.64 (95% CI 0.51-5-23) P = 0.41, I^2 = 93%, random-effect modeling] nor mortality [OR 0.78 (95% CI 0.50-1.21), I^2 = 0%, P = 0.26].[203]

Vitamin C

This is an antioxidant and anti-inflammatory. With few complications, it has been studied in sepsis with disappointing results.[204–206] A small case series (n = 17) suggested that vitamin C at 1,000 g IV every 8 hours lowered inflammatory markers, mechanical ventilation rates, and mortality.[207]

Vitamin D

Vitamin D has antiviral and anti-inflammatory properties, and low serum levels in hospitalized patients are associated with poor prognosis.[208] A retrospective study (n = 489) suggested that vitamin D deficiency was associated with increased COVID-19 risk.[209] In a small case series (n = 4), patients had improved outcomes after supplementation with cholecalciferol 1,000 IU daily or ergocalciferol 50,000 IU daily for 5 days.[210] A prospective study (n = 324) found that supplementation was not associated with hospitalization or in-hospital mortality, but a trend toward higher risk of death.[210] A recent multi-center double blinded RCT (n = 240) in Brazil showed patients given 200,000 IU of vitamin D3 vs placebo had no significant difference in in-hospital mortality ([7.6 vs 5.1%;95% CI −4.1 to 9.2%]; P = 0.43), admission to ICU ([16% vs 21.2%, 95% CI −15.1 to 4.7%]; P = 0.30), or need for mechanical ventilation ([9.6% vs 14.4% 95% CI −15.1% to 1.2%]; P = 0.09) despite improvement in 25-hydroxyvitamin D levels (44.4 ng/mL vs 19.8 ng/mL [95% CI 19.5-28.7]; p<0.001).[211]

Zinc

Zinc has an immune-modulator role with antibody and white blood cell production. Zinc deficiency can lead to increased pro-inflammatory cytokine production and decreased production antibodies while supplementation increases ability for polymorphonuclear cells to combat infection.[212–214] In vitro and cell culture studies on SARS-CoV-1 shows inhibition of viral RNA polymerase activity.[212–214] It has been suggested that zinc supplementation can be synergistic with chloroquine/hydroxychloroquine + azithromycin, at a dose of HCQ 200 mg twice a day, zinc 220 mg daily, and azithromycin 500 mg daily for 5 days.[215,216] A retrospective study with treatment (n = 141) with control (n = 377) showed that treatment group had 4 (2.8%) of 141 patients hospitalized compared to control 58 (15.4%) of 377 patients [OR = 0.16, 95% CI 0.06–0.5; P<0.001].[217]

REFERENCES

1. Yeu Y, Yoon Y, Park S. Protein localization vector propagation: a method for improving the accuracy of drug repositioning. *Mol Biosyst.* 2015;11:2096-2102.

2. Zhou Y, Wang F, Tang J, Nussinov R, Cheng F. Artificial intelligence in COVID-19 drug repurposing. *Lancet Digital Health.* 2020;2:e667-e676.

3. Ciliberto G, Mancini R, Paggi MG. Drug repurposing against COVID-19: Focus on anticancer agents. *J Exp Clin Cancer Res.* 2020;39:86.

4. Singh TU, Parida S, Lingaraju MC, Kesavan M, Kumar D, Singh RK. Drug repurposing approach to fight COVID-19. *Pharmacol Rep.* 2020;72(6):1479-1508.

5. Huang F, Zhang C, Liu Q, et al. Identification of amitriptyline HCl, flavin adenine dinucleotide, azacitidine and calcitriol as repurposing drugs for influenza A H5N1 virus-induced lung injury. *PLoS Pathog.* 2020;16(3):e1008341.

6. Cheng F, Desai RJ, Handy DE, et al. Network-based approach to prediction and population-based validation of in silico drug repurposing. *Nat Commun.* 2018;9:2691.

7. Dotolo S, Marabotti A, Facchiano A, Tagliaferri R. A review on drug repurposing applicable to COVID-19. *Brief Bioinform.* 2020:1-16.

8. Roschewski M, Lionakis MS, Sharman JP, et al. Inhibition of Bruton tyrosine kinase in patients with severe COVID-19. *Sci Immunol.* 2020;5(48):eabd0110.

9. Page TH, Urbaniak AM, Espirito Santo AI, et al. Bruton's tyrosine kinase regulates TLR7/8-induced TNF transcription via nuclear factor-κB recruitment. *Biochem Biophys Res Commun.* 2018;499:260-266.

10. Tatematsu M, Nishikawa F, Seya T, Matsumoto M. Toll-like receptor 3 recognizes incomplete stem structures in single-stranded viral RNA. *Nat Commun.* 2013;4:1833.

11. Byrne JC, Ní Gabhann J, Stacey KB, et al. Bruton's tyrosine kinase is required for apoptotic cell uptake via regulating the phosphorylation and localization of calreticulin. *J Immunol.* 2013;190:5207-5215.

12. Feng M, Chen JY, Weissman-Tsukamoto R, et al. Macrophages eat cancer cells using their own calreticulin as a guide: Roles of TLR and Btk. *Proc Natl Acad Sci USA.* 2015;112:2145-2150.

13. Liu X, Pichulik T, Wolz OO, et al. Human NACHT, LRR, and PYD domain-containing protein 3 (NLRP3) inflammasome activity is regulated by and potentially targetable through Bruton tyrosine kinase. *J Allergy Clin Immunol.* 2017;140:1054-1067.e10.

14. Ito M, Shichita T, Okada M, et al. Bruton's tyrosine kinase is essential for NLRP3 inflammasome activation and contributes to ischaemic brain injury. *Nat Commun.* 2015;6:7360.

15. Bittner ZA, Liu X, Shankar S, et al. BTK operates a phospho-tyrosine switch to regulate NLRP3 inflammasome activity. *bioRxiv.* 2020. Available at https://www.biorxiv.org/content/10.1101/864702v3.

16. Florence M, Krupa A, Booshehri LM, Davis SA, Matthay MA, Kurdowska AK. Inhibiting Bruton's tyrosine kinase rescues mice from lethal influenza-induced acute lung injury. *Am. J. Physiol Lung Cell Mol Physiol.* 2018;315:L52-L58.

17. Mehta N, Katra A, Nowacki AM, et al. Association of use of angiotensin-converting enzyme inhibitors and angiotensin II receptor blockers with testing positive for coronavirus Disease 2019 (COVID-19). *JAMA Cardiol*. 2020;5(9):1020-1026.

18. Li J, Wang X, Chen J, Zhang H, Deng A. Association of renin-angiotensin system inhibitors with severity or risk of death in patients with hypertension hospitalized for coronavirus disease 2019 (COVID-19) infection in Wuhan, China. *JAMA Cardiol*. 2020;5(7):825-830. Erratum in: *JAMA Cardiol*. 2020;5(8):968.

19. Fosbøl EL, Butt JH, Østergaard L, et al. Association of angiotensin-converting enzyme inhibitor or angiotensin receptor blocker use with COVID-19 diagnosis and mortality. *JAMA*. 2020;324(2):168-177.

20. Christiansen CF, Pottegård A, Heide-Jørgensen U, et al. SARS-CoV-2 infection and adverse outcomes in users of ACE inhibitors and angiotensin-receptor blockers: A nationwide case-control and cohort analysis. *Thorax*. 2020;thoraxjnl-2020-215768. [Online ahead of print.]

21. Hippisley-Cox J, Young D, Coupland C, et al. Risk of severe COVID-19 disease with ACE inhibitors and angiotensin receptor blockers: cohort study including 8.3 million people. *Heart*. 2020;106(19):1503-1511.

22. Zhou F, Liu YM, Xie J, et al. Comparative impacts of ACE (angiotensin-converting enzyme) inhibitors versus angiotensin II receptor blockers on the risk of COVID-19 mortality. *Hypertension*. 2020 Aug;76(2):e15-e17

23. Boriskin YS, Leneva IA, Pechaeur E-I, Polyak SJ. Arbidol: A broad-spectrum antiviral compound that blocks viral fusion. *Curr Med Chem*. 2008;15(10):997-1005.

24. Gao W, Chen S, Wang K, Chen R, et al. Clinical features and efficacy of antiviral drug, Arbidol in 220 nonemergency COVID-19 patients from East-West-Lake Shelter Hospital in Wuhan: A retrospective case series. *Virol J*. 2020; 14:162.

25. Wei R, Zheng N, Jiang X, Ma C, et al. Early antiviral therapy of abidor combined with lopinavir/ritonavir and re-combinant interferon a-2b in patients with novel coronavirus pneumonia in Zhejiang: A multicenter and prospective study. *Chinese J Clin Infect Dis*. March 2020;13:e010-e010.

26. Kanoh S, Rubin BK. Mechanisms of action and clinical application of macrolides as immunomodulatory medications. *Clin Microbiol Rev*. 2010;23(3):590-615.

27. Cramer CL, Patterson A, Alchakaki A, Soubani AO. Immunomodulatory indications of azithromycin in respiratory disease: A concise review for the clinician. *Postgrad Med*. 2017;129:493-9.

28. Parnham MJ, Haber VE, Giamarellos-Bourboulis EJ, Perletti G, Verleden GM, Vos R. Azithromycin: Mechanisms of action and their relevance for clinical applications. *Pharmacol Ther*. 2014;143:225-245.

29. Bosseboeuf E, Aubry M, Nhan T, et al. Azithromycin inhibits the replication of Zika virus. *J Antivir Antiretrovir*. 2018;10:6-11.

30. Retallack H, Di Lullo E, Arias C, et al. Zika virus cell tropism in the developing human brain and inhibition by azithromycin. *Proc Natl Acad Sci USA*. 2016; 113:14408-14413.

31. Madrid PB, Panchal RG, Warren TK, et al. Evaluation of Ebola virus inhibitors for drug repurposing. *ACS Infect Dis*. 2015;1(7):317-326.

32. Gielen V, Johnston SL, Edwards MR. Azithromycin induces anti-viral responses in bronchial epithelial cells. *Eur Respir J*. 2010;36(3):646-654.

33. Kakeya H, Seki M, Izumikawa K, et al. Efficacy of combination therapy with oseltamivir phosphate and azithromycin for influenza: A multicenter, open-label, randomized study. *PLoS One*. 2014;9:1-10.

34. Arabi YM, Deeb AM, Al-Hameed F, et al. Macrolides in critically ill patients with Middle East Respiratory Syndrome. *Int J Infect Dis*. 2019;81:184-190.

35. Rodriguez-Molinero A, Perez-Lopez C, Galvez-Barron C, et al. Observational study of azithromycin in hospitalized patients with COVID-19. *PLoS One*. 2020;15(9):e0238681.

36. Gautret P, LAgier JC, Parola P, et al. Hydroxychloroquine and azithromycin as a treatment of COVID-19: Results of an open-label non-randomized clinical trial. *Int J Antimicrob Agents*. Jul;56(1):105949.

37. Rosenberg ES, Dufort EM, Udo T, et al. Association of treatment with hydroxychloroquine or azithromycin with in-hospital mortality in patients with COVID-19 in New York State. *JAMA*. 2020;323(24):2493-2502.

38. Furtadao RHM, Berwanger O, Foseca HA, et al. Azithromycin in addition to standard of care versus standard of care alone in the treatment of patients admitted to the hospital with severe COVID-19 in Brazil (COALITION II): A randomized clinical trial. *Lancet*. 2020;396:959-967.

39. Cavalcanti AB, Zampieri FG, Rosa RG, et al. Hydroxychloroquine with or without azithromycin in mild to moderate COVID-19. *N Engl J Med*. 2020;383:2041-2052.

40. Cantini F, Niccoli L, MAtarrese D, Nicastri E, Stobbione P, Goletti D. Bacritinib therapy I COVID-19: A pilot study on safety and clinical impact. *Journal of J Infect*. 2020;81:318-356.

41. Richardson P, Griffin I, Tucker C, et al. Baricitinib as potential treatment for v2019-nCoV acute respiratory disease. *Lancet*. 2020;395:e30-1.

42. Kalil AC, Patterson TF, Mehta AK, et al. Baricitinib plus remdesivir for hospitalized adults with Covid-19. *N Engl J Med*. 2021;384(9):795-807.

43. Butkeviciute E, Jones CE, Smith SG. Heterologous effects of infant BCG vaccination: Potential mechanisms of immunity. *Future Microbiol*. 2018;13:1193-1208.

44. O'Neill LAJ, Netea MG. BCG-Induced trained immunity: Can it offer protection against COVID-19? *Nature Review: Immunology*. 2020:1-3.

45. Aaby P, Roth A, Ravn H, et al. Randomized trial of BCG vaccination at birth to low-birth-weight children: Beneficial nonspecific effects in the neonatal period? *J Infect Dis*. 2011; 204:245-252.

46. Stensballe LG, Nante E, Jensen IP, et al. Acute lower respiratory tract infections and respiratory syncytial virus in infants in Guinea-Bissau: A beneficial effect of BCG vaccination for girls community based case-control study. *Vaccine*. 2005;23:1251-1257.

47. Wardhana, Datau EA, Sultana A, Mandang VVV, Jim E. The efficacy of Bacillus Calmette-Guerin vaccinations for the prevention of acute upper respiratory tract infection in the elderly. *Acta Med Indones*. 2011;43;185-190.

48. Ohrui T, et al. Prevention of elderly pneumonia by pneumococcal, influenza and BCG vaccinations [Japanese]. *Nihon Ronen Igakkai Zasshi*. 2005;42:34-36.

49. Nemes, E. et al. Prevention of *M. tuberculosis* infection with H4:IC31 vaccine or BCG revaccination. *N Engl J Med.* 2018;379:138-149.

50. Spencer JC, Ganguly R, Waldman RH. Nonspecific protection of mice against influenza virus infection by local or systemic immunization with Bacille Calmette-Guerin. *J Infect Dis.* 1977;136:171-175.

51. Starr SE, et al. Effects of immunostimulants on resistance of newborn mice to herpes simplex type 2 infection. *Proc Soc Exp Biol Med.* 1976;152:57-60.

52. Ikeda S, Negishi T, Nishimura C. Enhancement of non-specific resistance to viral infection by muramyldipeptide and its analogs. *Antivir Res.* 1985;5:207-215.

53. Kleinnijenhuis J, Quintin J, Preijers F, et al. Bacille Calmette-Guerin induces NOD2- dependent nonspecific protection from reinfection via epigenetic reprogramming of monocytes. *Proc Natl Acad Sci USA.* 2012;109:17537-17542.

54. Netea MG, Joosten LA, Latz E, et al. Trained immunity: A program of innate immune memory in health and disease. *Science.* 352, aaf1098 (2016).

55. Escobar LE, Molina-Cruz A, Barillas-Mury C. BCG vaccine protection from severe coronavirus disease 2019 (COVID-19). *PNAS.* 2020;117(30): 17720-17726.

56. Urashima M, Otani K, Hasegawa Y, Akutsu T. BCG vaccination and morality of COVID-19 across 173 countries: An ecological study. *Int J Environ Res Public Health.* 2020,17.5589.

57. Moorlag SJCFM, van Deuren RC, van Werkhoven CH, et al. Safety and COVID-19 symptoms in individuals recently vaccinated with BCG: A retrospective cohort study. *Cell Rep Med.* 2020;1(5):100073.

58. Klinger D, Blass I, Rappoport N, Linial M. Significantly improved COVID-19 outcomes in countries with higher BCG vaccination coverage: A multivariable analysis. *Vaccines.* 2020;8(3):378.

59. Joy M, Malavika B, Asirvatham ES, Sudarsanam TD, Jayaseelan L. Is BCG associated with reduced incidence of COVID-19? A meta-regression of global data from 160 countries. *Clin Epidemiol Glob Health.* 2021;9:202-203.

60. Kumar A, Misra S, Verma V, et al. Global impact of environmental temperature and BCG vaccination coverage on the transmissibility and fatality rate of COVID-19. *PLoS One.* 2020;15(10):e0240710.

61. Molyvdas A, Matalon S. Cyclosporine: An old weapon in the fight against coronaviruses. *Eur Respir J.* 2020;56(5):2002484.

62. Li HS, et al. Effect of interferon alpha and cyclosporine treatment separately and in combination on Middle East Respiratory Syndrome Coronavirus (MERS-CoV) replication in a human in-vitro and ex-vivo culture model. *Antiviral Res.* 2018;155:89-96.

63. Hausenloy D, Boston-Griffiths E, D. Yellon D. Cyclosporin A and cardioprotection: From investigative tool to therapeutic agent. *Br J Pharmacol.* 2012;165(5):1235-1245.

64. Liddicoat AM, Lavelle EC. Modulation of innate immunity by cyclosporine A. *Biochem Pharmacol.* 2019;163:472-480.

65. Elgebaly SA, Elbayoumi T, Kreutzer DL. Cyclosporin H: A novel anti-inflammatory therapy for influenza flu patients. *J Egypt Soc Parasitol.* 2017;47(1):25-33.

66. Handschumacher RE, et al. Cyclophilin: A specific cytosolic binding protein for cyclosporin A. *Science*. 1984;226(4674):544-547.
67. Friedman J, Weissman I. Two cytoplasmic candidates for immunophilin action are revealed by affinity for a new cyclophilin: One in the presence and one in the absence of CsA. *Cell*. 1991;66(4):799-806.
68. Liu J, Farmer JD, Lane WS, et al. Calcineurin is a common target of cyclophilin-cyclosporin A and FKBP-FK506 complexes. *Cell*. 1991;66(4):807-815.
69. Li YJ, Wu HH, Weng CH, et al. Cyclophilin A and nuclear factor of activated T cells are essential in cyclosporine-mediated suppression of polyomavirus BK replication. *Am J Transplant*. 2012;12(9):2348-2362.
70. Guisado-Vasco P, Valderas-Ortega S, Carralon-Gonzalez MM, et al. Clinical characteristics and outcomes among hospitalized adults with severe COVID-19 admitted to a tertiary medical center and receiving antiviral, antimalarials, glucocorticoids or immunomodulation with tocilizumab or cyclosporine: a retrospective observational study. *EClinical Medicine*. 2020;28:100591.
71. Cavalcanti AB, Zampieri FG, Rosa RG, Azevedo LCP, et al. Hydroxychloroquine with or without azithromycin in mild to moderate COVID-19. *N Engl J Med*. 2020;383:2041-2052.
72. Ferner RE, Arons JK. Chloroquine and hydroxychloroquine in COVID-19. *BMJ*. 2020;369:m1432.
73. Salata C, Calistri A, Parolin C, Baritussio A, Palù G. Antiviral activity of cationic amphiphilic drugs. *Expert Rev Anti Infect Ther*. 2017;15(5):483-492.
74. Vincent MJ, Bergeron E, Benjannet S, et al. Chloroquine is a potent inhibitor of SARS coronavirus infection and spread. *Virol J*. 2005;2:69.
75. Yan Y, Zou Z, Sun Y, et al. Anti-malaria drug chloroquine is highly effective in treating avian influenza A H5N1 virus infection in an animal model. *Cell Res*. 2013;23:300-302.
76. Shiryaev SA, Mesci P, Pinto A, et al. Repurposing of the anti-malaria drug chloroquine for Zika virus treatment and prophylaxis. *Sci Rep*. 2017;7:15771.
77. Li X, Burton EM, Bhaduri-McIntosh S. Chloroquine triggers Epstein-Barr virus replication through phosphorylation of KAP1/TRIM28 in Burkitt lymphoma cells. *PLoS Pathog*. 2017;13:e1006249.
78. Li C, Zhu X, Ji X, et al. Chloroquine, an FDA-approved drug, prevents Zika virus infection and its associated congenital microcephaly in mice. *EBioMedicine*. 2017;24:189-194.
79. Dowall SD, Bosworth A, Watson R, et al. Chloroquine inhibited Ebola virus replication in vitro but failed to protect against infection and disease in the in vivo guinea pig model. *J Gen Virol*. 2015;96:3484-3492.
80. Falzarano D, Safronetz D, Prescott J, Marzi A, Feldmann F, Feldmann H. Lack of protection against Ebola virus from chloroquine in mice and hamsters. *Emerg Infect Dis*. 2015;21:1065-1067.
81. Roques P, Thiberville SD, Dupuis-Maguiraga L, et al. Paradoxical effect of chloroquine treatment in enhancing chikungunya virus infection. *Virus*. 2018;10:268.
82. Wang LF, Lin YS, Huang NC et al. Hydroxychloroquine-inhibited dengue virus is associated with host defense machinery. *J Interferen Cytokine Res*. 2015;35:143-156.

83. Gao J, Tian Z, Yang X. Breakthrough: chloroquine phosphate has shown apparent efficacy in treatment of COVID-19 associated pneumonia in clinical studies. *Biosci Trends*. 2020;14(1):72-73.

84. Skipper C, Pastick K, Engen N, Bangdiwala A, et al. Hydroxychloroquine in non-hospitalized adults with early COVID-19: A randomized control trial. *Annals of Internal Medicine*. 2020;173(8):623-631.

85. Recovery Group. Effect of hydroxychloroquine in hospitalized patients with COVID-19. *N Engl J Med*. 2020;383:2030-2040.

86. Boulware DR, Pullen MF, Bangidwala AS, Pastick KA, et al. A randomized trial of hydroxychloroquine as postexposure prophylaxis for COVID-19. *N Engl J Med*. 2020;383:517-525.

87. Arabi YM, Mandourah Y, Al-Hameed F, et al. Corticosteroid therapy for critically ill patients with Middle East Respiratory Syndrome. *Am J Respir Crit Care Med*. 2018;197:757-767.

88. Lee N, Allen Chan KC, Hui DS, et al. Effects of early corticosteroid treatment on plasma SARS-associated coronavirus RNA concentrations in adult patients. *J Clin Virol*. 2004;31:304-309.

89. Ni YN, Chen G, Sun J, Liang BM, Liang ZA. The effect of corticosteroids on mortality of patients with influenza pneumonia: A systematic review and meta-analysis. *Crit Care*. 2019,23:99.

90. RECOVERY Collaborative Group, et al. Dexamethasone in hospitalized patients with COVID-19 – Preliminary Report. *N Engl J Med*. 2021;384(8):693-704.

91. Salton F, Confalonieri P, Meduri GU, et al. Prolonged low-dose methylprednisolone in patients with severe COVID-19 pneumonia. *Open Forum Infect Dis*. 2020;7(10):ofaa421.

92. Keller MJ, Kitsis EA, Arora S, et al. Effect of systemic glucocorticoids on mortality or mechanical ventilation in patients with COVID-19. *J Hosp Med*. 2020;15(8):489-493.

93. Jernimo CMP, Farias ME, Val FFA, et al. Methylprednisolone as adjunct therapy for patients hospitalized with COVID-19 (Metcovid): A randomised, double-blinded, phase IIb, placebo-controlled trial. *Clin Infect Disc*. 2021;72:e373-e381.

94. Annane D, Heming N, Grimaldi-Bensouda L, et al. Eculizumab as an emergency treatment for adult patients with severe COVID-19 in the intensive care unit: A proof of concept study. *EClinical Medicine*. 2020;28:100590:1-9.

95. Sun S, Zhao G, Liu C, et al. Inhibition of complement activation alleviates acute lung injury induced by highly pathogenic avian influenza H5N1 virus infection *Am J Respir Cell Mol Biol*. 2013;49:221-230.

96. Jiang Y, Zhao G, Song N, et al. Blockade of the C5a-C5aR axis alleviates lung damage in hDPP4-transgenic mice infected with MERS-CoV. *Emerg Microbes Infect*. 2018;7:77.

97. Sun S, Zhao G, Liu C, et al. Treatment with anti-C5a antibody improves the outcome of H7N9 virus infection in African green monkeys. *Clin Infect Dis*. 2015;60:586-595.

98. Pang RT, Poon TC, Chan KC, et al. Serum proteomic fingerprints of adult patients with severe acute respiratory syndrome. *Clin Chem*. 2006;52:421-429.

99. Diurno F, Numis FG, Porta G, Cirillo F, et al. Eculizumab treatment in patients with COVID-19: Preliminary results from real life. *ASL Napoli 2 NORD Experience*. 2020;24:4040-4047.

100. Laurence J, Mulvey JJ, Seshadri M, Racanelli A, et al. Anti-complement C5 therapy with eculizumab in three cases of critical COVID-19. *Clin Immunol*. 2020;219:108555.

101. Giudice V, Pagliano P, Vatrella A, et al. Combination of ruxolitnib and eculizumab for treatment of severe SARS-CoV-2 related acute respiratory distress syndrome: A controlled study. *Front Pharmacol*. 2020;11:857.

102. Freedberg DE, Conigliaro J, Wang TC, et al. Famotidine use is associated with improved clinical outcomes in hospitalized COVID-19 patients: A propensity score matched retrospective cohort study. *Gastroenterology*. 2020;159:1129-1131.

103. Bourinbaiar AS, Fruhstorfer EC. The effect of histamine type 2 receptor antagonists on human immunodeficiency virus (HIV) replication: Identification of a new class of antiviral agents. *Life Sci*. 1996;59:PL365-370.

104. Wu C, Liu Y, Yang Y, Zhang P, et al. Analysis of therapeutic targets for SARS-CoV-2 and discovery of potential drugs by computational methods. *Acta Pharm Sin B*. 2020;10:766-788.

105. Anand K, Zicbuhr J, Wadhwani P, Wadhwani P, Mesters JR, Hilgenfeld R. Coronavirus main protenaise (3CLpro) structure: Basis for design of anti-SARS drugs. *Science*. 2003;300:1763-1767.

106. Malone RW, Tisdall P, Fremont-Smith P, et al. COVID-19: Famotidine, histamine,mast cells, andmechanisms. *Preprint Res Sq*. 2020;rs.3.rs-30934.

107. WuC, Liu Y, Yang Y, et al. Analysis of therapeutic targets for SARS-CoV-2 and discovery of potential drugs by computational methods. *Acta Pharm Sin B*. 2020;10(5):766-788.

108. Kritas SK, Ronconi G, Caraffa A, et al. Mast cells contribute to coronavirus-induced inflammation: New anti-inflammatory strategy. *J Biol Regul Homeost Agents*. 2020;34(1):9-14.

109. Giacomelli A, Pezzati L, Conti F, et al. Self-reported olfactory and taste disorders in SARS-CoV-2 patients: A cross-sectional study. *Clin Infect Dis*. 2020;71(15):889-890.

110. Eliezer M, Hautefort C, Hamel A, et al. Sudden and complete olfactory loss of function as a possible symptom of COVID-19. *JAMA Otolaryngol Head Neck Surg*. 2020;146:674-675.

111. Mather JF, Seip RL, McKay RG. Impact of famotidine use on clinical outcomes of hospitalized patients with COVID-19. *Am J Gastroenterol*. 2020;00:1-7.

112. Jean S, Hsueh P. Old and re-purposed drugs for the treatment of COVID-19. *Expert Rev Anti Infect Ther*. 2020;18(9):843-847.

113. Wang Y, Fan G, Salam A, et al. Comparative effectiveness of combined favipiravir and oseltamivir therapy versus oseltamivir monotherapy in critically ill patients with influenza virus infection. *J Infect Dis*. 2019;221(10):1688-1698.

114. Shiraki K, Daikoku T. Favipiravir, an anti-influenza drug against life-threatening RNA virus infections. *Pharamcol Ther*. 2020;209:107512.

115. Oestereich L, Ludtke A, Wurr S, Rieger T, Munoz-Fontela C, Gunther S. Successful treatment of advanced Ebola virus infection with T-705 (favipiravir) in a small animal model. *Anitviral Res*. 2014;105:17-21.

116. Sissoko D, Laouenen C, Folkesson E, et al. Experimental treatment with favipiravir for Ebola virus disease (JIKI Trial): A historically controlled, single-arm proof of concept trial in Guinea. *Plos Med*. 2016;13(3):e1001967.

117. Kerber R, Lorez E, Duraffour S, Sissoko D. Laboratory findings, compassionate use of favipiravir, and outcome in patients with Ebola virus disease, Guinea, 2015-A retrospective observational study. *J Infect Dis*. 2019;220(2):195.

118. Wang Y, Fan G, Salem A, et al. Comparative effectiveness of combined favipiravir and oseltamivir therapy versus oseltamivir monotherapy in critically ill patients with influenza virus infection. *J Infect Dis*. 2020;221(10):1698.

119. Ivashchenko AA, Dmitriev KA, Vostokova NV, et al. Avifavir for treatment of patients with moderate COVID-19: Interim results of phase II/III multicenter randomized clinical trial. *Clin Infect Dis*. Aug 2020.

120. Gozzo L, Viale P, Longo L, Vitale DC, Drago F. The potential role of heparin in patients with COVID-19: Beyond the anticoagulant effect. A review. *Front Pharmacol*. 2020;11:1307.

121. INSPIRATION Investigators. Effect of Intermediate-Dose vs Standard-Dose Prophylactic Anticoagulation on Thrombotic Events, Extracorporeal Membrane Oxygenation Treatment, or Mortality Among Patients With COVID-19 Admitted to the Intensive Care Unit: The INSPIRATION Randomized Clinical Trial. *JAMA*. 2021;325(16):1620-1630.

122. Al-Samkari H, Gupta S, Leaf RK, Wang W, et al. Thrombosis, bleeding, and the observational effect of early therapeutic anticoagulation on survival in critically ill patients with COVID-19. *Ann Intern Med*. 2021:M20-6739.

123. The REMAP-CAP, ACTIV-4a, ATTACC Investigators, Ryan Zarychanski. Therapeutic Anticoagulation in Critically Ill Patients with COVID-19. Preliminary Report. March 12, 2001.

124. Lawler PR, Golighe EW, Berger JS, et al. Therpaeutic Anticoagulation in Non-Critically Ill Patients withCOVID-19. MedRxiv. May 17, 2021. https://doi.org/1 0.1101/2021.05.13.21256846.

125. Xu X, Han M, Li T, Sun W, et al. Effective treatment of severe COVID-19 patients with tocilizumab. chinaXiv:202003.00026v1.

126. Stone JH, Frigault MJ, Serling-Boyd NJ, et al. Efficacy of tocilizumab in patients hospitalized with COVID-19. *N Engl J Med*. 2020:383:2333 2344.

127. Salvarani C, Dolci G, Massari M, et al. Effect of tocilizumab vs standard care on clinical worsening in patients hospitalized with COVID-19 pneumonia: A randomized clinical trial. *JAMA Intern Med*. 2021;181(1):24-31.

128. Salama C, Han J, Yan L, et al. Tocilizumab in patients hospitalized with COVID-19 pneumonia. *N Engl J Med*. 2021;384:20-30.

129. Rosas IO, Brau N, Waters M, et al. Tocilizumab in hospitalized patients with severe COVID-19 pneumonia. *N Engl J Med*. April 22, 2021;384(16):1503-1516.

130. Gordon AC, Mouncey PR, Al-Beidh F, et al. Interleukin-6 receptor antagonists in critically ill patients with COVID-19. *N Engl J Med*. 2021;384(16):1491-1502.

131. Horby PW, Gessoa-Amorim G, Peto L, et al. Tocilizumab in patients admitted to hospital with COVID-19 (Recovery):a randomised, controlled, open-label platform trial. Lancet 2021;397:1637-1645.

132. Sivapalasingam S, Lederer D, Bhore R et al. A Randomized Placebo-Controlled Trial of Sarilumab in Hospitalized Patints iwth COVID-19. MedRxiv. May 14, 2021. https://doi.org/10.1101/2021.05.13.21256973. Accessed May 16, 2021.

133. Davoudi-Monfared E, Rahmani H, Khalili H, et al. A randomized clinical trial of the efficacy and safety of interferon β-1a in treatment of severe COVID-19. *Antimicrob Agents Chemother*. 2020;64:e01061-20.

134. Su S, Jiang S. A suspicious role of interferon in the pathogenesis of SARS-CoV-2 by enhancing expression of ACE2. *Sig Transduct Target Ther*. 2020;5:71.

135. Cinat J, Morgenstern B, Bauer G, Chandra P, Rabenau H, Doerr HW. Treatment of SARS with human interferons. *Lancet*. 2003;362:293-294.

136. Arabi YM, Shalhoub S, Mandourah Y, et al. Ribavirin and interferon therapy for critically ill patients with Middle East respiratory syndrome: A multicenter observational study. *Clin Infect Dis*. 2020;70:1837-1844.

137. Hung IF, Lung KC, Tso EY, et al. Triple combination of interferon beta-1b, lopinavir-ritonavir, and ribavirin in the treatment of patients admitted to hospital with COVID-19: An open-label, randomised, phase 2 trial. *Lancet*. 2020;395:1695-1704.

138. Zhou Q, Chen V, Shannon CP, et al. Interferon-a2b treatment for COVID-19. *Front Immunol*. 2020;11:1061.

139. Rahmani H, Davoudi-Monfared E, Nourian A, et al. Interferon β-1b in treatment of severe COVID-19: A randomized clinical trial. *Int Immunopharmacol*. 2020;88:106903.

140. Cao B, Wang Y, Wen D, et al. A trial of lopinavir-ritonavir in adults hospitalized with severe COVID-19. *N Engl J Med*. 2020;382:1787-99.

141. Recovery Collaborative Group. Lopinavir-ritonavir in patients admitted to hospital with COVID-19 (RECOVERY): A randomized, controlled, open-label platform. *Lancet*. 2020;396:1345-1352.

142. Jans DA, Wagstaff KM. Ivermectin as a broad-spectrum host-directed antiviral: The real deal? *Cells*. September 2020;9:2100.

143. Heidary F, Gharebaghi R. Ivermectin: A systematic review from antiviral effects to COVID-19 complementary regimen. *J Antibiot (Tokyo)*. 2020;73(9):593-602.

144. Caly L, Druce JD, Catton MG, Jans DA, Wagstaff KM. The FDA approved drug ivermectin inhibits the replication of SARS-CoV-2 in vitro. *Antiviral Res*. 2020:104787.

145. Barrows NJ, Campos RK, Powell ST, et al. A screen of FDA approved drugs for inhibitors of Zika virus infection. *Cell Host Microbe*. 2016;20:259-270.

146. Ketkar H, Yang L, Wormser GP, Wang P. Lack of efficacy of ivermectin for prevention of a lethal Zika virus infection in a murine system. *Diagn Microbiol Infect Dis*. 2019;95:38-40.

147. Khalil AM, Abu Samrah HM. In vivo combined treatment of rats with ivermectin and aged garlic extract attenuates ivermectin induced cytogenotoxicity in bone marrow cells. *Res Vet Sci*. 2018;120:94-100.

148. Ji W, Luo G. Zika virus NS5 nuclear accumulation is protective of protein degradation and is required for viral RNA replication. *Virology*. 2020;541:124-135.

149. Tay MYF, Fraser JE, Chan WKK, et al. Nuclear localization of dengue virus (DENV) 1-4 non-structural protein 5; protection against all 4 DENV serotypes by the inhibitor ivermectin. *Antivir Res*. 2013;99:301-306.

150. Wagstaff KM, Sivakumaran H, Heaton SM, Harrich D, Jans DA. Ivermectin is a specific inhibitor of importin alpha/beta-mediated nuclear import able to inhibit replication of HIV-1 and dengue virus. *Biochem J*. 2012;443:851-856.

151. Surnar B, Kamran MZ, Shah AS, et al. Orally administrable therapeutic synthetic nanoparticle for Zika virus. *ACS Nano*. 2019;13:11034-11048.

152. Yang SNY, Atkinson SC, Wang C, et al. The broad spectrum antiviral ivermectin targets the host nuclear transport importin alpha/beta1 heterodimer. *Antivir Res*. 2020;177:104760.

153. Kosyna FK, Nagel M, Kluxen L, Kraushaar K, Depping R. The importin alpha/beta-specific inhibitor ivermectin affects HIF-dependent hypoxia response pathways. *Biol Chem*. 2015;396:1357-1367.

154. Mastrangelo E, Pezzullo M, De Burghgraeve T, et al. Ivermectin is a potent inhibitor of flavivirus replication specifically targeting NS3 helicase activity: New prospects for an old drug. *J Antimicrob Chemother*. 2012;67:1884-1894.

155. Fraser JE, Rawlinson SM, Wang C, Jans DA, Wagstaff KM. Investigating dengue virus nonstructural protein 5 (NS5) nuclear import. *Methods Mol Biol* 2014;1138:301-328.

156. Croci R, Bottaro E, Chan KWK, et al. Liposomal systems as nanocarriers for the antiviral agent ivermectin. *Int J Biomater*. v2016;2016:8043983.

157. Atkinson SC, Audsley MD, Lieu KG. et al. Recognition by host nuclear transport proteins drives disorder-to-order transition in Hendra virus. *V Sci Rep*. 2018;8:358.

158. Azeem S, Ashraf M, Rasheed MA, Anjum AA, Hameed R. Evaluation of cytotoxicity and antiviral activity of ivermectin against Newcastle disease virus. *Pak J Pharm Sci*. 2015;28:597-602.

159. Lundberg L, Pinkham C, Baer A, et al. Nuclear import and export inhibitors alter capsid protein distribution in mammalian cells and reduce Venezuelan equine encephalitis virus replication. *Antivir Res*. 2013;100:662-672.

160. Shechter S, Thomas DR, Lundberg L, et al. Novel inhibitors targeting Venezuelan equine encephalitis virus capsid protein identified using in silico structure-based-drug-design. *Sci Rep*. 2017;7:17705.

161. Varghese FS, Kaukinen P, Glasker S, et al. Discovery of berberine, abamectin and ivermectin as antivirals against chikungunya and other alphaviruses *Antivir Res*. 2016;126:117-124.

162. Gotz V, Magar L, Dornfeld D, et al. Influenza A viruses escape from MxA restriction at the expense of efficient nuclear vRNP import. *Sci Rep*. 2016;6:23138.

163. Lee YJ, Lee C. Ivermectin inhibits porcine reproductive and respiratory syndrome virus in cultured porcine alveolar macrophages. *Arch Virol*. 2016;161:257-268.

164. Wagstaff KM, Rawlinson SM, Hearps AC, Jans DA. An AlphaScreen(R)-based assay for high-throughput screening for specific inhibitors of nuclear import. *J Biomol Screen*. 2011;16:192-200.

165. Slonska A, Cymerys J, Skwarska J, Golke A, Banbura MW. Influence of importin alpha/beta and exportin 1 on equine herpesvirus type 1 (EHV-1) replication in primary murine neurons. *Pol J Vet Sci*. 2013;16:749-751.
166. Lv C, Liu W, Wang B, et al. Ivermectin inhibits DNA polymerase UL42 of pseudorabies virus entrance into the nucleus and proliferation of the virus in vitro and vivo. *Antivir Res*. 2018;159:55-62.
167. Berthomme H, Monahan SJ, Parris DS, Jacquemont B, Epstein AL. Cloning, sequencing, and functional characterization of the two subunits of the pseudorabies virus DNA polymerase holoenzyme: Evidence for specificity of interaction. *J Virol*. 1995;69(5):2811-2818.
169. Wang Y-P, Du W-J, Huang L-P, et al. The pseudorabies virus DNA polymerase accessory subunit UL42 directs nuclear transport of the holoenzyme. *Front Microbiol*. 2016;7:124.
170. Bennett SM, Zhao L, Bosard C, Imperiale MJ. Role of a nuclear localization signal on the minor capsid proteins VP2 and VP3 in BKPyV nuclear entry. *Virology*. 2015;474:110-116.
171. Rajter JC, Sherman MS, Fatteh N, Vogel F, Sacks J, Rajter JJ. Use of ivermectin is associated with lower mortality in hospitalized patients with coronavirus disease. 2019; The Icon Study. *CHEST*. 2021;159(1):85-92.
172. López-Medina E, López P, Hurtado IC, et al. Effect of ivermectin on time to resolution of symptoms among adults with mild COVID-19: A randomized clinical trial. *JAMA*. April 13, 2021;325(14):1426-1435.
173. Alamdari DH, Moghaddam AB, Amini S, et al. Application of methylene blue-vitamin C-N-acetyl cysteine for treatment of critically ill COVID-19 patients, report of a phase I clinical trial. *Eur J Pharmacol*. 2020;885: 1734949.
174. Eickmann M, Gravemann U, Handke W, et al. Inactivation of three emerging viruses – severe acute respiratory syndrome coronvirus, Crimean-Congo haemorrhagic fever virus and nipah virus – in platelet concentrates by ultraviolet C light and in plasma by methylene blue plus violet light. *Vox Sanguinis*. 2020;115:146-151.
175. Gendrot M, Andreani J, Duflot I, et al. Methylene blue inhibits replication of SARS-CoV-2 in vitro. *Int J Antimicrob Agents*. 2020;56:106202.
176. Sheahan TP, Sims AC, Leist SR, et al. Comparative therapeutic efficacy of remdesivir and combination lopinavir, ritonavir, and interferon beta against MERSCoV. *Nat Commun*. 2020;11:222.
177. Agostini ML, Andres EL, Sims AC, et al. Coronavirus susceptibility to the antiviral remdesivir (GS-5734) is mediated by the viral polymerase and the proofreading exoribonuclease. *mBio*. 2018;9(2):e00221-18.
178. Brown AJ, Won JJ, Graham RL, et al. Broad spectrum antiviral remdesivir inhibits human endemic and zoonotic deltacoronaviruses with a highly divergent RNA dependent RNA polymerase. *Antiviral Res*. 2019;169:104541.
179. Sheahan TP, Sims AC, Graham RL, et al. Broad-spectrum antiviral GS-5734 inhibits both epidemic and zoonotic coronaviruses. *Sci Transl Med*. 2017;9:eaal3653.

180. Wang M, Cao R, Zhang L, et al. Remdesivir and chloroquine effectively inhibit the recently emerged novel coronavirus (2019-nCoV) in vitro. *Cell Res.* 2020;30:269-271.

181. Grein J, Ohmagari N, Shin D, et al. Compassionate use of remdesivir for patients with severe COVID-19. *N Engl J Med.* 2020;382:2327-2336.

182. Goldman JD, Lye DCB, Hui DS, et al. Remdesivir for 5 or 10 days in patients with severe COVID-19. *N Engl J Med.* 2020;383:1827-1837.

183. Beigel JH, Tomashek KM, Dodd LE, et al. Remdesivir for the treatment of COVID-19 – Final report. *N Engl J Med.* 2020;383:1813-1826.

184. Pan H, Peto Karim QA, Alejandria M, et al. Repurposed antiviral drugs for COVID-19 – Interim WHO SOLIDARITY trial results. *N Engl J Med.* 2021;384:497-511.

185. Khalili JS, Zhu H, Yan Y, Zhu Y. Novel coronavirus treatment with ribavirin: Groundwork for an evaluation concerning COVID-19. *J Med Virol.* 2020;1-7.

186. Alfson KJ, Worwa G, Carrion R, Griffiths. Determination and therapeutic exploitation of Ebola virus spontaneous mutation frequency. *J Virol.* 90:2345-2355.

187. Soares-Weiser K, Thomas S, Thomas G, Garner P. Ribavarin for Crimean-Congo hemorrhagic fever: Systematic review and meta-analysis. *BMC Infect Dis.* 2010;10:207.

188. Hung IFN, Lung KC, Tso EYK, et al. Triple combination of interferon beta-1b, lopinavir-ritonavir, and ribavirin in the treatment of patients admitted to hospital with COVID-19: An open-label randomized phase 2 trial. *Lancet.* 2020;395:1695-1704.

189. Rosee FL, Bremer HC, Gehrke I, et al. The Janus kinase ½ inhibitor ruxolitinib in COVID-19 with severe hyperinflamation. *Leukemia.* 2020;34:1805-1815.

190. Ahmed A, Merrill SA, Alsawah F, et al. Ruxolitinib in adult patients with secondary haemophagocytic lymphohistiocytosis: An open-label, single-centre, pilot trial. *Lancet Haematol.* 2019;6:e630-e637.

191. Elfiky AA. Ribavirin, remdesivir, sofosbuvir, galidesivir, and tenofovir against SARS-CoV-2 RNA dependent RNA polymerase (RdRp): A molecular docking study. *Life Sciences.* 2020;253:117592.

192. de Freitas CS, Higa LM, Sacramento CQ, et al. Yellow fever virus is susceptible to sofosbuvir both in vitro and in vivo. *PLoS Negl Trop Dis.* 2019;13:e0007072.

193. Bullard-Feibelman KM, Govero J, Zhu Z, et al. The FDA-approved drug sofosbuvir inhibits Zika virus infection. *Antiviral Res.* 2017;137:134-140.

194. Ferreira AC, Reis PA, de Freitas CS, et al. Beyond members of the flaviviridae family, sofosbuvir also inhibits chikungunya virus replication. *Antimicrob Agents Chemother.* 2019;63:e01389-18.

195. Gan CS, Lim SK, Chee CF, et al. Sofosbuvir as treatment against dengue? *ChemBiol Drug Des.* 2018;91:448-455.

196. Sadeghi A, Asgari AA, Norouzi A, et al. Sofosbuvir and daclatasvir compared with standard of care in the treatment of patients admitted to hospital with moderate or severe coronavirus infection (COVID-19): A randomized controlled trial. *J Antimicrob Chemother.* 2020;75(11):3379-3385.

197. Fedson DS. Treating influenza with statins and other immunomodulatory agents. *Antiviral Res.* 2013;99(3):417-435.

198. Fedson DS, Jacobson JR, Rordam OM, Opal SM. Treating the host response to Ebola virus disease with generic statins and angiotensin receptor blockers. *mBio*. 2015;6(3):e00716.

199. Tan WYT, Young BE, Lye DC, et al. Statin use is associated with lower disease severity in COVID-19 infection. *Sci Rep*. 2020;10:17458.

200. Daniels LB, Sitapati AM, Zhang J, et al. Relation of statin use prior to admission to severity and recovery among COVID-19 inpatients. *Am J Cardiol*. 2020;136:149-155.

201. Zhang XJ, Qin JJ, Cheng X, et al. In-hospital use of statins is associate with a reduced risk of mortality among individuals with COVID-19. *Cell Metabolism*. 2020;32:177-187.

202. Saeed O, Castagna F, Agalliu I, et al. Statin use and in-hospital mortality in patients with diabetes mellitus and COVID-19. *J Am Heart Assoc*. 2020;9(24):e018475.

203. Hariyanto TIH, Kurniawan A. Statin therapy did not improve the in-hospital outcome of coronavirus disease 2019 (COVID-19) infection. *Diabetes Metab Syndr*. 2020;14:1613-1615.

204. Hwang SY, Ryoo SM, Park JE, et al. Combination therapy of vitamin C and thiamine for septic shock: a multi-centre, double-blinded randomized, controlled study. *Intensive Care Med*. 2020;46(11):2015-2025.

205. Fujii T, Luethi N, Young PJ, et al. Effect of vitamin C, hydrocortisone, and thiamine vs hydrocortisone alone on time alive and free of vasopressor support among patients with septic shock: The VITAMINS randomized clinical trial. *JAMA*. 2020;323(5):423-431.

206. Fowler AA 3rd, Truwit JD, Hite RD, et al. Effect of vitamin C infusion on organ failure and biomarkers of inflammation and vascular injury in patients with sepsis and severe acute respiratory failure: The CITRIS-ALI randomized clinical trial. *JAMA*. 2019;322(13):1261-1270. [Published correction appears in JAMA. 2020;323(4):379.]

207. Hiedra R, Lo KB, Elbashabsheh M, et al. The use of IV vitamin C for patients with COVID-19: a case series. *Expert Rev Anti Infect Ther*. 2020;18(12):1259-1261.

208. Meltzer DO, Best TJ, Zhang H, Vokes T, Arora V, Solway J. Association of vitamin D status and other clinical characteristics with COVID-19 test results. *JAMA Netw Open*. 2020;3(9):e2019722.

209. Ohaegbulam KC, Swalih M, Patel P, Smith MA, Perrin R. Vitamin D supplementation in COVID-19 patients: A clinical case series. *Am J Ther*. 2020;27(5):e485-e490.

210. Cereda E, Bogliolo L, Lobascio F, et al. Vitamin D supplementation and outcomes in coronavirus disease 2019 (COVID-19) patients from the outbreak area of Lombardy, Italy. *Nutrition*. 2020;82:111055.

211. Murai IH, Fernandes AL, Sales LP, et al. Effect of a single high dose of vitamin D3 on hospital length of stay in patients with moderate to severe COVID-19: A randomized clinical trial. *JAMA*. 2021;325(11):1053-1060.

212. Bauer SR, Kapoor A, Rath M, Thomas SA. What is the role of supplementation with ascorbic acid, zinc, vitamin D, or N-acethylcysteine for prevention or treatment of COVID-19? *Cleveland Clinic Medicine*. June 8, 2020.

213. te Velthuis AJW, van den Worm SHE, Sims AC, Baric RS, Snijder EJ, van Hemert MJ. Zn2+ inhibits coronavirus and arterivirus RNA polymerase activity in vitro and zinc ionophores block the replication of these viruses in cell culture. *PLoS Pathog.* 2010;6(11):e1001176.

214. Singh M, Das RR. Zinc for the common cold. *Cochrane Database Syst Rev.* 2013;2013(6):CD001364.

215. Derwand R, Scholz M. Does zinc supplementation enhance clinical efficacy of chloroquine/hydroxychloroquine to win today's battle against COVID-19? *Med Hypotheses.* 2020;142:109815.

216. Arentz S, Hunter J, Yang G, et al. Zinc for the prevention and treatment of SARS-CoV-2 and other acute viral respiratory infections: A rapid review. *Adv Integr Med.* 2020:252-260.

217. Derwand R, Scholz M, Zelenko V. COVID-19 outpatients: Early risk stratified treatment with zinc plus low dose hydroxychloroquine and azithromycin: A retrospective case series study. *Int J Antimicrob Agents.* 2020;56:106214:1-11.

PERSONAL PROTECTIVE EQUIPMENT 5

Avalon Mertens, DO and Ronaldo C. Go, MD

INTRODUCTION

Personal protective equipment (PPE) is necessary to ensure the safety of the health care provider while providing high quality patient care. In a crisis, there should be a concern for shortages on PPE. Understanding the etiology of the crisis and level of PPE is paramount. Then, mobilization of the health care facility to focus on the crisis, limiting non-emergent entry into the patient room, and recycling mitigate PPE shortages. This chapter will discuss levels of PPE and the requirements for various pathogens. Due to the immense increase in use of PPE during the COVID-19 pandemic, techniques for recycling different aspects of PPE were revisited, analyzed, and examined anew. We review the types of PPE, mechanisms, and safety of reusing PPE, as well as other techniques to minimize PPE and to keep front-line health care workers safe.

BIOSAFETY

Biocontainment refers to the safety measures on research and laboratory staff who work with infectious agents to prevent contamination and outbreaks. The level of safety is determined by several factors of the infectious agent including its infectivity, transmissibility, virulence, the type of work being conducted, and whether there are existing protective measures for said agent including vaccination or treatment. These levels are referred to as biosafety levels and have been outlined by the Centers for Disease Control (CDC).[1,2] (See Table 5-1.)

TYPES OF PRECAUTIONS

The CDC outlines four basic levels of isolation precautions: standard, contact, droplet, and airborne. Standard precautions are meant to reduce

Table 5-1	BIOSAFETY LEVELS AS DEFINED BY THE CDC		
Biosafety Level	**Risk**	**Characteristics**	**Example**
1	Minimal	Unlikely to cause human disease	Escherichia coli K12, lactobacillus
2	Moderate	Cause treatable disease, difficult to contract	Salmonella, measles
3	High	Cause serious diseases, contagious	Mycobacterium tuberculosis
4	Very high	Lethal disease, very contagious	Ebola virus, Lassa fever virus

transmission from blood borne pathogens or known or unknown sources. This includes hand hygiene, the use of PPE (such as masks, gloves, and gowns based on risk assessment), and respiratory hygiene/cough etiquette.

Contact precautions are additional precautions for diseases that are epidemiologically important or multi-drug resistant that can easily be transmitted through the patient's intact skin or contaminated surfaces. Droplet precautions are additional precautions to prevent contact with respiratory secretions, usually within 6 feet of the patient. Surgical masks may be sufficient. Airborne precautions are additional precautions for pathogens that can remain suspended in air.[3] The following tables list the level of precautions and necessary PPE for the different types of pandemics (Table 5-2) and pathogens for bioterrorism (Table 5-3).

▌CONSERVATION

The National Center for Immunization and Respiratory Disease (NCIRD) and CDC offered guidelines describing the preservation of PPE in preparation for PPE shortages.[9] They advised during periods of anticipated PPE shortages (contingency capacity) to selectively cancel elective and non-urgent procedures, discharge medically stable patients with SARS-CoV-2, exclude visitors, cohort patients, use of cloth gowns, and extend use of N95-filtering facepiece respirators (FFRs) by wearing the same one for multiple encounters. In a time of crisis capacity when supplies are

Table 5-2 PRECAUTIONS AND PPE REQUIRED FOR A NUMBER OF COMMON AND RARE PATHOGENS, AS OUTLINED BY THE CDC[3-5]		
Agent	**PPE Required**	**Notes**
SARS	Airborne/droplet/ contact/standard (Gloves, gown, eye-protection, respirator)	
MERS	Airborne/droplet/ contact/standard (Gloves, gown, eye-protection, respirator)	
SARS-CoV-2	Airborne/droplet/ contact/standard (Gloves, gown, eye-protection, respirator)	
Influenza	Droplet/standard (Surgical mask)	
Plague	Standard	Droplet precautions until 48 hours of treatment
Tularemia	Standard	
Ebola	Droplet/contact/ standard (Gloves, gown, eye-protection, surgical mask)	N95 during aerosolizing procedures*
Hemorrhagic fevers (Lassa, Crimean-Congo-Hemorrhagic, Dengue, Yellow, and Chikungunya)	Droplet/contact/ standard (Gloves, gown, eye-protection, surgical mask)	N95 during aerosolizing procedures
	Standard for dengue fever and yellow fever.	
Encephalitis (Nipah virus, Hendra virus, and Rift Valley Fever)	Standard	
	Nipah is standard/ contact/droplet	
Agents of bioterrorism	See below	

*Intubation, bronchoscopy, suctioning, autopsy with oscillating saw.

Table 5-3   PRECAUTIONS AND PPE REQUIRED FOR BIOTERRORISM PATHOGENS, AS OUTLINED BY THE CDC[3,5-8]

Agent	PPE Required	Notes
Anthrax	Standard	Contact if copious drainage, airborne if in powder form
Botulism	Standard	
Plague	Standard	Droplet precautions until 48 hours of treatment
Smallpox	Airborne/contact/ standard (Gloves, gown, respirator)	
Tularemia	Standard	
Viral hemorrhagic fevers	Droplet/contact/ standard (Gloves, gown, eye-protection, surgical mask)	
Brucellosis	Standard	
Clostridium perfringens	Standard	Contact if wound drainage extensive
Salmonella	Standard	Use contact for diapered or incontinent patients
E. coli 0175:H7	Standard	Use contact for diapered or incontinent patients
Shigella	Standard	Use contact for diapered or incontinent patients
Glanders (*burkholderia mallei*)	Standard/airborne (Respirator)	
Meliodosis	Standard	
Psittacosis	Standard	
Q-fever	Standard/airborne (Respirator)	

Table 5-3 PRECAUTIONS AND PPE REQUIRED FOR BIOTERRORISM PATHOGENS, AS OUTLINED BY THE CDC[3,5-8] (CONTINUED)		
Agent	**PPE Required**	**Notes**
Ricin toxin	Chemical, biological, radiological, nuclear (CBRN) self-contained breathing apparatus (SCBA) with a Level A protective suit	
Staphylococcal enterotoxin B	Standard	
Typhus fever	Standard	
Viral encephalitis	Standard	
Vibrio cholerae	Standard	Use contact for diapered or incontinent patients
Cryptosporidium parvum	Standard	Use contact for diapered or incontinent patients
Nipah virus	Standard/contact/droplet (Gloves, gown, surgical mask)	
Hanta virus	Standard	

not enough to meet demands, they recommended additionally canceling elective and non-urgent procedures, using respirators beyond their recommended shelf-life and reusing respirators between patients, as well as extending the life of isolation gowns and reusing cloth isolation gowns.[9]

Minimizing Patient Contact

To preserve PPE, nurses and other staff minimized their entry into patient rooms. Often just one member of the physician team would enter, and specialists not requiring a direct physical examination would forego entry altogether. Pharmacists at one hospital put together recommendations that addressed not only medication recommendations but the bundling of medication administration and therapeutic drug monitoring to minimize patient contact by nurses to encourage both the safety of staff and the preservation of PPE.[10] Medications and doses were optimized to prevent multiple re-entries in the patient's room. These are low impact changes that any hospital could consider to minimize entry into patient rooms.

MASKS

Surgical Masks

Surgical masks, worn regularly to prevent transmission of respiratory infections, are typically made up of three layers (Figure 5-1). The outer layer serves to repel fluids. The middle layer is a filter that prevents particles from passing through, and the inner layer is absorbent and serves to trap droplets and absorb moisture from the wearer's mouth.[11] Surgical masks are assigned a protection level by the American Society of Testing and Materials (ATSM) F2100 Standard, based on their performance in the five necessary categories: particulate filtration efficiency, bacterial filtration efficiency, fluid resistance, differential pressure, and flammability. Level 1 is suggested for use during procedures where low levels of aerosols, sprays, and fluids are produced. Level 2 is recommended for light to moderate levels, and Level 3 is recommended for heavy levels.[11] N95 masks are superior in all categories.

N95

N95 respirators contain a layer of meltblown fabric formed by high velocity air to make a web shaped crisscross of fibers designed to stop small viral and bacterial particles, accentuated by an electrostatic charge[12] (Figure 5-2). They are recommended for use when exposure to airborne particles is expected.

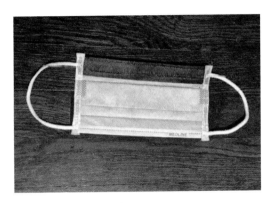

Figure 5-1 • Example of a surgical mask.

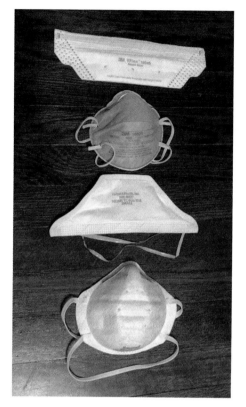

Figure 5-2 • Various types of N95-FFRs.

PAPRs

Another option for respiratory protection against airborne pathogens is a powered air-purifying respirator (PAPR), which comes in several forms but includes a tight fitting respirator that covers the whole face and a loose fitting hood, and filter air by way of a high efficiency particular air (HEPA) filter.[13] PAPRs have a higher level of protection than a disposable N95-FFR, and have been found to have a high level of comfort for health care workers, although they may cause decreased mobility, dexterity, and ability to communicate.[13] Despite their superiority in protection, there was no difference in infection rate in workers wearing PAPRs versus the typical N95-FFR. They must be decontaminated after each use but can be reused many times, which could save hospitals money in the long run over replacing N95-FFRs.[13]

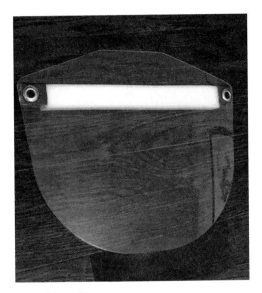

Figure 5-3 • Example of a face shield.

Face Shields

Face shields are an easily decontaminated aspect of PPE used as eye protection in highly contagious respiratory viruses (Figure 5-3). There are various designs, but typically they consist of a clear plastic shield held together with an adjustable or elastic strap.

FIT TESTING

There are many styles and brands of N95-FFRs, and the fit is of utmost importance to maintaining airborne protection. Fit testing is the process by which mask fit is established for each individual. There are several OSHA approved fit testing procedures, following the selection of the mask and ensuring it feels comfortable on the face. After mask placement, the user should perform a user seal check by moving their face side to side and up and down while taking deep breaths to see if they can detect a leak. The user should then undergo either a qualitative or quantitative fit test, during which they must prove a good seal by taking deep breaths, turning the head side to side, moving the head up and down, talking, smiling/frowning, and jogging in place.[14]

The most common tests are qualitative fit tests, with several described below. The isoamyl acetate (IAA) protocol involves testing a user's ability smell the banana like odor of an IAA solution on a wetted paper towel or other material, hung within a fit test chamber. If they can detect the odor, it is considered a failure.[14]

The saccharin solution aerosol protocol involves testing a user's ability to taste a 0.83 g sodium saccharin solution in 100 ml of warm water aerosolized into the fit test enclosure placed around their head. If the user tastes something sweet before 10 squeezes of the nebulizer bulb, it is a failure, but if they taste it after 10 squeezes, then they have passed the test.[14]

The Bitrex™ (denatonium benzoate) solution is identical to the saccharin solution protocol, but it tests the ability to taste a bitter substance (13.5 mg of Bitrex to 100 ml of 5% salt solution in distilled water) aerosolized into the fit test enclosure.[14]

The final qualitative fit test protocol involves exposing the user to an irritant smoke (stannic chloride) and assessing their ability to detect the irritant, which would be considered a failure.[14]

▌METHODS OF RE-USING MASKS

Surgical Masks over N95

During previous outbreaks, the CDC and the Institute of Medicine have suggested the possibility of wearing a surgical mask over an N95-FFR to extend its usable lifetime, which is a technique that has been observed frequently during the COVID-19 pandemic.[15] Few studies exist discussing the feasibility or safety of this technique, and it is important to remember that bioaerosols that pass easily through surgical masks may remain on the N95 surface and pose a threat as a potential contaminant to the wearer (Roberge effect).[15] One study did evaluate the comfort of two masks at once.[15,16] Surgical masks were worn over N95-FFRs for one hour and the wearers' vital signs, tidal volume, minute volume, and other variables were measured, with the conclusion that there was no physiological burn to health care workers should they choose to wear a surgical mask concordantly over their N95-FFR.[16] No specific study could be found evaluating the presence of infectious material on an N95-FFR after exposure to a pathogen while wearing a surgical mask as a barrier, but it is recommended that the wearer continue to treat the N95-FFR as contaminated even after removing the surgical mask.

Recycling

In 2009 following the H1N1 pandemic, the CDC recommended that health care facilities investigate means of reusing decontaminated respirators, and the Institute of Medicine (IOM) acknowledged the lack of research in this area.[17] Thus, there exist a number of studies past this date that begin to evaluate techniques for decontamination of respirators. Following the start of the pandemic in 2019, researchers continued this work and extended it to apply specifically to SARS-CoV-2.

The most studied techniques for recycling N95 are ultraviolet decontamination, moist heat decontamination in the form of microwave generated steam or incubation with a water reservoir, dry heat, and hydrogen peroxide vapor (HPV)[18,19] (Table 5-4). The studies' goals include maintenance of mask architecture after reprocessing, filter efficiency, microbicidal efficacy, continued fit for providers, and general acceptance by providers based on appearance, comfort, and smell.[18,20] The caveat to the studies is that surrogate pathogens were occasionally used instead, and not the actual pathogen the study was intended for. The FDA considers a $\geq$ 3-log reduction in non-enveloped virus or two gram positive and two gram negative vegetative bacteria an effective viral reduction in the setting of Sars-CoV-2 mask decontamination.[21]

UVGI

Ultraviolet germicidal irradiation (UVGI) cross-links thymidine nucleotides in DNA and uracil nucleotides in RNA, blocking replication of bacteria and viruses.[17] However, there is a concern for degradation of the mask filter material and maintaining fit.[17]

One 2020 meta-analysis of 13 studies performed prior to the COVID-19 pandemic found that after UV decontamination, N95 masks maintained their certification standards with regards to aerosol penetration, airflow resistance, and recommended ideally a dose of 4 J/cm^2 to achieve a $\geq$ 3log reduction in virus.[20] Due to variety in protocols and mask style, there was variability in results, and maximum number of reusability could not be determined.[20,23,24]

With regards to increasing UV irradiation dosage, particle penetration, flow resistance, and bursting strength of four different N95 masks were studied, and it was found that even up to 950 J/cm^2 there was little change in the first two variables. The penetrance did increase slightly; however, it remained at the < 5% level required for these masks to be deemed effective, concluding that UVIG even at high doses is a safe and effective method of decontamination.[17] In this particular study, 3–4 circular pieces were punched out from each mask, loaded into holders so that both sides were exposed, placed in a custom made black felt lined chamber equipped with two UV-C 15 watt lamps, and exposed to variable levels of UV light. The mask straps were tested similarly. Due to the variability of each N95-FFR, each mask model should be tested in preparation

Table 5-4 METHODS OF STERILIZATION OF N95 MASKS

Methods	Description
Hydrogen peroxide vaporization	• Only on N95 without cellulose • Via Battelle, Sterrad, or Steris • Maintains efficacy and structure up to 20 cycles[19] • Inactivates Geobacillus stearothermophilus spores[19]
UV treatment	• UVC (254 nm) irradiation, variable dose, but at < 2 J/cm², at 1–45 minutes[19] • Assessed for 1–3 cycles at 15–30 minutes per cycle[19] • Inactivates influenza, H5N1, H1N1, Bacillus subtilis spores[19] • Inactivates MERS-CoV, SARS-CoV-1, Ebola, Crimean Congo hemorrhagic virus, Nipah virus
Moist heat	• Heating at 75°C for 30 minutes or 85°C for 20 minutes at 100% relative humidity[12] • Inactivates bacteriophage MS2, SARS-COV-1, H5N1, H1N1 • Assessed for up to 3 cycles[12]
Dry heat	• 80–120 degrees for 1 hour[18] • Inactivates SARS-CoV-2 • Least likely to reduce efficiency • Only one cycle[22] • More likely to have physical changes[18]

for a mass decontamination program, and the dosage of UV irradiation should be specified to said pathogen.[17] Two separate literature reviews found UVGI is an effective method of decontamination that maintains mask filtration and structural integrity.[18,19]

Heat

Microwaves and autoclaves are ubiquitously available in health care clinics and/or hospitals and moist heat was overall more effective than dry heat.[18]

In the review by Paul et al., researchers found four studies evaluating dry heat via microwave, hot air oven, and electric rice cooker, and based on visible damage to masks via dry microwave, alteration in filter efficiency and physical structure via hot air oven, and reduced decontamination efficacy via rice cooker, these methods were not recommended. Moist heat via microwave generated steam (MGS) was evaluated in seven separate studies. Their conclusion was that moist heat retained efficacy of filtration, appropriate airflow resistance, and appropriate microbicidal efficacy for variable viruses and phages with $\geq 3\log_{10}$ reduction or more, and no alteration in fit.[18] Protocols for moist heat via MGS included exposing masks to steam by using a water reservoir or commercial steam bags in an incubator with a water reservoir. Five studies evaluated moist heat via lab incubator of about 60° for varying amounts of time with overall effective filter efficiency, appropriate microbicidal efficacy, and no change in respirator fit.[18]

Three studies involving viruses including SAR-CoV-2 concluded that heat treatments of 75°C for 30 minutes or 85°C for 20 minutes at 100% relative humidity resulted in decontamination of all three viruses without lowering filtering efficiency and recommended this technique as a cheap and effective method for reusing N95 masks.[12] Another study compared dry and moist heat decontamination of both N95 masks and surgical masks on oropharyngeal bacteria and viruses. They used either dry heat via a tumble dryer at 70°C or moist heat in a constant climate chamber and used infrared spectroscopy to evaluate the molecular integrity of the mask fibers following each procedure. The protocol describes full masks, which were placed in sterilization bags and heated in a constant climate chamber at 70°C for one hour at 75% humidity.[25] The tumble dryer (dry heat) did not effectively decontaminate the mask, while the moist heat climate chamber was successful, and preserved the structure of the mask.[25] This trial did not evaluate fit or filtration efficacy following decontamination.

One Canadian hospital carried out a novel evaluation of N95-FFRs that had been worn by health care providers during a normal workday for 2–8 hours (not interacting with COVID-19 patients) and tested them for fit based on quantitative fit test scoring after 30 minutes of autoclaving at 121°C. They found that the fit remained effective after one use and sterilization, but was not maintained after a second cycle.[22] Cadnum et al., found that dry heat at 70° for 30 minutes was not effective for disinfection, but did not evaluate moist heat.[26]

Ultimately moist heat in the form of microwave generated steam and lab incubator were effective at decontamination while retaining the masks' integrity, and seem to be a viable and affordable option.[18,19,25]

Hydrogen Peroxide

Hydrogen peroxide works by generating free radicals, without harmful degradation products.[18] The meta-analysis by Paul et al., reviewed one study utilizing vaporized hydrogen peroxide and yielded appropriate levels of filter aerosol penetration and resistance, although fit was not assessed,[18] and another review of studies performed prior to the pandemic also found vaporized hydrogen peroxide to have effective decontamination while maintaining filtration and physical structure.[19] The protocol of the former study involved a portable hydrogen peroxide vapor (HPV) generator within a closed room generating a room concentration of 8 g/m^3, with a 15 minute dwell time and 125 minute total cycle time, with N95-FFRs hung across the room on a string. An aeration unit then ran overnight to convert the vapor into oxygen and water vapor, and the cycle was repeated twice more.[23] Other HPV studies involved similar protocols involving an HPV generator with 30% or 35% hydrogen peroxide solution, with N95 masks on wire racks, and they were gassed for 25 and 40 minutes with dwell times of 15, 20, and 25 minutes, followed by an aeration period of at least four hours.[19]

One 2020 study tested four methods specifically for inactivation of SARS-CoV-2 and found both vaporized hydrogen peroxide and UV light to have rapid inactivation of virus while maintaining N95 respirator integrity and fit.[27] One hydrogen peroxide vaporizing system was granted emergency FDA approval for use during the COVID-19 pandemic and seems quite promising, but is unlikely to be available in resource poor settings, in which case the moist heat techniques could be most feasible.[18]

Although there is a plethora of studies evaluating decontamination techniques for N95-FFRs, one systematic review found only one study evaluating the same for surgical masks.[28] The study found that dry heat was the best technique to preserve the masks' filtering effect, but the germicidal effect was not evaluated. Several studies evaluated pretreating the masks with several substances, and germicidal effect was noted in salt, N-thalamine, and nanoparticle coated masks, but the techniques were heterogeneous, and it remains unclear how long the germicidal effect would last before the mask would need a fresh decontamination.[28] There need to be further studies performed on decontamination of surgical masks.

GOWNS

Isolation gowns, designed to protect health care personnel from body fluid and transfer of microorganisms, also were in short supply due to the COVID-19 pandemic. In the United States, disposable gowns are typically more widely used and more available for purchase than reusable fabric gowns.

One recent study evaluated the performance of disposable and reusable gowns with regards to the requirements set by the Association of Advancement Instrumentation (AAMI): water resistance and hydrostatic pressure, which reflect liquid barrier performance at different levels of force. They performed evaluation on Level I, II, and III gowns (levels are assigned by predetermined requirements of water resistance and hydrostatic pressure) and found that reusable gowns of all levels met said requirements and had no change in performance after 1, 25, 50, and 75 launderings. Disposable gowns were not laundered. One can conclude from this study that reusable gowns are a favorable option certainly in terms of reusability and decontamination in the setting of PPE shortage.[29]

One hospital, in preparation for a shortage of protective gowns, tested durability of single-use surgical gowns after laundering, and found that degradation was noted after four or more cycles. The gowns were not tested for water resistance nor hydrostatic pressure, but instead inspected visually after each wash. Although the gowns were not used clinically or fully evaluated for level of protection, the study suggests the possibility of laundering to reuse single use gowns to increase the supply. As gown models and components differ, it would be prudent for hospitals looking to initiate a mass gown recycling program to check the durability of their particular model of gown before proceeding.[29]

There does not currently appear to exist a study examining both structural integrity of disposable gowns after laundering as well as fluid resistance for protection of health care personnel. There is a wide variety of disposable gowns, and it is likely that each hospital system would need reference a study that examines their model of gown.

▌GLOVES

There are several types of disposable gloves including latex, nitrile, and vinyl gloves, among others. Latex has long been used in the medical field but is going out of style due to its propensity for allergic reaction due to proteins it contains. Latex is made from a natural rubber, has an elastic quality, and is strong and durable.[31] Nitrile has no allergic component, is resistant to punctures and tears, and fits well with an elastic quality. Vinyl also contains no allergic components, but is weaker, and breaks and punctures more easily with use, with typically poor fit.[31]

Although less publicized than masks, nitrile and vinyl gloves are also in shortage, and a report from the U.S. Accountability Office recently calculated the number of gloves in the national stockpile to be 2 million in October 2020, down from 16.9 million in December 2019.[32] One recently published study evaluated the effectiveness of decontamination of nitrile and vinyl gloves and found that the gloves maintained their structure and surface morphology up to 20 cycles of decontamination with alcohol, UV radiation, and heat treatment.[33]

BLEACH SOLUTION

Faced with a shortage of disinfectant and bleach wipes, the CDC released guidance for making bleach solution at home:

> *Mix 5 tablespoons (1/3 cup) of household bleach containing 5–9% of sodium hypochlorite with one gallon of room temperature water or 4 tablespoons of bleach with one quart of room temperature water to form a dilute bleach solution. Be sure to open windows or mix solution in a well ventilated area. The solution will lose efficacy over time so it should be used within 24 hours, and a new solution can be prepared. This solution can be applied to surfaces (and left for at least one minute of contact time before wiping off), or used to saturate paper or fabric towels then used to wipe surfaces.[34]*

HAND SANITIZERS

Soap and water is very effective against SARS-CoV-2, and hands should be washed for at least 20 seconds. Alternatively alcohol-based hand cleanser of 60% or more alcohol can be used for hand hygiene.[35]

Another shortage faced during the COVID-19 was that of hand sanitizer, and during the pandemic even breweries were repurposed to produce alcohol-based hand rubs. The WHO released a guide for local production of hand rub formulations in 2010 with two simple formulations. In order to make a 10-liter preparation, the following steps were recommended to produce either an 80% ethanol solution or a 75% isopropyl alcohol solution:[36]

1. Pour either 8333 ml of ethanol 96% or 7515 ml of isopropyl alcohol 99.8% into the mixing tank.
2. Add 417 ml of hydrogen peroxide.
3. Add 145 ml of glycerol 98%, rinsed from its measuring cylinder by sterile distilled water or cold boiled water.

4. Fill the remaining space in the tank to the 10 L mark with sterile distilled or cold boiled water, and place the lid on the bottle rapidly to prevent evaporation.
5. Shake gently or mix with a paddle.
6. Place the solution into its containers and wait 72 hours before distributing.

These instructions could be easily utilized by health care facilities, and safety guidelines found in the 2010 WHO guideline should be closely followed.[36]

▌DECONTAMINATION OF HEALTH CARE WORKERS

Although no consensus statement or guidelines have been published by the CDC, the Journal of Primary Care & Community Health put forth a set of suggested guidelines for health care workers concerning general protective actions and personal decontamination.[35] They suggest that health care workers change into travel clothes to be worn on the way home from a hospital/clinic shift. Any potentially contaminated clothes should be washed at the highest heat (56°C or 132.8°F inactivates SARS-CoV-2) and dried in an electric or gas dryer at the maximum heat setting. Soap is an effective tool as its surfactant destroys the lipid capsid surrounding SARS-CoV-2 and thus they recommend showering following each shift, ideally at the hospital but this may not be possible. Phones should be cleaned after each shift and at least once daily with either a disinfectant wipe or a microfiber cloth. Workers should be aware that due to its small size, SARS-CoV-2 can penetrate the disposable bouffant caps often supplied in hospitals and are recommended to wash head and facial hair after shifts. Workers should wear one pair of shoes at the hospital, and wipe them down each day, as virus has been isolated from the soles of shoes. Work shoes should be kept at work or in a plastic or paper bag, and ideally a pair of travel shoes is worn for the journey home and left outside or in a garage. Virus has also been isolated from the upholstery of vehicles, and car surfaces should be wiped daily, and cars can be parked in sunlight if possible, which serves as a disinfectant (not tested for SARS-CoV-2).[35] One journalist interviewed several physicians who reported changing their clothes before leaving the hospital or changing immediately upon arriving home and showering before touching anything in the house. There exist no official guidelines on shoe covers (not routinely recommended by the CDC), but some health care workers choose to leave their hospital shoes outside or in the hospital.[37]

REFERENCES

1. Kraus AA, Mirazimi A. Laboratory biosafety in containment laboratories. In: Weidmann M, Silmann N, Butaye P, Elschner M, eds. *Working in Biosafety Level 3 and 4 Laboratories: A Practical Introduction.* Wiley-VCH Verlag GmbH & Co. KGaA; 2013:1-4.
2. Ta L, Gosa L, Nathanson DA. Biosafety and biohazards: Understanding biosafety levels and meeting safety requirements of a biobank. In: Yong W, ed. *Biobanking. Methods in Molecular Biology.* New York, NY: Humana Press; 1897.
3. Siegel JD, Rhinehard E, Jackson M, Chiarello L. 2007 guideline for isolation precautions: Preventing transmission of infectious agents in healthcare settings. cdc.gov. Updated July 2019.
4. CDC. Interim infection prevention and control recommendations for hospitalized patients with Middle East Respiratory Syndrome Coronavirus (MERS-CoV). cdc.gov. Updated June 2015.
5. Sazzad HMS, Luby SP, Stroher U, et al. Exposure-based screening for Nipah virus encephalitis. *Emerg Infect Dis.* 2015;21(2):349-351.
6. CDC. Glanders. cdc.gov. https://www.cdc.gov/glanders/index.html. Updated October 2017.
7. CDC: Q-fever. cdc.gov. https://www.cdc.gov/qfever/index.html. Updated January 2019.
8. CDC. Ricin: Biotoxin. cdc.gov. https://www.cdc.gov/nish/ershdb/emergencyresponsecard_29750002.html. January 2019.
9. National Center for Immunization and Respiratory Diseases (NCIRD), Division of Viral Diseases. Summary for healthcare facilities: Strategies for optimizing the supply of PPE during shortages. cdc.gov. https://www.cdc.gov/coronavirus/2019-ncov/hcp/ppe-strategy/strategies-optimize-ppe-shortages.html. Updated July 2020.
10. Dzierba AL, Pedone T, Patel MK, et al. Rethinking the drug distribution and medication management model: How a New York City hospital pharmacy department responded to COVID-19. *J Am Coll Clin Pharm.* 2020. Online ahead of print.
11. Chua MH, Cheng W, Goah SS, et al. Face masks in the new COVID-19 normal: Materials, testing, and perspectives. *AAAS Research.* 2020.
12. Campos RK, Jin J, Rafael GH, et al. Decontamination of SARS-CoV-2 and other RNA viruses from N95 level meltblown polypropylene fabric using heat under different humidities. *ACS Nano.* 2020;14(10):14017-14025.
13. Licina A, Silvers A, Stuart R. Use of powered air-purifying respirator (PAPR) by healthcare workers for preventing highly infectious viral diseases – A systematic review of evidence. *Syst Rev.* 2020;9(1):173.
14. OSHA. Fit Testing Procedures. *OSHA Laws & Regulations.* August 2004.
15. Roberge R. Effect of surgical masks worn concurrently over N95 Filtering Facepiece Respirators: Extended service life versus increased user burden. *Journal of Public Health Management Practice.* 2008;14(2):E19-E26.
16. Roberge R, Coca A, Williams WJ, et al. Surgical mask placement over N95 filtering facepiece respirators: Physiological effects on healthcare workers. *Respirology.* 2010;15(3):516-521.

17. Lindsley WG, Martin SB, Thewlis RE, et al. Effects of ultraviolet germicidal irradiation (UVGI) on N95 respiratory filtration performance and structural integrity. *J Occup Environ Hyg*. 2015;12(8):509-517.

18. Paul D, Gupta A, Maurya AK. Exploring options for reprocessing of N95 Filtering Facepiece Respirators (N95-FFRs) amidst COVID-19 pandemic: A systematic review. *PLoS One*. 2020;15(11):e0242474.

19. Seresirikachorn K, Phoophiboon V, Chobaroporn T, et al. Decontamination and reuse of surgical masks and N95 filtering facepiece respirators during the COVID-19 pandemic: A systematic review. *Infect Control Hosp Epidemiol*. 2021;42(1): 25-30.

20. O'Hearn K, Gertsman S, Sampson M, et al. Decontaminating N95 and SN95 masks with ultraviolet germicidal irradiation does not impair mask efficacy and safety. *J Hosp Infect*. 2020;106(1):163-175.

21. FDA. Recommendations for sponsors requesting EUAs for decontamination and bioburden reduction systems for surgical masks and respirators during the coronavirus disease 2019 (COVID-19) public health emergency. U.S. Department of Health and Human Services Food and Drug Administration. May 2020.

22. Czubryt MP, Stecy T, Popke E, et al. N95 mask reuse in a major urban hospital: COVID-19 response process and procedure. *J Hosp Infect*. 2020;106: 211-282.

23. Bergman MS, Viscusi DJ, Palmiero AJ, Power JB, Shaffer RE. Impact of three cycles of decontamination treatments on filtering facepiece respirator fit. *J Int Soc Resp Prot*. 2011;28:48-59.

24. Fisher RJ, Morris DH, van Doremalen N, et al. Effectiveness of N95 decontamination and reuse against SARS-CoV-2 virus. *Emerg Infect Dis*. 2020;26(9): 2253-2255.

25. Bernard L, Desoubeaux G, Boder-Montagutelli E, et al. Controlled heat and humidity-based treatment for the reuse of personal protective equipment: A pragmatic proof-of-concept to address the mass shortage of surgical masks and N95/FFP2 respirators and to prevent the SARS-CoV2 transmission. *Front Med (Lausanne)*. 2020;7:584036.

26. Cadnum JK, Li DF, Redmond SN, Joh AR, Pearlmutter B, Donskey CJ. Effectiveness of ultraviolet-C light and a high level disinfection cabinet for decontamination of N95 respirators. *Pathog Immun*. 2020;1(5):52-67.

27. Fisher EM, Shaffer RE. A method to determine the available UV-C dose for the decontamination of filtering facepiece respirators. *J Appl Microbiol*. 2011;11:287-295.

28. Zorko DJ, Gertsman S, O'Hearn K, et al. Decontamination interventions for the reuse of surgical mask personal protective equipment: A systematic review. *The J Hosp Infect*. 2020;106(2):283-294.

29. McQuerry M, Easter E, Cao A. Disposable versus reusable medical gowns: A performance comparison. *Am J Infect Cont*. 2020;S0196-6553(20):30929-9.

30. Poller B, Lynch C, Ramsden R, et al. Laundering single-use gowns in the event of critical shortage: Experience of a UK acute trust. *J Hosp Infect*. 2020;106(3):629-630.

31. Korniewicz D. Advantages and disadvantages of non-latex surgical gloves. *Business Briefing: Global Surgery 2004.*

32. Zubrow K. US faces nitrile glove shortage ahead of national COVID-19 vaccination effort. *CBS News.* Dec 2020.

33. Esmizadeh E, Chang BP, Jubinville D, et al. Can medical-grade gloves provide protection after repeated disinfection? *ACS Applied Polymer Materials.* December 2020.

34. CDC. Cleaning and disinfecting your home. cdc.gov. December 2020.

35. Baker TL, Greiner JV, Maxwell-Schmidt E, Lamothe PH, Vesonder M. Guidelines for frontline health care staff safety for COVID-19. *J Prim Care Community Health.* 2020(11):1-10.

36. WHO. Guide to local production: WHO-recommended handrub formulations. who.int. April 2010.

37. Landsverk G. How medical workers decontaminate their clothes when they get home from treating coronavirus patients. Online: *Insider.com.* April 2020.

6 THROMBOSIS AND TRANSFUSIONS

Alina Dulu, MD, Padmastuti Akella, MD, Mustapha Serhan MD, and Stephen M. Pastores, MD

INTRODUCTION

There is increasing evidence that the activation of coagulation and inflammation are essential responses for host defense during critical illnesses such as sepsis, severe trauma, and in the current era of pandemic respiratory viruses. Venous thromboembolism (VTE), pulmonary microvascular thrombosis, and arterial thrombosis have been associated with influenza A virus and most recently with the severe acute respiratory syndrome-coronavirus-2 (SARS-CoV-2). Similarly, there have been significant advances in transfusion medicine with the establishment of appropriate thresholds for blood product support in critically ill patients, enhanced understanding of transfusion-related complications, and use of blood alternatives. This chapter will discuss the pathophysiology of thrombosis during critical illness, and review the thrombotic complications and issues surrounding anticoagulation management particularly in patients with coronavirus disease-19 (COVID-19) and anticoagulant reversal agents. Indications for red blood cell, platelet, and plasma transfusion in critically ill and trauma patients will be reviewed as well as the indications for massive transfusion, complications of blood product support, and strategies to minimize blood loss and optimize hematopoiesis.

PATHOPHYSIOLOGY OF THROMBOSIS DURING CRITICAL ILLNESS

The coagulation system is a highly regulated cascade that ultimately leads to blood clot formation. The primary purpose of coagulation is hemostasis. In recent years, coagulation factors have been implicated in tissue repair and inflammatory responses in sepsis, major trauma, and other critical illnesses. During sepsis, activation of the coagulation cascade is important in the process of isolation of invading microorganisms. Coagulation abnormalities are present in virtually all patients with sepsis, and when exaggerated and dysregulated can lead to disseminated intravascular coagulation (DIC), associated with microvascular and macrovascular thrombosis, multi-organ dysfunction, and/or hemorrhage.[1]

Host-released proinflammatory molecules freed into the extracellular environment following tissue injury (histones, nucleosomes, cell-free chromosomal and mitochondrial DNA, high-mobility group box 1 protein [HMGB-1], and heat shock protein) are known as damage-associated molecular patterns (DAMPs) and play key roles in the immune system and tissue repair. DAMPs are released from dying cells or secreted from immune cells in response to infection or tissue injury. When DAMPs are recognized by monocytes, they deliver tissue factor (TF), a transmembrane glycoprotein, to the sites of pathogen exposure. The complex pathophysiology of sepsis-induced coagulopathy is mediated by pathogen-associated molecular patterns (PAMPs). PAMPs are exogenous substances associated with pathogens that are recognized by specific toll-like and complement receptors known as pattern recognition receptors (PRRs). This intracellular signaling results in the synthesis of proinflammatory cytokines, which are key mediators of inflammation and vascular dysfunction. Interleukin-6 (IL-6), monocyte chemotactic protein-1 (MCP-1), and tumor necrosis factor-alpha (TNF-α) can induce the upregulation of TF on monocytes and macrophages with initiation of anticoagulation and fibrinolysis. TF can circulate in the blood in soluble form or associated with extracellular vesicles (EVs). EVs are submicron sized spherical particles that are enclosed by bilayer phospholipid membranes released from inflammatory cells into plasma that initiate coagulation with the expression of TF on their surfaces. Although platelet derived EVs were reported to be the main type in sepsis-induced coagulopathy, endothelial cells, leukocytes, and other cell types contribute to proinflammatory and procoagulant reactions during sepsis. TF has been recognized as the main initiator of coagulation together with FVII, FX, thrombin, and fibrin. In meningococcal sepsis, the level of TF on monocytes at presentation may be predictive of survival. TF expression is increased in endothelial cells infected with herpes simplex virus (HSV) and dengue virus, and in macrophages and circulating blood cells during Ebola virus infection.

Dysregulation of endothelial cell functions can cause a wide range of vascular effects that lead to changes in vascular permeability and activation of coagulation. Several microbial diseases such Rocky Mountain spotted fever and Nipah virus infection are characterized by severe vascular lesions attributed to direct microbial replication and induced damage to endothelial cells. Systemic endothelial immune activation results in multiple changes including the exocytosis of large von Willebrand factor (VWF) multimers, loss of heparan sulfate on the endothelial surface, platelet activation, expression of TF, downregulation of thrombomodulin, and production of nitric oxide. This generalized endothelial dysfunction and thrombo-inflammation in the microvasculature may lead to multiorgan dysfunction.[2]

Platelets are activated at the site of vascular endothelial cells injury to form a platelet plug. There are several physiologic platelet stimuli including adenosine diphosphate (ADP), thrombin, and collagen. The integrin glycoproteins GPIa/IIa and GPVI are the two major platelet collagen receptors, playing important roles in platelet adhesion and activation. Platelets have a dual receptor system for thrombin, with two distinct receptors: protease-activated receptor-1 (PAR-1) and PAR-4. ADP binds to two G-protein coupled purinergic receptors, P2Y1 and P2Y2, and functions in a paracrine/autocrine fashion to recruit additional platelets and amplify platelet aggregation. Platelet adhesion is primarily mediated by the binding of platelet surface receptor GPIb/IX/V complex to VWF in the subendothelial matrix. Platelets secrete a variety of substances from their granules upon cell stimulation, including HMGB-1 that trigger neutrophil recruitment-mediated amplification of injury through the activity of its receptor. Platelet procoagulant activity results from the exposure of procoagulant phospholipids and the subsequent assembly of enzyme complexes of the clotting cascade on the platelet surface. The initiation phase of coagulation is largely mediated by the activation of factor X (FX) by TF/ FVIIa, giving rise to a small amount of thrombin, which in turn activates more platelets and FV, VIII, and XI.[3]

Neutrophil extracellular traps (NETs) are web-like structures composed of decondensed chromatin coated with a variety of cellular proteins (myeloperoxidase, neutrophil elastase, histones, and HMGB-1). NETs are released from dead or dying neutrophils. Coagulation activation induced by NETs represents an important host defense mechanism that can contribute to the isolation and destruction of microorganisms. NET formation (NETosis) is a complex process in which nuclear chromatin becomes condensed and released into the cytoplasm, followed by rupture of the plasma membrane and expulsion of the cellular contents into the extracellular space. NETosis is highly procoagulant and distinct from apoptosis and necrosis. Serine proteases such as elastase and cathepsin G, which are components of NETs, activate PARs that are followed by the mobilization of Weibel–Palade bodies and release of VWF, and P-selectin expression by platelets and endothelial cells. P-selectin is a key component for platelet and leukocyte adhesion. In a study involving 199 patients with DIC and 20 healthy controls, elevated plasma levels of DNA-histone complexes and double-stranded DNA, considered to be in vivo markers of NETosis, correlated with the severity of coagulopathy in DIC and were independent prognostic factors. Monocytes and neutrophils have evolved cell-specific mechanisms to potentiate coagulation by expressing TF, releasing microparticles, and ejecting NETs. D-dimers and fibrin fragment E induce synthesis and release of IL-6 from monocytes and macrophages. Thrombin can also stimulate the release of chemokines including IL-6, IL-8, and MCP-1 by monocytes and endothelial cells likely through the activation of PARs.[3] In sepsis the diffuse microthrombi formation is intended to serve a protective purpose, promoting pathogen recognition and creating a sterile barrier against further pathogen invasion, but when dysfunctional leads to multiorgan failure.

THROMBOSIS ASSOCIATED WITH PANDEMIC RESPIRATORY VIRUSES

In the last century, several new viruses have emerged, including different strains of influenza virus—A virus (1918 H1N1 Spanish flu, 1957 H2N2 Asian flu, 1968 H3N2 Hong Kong flu, and 2009 H1N1), severe acute respiratory syndrome-coronavirus (SARS-CoV, 2002–2004), Middle East Respiratory Syndrome-Coronavirus (MERS-CoV, 2012), and most recently in December 2019, SARS-CoV-2—that have caused epidemics and pandemics.

VTE, pulmonary microvascular thrombosis, and arterial thrombosis have been associated with influenza A virus and pandemic coronavirus infections. Severe H1N1 influenza infection resulted in systemic and pulmonary activation of coagulation, as reflected by elevated plasma and lung levels of thrombin-antithrombin complexes and fibrin degradation products. These procoagulant changes were accompanied by inhibition of the fibrinolytic response due to enhanced release of plasminogen activator inhibitor-1 (PAI-1). One study reported 7 (5.9%) thrombotic vascular events (4 venous and 3 arterial) in 119 hospitalized patients[4] while another study observed a higher rate of VTE (44%) in H1N1 patients (n=36) with severe acute respiratory distress syndrome (ARDS) compared with 29% in non-H1N1 patients with ARDS.[5] Thrombotic complications including arterial ischemic strokes were also observed in SARS-CoV patients, while approximately 30% of critically ill patients had VTE.[6]

During the SARS-CoV-1 outbreak, there were few hematologic and coagulation abnormalities described.[7,8] In a cohort of 138 hospitalized patients in Hong Kong, the most common findings were leukopenia in 34% of patients, thrombocytopenia in 45%, elevated D-dimer in 45%, and a prolonged activated partial-thromboplastin time (aPTT) in 43%.[7] Thrombi were identified in pulmonary, bronchial, and small lung veins of postmortem SARS-CoV-1 infected lung autopsies, suggesting a pro-thrombotic effect of the SARS-CoV-1 virus on the pulmonary vasculature. The damaged lung tissue and pulmonary endothelial cells result in platelet activation and aggregation with thrombi formation within the pulmonary vasculature. In another cohort study of 157 SARS-CoV-1infected heath care workers, the most common hematologic abnormalities were lympho-penia in 98%, thrombocytopenia in 55%, thrombocytosis in 49%, isolated aPTT in 63%, and overt DIC in 2.5%.[8] Majority had mild thrombocyto-penia with only 2% of patients with a platelet count below 50,000/μL.

Most cases of MERS infection in 2012 occurred in Saudi Arabia and the United Arab Emirates, but cases were also reported in the United States, Europe, and Asia in people who traveled from the Middle East or their contacts. Thrombocytopenia was noted in 36% of 47 laboratory confirmed MERS-CoV cases in Saudi Arabia. Mild thrombocytopenia was as a common finding during the first week, without any difference between patients with mild or severe disease.[9]

Most recently, with COVID-19, several studies have reported VTE rates ranging from 0.9% to 6.5% for noncritically ill hospitalized patients and 8% to 69% in COVID-19 patients in the ICU.[10–20] Rates of PE were between 16.7% and 35% in severely ill COVID-19 patients, and rates of DVT were between 0% and 46.1% for not severely ill patients. Rates of arterial thrombotic events were between 2.8% and 3.8%.[21] Differences in clinical practice, including whether venous ultrasound is performed as a screening strategy or if thromboprophylaxis is routinely used, reporting of symptomatic versus asymptomatic VTE, and differences in patient populations may account for the wide variation in thrombosis rates in the different studies.

The immune dysregulation characteristic of severe COVID-19 may be initiated by a particularly proinflammatory form of apoptosis initially described in macrophages with rapid viral replication leading to massive release of proinflammatory mediators. Several studies have suggested that SARS-CoV-2 infection leads to a dysregulated immune response with increased IL-6, IL-1, IL-8, and TNF-α levels that is responsible for pro-gressive lung injury (ARDS) and multiorgan failure. Thromboembolic events are the result of at least two distinct mechanisms: a microvascu-lar thrombotic process initiated in the lungs (immunothrombosis) and an independent hospital-associated macrovascular VTE, which can be more exaggerated in severely ill, immobilized, mechanically ventilated patients exposed to high doses of sedative and paralytic agents in the ICU set-ting. Immunothrombosis is the process where the inflammatory reaction, along with hypoxia, results in pulmonary microvascular thrombosis.[22] Hypoxemia can stimulate thrombosis not only by increasing blood viscosity, but also via a hypoxia-inducible transcription factor-dependent mechanism, that activates TF and PAI-1. Histopathology of lung specimens from COVID-19 patients with early disease shows characteristic findings of ARDS and evidence of small vessel occlusion with microvascular thrombi containing numerous neutrophils consistent with NETs.[15,20] Thromboelastography in ICU patients with COVID-19 shows a hypercoagulable state with clot formation that is extremely rapid and resistant to breakdown likely related to reduced fibrinolysis due to increased production of PAI-1.[23]

SARS-CoV2 induces a unique form of coagulopathy, characterized by increased levels of D-dimer and fibrin degradation products (FDP) without severe thrombocytopenia or hypofibrinogenemia. The coagulation abnormalities reported in COVID-19 patients are listed in Table 6-1. The increase in D-dimer was the most significant alteration observed in COVID-19 patients and occurred more frequently than other coagulation parameters. Fibrinogen appears to increase early and may be used as a

Table 6-1 COAGULATION ABNORMALITIES IN PATIENTS WITH COVID-19

Normal or slight prolongation of PT and aPTT

Mild thrombocytopenia (platelet count < 100,000/μL); in severe cases, platelet count < 50,000/μL (rarely)

Elevated D-dimer (markedly elevated in severe cases)

Elevated fibrinogen (majority); in rare cases can mimic DIC with decreased fibrinogen (< 1.0 g/L)

Elevated fibrin degradation products

Positive lupus anticoagulant

Elevated FVIII and VWF antigen

Mild decrease in antithrombin level

Elevated PAI-1

TEG findings

- Reaction time (R) shortened consistent with increased early thrombin burst (50%)

- Clot formation time (K) shortened, consistent with increased fibrin generation (83%)

- Maximum amplitude (MA) increased, consistent with greater clot strength (83%)

- Clot lysis at 30 minutes (LY30) reduced, consistent with reduced fibrinolysis (100%)

aPTT = activated partial thromboplastin time; DIC = disseminated intravascular coagulation; FVIII = factor VIII; PAI-1 = plasminogen activator inhibitor-1; PT = prothrombin time; TEG = thromboelastography; VWF = von Willebrand factor.

risk stratification marker for increased risk to develop ARDS. At hospital admission, COVID-19 patients showed statistically significant increased levels of fibrinogen (> 400 mg/dL), particularly in those patients who developed ARDS.[17] Zhou et al. reported abnormally elevated D-dimer levels in 46.4% of patients with a prevalence of 43% in non-severe patients versus 60% in critically ill patients.[18] Tang et al. similarly reported increased D-dimers and FDP and mild to moderately increased PT and aPTT in COVID-19 patients. D-dimer levels greater than 2.0 mg/L were shown to predict mortality with a sensitivity of 92.3% and a specificity of 83.3%.[19]

Currently, the optimal antithrombotic prophylactic strategy for patients with COVID-19 is unclear. In a cross-sectional study of 81 ICU patients in China, with no routine thromboprophylaxis as standard of care, 25% of patients were diagnosed with DVT.[11] In a retrospective study of 184 ICU patients in three Dutch hospitals, where routine low molecular weight heparin (LMWH) prophylaxis was used, the VTE incidence was 27%.[10] Similar observations are reported in ICU patients in France and Italy.[16] In a study of 2,700 patients admitted to the Mount Sinai Health System in New York City, compared to no anticoagulation, both prophylactic and therapeutic anticoagulation were associated with decreased mortality and intubation.[20] In those who began anticoagulation < 48 h of hospital admission, there was no statistically significant difference in outcomes between therapeutic and prophylactic anticoagulation. Clinical trials are underway to address the optimal antithrombotic prophylactic strategy in hospitalized COVID-19 patients.

With regards to acute ischemic strokes, one study of 214 patients in Wuhan, China, reported the incidence of arterial ischemic events at 2.34%–3.67%. In a systematic review including 39 studies comprising 135 patients with a mean age of 63.4 ± 13 years, the pooled incidence of acute ischemic strokes in COVID-19 patients was 1.2% (range 0.9%–2.7%).[21] Laboratory findings were elevated D-dimer and fibrinogen levels and positive lupus circulating anticoagulant. The majority of neuroimaging patterns observed were large vessel thrombosis, embolism, or stenosis, followed by multiple vascular territory.

▌HEMORRHAGIC FEVER VIRUSES

Viral hemorrhagic fevers are a group of febrile illnesses caused by RNA viruses from several viral families including filoviruses (Ebola and Marburg), arenaviruses (Lassa and New World arenaviruses), bunyaviruses (Congo-Crimean Hemorrhagic Fever and Rift Valley Fever), and flaviviruses (yellow fever).[24] They are all associated with fever, malaise, vomiting, mucosal and gastrointestinal bleeding, edema, and hypotension.

Dengue Virus

The dengue virus is found in tropical and subtropical climates worldwide, mostly in urban and semi-urban areas. There are three types of symptomatic dengue infection: dengue fever (DF), dengue hemorrhagic fever (DHF), and dengue shock syndrome (DSS). People of all ages who are exposed to infected mosquitoes are at risk for dengue fever.

The pathophysiological basis of hemorrhage in dengue virus infection remains incompletely understood. Bleeding can manifest as petechiae, ecchymoses, purpura, diffuse mucosal bleeding, hematemesis, and melena. One pathogenetic mechanism is molecular mimicry between dengue viral proteins and human coagulation factors. DHF may be caused by an autoimmune reaction against thrombin and other components of the coagulation cascade leading to an antithrombotic and profibrinolytic state.[25] Dengue virus proteins show sequence homologies to coagulation proteases. In vitro, DENV isolates can bind to and activate plasminogen directly and the plasmin generated can degrade both fibrin and fibrinogen. Antibody responses to homologous peptides derived from the dengue virus E protein have been shown to cross-react and bind to human plasminogen. They can either inhibit plasmin activity or enhance plasminogen activation. The presence of plasminogen cross-reactive antibodies in acute phase and convalescent-phase serum samples from patients with DF positively correlates with petechiae and hemorrhage. Thrombomodulin levels suggestive of endothelial activation correlate with increasing shock severity. Rather than causing true DIC, the dengue virus may activate fibrinolysis primarily, degrading fibrinogen directly.[24]

IgM antiplatelet antibodies causing the destruction of platelets is a predictor for the development of thrombocytopenia. An increased level of PA IgM was associated with the development of DHF. Marked thrombocytopenia ($< 100,000$ platelets/ μL) is one of the criteria used to define DHF. The formation of platelet associated immunoglobulins may play a role in the mechanism of thrombocytopenia and the accompanying increased vascular permeability.

In DSS, there is increased cytokine expression and capillary leakage. Clinically, serum IL-6 levels appear to correlate with mortality of patients with DSS. The dengue virus induces endothelial production of TF as well as IL-6. Hemoconcentration, hypoalbuminemia, and anasarca are frequent due to capillary leakage and correlate with severity. The coagulation proteins that have molecular weights of 30,000–70,000 Da, close to the molecular weight of albumin, leak out of the intravascular compartment. There are minor prolongations of PT and aPTT, moderate hypofibrinogenemia, low concentrations of proteins C, S, and antithrombin III. The most important pathophysiologic abnormality seen in DHF/DSS is an acute increase in vascular permeability that leads to plasma leakage into extravascular compartment and a consumptive coagulopathy that leads to diffuse bleeding mimicking DIC.[26,27]

Ebola Virus

Ebola virus is the most notorious of the hemorrhagic fever viruses. During the 2014–2016 Ebola epidemic in West Africa, there were nearly 29,000 total cases suspected, 15,000 laboratory-confirmed cases, and 11,000 deaths. The infection is characterized by extensive virus replication, dysregulated immune responses, extensive tissue damage, and disordered coagulation.[28,29] Lymphopenia and elevated proinflammatory cytokines in plasma are typical, especially in fatal infections. Extensive apoptosis of bystander T lymphocytes appears to be a prominent feature. Large numbers of T lymphocyte-derived microparticles also contribute to the observed vascular and coagulation complications. Virus-infected macrophages synthesize TF, triggering the coagulation pathway. The coagulation abnormalities are generally consistent with DIC and manifest as petechiae, ecchymoses, and mucosal hemorrhages. Massive loss of blood is atypical and restricted to the gastrointestinal tract.

Yellow Fever

Yellow fever virus causes a systemic illness characterized by high viremia; hepatic, renal, and myocardial injury; hemorrhage and high mortality.[30] Yellow fever is found in tropical South America and sub-Saharan Africa. Hemorrhagic manifestations include coffee-ground hematemesis ("black vomit"), melena, hematuria, metrorrhagia, petechiae, ecchymoses, bleeding from the gums and nose, and prolonged bleeding at needle puncture sites. Laboratory findings include thrombocytopenia, prolonged clotting and prothrombin times, and reductions in clotting factors synthesized by the liver. Tests indicating DIC include diminished fibrinogen and FVIII and elevated FDP. There is damage to endothelial cells and plasma leakage from capillaries. Gross findings at autopsy include widespread petechial hemorrhages of skin and mucosae, moderate pleural and peritoneal effusions, and pulmonary edema.

Lassa Fever

Lassa fever is caused by the Lassa virus, an Old World arenavirus that is mainly transmitted by contact with excretions and secretions of infected rats via foods and water and through exposure to other contaminated items.[31] It is endemic in parts of West Africa, primarily Sierra Leone, Guinea, Liberia, and Nigeria. Hemorrhagic manifestations result from endothelial dysfunction, abnormal platelet aggregation, and severe thrombocytopenia. The presence of a circulating inhibitor of platelet aggregation is strongly associated with the occurrence of hemorrhage and a high mortality. Unlike Ebola where the bleeding is mostly due to DIC-induced cytokine storm, fatal cases of Lassa fever are associated with poor cellular response by monocytes and macrophages to the virus, which allows the Lassa virus to replicate unchecked. Ribavirin has been used with success in Lassa fever patients and is most effective when given early in the course of the illness.

Crimean-Congo Hemorrhagic Fever Virus

Crimean-Congo hemorrhagic fever virus is a widely distributed hemorrhagic fever virus and the cause of hemorrhagic disease in Africa, Southern and Eastern Europe, the Middle East, India, and Asia. The main vector and reservoir are hard-body ticks principally of the *Hyalomma* genus.[32] Domestic livestock and wild animals such as hares serve as amplifying hosts, with uninfected ticks becoming infected during feeding on viremic animals or during co-feeding with an infected tick. Humans can become infected via tick bites and butchering of infected livestock and in the health care setting during the care of infected patients. High viral loads, absence of early antibody responses, and high levels of alanine aminotransferase and aspartate aminotransferase predict poor outcome. Thrombocytopenia, prolonged clotting times, and elevated levels of inflammatory cytokines are also observed in severe cases. The coagulopathy seems to be the result of DIC and loss of clotting factors due to endothelial dysfunction and increased permeability.

▌ MANAGEMENT OF VENOUS THROMBOEMBOLISM IN THE ACUTE CARE SETTING

Critically ill patients exhibit a 5% to 10% rate of VTE (DVT or PE) despite thromboprophylaxis.[33] The presentation of PE can range from asymptomatic to sudden death. The severity of PE and the acute risk of death is based on its acute hemodynamic effects and the presence of right heart failure. Supplemental oxygen is indicated in patients with PE and arterial oxygen saturation of less than 90% with consideration of high-flow nasal cannula and mechanical ventilation in cases of extreme instability. The cornerstone of treatment is anticoagulation. Patients with low risk VTE can be managed with anticoagulation alone. High and intermediate-risk PE patients have a very high mortality and should be treated with therapeutic escalation with systemic thrombolysis, catheter-directed therapies, or surgical embolectomy if appropriate candidates.

In patients with high or intermediate clinical probability of PE, anticoagulation with subcutaneous, weight-adjusted low-molecular weight heparin (LMWH) or fondaparinux, or IV unfractionated heparin (UFH) should be initiated while awaiting the results of diagnostic tests.[34] LMWH and fondaparinux are preferred over UFH for initial anticoagulation in PE, as they have a lower risk of major bleeding and heparin-induced thrombocytopenia. Neither LMWH nor fondaparinux need routine monitoring of anti-Xa levels. UFH is recommended for patients with overt hemodynamic instability or imminent hemodynamic decompensation in whom primary reperfusion treatment will be necessary, for patients with severe renal impairment (creatinine clearance [CrCl] < 30 mL/min) or severe obesity. If LMWH is used in patients with CrCl 15–30 mL/min, an adapted dosing scheme should be used.

Based on pharmacokinetic data, an equally rapid anticoagulant effect can also be achieved with direct oral anticoagulants (DOACs), including the direct thrombin inhibitor dabigatran and the factor Xa inhibitors rivaroxaban, apixaban, and edoxaban.[30] DOACs were shown to be non-inferior when compared with vitamin K antagonists (VKA) for the treatment of non-cancer VTE, with similar or lower rates of major bleeding.[35-39] DOACs are also approved for the stroke prevention in patients with nonvalvular atrial fibrillation.

Dabigatran is the only oral direct thrombin inhibitor. It is rapidly absorbed, reaching its peak plasma concentration in under 2 h, with a half-life of approximately 14–17 h. It is 80% renally excreted and, thus, renal impairment can increase the half-life up to 34 h. The dose of dabigatran for the treatment and secondary prevention of VTE is 150 mg orally twice daily after 5 to 10 days of parenteral anticoagulation in patients with CrCl > 30 mL/min. In the RE-COVER trial,[35] the composite endpoint of major or clinically relevant nonmajor bleeding was lower in the dabigatran group compared to warfarin (5.0% vs. 7.9%). However, there was a trend to higher incidence of gastrointestinal hemorrhage in the dabigatran group.

Rivaroxaban has very high oral bioavailability and rapid absorption rate, reaching a peak plasma concentration between 2 and 8 h with a half-life ranging from 5 to 13 h. Elimination of rivaroxaban occurs via both the kidney and liver. Apixaban also has a predictable bioavailability, reaching a peak plasma concentration in approximately 3 h, with a half-life of up to 12 h. It is metabolized by multiple different pathways including cytochrome P450, intestinal excretion, and renal elimination. The half-life of apixaban is increased up to 17 h in patients with severe renal impairment (CrCl < 30 mL/min). Edoxaban is rapidly absorbed reaching a peak plasma concentration between 1 and 3 h, an oral bioavailability of 62%, half-life of 10–14 h, and metabolized by both the kidney and liver.

The choice of one DOAC over another is based on different treatment regimens, patient characteristics, and patient preference. DOACs are recommended by several international guidelines for first-line treatment of VTE in the general population.[30] DOACs have several advantages over VKAs, including their predictable bioavailability and pharmacokinetics, which allows to be administered at fixed doses without routine laboratory monitoring, and fewer interactions when given concomitantly with other drugs. DOACs are not recommended in patients with severe renal impairment, patients with concomitant use of potent P-glycoprotein inhibitors or cytochrome P4503A4 inhibitors or inducers, including azole antimycotics (e.g., ketoconazole), several protease inhibitors used for HIV treatment, and antiepileptic drugs (phenytoin, carbamazepine).

In high-risk PE patients and non-high-risk patients with hemodynamic deterioration despite receiving anticoagulation therapy, systemic thrombolysis is recommended. Thrombolytic therapy leads to faster improvement in pulmonary obstruction and hemodynamics compared with UFH alone. The greatest benefit is observed when treatment is initiated within 48 h of symptom onset, although it can still be useful in patients who have had symptoms for 6–14 days.[34] A systematic review and meta-analysis of thrombolysis trials showed a significant reduction in the combined outcome of mortality and recurrent PE, with a 9.9% rate of severe bleeding and a 1.7% rate of intracranial hemorrhage. In normotensive patients with intermediate-risk PE, defined as the presence of RV dysfunction and elevated troponin levels, thrombolytic therapy was associated with a significant reduction in the risk of hemodynamic decompensation or collapse, but with an increased risk of severe extracranial and intracranial bleeding.[40] Accelerated IV recombinant tissue type plasminogen activator (rtPA; 100 mg over 2 h) is preferable to prolonged infusions of streptokinase and urokinase. The efficacy and safety of reduced dose rtPA need further confirmation. In patients with high-risk PE in whom thrombolysis is contraindicated or has failed, percutaneous catheter-directed treatment or surgical embolectomy should be considered.[34,41] Vena cava filters are indicated in patients with VTE and absolute contraindication to anticoagulation, recurrent PE despite adequate anticoagulation, and primary prophylaxis in patients with a high risk of VTE.

Reversal of DOACs

Two specific DOAC reversal agents are approved by the U.S. Food and Drug Administration: idarucizumab (Praxbind®) for reversal of dabigatran and andexanet alfa (Andexxa®) for reversal of apixaban and rivaroxaban.[42] Idarucizumab is a humanized monoclonal antibody fragment that binds free and thrombin-bound dabigatran and neutralizes its activity. It is rapidly cleared and does not induce a prothrombotic state. It is catabolized with 32% of the dose being excreted in the urine within 6 h of infusion. The recommended dose is 5 g IV provided as two separate vials each containing 2.5 g/50 mL idarucizumab.

Andexanet alfa is a modified recombinant factor Xa, which is catalytically inactive and binds to factor Xa inhibitors, neutralizing its anticoagulant effects by preventing the inhibitors from binding to endogenous factor Xa. It was approved in 2018 for the management of life-threatening or uncontrolled bleeding due to apixaban and rivaroxaban. The recommended dose is based on the specific FXa inhibitor, dose of the inhibitor, and the time from last dose. A low dose of andexanet alfa (400 mg bolus given over 15 to 30 min followed by a continuous infusion of 4 mg/min for 120 min) is recommended for patients on apixaban and those who had last taken rivaroxaban > 7 h ago. A high dose (800 mg bolus given over 30 min followed by a continuous infusion of 8 mg/min for 120 min) is recommended for patients who had taken rivaroxaban within the last 7 h, or at an unknown time.[42] Additional studies are needed regarding the hemostatic efficacy and prothrombotic risk of andexanet alfa.

Non-specific prohemostatic agents have also been used off-label for DOAC reversal including prothrombin complex concentrate (PCC) and activated prothrombin complex concentrate (APCC) [FEIBA]. PCCs are plasma-derived concentrates of the vitamin K-dependent clotting factors in their inactive form. Four-factor PCC contains factors II, VII, IX, and X, whereas three-factor PCC contains predominantly factors II, IX, and X, and no or trivial concentrations of factor VII. The recommended dose of 4-F PCC to achieve hemostasis is 50 units/kg in bleeding patients. In settings where 4-F PCC is not available, supplementing 3-F PCC with fresh frozen plasma to provide factor VII has been suggested. APCC is a plasma-derived concentrate of the vitamin K-dependent clotting factors in which a fraction of the clotting factors has been activated by proteolytic cleavage.

Activated charcoal may be effective in reducing factor Xa inhibitor absorption up to 6 h after ingestion especially in overdose cases and can be used unless there are contraindications (unprotected airway, non-intact gastrointestinal tract, intestinal obstruction). Renal replacement therapy (hemodialysis or CRRT) has been used only for dabigatran reversal in patients with bleeding associated with overdose or acute renal impairment. Two other reversal agents, ciraparantag and FXaI16L, are undergoing further investigation.

Anticoagulation Therapy in COVID-19

The International Society on Thrombosis and Hemostasis recommends standard prophylactic dose anticoagulation (LMWH or UFH) for hospitalized patients with COVID-19 in the absence of any contraindications such as active bleeding and severe thrombocytopenia (platelet count < 30,000/mm^3).[43] Therapeutic anticoagulation with LMWH or UFH should be administered in patients with COVID-19 who have confirmed VTE. Several clinical trials are underway to determine the appropriate type, dose, and timing of anticoagulation especially for those patients with COVID-19 in whom PE is highly likely but imaging is not feasible. The use of VKA and DOACs in these patients has generated less interest due to potential drug–drug interactions with antiviral therapies.

Anticoagulation Therapy for Sepsis

The efficacy of anticoagulant therapy including UFH, antithrombin and thrombomodulin for sepsis-associated coagulopathy (SAC) remains controversial despite multiple RCTs.[1] A recent updated meta-analysis reported a statistically significant reduction in mortality of 13% in the subgroup of septic patients with INR > 1.4 and platelet count > 30,000 when the first dose of recombinant human soluble thrombomodulin was administered.[44] Although platelet activation, aggregation and composite thrombus formation with leukocytes are crucial events during sepsis, attempts to suppress platelet activation have not yielded a favorable effect.[2]

Antiplatelet Therapy

Aspirin inhibits platelet cyclooxygenase-1 and the synthesis of prostaglandin G2 and subsequent transformation into prostaglandin H2 that is required for the production of thromboxane A2, a powerful promoter of platelet aggregation and vasoconstriction. The benefits of aspirin are well established for patients with cardiovascular conditions, such as acute coronary syndrome and stroke prevention in patients with atrial fibrillation. However, the benefits of aspirin are less clear for the primary prevention of VTE after major orthopedic surgery.[45]

▌ TRAUMA-INDUCED COAGULOPATHY

Up to 25% of trauma patients develop trauma-induced coagulopathy (TIC). TIC is caused by multiple factors, such as hemorrhagic shock, hemodilution, hypothermia, acidosis, and DIC.[46-48] Tissue damage, hypoperfusion, and massive bleeding are the main drivers of the inflammatory and neurohormonal response with a significant increase in thrombin generation, catecholamines, hormones, and cytokines (TNF-α, IL-1β, and IL-6). Primary predisposing conditions for TIC are based on four pillars: endogenous anticoagulation in the form of DIC or acute coagulopathy induced by trauma and shock; fibrinogen depletion, hyperfibrinolysis and fibrinolytic shutdown; platelet dysfunction; and endotheliopathy.[46]

Management of TIC includes hypothermia prevention, acid–base balance control, maintenance of fluid balance, and transfusion therapy. Hypovolemic resuscitation with permissive hypotension is useful in minimizing the risk of fibrinogen and platelet dysfunction and hemodilution.

▌ TRANSFUSIONS

How Blood Products Are Prepared from Whole Blood to Its Products

The technology of blood transfusions has tremendously evolved from the transfusion of whole blood to using individual components.[49,50] Primarily, the goal of individual components is to produce high quality blood products that cause minimal risk to the recipient and the donor. Obtaining individual components such as packed red blood cells (RBC), platelet concentrates, and plasma consists of filtering to reduce the number of immune cells, which may induce adverse effects and transfer DNA from donor to recipient.[50] Blood products are scarce resources, even more so when pandemics afflict the world. Liberal use of blood products increases health care expenditure worldwide. In the critical care setting, administering blood products judiciously is paramount. First, the need for a blood product should be established, then the etiology should be identified and finally clinicians should use evidence-based protocols to choose and administer needed products based on patient category.

In the ICU, multiple units of blood products are used routinely for patients and different products are often given to the same patient. Red cell concentrates in plasma are prepared by removing part of the plasma from centrifuged whole blood. Storage medium is added to preserve RBC concentrates. During storage, the RBC changes shape and function, and substances are leaked from the cell into the storage medium—changes that combined are called the "storage lesion."[51] In the ICU, RBC concentrates are usually used to correct anemia and bleeding. Fresh frozen plasma contains proteins such as albumin, coagulation factors (most notably FVIII), and immunoglobulins.

Blood donors worldwide put themselves at risk when they choose to donate. Up to one-third of donors may experience adverse effects such as vasovagal episodes, iron deficiency, and local symptoms.[51]

Transfusion Goals for Red Blood Cells, Plasma, and Platelets

Anemia is common in the critically ill and can be associated with significant morbidity and mortality.[52] The etiology of anemia in these patients is multifactorial and may include acute blood loss, diagnostic blood sampling, inappropriately low circulating erythropoietin concentrations, reduced RBC production and survival, functional iron deficiency, and nutritional deficiencies. With the advent of improved individual components of blood products, anemia can be easily treated with packed RBCs. Indications for RBC transfusions in the general ICU population include acute bleeding with hemodynamic instability and anemia with a hemoglobin level of less than 7 g/dL.

Two large RCTs firmly established the safety and benefits of using a restrictive transfusion strategy in ICU patients. The TRICC (Transfusion Requirements in Critical Care) trial conducted in a general, Canadian ICU population showed effectiveness and safety of using a restrictive transfusion strategy (Hb level 7.0 g/dL) and even signs of superiority in some subgroups of patients (younger and less critically ill) than a liberal transfusion strategy (9.0 g/dL).[53] Among those patients who received a liberal transfusion goal, there were significantly worse outcomes during hospitalization, and in rates of cardiac complications and organ dysfunction. In 2013, the TRISS (Transfusion Requirements in Septic Shock) trial used the same threshold levels as for transfusion in patients with septic shock and showed that the lower hemoglobin transfusion strategy resulted in fewer patients and RBCs transfused, with outcomes similar to those who were on the higher hemoglobin threshold.[54]

Another trial published in 2013 demonstrated lower mortality with the restrictive transfusion strategy in patients with upper acute gastrointestinal bleeding.[55] In patients with ongoing acute coronary syndrome or chronic cardiovascular disease, a recent systematic review and meta-analysis concluded that a more liberal transfusion threshold (Hb greater than 8 g/dL) should be advocated until the safety of a more restrictive threshold is shown.[56] Similarly, in patients with traumatic brain injury, RBC transfusion at higher Hb levels (greater than 10 g/dL) was associated with higher brain tissue oxygenation.[57] To further minimize the blood product use, all nonbleeding patients should be treated with single-unit transfusions followed by assessment of the patient's clinical status and repeat Hb level.[51]

Plasma transfusions are indicated for correction of major bleeding or in preparation for invasive procedures when the international normalized ratio (INR) is substantially elevated due to vitamin K antagonist therapy, vitamin K deficiency, or a deficiency of multiple coagulation factors (e.g., liver disease, disseminated intravascular coagulation), and as components of massive transfusion protocols.[58] Mildly abnormal laboratory coagulation values are not predictive of clinical bleeding and should not be corrected with plasma. Platelet transfusions are indicated for patients who are bleeding with a platelet count < 50,000/μL (100,000/μL for central nervous system or ocular bleeding), or in any patient with an acquired or inherited platelet function defect regardless of platelet count. Platelet transfusion may also be indicated in thrombocytopenic patients undergoing invasive procedures, depending on the procedure and the platelet count or prophylactically to prevent spontaneous bleeding in those with a platelet count < 10,000/μL.[59]

Blood Product Transfusions in Trauma

The approach to resuscitation in trauma has advanced in the last twenty years. Until 2006 few trauma centers worldwide had well-defined protocols to address the preparation, process, and monitoring of a massive transfusion. In the early hours of a traumatic injury, death by exsanguination is a leading cause of mortality. In the review of U.S. combat deaths from Iraq and Afghanistan, hemorrhage accounted for 90% of deaths from potentially survivable trauma.[60] Providing blood at the times of national emergencies and war-like scenarios is a challenge to the blood transfusion services. For the successful implementation of its role, military frontline transfusion services should be fully mobile with integral transportation and communication systems. Supplementation of blood supplies must be prompt, and for this adequate air transport facilities must be established.

A rational approach to using blood products in patients with bleeding requires an understanding of the principles of managing hemorrhagic shock. The main priorities are controlling hemorrhage and restoring adequate oxygen delivery to the tissues. Surgical control and treatment of coagulopathy are required to stop hemorrhage in these patients.[61] The "damage control resuscitation" approach stemming out of combat operations in Southwest Asia has allowed for management of life-threatening hemorrhage with higher ratios of plasma to RBC transfusion. Practices such as aggressive crystalloid resuscitation and only RBC transfusions appear to be associated with worse outcomes when compared to the practice of early blood product resuscitation with a ratio of plasma to platelets to RBCs approaching 1:1:1.[61]

Finally, the approach in trauma resuscitation using the "deadly triad" of acidemia, coagulopathy, and hypothermia as targets for resuscitation strategies have improved outcomes.[57] Traumatically injured patients should be transported quickly and treated by a specialized trauma/military center whenever possible. Measures to monitor and support coagulation should be initiated as early as possible and used to guide a goal-directed treatment strategy. A damage-control approach to surgical intervention should guide patient management. Coagulation support and thrombo-prophylactic strategies should be considered in trauma patients who have been pre-treated with anticoagulants or platelet inhibitors. Local adherence to a multidisciplinary, evidence-based treatment protocol should serve as the basis of patient management and undergo regular quality assessment.

Indications for Massive Transfusion Protocol

Massive transfusion is traditionally defined as transfusion of 10 units of packed RBCs within a 24-h period. This process requires the consideration of multiple physiologic parameters such as volume status, tissue oxygenation, management of bleeding and coagulation abnormalities, and acid-base balance. Indications for massive transfusion protocols (MTP) include bleeding due to trauma, obstetrical catastrophes, surgery, and gastrointestinal bleeding. In most patients requiring MTP, blood products need to be given rapidly and therefore, catheters larger in diameter and shorter in length that can provide higher flow rates are more desirable. Institution-specific protocols facilitate ordering of blood products and receiving them expeditiously from the blood bank. Targets of resuscitation in the setting of massive transfusion include mean arterial pressure of 60–65 mm Hg, hemoglobin > 7 g/dL, INR < 1.5, fibrinogen > 1.5 to 2 g/L, platelets > 50,000/μL, pH 7.35 to 7.45, and core temperature >35°C.[62] Potential complications of massive transfusion include metabolic alkalosis, hypocalcemia, hypothermia, and hyperkalemia.

Transfusion Support in Burn Injuries

Patients with burn injuries are fundamentally different from other critically ill patients. The burn wound represents loss of skin, the major infection and inhalation injury has systemic and local effects. Burn injury results in hypermetabolism associated with sustained increased temperature and tachycardia; cardiac dysfunction, immunosuppression, sepsis, iron deficiency, open or granulating wounds, hemodilution during resuscitation, escharotomies, donor site loss, coagulopathy, and bone marrow suppression. Burn treatment also differs due to multiple operations, frequent dressing changes, topical and systemic antibiotics, and prolonged stays with extensive rehabilitation needs. The TRIBE trial compared outcomes using a restrictive blood transfusion policy (maintaining Hb level 7–8 g/dl) to a traditional transfusion policy (maintaining Hb level 10–11 g/dl) in patients with a burn injury greater than 20% of total body surface area.[63] They showed that a restrictive transfusion strategy markedly reduced the number of blood transfusions but found no statistically significant differences in the primary outcome of bloodstream infection or in the secondary outcome measures, including mortality, pneumonia, urinary tract infection, wound infection, hospital length of stay, ICU length of stay, organ dysfunction, or wound healing.

Blood Product Transfusions in Various Pandemics

Passive immunization for the prevention and treatment of human infectious diseases can be traced back to the 20th century. Convalescent blood products (CBP), obtained by collecting whole blood or plasma from a patient who has survived a previous infection and developed humoral immunity against the pathogen responsible for the disease in question, is a possible source of specific antibodies of human origin. The transfusion of CBP can neutralize the pathogen and eventually lead to its eradication from the blood circulation. Prior to COVID-19, transfusion of CBP, especially convalescent plasma, was utilized in a variety of pandemic outbreaks, including influenza, Ebola virus, SARS, and MERS (Table 6-2).

COVID-19 Convalescent Plasma

Human convalescent plasma has been used to treat patients with COVID-19, but the efficacy remains uncertain. In a multicenter open-label, expanded access program that enrolled 35,322 patients with COVID-19 (including 52% who were critically ill in the ICU), early administration of convalescent plasma had a marked effect on mortality. Patients who

		Table 6-2 BLOOD PRODUCT TRANSFUSIONS USED IN VARIOUS PANDEMICS	
Pandemic	Year	Products Under Investigation	Convalescent Plasma Used
Ebola	2013–2014	ZMapp, recombinant human activated protein C, RNA interference with oligonucleotides	+
Spanish influenza (H1N1)	1918	N/A	+
Avian influenza (H5N1)	2005–2008	Serum or hyperimmune immunoglobulin	+
Severe acute respiratory syndrome (SARS)-coronavirus (SARS-CoV)	2003	Serum or hyperimmune immunoglobulin	+
Middle East Respiratory Syndrome (MERS) MERS-CoV	2012	N/A	+
Pandemic influenza A (H1N1)	2009	Serum or hyperimmune immunoglobulin	+
SARS-CoV2/ COVID-19	2019–2020	Hyperimmune immunoglobulin	+
Zika virus	2015–2016	Pathogen reduction systems in plasma	-
Crimean–Congo hemorrhagic fever virus (CCHFV)	1999–2000	THERAFLEX Ultraviolet (UV)-Platelets and THERAFLEX Methylene blue (MB)-Plasma pathogen inactivation systems	-

(*Continued*)

		Products Under	Convalescent
Table 6-2 BLOOD PRODUCT TRANSFUSIONS USED IN VARIOUS PANDEMICS (CONTINUED)			
Pandemic	**Year**	**Investigation**	**Plasma Used**
Nipah virus	1998	THERAFLEX Ultraviolet (UV)-Platelets and THERAFLEX Methylene blue (MB)-Plasma pathogen inactivation systems	-

received convalescent plasma within three days of diagnosis had a 7-day mortality rate of 8.7% versus 11.9% (p<0.001) in patients transfused 4 or more days after COVID-19 diagnosis.[64] Additionally, the use of convalescent plasma with higher IgG antibody levels (>18.45 S/Co) was associated with reduced 7-day and 30-day mortality. There are 138 ongoing studies evaluating convalescent plasma and hyperimmune immunoglobulin, of which 73 are RCTs (three already completed).[65]

Transfusion Complications

Blood transfusions can cause febrile or allergic reactions and sometimes fatal adverse events such as transfusion-related acute lung injury (TRALI), transfusion associated circulatory overload (TACO), anaphylaxis, and alloimmunization to red cell, platelet, and plasma antigens.[52] Blood transfusions can also lead to hospital-acquired infections, multiorgan failure, thrombosis and transfusion-associated graft-versus-host disease. Presently, the two main causes of transfusion associated mortality in the United States are TRALI and ABO and non-ABO hemolytic reactions.[66] Leukoreduction, use of autologous transfusions, and restrictive transfusion strategies have helped mitigate the more serious complications of transfusion.

Human error is one of the most preventable risks of transfusions. In the United States, death due to ABO incompatibility is estimated to occur at a rate of 1 in 600,000 RBC transfusions. This is can due to either wrong specimen labeling, incorrect blood type for the patient, or incorrect patient identification information. There are several policies and precautions that have been implemented to reduce the risk of such reactions such as requiring two patient identifiers or requiring the presence of two nurses at the time of blood collection and during infusion.

Febrile transfusion reactions occur in ~1% of transfusions. Prestorage leukocyte reduction has resulted in a decrease in febrile transfusion reactions, particularly for RBC transfusions. It is believed that pre-storage LR decreases inflammatory cytokine release that typically occurs during blood component storage. Allergic transfusion reactions (rash, urticaria) are typically attributable to plasma proteins, dietary or environmental antigens, or proteins bound to the RBC or platelet membrane. These are usually donor specific; however, patients who have multiple allergic reactions (usually atopic individuals) to different donors can be provided with washed platelet or RBC components. Patients may also develop anaphylactic reactions to blood components. These individuals should be evaluated for IgA deficiency; however, only ~5% of patients who are IgA deficient develop anti-IgA and are at risk for such reactions. IgE-mediated histamine release from mast cells is the cause of many anaphylactic transfusion reactions.

The rate of TACO is about 1%. The high osmotic load of blood products draws volume into the intravascular space over the course of hours, which can cause TACO in susceptible patients such as those with cardiac or renal insufficiency. In most cases, TACO is preventable by reducing the transfusion rate or volume and/or with possible concomitant use of diuretics. Other strategies to reduce the incidence of TACO (as well as TRALI) are implementation of universal leukoreduction and removal of supernatant from cellular transfusions by washing.

TRALI is defined as acute lung injury, or worsening lung injury, occurring within 6 h of blood transfusion. It is caused in many instances by HLA antibodies present in the blood component that recognize the recipient and/or by antineutrophil antibodies. Bioactive substances such as lysophosphatidylcholine, nonpolar lipids, and CD40 ligand accumulate during storage of RBCs or platelets and can induce lung injury in animal models and in humans. To mitigate TRALI and febrile transfusion reaction risk, apheresis platelets are also available with reduced plasma composition that have platelet additive solution instead, and the use of pooled plasma components can be also used.

Acute hemolytic transfusion reaction (AHTR) usually results from recipient plasma antibodies to donor RBC antigens. ABO incompatibility is the most common cause of AHTR. Antibodies against blood group antigens other than ABO can also cause AHTR. Mislabeling the recipient's pretransfusion sample at collection and failing to match the intended recipient with the blood product immediately before transfusion are the typical causes.

Prior to the advent of DNA-/RNA-based testing, the majority of transfusion-acquired diseases included hepatitis B virus and hepatitis C virus (HCV) infections. Hepatitis B, HCV, human immunodeficiency virus (HIV), West Nile virus (WNV), Zika virus, bacterial, parasitic, and prion diseases formed the majority of transfusion-acquired infections.[67] Bacterial contaminants such as *Staphylococcus epidermidis* and *Staphylococcus aureus* were the most common infections transmitted with platelet transfusions due to their storage at room temperature. Gram-negative bacterial transmission is more common with RBC transfusions. Currently, although blood is routinely tested for HIV, HBV, HCV, WNV, and Zika virus, the rates of transmission of these infections vary by country. Furthermore, blood is not routinely tested for infections like malaria or Babesia since there are no FDA approved tests and/or the costs of screening are huge.

Transfusion-Related Immunomodulation (TRIM)

Transfusion of blood components causes suppression of T cell and natural killer cell effector functions and dysregulates innate immunity toward proinflammatory profile in many animal models and clinical settings.[68] The strongest evidence for the clinical importance of these effects are randomized trials demonstrating that leukoreduction mitigates the effect of RBC transfusion in promoting postoperative infection. Transfusion immunomodulation is comprised of complex immunosuppressive and proinflammatory effects that are mediated by leukocytes, apoptotic cells, cytokines, soluble mediators, soluble HLA peptides, cell-derived microparticles, and free hemoglobin. Immunomodulation after blood transfusion leads to release of endogenous recipient cytokines including IL-6, IL-8, and other acute phase proteins that play a role in impaired host defense, organ dysfunction, and mortality.

Blood Alternatives

During the influenza A virus subtype H1N1 pandemic, there was a major impact on the blood supply due to donors' fear of exposure to the virus at a hospital or a free-standing donor facility.[69] However, despite the usual decrease in surgeries, the demand was almost the same due to blood utilization for urgent and emergent interventions and due to chronically transfusion dependent patients such as patients with hematologic disorders and malignancies.

With the current COVID-19 pandemic, more than 4,000 American Red Cross blood drives were canceled across the United States resulting in about 130,000 fewer blood donations in a span of a few weeks. Other reasons for the reduced blood supply include potential donors becoming sick, interruption in the supply chain, and the fear of possible virus transmission with blood transfusion. To this end, the Patient Blood Management guidelines created in Australia and endorsed by the World Health Organization in 2010 have been strongly recommended during the COVID-19 pandemic.[70] Correction of iron, folic acid, and vitamin B12 deficiencies can lead to reduction in blood utilization and improve patient outcomes.[71]

Erythropoiesis-stimulating agents (ESAs), commonly used in the management of anemia in patients with chronic kidney disease and chemotherapy-induced bone marrow suppression, can also be used short-term in patients with preoperative anemia, particularly when anemia is deemed secondary to anemia of inflammation. In preoperative patients and in the critically ill, ESA utilization with either 100,000 units weekly in the ICU or 600 units/kg in the preoperative period resulted in higher hemoglobin concentrations and reduced transfusion utilization.[72]

Intraoperative autologous transfusions (also known as intraoperative cell salvage) involve the collection of a patient's own blood loss, filtering and washing to ensure the removal of impurities, and direct return of the autologous component to the patient. It has been associated with reductions in allogeneic blood component utilization and is recommended for all procedures with moderate-to-large volume blood loss such as cardiac, trauma, and orthopedic surgery.[73–75] Rapidly identifying and correcting issues related to coagulation and hemostasis perioperatively can limit the needs for transfusion in the perioperative period.

Perioperative blood conservation can also be achieved with acute normovolemic hemodilution (ANH), the process by which a controlled volume of a patient's own blood is removed before the surgical insult followed by replacement with crystalloids or colloids.[76] In adults, this has been shown to result in less RBC loss during the surgical procedure and allows for the reinfusion of autologous blood, rich in red blood cells, platelets, and clotting factors, when it is needed intraoperatively or postoperatively.[63] Early therapy with tranexamic acid (TXA) appears beneficial by stabilizing clot formation and preventing fibrinolysis. The CRASH-2 trial evaluated TXA versus placebo in over 20,000 trauma patients at 274 hospitals within 40 different countries. Patients who received TXA within 3 h of trauma had a statistically significant reduction in overall mortality and morbidity.[77]

Recombinant activated factor VII (rFVIIa) replaces endogenous factor VII, which is rapidly consumed when massive amounts of tissue factor are expressed in response to trauma, and factor VII is also used to treat hemophilia and promotes platelet aggregation. However, the American College of Surgeons does not recommend the routine use of rFVIIa in trauma.

In patients with trauma-induced coagulopathy, the administration of 4-factor prothrombin complex concentrate (4-factor PCC), alone or in combination with fibrinogen concentrate or fresh frozen plasma, can reduce transfusion of RBCs and other blood components.[78] 4-factor PCC has clotting factors II, V, VII, and IX and is indicated for reversal of coagulopathy associated with vitamin K antagonists. PCC is superior to fresh frozen plasma, as it can be administered rapidly in a small volume, resulting in more rapid reversal of the anticoagulant effect and avoidance of volume overload and transfusion reactions.

Thromboelastography (TEG) and Rotational Thromboelastometry (ROTEM)

Rotational thromboelastometry (ROTEM) and thromboelastography (TEG) are viscoelastic assays that evaluate both platelet function and coagulation by assaying several parameters of clot formation dynamically in whole blood. They provide detailed information on clotting kinetics from clot formation through degradation. Traditionally the standard was to use the routine coagulation tests including PT and aPTT. However, these coagulation tests had limited utility in the diagnosis and management of trauma-associated coagulopathies.

Despite the availability of multiple systematic reviews,[79–81] the data on using TEG and ROTEM is limited due to the lack of RCTs evaluating their utility. In civilian and military trauma settings, they showed superiority to routine testing in detecting early trauma coagulopathy, including hypocoagulability, hyperfibrinolysis, hypercoagulability, and platelet dysfunction. In addition, abnormal TEG and ROTEM results were able to predict the need for massive transfusion and predict death although most studies failed to show any mortality benefit. Some studies demonstrated a reduction in the amount of blood products transfused especially platelets and FFP. In facilities where TEG and ROTEM are available, it is rational to utilize TEG- and ROTEM-based goal directed transfusion for trauma patients who require massive transfusion, in conjugation with the routine coagulation tests.

During the COVID-19 pandemic, a few centers attempted to utilize TEG and ROTEM to assist in the management of COVID-related hypercoagulopathy.[23,82] However, further prospective RCTs are needed to determine the use of TEG or ROTEM in guiding therapy in patients with COVID-19.

▌MINIMIZING BLOOD DRAWS

The most frequent and probably the most important reason for mild to moderate blood loss in the ICU is the "standard" blood tests that are usually drawn on a regular basis every day in the ICU. It has been demonstrated that after two weeks in the ICU, more than 1L of blood will be drawn depending on the patient's underlying disease and hospital policy for blood drawing.

The relationship between blood draws and outcomes of critically ill patients have been extensively studied.[83] In patients with major gastrointestinal bleeding, hemoglobin levels were measured every 8 h in the first 2 days and thereafter 1–2 times daily for each patient.[55] In hemodynamically stable patients who have developed an episode of bleeding requiring blood transfusion, the least frequent interval for blood draws would be 6–8 h. Anemia due to phlebotomy results in greater rates of sepsis, transfusion-related reactions, circulatory overload, and longer durations of hospital stay. It is important to use low-volume sampling tubes during phlebotomy and hospital-wide restrictive transfusion policies to reduce RBC transfusion.[84]

▌REFERENCES

1. Iba T, Levi M, Levy JH. Sepsis-induced coagulopathy and disseminated intravascular coagulation. *Semin Thromb Haemost*. 2020;46(01):089-095.
2. Iba T, Levy JH. Inflammation and thrombosis: roles of neutrophils, platelets and endothelial cells and their interactions in thrombus formation during sepsis. *J Thromb Haemost*. 2018;16(2):231-241.
3. Göbel K, Eichler S, Wiendl H. The coagulation factors fibrinogen, thrombin, and factor XII in inflammatory disorders - A systematic review. *Front Immunol*. 2018;9:1731.
4. Bunce PE, High SM, Nadjafi M, et al. Pandemic H1N1 influenza infection and vascular thrombosis. *Clin Infect Dis*. 2011;52:e14-e17.
5. Obi AT, Tignanelli CJ, Jacobs BN, et al. Empirical systemic anticoagulation is associated with decreased venous thromboembolism in critically ill influenza A H1N1 acute respiratory distress syndrome patients. *J Vasc Surg Venous Lymphat Disord*. 2019;7:317-324.
6. Umapathi T, Kor AC, Venketasubramanian N, et al. Large artery ischaemic stroke in severe acute respiratory syndrome (SARS). *J Neurol*. 2004;251(10):1227-1231.

7. Lee N, Hui D, Alan Wu, et al. A major outbreak of severe acute respiratory syndrome in Hong Kong. *N Engl J Med*. 2003;348(20):1986-1994.

8. Wong RSM, Wu A, To KF, et al. Haematological manifestations in patients with severe acute respiratory syndrome: Retrospective analysis. *BMJ*. 2003;326(7403):1358-1362.

9. Giannis D, Ziogas IA, Gianni P. Coagulation disorders in coronavirus infected patients: COVID-19, SARS CoV-1, MERS-CoV and lessons from the past. *J Clin Virol*. 2020;127:104362.

10. Klok FA, Kruip M, van der Meer NJM, et al. Incidence of thrombotic complications in critically ill ICU patients with COVID-19. *Thromb Res*. 2020;191:145-147.

11. Cui S, Chen S, Li X, et al. Prevalence of venous thromboembolism in patients with severe novel coronavirus pneumonia. *J Thromb Haemost*. 2020;18:1421-1424.

12. Middeldorp S, Coppens M, van Haaps TF, et al. Incidence of venous thromboembolism in hospitalized patients with COVID-19. *J Thromb Haemost*. 2020;18(8):1995-2002.

13. Llitjos JF, Leclerc M, Chochois C, et al. High incidence of venous thromboembolic events in anticoagulated severe COVID-19 patients. *J Thromb Haemost*. 2020;18(7):1743-1746.

14. Poissy J, Goutay J, Caplan M, et al. Pulmonary embolism in COVID-19 patients: Awareness of an increased prevalence. *Circulation*. 2020;142:184-186.

15. Mackman N, Antoniak S, Wolberg AS, et al. Coagulation abnormalities and thrombosis in patients infected with SARS-CoV-2 and other pandemic viruses. *Arterioscler Thromb Vasc Biol*. 2020;40(9):2033-2044.

16. Lodigiani C, Iapichino G, Carenzo L, et al. Venous and arterial thromboembolic complications in COVID-19 patients admitted to an academic hospital in Milan, Italy. *Thromb Res*. 2020;191:9-14.

17. Tang N, Li D, Wang X, Sun Z. Abnormal coagulation parameters are associated with poor prognosis in patients with novel coronavirus pneumonia. *J Thromb Haemost*. 2020;18(4):844-847.

18. Zhou F, Yu T, Du R, et al. Clinical course and risk factors for mortality of adult inpatients with COVID-19 in Wuhan, China: A retrospective cohort study. *Lancet*. 2020;395(10229):1054-1062.

19. Tang N, Bai H, Chen X, Gong J, Li D, Sun Z. Anticoagulant treatment is associated with decreased mortality in severe coronavirus disease 2019 patients with coagulopathy. *J Thromb Haemost*. 2020;18(5):1094-1099.

20. Nadkarni GN, Lala A, Bagiella E, et al. Anticoagulation, mortality, bleeding and pathology among patients hospitalized with COVID-19: A single health system study. *J Am Coll Cardiol*. 2020;76(16):1815-1826.

21. Tan YK , Goh C, Leow AST, et al. COVID-19 and ischemic stroke: a systematic review and meta-summary of the literature. *J Thromb Thrombolysis*. 2020;50(3):587-595.

22. Varga Z, Flammer AJ, Steiger P, et al. Endothelial cell infection and endotheliitis in COVID-19. *Lancet*. 2020;395(10234):1417-1418.

23. Panigada M, Bottino N, Tagliabue P, et al. Hypercoagulability of COVID-19 patients in intensive care unit. A report of thromboelastography findings and other parameters of hemostasis. *J Thromb Haemost*. 2020;18:1738-1742.

24. Pigott DC. Hemorrhagic fever viruses. *Crit Care Clin.* 2005;21:765-783.

25. Chuang YC, Lin YS, Liu HS, et al. Antibodies against thrombin in dengue patients contain both anti-thrombotic and pro-fibrinolytic activities. *Thromb Haemost.* 2013;110(2):358-365.

26. Chuang YC, Lin YS, Liu CC, et al. Factors contributing to the disturbance of coagulation and fibrinolysis in dengue virus infection. *J Formos Med Assoc.* 2013;112(1):12-17.

27. Wills BA, Oragui EE, Stephens AC, et al. Coagulation abnormalities in dengue hemorrhagic Fever: Serial investigations in 167 Vietnamese children with Dengue shock syndrome. *Clin Infect Dis.* 2002;35(3).

28. Hensley LE, Geisbert TW. The contribution of the endothelium to the development of coagulation disorders that characterize Ebola hemorrhagic fever in primates. *Thromb Haemost.* 2005;94(2):254-261.

29. Basler CF. Molecular pathogenesis of viral hemorrhagic fever. *Semin Immunopathol.* 2017;39(5):551-561.

30. Gardner C, Ryman KD. Yellow fever: a reemerging threat. *Clin Lab Med.* 2010;30(1):237-260.

31. McCormick JB, Fisher-Hoch SP. Lassa fever. *Curr Top Microbiol Immunol.* 2002;262:75-109.

32. Hawman DW, Feldmann H. Recent advances in understanding Crimean–Congo hemorrhagic fever virus. F1000Res 2018;7:F1000 Faculty Rev-1715.

33. Cook DJ, Crowther MA. Thromboprophylaxis in the intensive care unit: focus on medical-surgical patients. *Crit Care Med.* 2010;38(2 Suppl):S76-82.

34. Konstantinides SV, Meyer G, Becattini C, et al. 2019 ESC guidelines for the diagnosis and management of acute pulmonary embolism developed in collaboration with the European Respiratory Society (ERS). *Eur Respir J.* 2019;54:1901647.

35. Schulman S, Kearon C, Kakkar AK, et al. Dabigatran versus warfarin in the treatment of acute venous thromboembolism. *N Engl J Med.* 2009;361:2342-2352.

36. EINSTEIN Investigators. Bauersachs R, Berkowitz SD, Brenner B, et al. Oral rivaroxaban for symptomatic venous thromboembolism. *N Engl J Med.* 2010;363(26):2499-2510.

37. EINSTEIN–PE Investigators. Büller HR, Prins MH, Lensing AWA, et al. Oral rivaroxaban for the treatment of symptomatic pulmonary embolism. *N Engl J Med.* 2012;366(14):1287-1297.

38. Agnelli G, Buller HR, Cohen A, et al. Oral apixaban for the treatment of acute venous thromboembolism. *N Engl J Med.* 2013;369(9):799-808.

39. Hokusai-VTE Investigators. Büller HR, Décousus H, Grosso MA, et al. Edoxaban versus warfarin for the treatment of symptomatic venous thromboembolism. *N Engl J Med.* 2013;369(15):1406-1415.

40. Meyer G, Vicaut E, Danays T, et al. Fibrinolysis for patients with intermediate-risk pulmonary embolism. *N Engl J Med.* 2014;370:1402-1411.

41. Giri J, Sista AK, Weinberg I, et al. Interventional therapies for acute pulmonary embolism: Current status and principles for the development of novel evidence: A scientific statement from the American Heart Association. *Circulation.* 2019;140(20):e774-e801.

42. Cuker A, Burnett A, Triller D, et al. Reversal of direct oral anticoagulants: guidance from the anticoagulation forum. *Am J Hematol.* 2019;94(6):697-709.

43. Thachil J, Juffermans NP, Ranucci M, et al. ISTH DIC subcommittee communication on anticoagulation in COVID-19. *J Thromb Haemost.* 2020;18:2138-2144.

44. Yamakawa K, Levy JH. Iba Recombinant human soluble thrombomodulin in patients with sepsis-associated coagulopathy (SCARLET): An updated meta-analysis. *Crit Care.* 2019;23(1):302.

45. Cohen AT, Imfeld S, Markham J, Granziera S. The use of aspirin for primary and secondary prevention in venous thromboembolism and other cardiovascular disorders. *Thromb Res.* 2015;135:217-225.

46. Giordano S, Spiezia L, Campello E, Simioni P. The current understanding of trauma-induced coagulopathy (TIC): A focused review on pathophysiology. *Intern Emerg Med.* 2017;12(7):981-991.

47. Simmons JW, Powell MF. Acute traumatic coagulopathy: pathophysiology and resuscitation. *Br J Anaesth.* 2016;117(suppl 3):iii31-iii43.

48. Peralta R, Thani HA, Rizoli S. Coagulopathy in the surgical patient: trauma-induced and drug-induced coagulopathies. *Curr Opin Crit Care.* 2019;25(6):668-674.

49. Devine DV, Serrano K. Preparation of blood products for transfusion: Is there a best method? *Biologicals.* 2012;40:187-190.

50. Devine D, Howe D. Processing of whole blood into cellular components and plasma. *ISBT Science Series.* 2010;5:78-82.

51. Rygard SL, Holst LB, Perner A. Blood product administration in the critical care and perioperative settings. *Crit Care Clin.* 2018;34:299-311.

52. Corwin HL, Gettinger A, Pearl RG, et al. The CRIT Study: Anemia and blood transfusion in the critically ill—Current clinical practice in the United States. *Crit Care Med.* 2004;32:39-52.

53. Hebert PC, Wells G, Blajchman MA, et al. A multicenter, randomized, controlled clinical trial of transfusion requirements in critical care. Transfusion Requirements in Critical Care Investigators, Canadian Critical Care Trials Group. *N Engl J Med.* 1999;340:409-417.

54. Holst LB, Petersen MW, Wetterslev J, et al. Lower versus higher hemoglobin threshold for transfusion in septic shock. *N Engl J Med.* 2014;371(15):1381-1391.

55. Villanueva C, Colomo A, Bosch A, et al. Transfusion strategies for acute upper gastrointestinal bleeding. *N Engl J Med.* 2013;368:11-21.

56. Docherty AB, O'Donnell R, Brunskill S, et al. Effect of restrictive versus liberal transfusion strategies on outcomes in patients with cardiovascular disease in a non-cardiac surgery setting: Systematic review and meta-analysis. *BMJ.* 2016;352:i1351.

57. Zygun DA, Nortje J, Hutchinson PJ, et al. The effect of red blood cell transfusion on cerebral oxygenation and metabolism after severe traumatic brain injury. *Crit Care Med.* 2009;37(3):1074-1078.

58. O'Shaughnessy DF, Atterbury C, Bolton Maggs P, et al. British Committee for Standards in Haematology, Blood Transfusion Task Force. Guidelines for the use of fresh-frozen plasma, cryoprecipitate and cryosupernatant. *Br J Haematol.* 2004;126(1):11.

59. Kumar A, Mhaskar R, Grossman BJ, et al. Platelet transfusion: A systematic review of the clinical evidence. *Transfusion*. 2015;55:1116.

60. Borgman MA, Spinella PC, Perkins JG, et al. The ratio of blood products transfused affects mortality in patients receiving massive transfusions at a combat support hospital. *J Trauma*. 2007;63(4):805.

61. Bell DG, McCann ET. Transfusions in trauma. *Curr Pulm Reports*. 2016;5:94-100.

62. Foster, JC, Sappenfield JW, Smith RS, Kiley SP. Initiation and termination of massive transfusion protocols: current strategies and future prospects. *Anesth Analg*. 2017;125(6):2045-2055.

63. Palmieri TL, Holmes JH, Arnoldo B, et al. Transfusion requirement in burn care evaluation (TRIBE): A multicenter randomized prospective trial of blood transfusion in major burn injury. *Ann Surg*. 2017;266(4):595-602.

64. Joyner MJ, Senefeld JW, Klassen SA, et al. Effect of convalescent plasma on mortality among hospitalized patients with COVID-19: Initial three-month experience. medRxiv. 2020:2020.08.12.20169359.

65. Chai KL, Valk SJ, Piechotta V, et al. Convalescent plasma or hyperimmune immunoglobulin for people with COVID-19: A living systematic review. *Cochrane Database Syst Rev*. 2020;10:CD013600.

66. Food and Drug Administration. *Fatalities reported to FDA following blood collection and transfusion: Annual Summary for Fiscal Year 2018*. Silver Spring, MD: US Food and Drug Administration; 2018.

67. Bihl F, Castelli D, Marincola F, Dodd RY, Brander C. Transfusion-transmitted infections. *J Transl Med*. 2007;5:25.

68. Youssef LA, Spitalnik SL. Transfusion-related immunomodulation: A reappraisal. *Curr Opin Hematol*. 2017;24(6):551-557.

69. Shander A, Goobie SM, Warner MA, et al. International Foundation of Patient Blood Management (IFPBM) and Society for the Advancement of Blood Management (SABM). Essential role of patient blood management in a pandemic: A call for action. *Anesth Analg*. 2020;131(1):74-85.

70. Patient Blood Management Guidelines: Module 4 - Critical Care. 2012. Canberra, Australia: National Blood Authority. http://www.blood.gov.au/pbm-module-4. Accessed October 22, 2020.

71. Spahn DR, Schoenrath F, Spahn GH, et al. Effect of ultra-short-term treatment of patients with iron deficiency or anaemia undergoing cardiac surgery: A prospective randomised trial. *Lancet*. 2019;393:2201-2212.

72. Cho BC, Serini J, Zorrilla-Vaca A, et al. Impact of preoperative erythropoietin on allogeneic blood transfusions in surgical patients: Results from a systematic review and meta-analysis. *Anesth Analg*. 2019;128(5):981-992.

73. Frank SM, Sikorski RA, Konig G, et al. Clinical utility of autologous salvaged blood: A review. *J Gastrointest Surg*. 2020;24(2):464-472.

74. Li J, Sun SM, Tian SM, et al. Cell salvage in emergency trauma surgery. *Cochrane Database Syst Rev*. 2015;1:CD007379.

75. Wang G, Bainbridge D, Martin J, Cheng D. The efficacy of an intraoperative cell saver during cardiac surgery: A meta-analysis of randomized trials. *Anesth Analg*. 2009;109(2):320-330.

76. Zhou X, Zhang C, Wang Y, Yu L, Yan M. Preoperative acute normovolemic hemodilution for minimizing allogeneic blood transfusion: A meta-analysis. *Anesth Analg*. 2015;121:1443-1455.

77. Roberts I, Shakur H, Coats T, et al. The CRASH-2 trial: A randomised controlled trial and economic evaluation of the effects of tranexamic acid on death, vascular occlusive events and transfusion requirement in bleeding trauma patients. *Health Technol Assess Rep*. 2013;17:1-79.

78. Jehan F, Aziz H, O'Keefe T, et al. The role of four-factor prothrombin complex concentrate in coagulopathy of trauma: A propensity matched analysis. *J Trauma Acute Care Surg*. 2018;85(1):18.

79. Da Luz LT, Nascimento B, Shankarakutty AK, et al. Effect of thromboelastography (TEG®) and rotational thromboelastometry (ROTEM®) on diagnosis of coagulopathy, transfusion guidance and mortality in trauma: Descriptive systematic review. *Crit Care*. 2014;18:518.

80. Hunt H, Stanworth S, Curry N, et al. Thromboelastography (TEG) and rotational thromboelastometry (ROTEM) for trauma-induced coagulopathy in adult trauma patients with bleeding. *Cochrane Database Syst Rev*. 2015;2:CD010438.

81. Afshari A, Wikkelsø A, Brok J, et al. Thrombelastography (TEG) or thromboelastometry (ROTEM) to monitor haemotherapy versus usual care in patients with massive transfusion. *Cochrane Database Syst Rev*. 2011;3:CD007871.

82. Pavoni V, Gianesello L, Pazzi M, et al. Evaluation of coagulation function by rotation thromboelastometry in critically ill patients with severe COVID-19 pneumonia. *J Thromb Thrombolysis*. 2020;50:281-286.

83. Dolman HS, Evans K, Zimmerman LH, et al. Impact of minimizing diagnostic blood loss in the critically ill. *Surgery*. 2015;158:1083-1087; discussion 7-8.

84. Napolitano LM, Kurek S, Luchette FA, et al. Clinical practice guideline: Red blood cell transfusion in adult trauma and critical care. *J Trauma*. 2009;67:1439-1442.

SHOCK 7

Sung Hong, MD and Karan Omidvari, MD

INTRODUCTION

Shock is defined as a life-threatening condition of acute circulatory failure leading to hypotension and mean arterial pressure (MAP) of less than 65 mm Hg. Due to its high mortality rate, shock should be intervened as soon as recognized as it can progress to irreversible organ failure.

Shock is classified as four major categories, namely vasodilatory (distributive), cardiogenic, hypovolemic, and obstructive. Some degree of overlap exists between each type of shock. Any sustained hypotension should be considered for diagnosis of shock, especially when the MAP is consistently less than 65 mm Hg, which increases risk of end organ damage leading to multi-organ failures.[1-3]

Large volume fluid resuscitation has been traditionally thought to be the cornerstone for treatment of shock but was later shown to increase mortality and morbidity. Over time, a more conservative approach has been established that is thought to be life-saving and critical in decreasing mortality in patients with shock.[4]

PREVALENCE OF SHOCK DURING WAR

It was not until the 19th century that shock was described as a distinct entity from specific injuries themselves and more efforts were made to direct treatment for the shock.[5] In addition to hemorrhagic shock,[5] septic shock, disseminated intravascular coagulation, and multi-organ failure have been discussed from studies during World War II, the Korean War, and the Vietnam War.[5,6]

Trauma has been linked to war and the first trauma care center in the United States was started in 1966.[6] Since then, improved understanding of hemodynamics have led to improved outcomes.[7-9]

▌ PREVALENCE OF SHOCK DURING PANDEMICS

In the known pandemics such as SARS, MERS-CoV, COVID-19, influenza, plague, tularemia, and hemorrhagic fevers, there are various mechanisms of shock and they are associated with poor prognosis.[10–26]

▌ PREVALENCE OF SHOCK IN NATURAL DISASTERS

A disaster is defined by the Centre of Research on the Epidemiology of Disasters (CRED) as "a situation or event which overwhelms local capacity, necessitating a request to a national or international level for external assistance; an unforeseen and often sudden event that causes great damage, destruction and human suffering."[27] WHO defines sudden-onset disasters (SODs) as disasters "for which there is little or no warning."[28]

In the last 10 years, natural disasters have killed 760,000 people, injured 2 million, and affected more than 2 billion.[29] On the average, 68,000 lives per year are lost due to natural disaster, or 0.1% of all the world's population. Natural disasters are subdivided into two main categories: slow-onset natural disasters (SODs) and slow-onset natural disasters.

The true prevalence of shock in any specific natural disaster is extremely variable, and depends on the nature and ferocity of the disaster and on the sequelae of the disaster. Shock can develop rapidly, such as in a traumatic injury, or later as a consequence of injury or infection. It is important to note the sequelae of each natural disaster to anticipate the development of shock.

Tornados

A study of the immediate effects of tornado demonstrated that the all-cause admission among older adults was increased by 4% (incidence rate ration 1.04; 95% confidence interval 1.01 to 1.07). Eliminating the first 3 days after the disaster when admission may have been due to injuries, hospitalizations for any cause was still higher than when compared with the other 11 months of the year (incidence rate ratio 1.04; 95% confidence interval 1.01 to 1.07). There was a 9% increase in both hospitalizations and ICU admissions.[30]

Sepsis is not uncommon and may have rare pathogens. *Apophysomyces trapeziformis* was observed after 12 days among wound-injured victims from the tornado that struck Joplin, Missouri (USA) on May 22, 2011.[31] The disease is caused by fungi of the order Mucorales, which are typically found in soil and decaying wood. The disease has a high fatality rate (29–83%) and is often associated with immunocompetent hosts after traumatic penetration of fungal spores.[32,33]

Wildfires

Studies on adverse health events among firefighters during wildfires show that they probably have an increased risk of mortality, mostly because of inhalation injuries.[34,35] In a study of hospital visits related to a big urban wildfire in California in 1991, a total of 4% presented with burns, 1% major trauma, 7% minor trauma, and 4% simple fractures. In contrast, bronchospastic and irritating smoke reactions were significantly more common, constituting 31% and 20% of the total patient visits, respectively.[36]

Landslides

Landslides are one of the deadliest natural disasters, with a death-injury ratio of 4,5:1.[37] Little is known about specific injury patterns following landslides as few studies have been conducted.[38] Probably the most common cause of death during landslides is suffocation, with some additional deaths are caused by injuries from debris and rockfalls.[37,38]

Volcanic Eruptions

There are few studies on mortality causes and morbidity from volcanic eruptions. In one study following two volcanic eruptions in 1994 and 2010 on Java, out of 106 admitted patients, 44% and 16% of the patients, respectively, sustained burn injuries with a total body surface area of more than 80%. Of all the burn-injured patients, only 29% in 1994 and 37% in 2010 survived to discharge.[39] A study done during a 1989 ashfall in the USA showed increases in asthma and acute bronchitis. Of 25 people found dead, the cause of death was suffocation in 76% and thermal injury or head trauma in 12%.[40]

Extreme Temperatures

Very little is known about injuries during extreme cold. A few studies done about ice storms in Canada and the USA have not necessarily shown lower than normal temperatures. Ice storms seem to cause falls leading to contusions and fractures.[41] However, studies have not been able to show an absolute increase in these injuries compared to similar winter periods.[42]

Heatwaves increase the amount of emergency department visits and have been shown to increase overall mortality, especially in the elderly population.[43] A 10-day heatwave in Greece 1987 resulted in 2,960 heat-related admissions with a 31% mortality rate. In terms of excess trauma and injuries, there are no available data.[44]

Earthquakes

Earthquakes kill more people on an annual basis than any other natural disasters. About 35,000 people die and more than 100,000 people are injured annually from earthquakes.[29] Earthquakes also generate tsunamis, which increase the death toll.[45]

Earthquakes seem to have an approximate average death-injured ratio of 1:3–4.[29] High-magnitude earthquakes might cause more crush injuries and burying than low magnitude.[46] Building damage is a major cause of death and injury in earthquakes.[47] Among the instant deaths, severe trauma with head injury, asphyxiation, and/or shock is reportedly the most common cause of mortality.[45–47] These injuries are under-reported as many of them lead to death prior to arrival at hospital.

Floods

Flood is the most common natural disaster worldwide.[29] The most common cause of death in a flood is drowning.[48–50] Communicable disease and wound infections are common after floods because of contaminated water and malfunctioning air-conditioning and heating.[48]

Storms

One study assessed emergency visits following two 2008 hurricanes in the USA. Out of the 3,863 patient visits, less than 10% were labeled as injuries. A study of Hong Kong's tropical cyclone-related database found 460 cyclone-related injuries from 15 emergency departments between 2004 and 2009. They concluded that the most common injuries were contusions/abrasions and lacerations. Most injuries were minor, with only 2.8% triaged as high category.[51]

In 2013, a study revealed that direct deaths during storms accounted for 56% of the total deaths, and the rest were due to indirect causes. The most common causes of direct death were drowning (59%) and trauma (39%). Indirect death was mostly due to trauma including vehicle accidents, burns, and electrocution.[52]

In contrast, in one study based on a household survey in Indian Sundarbans hit by tropical cyclone Aila in May 2009, the prevalence of health shock was as high as 25%.[53] Most of the natural disasters have sequelae that last well beyond their initial impact. Bodily injury, combined with poor water access, poor access to health care especially in developing countries, lack of coping mechanisms, and slow recovery, all lead to long-term effects, such as shock, infections, and poor nutrition.

INFECTIOUS SEQUELAE OF NATURAL DISASTERS LEADING TO SHOCK

The risk of outbreaks after natural disasters is low, but the consequences of shock, when it develops, are catastrophic. The type of shock depends on the nature of the natural disaster itself. Diarrheal disease outbreaks can occur after drinking water has been contaminated and have been reported after flooding disasters. Hepatitis A and E are also transmitted by the fecal-oral route, in association with lack of access to safe water and sanitation. Hepatitis A is endemic in most developing countries, and most children are exposed and develop immunity at an early age. As a result, the risk for large outbreaks is usually low in these settings. Leptospirosis is also prevalent after flooding disasters because of the proliferation of rodents.[54]

After the tsunami in Aceh, a cluster of measles involving 35 cases occurred in Aceh Utara district, and continuing sporadic cases and clusters were common despite mass vaccination campaigns. *Neisseria meningitidis*, transmitted from person to person, caused many deaths from meningitis among those displaced in Aceh and Pakistan.[54]

Acute respiratory infections (ARI) are a major cause of illness and death among displaced populations, particularly in children < 5 years of age. An outbreak was reported in Nicaragua in the 30 days after Hurricane Mitch in 1998, and ARI accounted for the highest number of cases and deaths among those displaced by the tsunami in Aceh in 2004 and by the 2005 earthquake in Pakistan.

Malaria outbreaks in the wake of flooding are a well-known phenomenon. An earthquake in Costa Rica's Atlantic Region in 1991 was associated with changes in habitat that were beneficial for mosquito breeding and preceded an extreme rise in malaria cases.[54]

Many of these diseases can develop into shock with catastrophic consequences, both in terms of lives lost and economically.

DIAGNOSIS

Shock should be considered when presented with clinical features that include hypotension, tachycardia, oliguria, altered mental status, tachypnea, and cool, clammy, cyanotic skin. Additionally, metabolic acidosis and/or lactic acidosis can be a manifestation of tissue hypoperfusion.[55] Most of the mentioned clinical features when presented as a single feature are neither specific nor sensitive for the diagnosis of shock, but when multiple features are present, concerns for shock should be investigated early to be able to narrow down the differential diagnosis for appropriate and timely intervention. For instance, hypotension demonstrated low sensitivity (range 0.05–0.12), but high specificity (range 0.95–0.99) for ICU admission in one study. Combining hypotension and tachycardia did not change the predictive value for ICU admission. Similar results were found for hospitalization.[55]

Clinicians have therefore searched for a bedside parameter that can quickly and non-invasively identify shock. Shock index (SI), heart rate divided by systolic blood pressure, is a more sensitive and specific indicator of presence of shock. Normally 0.5 to 0.7, the presence of shock is greatly suspected when the shock index is above 0.8 and the correlation increases as does the SI.[56] However, like all the other parameters, the sensitivity and specificity of SI varies in different types of shock, and it is mostly helpful when taken into account along with the other parameters.[56]

The choice of body site where blood pressure is measured and the mechanism by which it is measured has been debated. However, more recent studies seem to indicate that it is not so. For instance, in one study, arm noninvasive MAP readings were accurate, and either the ankle or the thigh was a reliable alternative to detect hypotension and guide treatment in therapy-responding patients.[57,58] Additionally, there was no significant difference between manual vs electronic vs arterial catheter in monitoring blood pressure.[57,58]

ACCESS: VASCULAR AND INTRAOSSEOUS

Establishing good access for fluid resuscitation is crucial in treatment of shock. Obtaining a large bore intravenous (IV) access (>18G) is recommended for large volume rapid infusion of fluids.[49,59] Flow rates on IV catheters follow Poiseuille's law ($V = \prod p\ r^4 / 8\ \acute{\eta}\ l$), which defines that flow is directly proportional to the pressure of the fluid and to the radius of the catheter being used to the fourth power and inversely proportional to the length of the catheter and to the viscosity of the fluid. In summary, an IV catheter with the largest radius and shortest length will therefore allow the most rapid infusion (Table 7-1).[60]

Whether the patient will need a peripheral vs central venous catheter is determined by indication for patients to have a central venous catheter. Inadequate peripheral access, peripherally incompatible infusions such as long-term antibiotics or vasopressors, hemodynamic monitoring,

Table 7-1 VASCULAR AND INTRAOSSEUS ACCESS		
Types of vascular access	Flow rates via gravity	Flow rates via pressure
14G 59 mm cannula	240 mL/min	384 mL/min
14G 14 cm Abbocath	197 mL/min	366 mL/ min
16G	180 mL/min	334 mL/min
18G	90 mL/min	153 mL/min
20G	60 mL/min	105 mL/min
22G	36 mL/min	71 mL/min
Central catheter		
Distal port (16G)	52 mL/min	110 mL/min
Proximal port (18G)	26 mL/min	55 mL/ min
IO	70 mL/min	140 mL/min
Introducer	126 ml/min	333 mL/min

and patients on hemodialysis are some of the indications for using central venous catheters (Table 7-1).

Intraosseous (IO) infusion, another option for vascular access, was described first in 1922 and was widely used for drug administration in the 1940s.[61,62] After showing effectiveness of vascular access via IO, the use has since increased and is typically reserved for acute, life-threatening, or medically necessary situations when standard venous access methods cannot be rapidly achieved and as the first attempt at vascular access in cardiopulmonary arrest or severe shock in selected patients.[58,63] Typical sites used are the proximal tibia and femur.

It is not necessary to obtain central venous access in hemorrhagic shock patients. Rather, large-bore IV access should be established as soon as possible and if difficult vascular access, intraosseous access should be established. Rapid transfusers can easily be accommodated by such access.[64,65]

RESUSCITATION

Fluids

Hypovolemia is frequently seen in patients due to decreased intake and increased insensible losses. Additionally, there are inflammatory processes that alter vascular resistance and overall effects of these findings causes low cardiac output and stroke volume, precipitating tissue hypoxia, anaerobic metabolism, and lactic acidosis.[4–7]

Assessment of Fluid Responsiveness

Passive leg raise can transiently increase venous return in hypovolemic patients who are pre-load depended and can be a useful diagnostic test and predict fluid responsiveness. Unfortunately, the effects are short-lived, such as after fluid is returned, and have a very little therapeutic role.[66–68]

The Trendelenburg position (TP) is defined as a body tilt where the head is lower than the body or legs in the supine position. The modified Trendelenburg position (mTP) is when the head is level with the body and legs are passively raised in the supine position. This is an attempt to increase venous return to the heart and therefore cardiac output. It is used as an immediate intervention to improve hypotension and hypovolemic shock. However, evidence is lacking that these maneuvers are helpful, and recent reviews reveal that neither TP nor mTP increase the cardiac output or blood pressure in any clinically significant way.[69,70]

Fluid Resuscitation

Fluid resuscitation in sepsis is to restore intravascular volume, which in turn would restore cardiac output and overall oxygen delivery to vital organs.[5] Measurement of central venous pressure, inferior vena cava filling, monitoring mixed venous oxygen saturation, and trending of lactate have been used to monitor oxygen demand and supply.

Selection of colloids over crystalloids was initially thought to optimize volume expansion through colloid retention in the intravascular space. However, recent studies show that membrane permeability and endothelial damage play a large role in alteration of response to fluid resuscitation in sepsis. Due to many intricate interactions of mean systemic filling pressure, right atrial pressure, venous resistance, and ventricular compliance, predicting a critically ill patient's response to fluid is more challenging than approaching fluid resuscitation with dose and choice of fluids.

Standard therapy for fluid resuscitation include targeting CVP of 8–12 mmHg, MAP of at least 65 mmHg, and urine output at least 0.5 ml/kg/hr.[1] Early Goal Directed Therapy (EGDT), when implemented, showed much improved mortality and included all elements of standard therapy in addition to a catheter measuring central venous oxygen saturation (SvO$_2$), along with early rapid fluid challenge to meet the above goal as written.[4–7]

The Surviving Sepsis Campaign (SSC) promotes goal-directed fluid resuscitation into early sepsis management. The most recent version of the

SSC guidelines recommends "protocolized, quantitative resuscitation of patients with sepsis induced tissue hypoperfusion" beginning with an "initial fluid challenge to achieve a minimum of 30 mL/kg of crystalloids" targeting CVP, blood pressure, urine output, and venous oxygen saturation goals.[1]

Intravenous Fluids

Shock is a state of systemic arterial hypotension and hypoperfusion to vital organs that can lead to multi-organ failure if not adequately resuscitated with large volume repletion of fluids in most cases. Regardless of the underlying cause of shock, the initial response for the hypotensive patient is almost always to administer a bolus fluid.[71] The choice of which fluid to administer, the timing, and the amount have long been a controversy.

IV fluid therapy infuses fluid, electrolytes, and buffers directly into the extracellular fluid volume, and their appropriate use requires reverence for the fine balance that constitutes human homeostasis.[72,73] In this section, we will discuss the different types of fluids widely used by clinicians and its contents.

Fluids have long been categorized as crystalloid or colloid, terms introduced by Thomas Graham (Professor of Chemistry, University College London, 1836–1855) long before intravenous fluids were widely used in clinical practice.[71]

Crystalloids are solutions containing salt, sugar, and urea that can crystallize and can pass through the semipermeable membrane. Colloid on the other hand are non-crystallizable solutions such as, gelatin, gum, egg albumen, starch, and dextrin that form masses when evaporated to dryness, diffuse with extreme slowness, and do not pass through membranes.[71–73] Commonly used crystalloids and colloids along with their chemical compositions are described in Tables 7-2 and 7-3, respectively.

Crystalloids

Crystalloid fluids are the most commonly used fluids worldwide, are inexpensive, and produce equivalent outcomes to colloid preparations. They are considered as a first-line choice for fluid resuscitation in patients with shock (Table 7-2).

Crystalloid fluids are classified further by their tonicity and chemical contents. Isotonic crystalloid solutions are saline (0.9% sodium chloride) and a group of balanced solution, which consist of lactated Ringer's, Hartmann's solution, Plasma-Lyte, and Isolyte. Saline contains a greater amount of sodium and chloride than extracellular fluid, whereas balanced crystalloids contain chemical composition more similar to that of extracellular fluid, as seen in Table 7-2. Balanced crystalloids achieve this by replacing

Table 7-2	COMPOSITION OF COMMONLY USED CRYSTALLOID INTRAVENOUS FLUIDS[72]						
	Osmolarity	Tonicity	Na^+	Cl^-	K^+	Mg^{2+}	Ca^{2+}
Plasma	288	Reference	140	103	4.5	1.25	2.5
0.9% NaCl	308	Isotonic	154	154	0	0	0
Lactated Ringer's	279	Hypotonic	130	111	4.0	0	2.7
PlasmaLyte	N/A	Isotonic	140	98	5.0	1.5	0
Sterofundin	309	Isotonic	140	127	4.0	1.0	2.5
5% Glucose	278	Hypotonic	0	0	0	0	0
1.4% $NaHCO_3$	333	Hypertonic	167	0	0	0	0

Source: Hoorn EJ. Intravenous fluids: Balancing solutions. *J Nephrol.* 2017;30(4):485-492. Erratum in: *J Nephrol.* 2020;33(2):387.

chloride anions with buffers that are rapidly metabolized into bicarbonate (e.g., lactate and acetate) or excreted (e.g., gluconate).[75] Historically, a debate on which fluid to use for maximal safety has been raised.

Numerous studies have surfaced that showed decreased mortality and complications and less toxicity in patients being treated with balanced solutions.[76–79] Additional research is needed to determine (i) the mechanism by which crystalloid composition may affect clinical outcomes and (ii) the patient characteristics (comorbidities, acute conditions, hemodynamic and laboratory values, and markers of organ function) that identify patients most likely to benefit from balanced crystalloids versus saline.[75]

Bicarbonate containing fluids have been used in the recent past to keep body pH above 7.3 to avoid severe metabolic acidosis. However, a recent study did not improve mortality and rate of organ failure in critically severe acidotic patients who were given bicarbonate fluid therapy to keep the pH above 7.3 in but did have 16.7% absolute reduction in receipt of renal replacement therapy (Table 7-2).[79]

Colloids

Commonly administered colloids include derivatives of human plasma (albumin) and semisynthetic colloids (starches, gelatins, and dextrans) (Table 7-3). Compared with crystalloids, the theoretical benefit of colloid solutions is improved volume expansion due to retention in the intravascular space. Recent evidence suggests, however, that the "volume-sparing" effect of colloids compared to crystalloids is less than anticipated for critically ill adults.[80,81]

Table 7-3	COMPOSITION OF COMMONLY USED COLLOID INTRAVENOUS FLUIDS[74]
Type of colloid fluid	**Chemical Content**
Albumin 4%	• Osmolarity: 250 mOsm/l (calculated) • Osmolality: 260 mOsm/kg (measured) • pH 6.7–7.3 • Na^+ 140 mmol, Cl^- 128 mmol and octanoate 6.4 mmol
Albumin 5%	• Osmolarity: 309 mOsm/l (calculated) • Osmolality: 309 mOsm/kg (measured) • pH 6.4–7.4 • Na^+ 130–160 mmol, K^+ <2 mmol, Cl^- ~130 mmol, sodium caprylate 4 mmol and sodium N-acetyl tryptophanate 4 mmol
Albumin 20%	• Osmolarity: 130 mOsm/l (calculated) • Osmolality: 130 mOsm/kg (measured) • pH 6.7–7.3 • Na^+ 48–100 mmol and octanoate 32 mmol
Albumin 25%	• Osmolarity: 312 mOsm/l (calculated) • Osmolality: 312 mOsm/kg (measured) • pH 6.4–7.4 • Na^+ 130–160 mmol, K^+ <1 mmol, Cl^- ~130 mmol, sodium caprylate 4 mmol and sodium N-acetyl tryptophanate 4 mmol
6% HES (130/0.4) in normal saline	• Osmolarity: 308 mOsm/l (calculated) • Osmolality: 304 mOsm/kg (measured) • pH 4.0–5.5 • Na^+ 154 mmol and Cl^- 154 mmol
6% HES (130/0.42) in Ringer's acetate	• Osmolarity: 296 mOsm/l (calculated) • Osmolality: NK • pH 5.6–6.4 • Na^+ 140 mmol, K^+ 4 mmol, Cl^- 118 mmol, Ca^{2+} 2.5 mmol, acetate 24 mmol, malate 5 mmol and Mg^{2+} 1.0 mmol
6% HES (130/0.4) in buffered salt solution	• Osmolarity: 286 mOsm/l (calculated) • Osmolality: 283 mOsm/kg (measured) • pH 5.7–5.5 • Na^+ 137 mmol, K^+ 4 mmol, Cl^- 110 mmol, acetate 34 mmol and Mg^{2+} 1.5 mmol

Source: Data from Quinlan GJ, Martin GS, Evans TW. Albumin: Biochemical properties and therapeutic potential. *Hepatology*. 2005;41(6):1211-1219.

Albumin is a protein synthesized by the liver, provides 75% of plasma colloid oncotic pressure, binds nitric oxide, and regulates inflammation.[74] A randomized trial comparing use of 4% albumin versus 0.9% sodium chloride among nearly 7,000 critically ill adults found that the albumin group received slightly less fluid but experienced no difference in 28-day mortality.[80] The high cost of albumin relative to crystalloid solutions suggests that, while albumin may be appropriate therapy for select subgroups, such as those with cirrhosis and those undergoing liver transplantation, more research is needed before clinicians can consider albumin to be used as a primary fluid for resuscitation.[75]

The semisynthetic colloid solutions, which contain hydrolyzed bovine collagen (gelatins), glucose polymers (dextrans), or the maize-derived d-glucose polymer amylopectin (hydroxyethyl starches) have been synthetically created due to the high cost of albumin.[75]

Hydroxyethyl starch (HES) is the only semisynthetic colloid that has been studied among critically ill adults. Several studies indicated that when HES was compared with saline for IVF resuscitation, there was no significant difference in mortality, except for small difference in volume delivered.[48] Additionally, subsequent studies have shown HES increases risk of acute kidney injury, renal replacement therapy and mortality in critically ill patient populations.[82–85] Such findings should encourage clinicians to avoid colloid solutions when deciding first line fluid solutions in patients with shock.

▌VASOPRESSORS AND INOTROPES

Push dose vasopressors were first used by anesthesiologists when planning for intubation as a temporary means of increasing blood pressure to prevent transient hypotension.[86] Push dose vasopressors are now also very frequently used in the setting of transient hypotension or during resuscitation in the ICU or ED setting prior to central line establishment in an urgent setting. The most common push vasopressors used are epinephrine and phenylephrine. Push dose epinephrine is given in 1 mL dose every 3–5 minutes during a cardiac arrest resuscitation. Typical push dose phenylephrine ranges from 50 to 100 mcg every 2–5 minutes.

Vasopressors are drugs that induce vasoconstriction and a mainstay of treatment in patients with prolonged shock state to restore perfusion. Inotropes are a class of drugs that increases cardiac contractility. Many of the drugs have both vasopressor and inotropic effects and the use of different kind of drugs differ on the causes of shock and side effect profile. Table 7-4 lists commonly utilized catecholamine and phosphodiesterase 3 inhibitor (PDI).

Table 7-4   COMMON VASOPRESSORS AND INOTROPES[85]

Drug	Indication	Receptor Binding				Major Side Effects
		α 1	β 1	β 2	DA	
Catecholamines						
Dopamine	Shock (cardiogenic, vasodilatory) HF symptomatic bradycardia unresponsive to atropine or pacing	+++	++++	++	+++++	Severe hypertension (especially in patients taking nonselective β-blockers), Ventricular arrhythmias, Cardiac ischemia Tissue ischemia/gangrene (high doses or due to tissue extravasation)
Dobutamine	Low CO (decompensated HF, cardiogenic shock, sepsis-induced myocardial dysfunction) Symptomatic bradycardia unresponsive to atropine or pacing	+	+++++	+++	N/A	Tachycardia Increased ventricular response rate in patients with atrial fibrillation, Ventricular arrhythmias, Cardiac ischemia Hypertension (especially nonselective β-blocker patients) Hypotension
Norepinephrine	Shock (vasodilatory, cardiogenic)	+++++	+++	++	N/A	Arrhythmias Bradycardia Peripheral (digital) ischemia Hypertension (especially nonselective β-blocker patients)
Epinephrine	Shock (cardiogenic, vasodilatory), Cardiac arrest Bronchospasm/ anaphylaxis Symptomatic bradycardia or heart block unresponsive to atropine or pacing	+++++	++++	+++	N/A	Ventricular arrhythmias; Severe hypertension resulting in cerebrovascular hemorrhage Cardiac ischemia Sudden cardiac death

(Continued)

Table 7-4   COMMON VASOPRESSORS AND INOTROPES[85] (CONTINUED)

Drug	Indication	Receptor Binding				Major Side Effects
		α1	β1	β2	DA	
Phenylephrine	Hypotension (vagally mediated, medication-induced) Increase MAP with AS and hypotension Decrease LVOT gradient in HCM	+++++	0	0	N/A	Reflex bradycardia Hypertension (especially with nonselective β-blockers) Severe peripheral and visceral vasoconstriction Tissue necrosis with extravasation
Milrinone	Low CO (decompensated HF, after cardiotomy)	NA	NA	NA	N/A	Ventricular arrhythmias Hypotension Cardiac ischemia Torsade des pointes
Vasopressin	Shock (vasodilatory, cardiogenic) Cardiac arrest	V₁ receptors (vascular smooth muscle) V₂ receptors (renal collecting duct system)				Arrhythmias Hypertension Decreased CO (at doses >0.4 U/min) Cardiac ischemia Severe peripheral vasoconstriction causing ischemia (especially skin) Splanchnic vasoconstriction

Source: Data from Lewis SR, Pritchard MW, Evans DJ, et al. Colloids versus crystalloids for fluid resuscitation in critically ill people. *Cochrane Database Syst Rev.* 2018;8:CD000567.

Alpha-1 adrenergic receptors are present in the vascular walls in myocardium and can cause significant vasoconstriction and increased contractility. Beta-1 adrenergic receptors are mainly located in myocardium and when activated can induce increased contractility and chronotropy. Beta-2 adrenergic receptors induce blood vessel vasodilation. Dopamine receptors are mainly located in the renal vasculature and splanchnic as well as coronary vasculature. There are two types of dopamine receptors, D1 and D2. Stimulation of D1 receptors causes vasodilation while stimulation of D2 receptors causes release of norepinephrine, which in turn will cause vasoconstriction.

Norepinephrine

Norepinephrine is a hydroxylated derivative of dopamine that stimulates both the alpha and beta receptors and is considered as the first-line vasopressor in patients with sepsis or septic shock.[1,83–86] Its alpha-1 effects predominate at therapeutic doses and induce vasoconstriction. Norepinephrine also increases the mean systemic filling pressure, which assists in increased blood return to the heart. Its beta 1 activity also induces increased contractility of the heart.[87]

Phenylephrine

Phenylephrine is a pure alpha-1 agonist. It is mainly used as an adjunct to inotropic agents in situations where the SVR needs to be increased without significant alterations in other cardiac parameters.[88] Surviving Sepsis Guidelines state that phenylephrine is contraindicated in patients with septic shock except when septic shock persists despite the use of two or more inotrope/vasopressor agents along with low-dose vasopressin cardiac output is known to be high, or norepinephrine is considered to have already caused serious arrhythmias.[1,88]

Epinephrine

Epinephrine is a nonselective agonist of alpha and beta receptors. Epinephrine is recommended for patients in septic shock as either a first alternative or in conjunction with norepinephrine.[1] Epinephrine is also used as a first line vasopressor in cardiac arrest. Alpha-1 receptor stimulation induces vasoconstriction, and beta-1 stimulation acts to increase contractility of the heart. Epinephrine is also useful for the treatment of acute left ventricular failure during cardiac surgery because it predictably increases cardiac output. It is most useful as an inotrope in patients who are hypotensive with no myocardial ischemia, especially following cardiac surgery.[89,90]

Angiotensin II

Angiotensin II (ATII) is a vasoconstrictor that is part of the renin-aldo-sterone-angiotensin (RAAS) system. ATII has been recently approved to be used as a vasopressor in patients with refractory shock despite the use of mainstay vasopressors. The major physiologic effects are mediated by the AT-1 receptor, which is located in the kidneys, vascular smooth muscle, lung, heart, brain, adrenal gland, pituitary gland, and liver.[91] These effects include direct vasoconstriction (via receptors located in the endothelium of peripheral vessels), inotropy and cardiac remodeling (via receptors located in the myocardium), potentiation of the sympathetic nervous system, vasopressin release, regulation of the thirst mechanism (via receptors in the brain, sympathetic ganglia, and pituitary), and regulation of aldosterone release (via receptors in the adrenal gland).[91]

Vasopressin

Vasopressin, also known as antidiuretic hormone (ADH), is a non-adrenergic vasopressor that acts on the ubiquitous V1 and V2 receptors in vascular beds that induced vasoconstriction. It is primarily used as an adjunct vasopressor for sepsis-associated hypotension.[1] Vasopressin at low doses can also cause vasodilation in the pulmonary capillaries due to release of nitric oxide, which may help in patients with acute right ventricular failure.[88,89]

Dobutamine

Dobutamine is a predominant beta-1 receptor agonist with lesser beta-2 receptor agonist and also a mild alpha-1 agonist.[88,89] Dobutamine is a first line inotropic drug in septic patients with high filling pressures or impaired cardiac output.[1,56] Dobutamine increases cardiac output in patients in shock and heart failure by increasing stroke volume and decreasing SVR. It also increases cerebral oxygenation during hypoxia and/or anemia and may be effective in improving neurological outcomes in ischemic cerebral injury via its action on β1-receptors.[88]

Dopamine

Dopamine predominantly binds to dopamine receptors and is dose dependent on the effects of vasoconstriction. At low doses, dopamine inhibits the release of norepinephrine in peripheral blood vessels, thereby acting as a mild vasodilator, but also inhibits the re-uptake of norepinephrine in presynaptic sympathetic nerve terminals resulting in an indirect increase in cardiac contractility and heart rate.[88] Combined effects include increased contractility, heart rate, and a mild increase in SVR.[88] At high doses, α1-adrenergic receptor–mediated vasoconstriction dominates the peripheral response and further increases blood pressure.[88]

Hypothermia and Vasopressors

Current guidelines for post-cardiac arrest with primary rhythm of ventricular fibrillation and ventricular tachycardia recommend therapeutic hypothermia to improve neurological outcomes.[88,89] Given that cardiac diseases are the most common causes of cardiac arrest in this patient population, hemodynamic instability and cardiogenic shock is a major concern. Therapeutic hypothermia increases systemic vascular resistance and lowers cardiac index.[90–93] Vasopressors are frequently used to maintain hemodynamic stability, and studies show that therapeutic hypothermia did not increase the need for vasopressors but instead was less likely to require vasopressor support when compared to normothermic patients.[92,93]

Acidosis and Vasopressors

Vasopressors, especially epinephrine and norepinephrine, have shown to be less efficacious in the presence of acidosis.[91] Although acidosis reduces the effect of the vasopressors, significant drop in the efficacy of the vasopressors was predominant when pH was less than 6.8.[92] Acid-base status of critically ill patients should be closely monitored especially when there is an increasing requirement for vasopressors in patients with shock.

Route of Vasopressor Administration

Central venous catheters should be used when there is a prolonged need for vasopressors or inotropic agents.[91,92,94–96] A central venous catheter can deliver the drug more rapidly for faster distribution to the systemic circulation. In urgent situations or if central venous catheters are not available, these agents can be administered through peripheral intravenous catheters until a central venous line can be established.[59,63] Other route of administration such as intramuscular or intratracheal are not appropriate for vasopressors.

▌RESUSCITATION AND MONITORING

Fluid Responsiveness

Aggressive intravenous fluid resuscitation is the main treatment modality in patients with shock, but how much fluid is enough? Fluid overload as a consequence of overly aggressive treatment does come with consequences such as prolonged mechanical intubation and acute respiratory distress syndrome.[97,98]

The risk of aggressive fluid administration has been clearly established, and volume expansion does not always increase cardiac output as one expects, which is why after the very initial phase and/or if fluid losses are not obvious, predicting fluid responsiveness should be the first step of fluid strategy.[99]

Hemodynamic Monitoring

Monitoring hemodynamics in patients with shock, especially if the patient is on vasopressors, requires close monitoring in the intensive care units (ICUs) to maintain appropriate blood pressure for adequate perfusion to vital organs.

Monitoring can often be done with clinical examination and monitoring basic vital parameters (heart rate, blood pressure, central venous pressure [CVP], peripheral and central venous oxygen saturation, and respiratory variables) and urine output.[100] The ultimate goal for blood pressure when treating patients with hemodynamic instability whether from a septic shock or cardiogenic shock is always a MAP > 65 mm Hg.[1]

Serial Lactic Acid

Serial blood lactic acid measurements are good predictors for the development of MSOF and death in patients with septic shock. Furthermore, the duration of lactic acidosis is more important than the initial lactate value. Many factors contribute to hyperlactatemia, but these observations demonstrate a direct role of prolonged tissue hypoxia in the development of complications following septic shock.[101] During the first 12 hours following shock development, the optimal time point of repeated blood lactate measurement was 6 hours, which was the greatest prognostic value for mortality.

Permissive Hypotension

Permissive hypotension is the technique of non-aggressive fluid resuscitation in order to sustain a goal systolic or MAP below normal physiological conditions in the setting of volume loss. This technique is commonly employed in the trauma setting for patients experiencing acute hemorrhagic volume depletion. The existing data suggests a quicker recovery, and a decrease in postoperative recovery time is achieved when permissive hypotension is employed.

Based upon retrospective data collection studies in the trauma setting, reports have suggested that permissive hypotension can generally be achieved in many patients, if the MAP is close to the target number of 50 mm Hg, or if the systolic pressures are between 80 mm Hg and 90 mm Hg.[102–104]

PATHOGENESIS

Distributive Shock

Distributive shock is defined by severe vasodilation or by vasoplegic state. Cytokine release during distributive shock plays a critical role in the pathogenesis of the disease. In septic shock, endotoxins, exotoxins, and cell wall glycopeptides of bacteria can induce the release of cytokines, which is neither specific nor unique to infection.[105,106] Other inducers of cytokines include trauma, ischemia-reperfusion injury, and other acute inflammatory states that result in both local and systemic inflammatory processes.[105] Physiologic changes, if not treated, lead to hypovolemia, progressive failure of multiple organ system, and death.

The most common form of distributive shock is septic shock, which occurs due to unregulated response to bacterial, viral, or fungal infection resulting in life threatening organ dysfunction or organ failure. Septic shock is associated with significant mortality ranging from 40% to 50%.[3]

Neurogenic Shock

Traumatic brain injury and spinal cord injuries can lead to hypotension and overt shock due to interruption of autonomic pathways, causing decrease in vascular resistance and altered vagal tone.[3]

Anaphylactic Shock

Shock from anaphylaxis can occur in patients with severe allergic reactions. Commonly encountered allergies include food, bee stings, drugs, exercise, contrast media, and latex. These can cause acute reactions that can directly release mediators from mast cells and basophils, which can also contribute to anaphylactic shock.[3]

Adrenal Insufficiency

Due to mineralocorticoid deficiency, vasodilation can occur due to dysregulation in vascular tone and aldosterone deficiency mediated hypovolemia. Thyroid hormones can also play a role in blood pressure, but there is an unclear mechanism of vasodilation leading to shock in patients with myxedema.[3]

The hypothalamic-pituitary-adrenal (HPA) axis in conjunction with the sympathetic system is largely responsible for mediating the homeostasis of the body's response to stress. Cortisol, the end-product of this HPA axis released from the adrenal glands, must be kept tightly regulated, especially in times of shock to prevent progression to multiorgan failure. The main components of the stress system are the hypothalamic corticotropin releasing hormone (CRH), norepinephrine autonomic system, and their peripheral effectors, HPA axis.[1] Damage anywhere along this stress response that results in alteration of the level of cortisol release from the HPA axis subsequently would lead to adrenal insufficiency and subsequent shock.

Acute adrenal insufficiency or adrenal crisis is the shock caused by decreased levels of cortisol or inadequate cortisol response to a physiological stress, which can also commonly occur in patients with septic shock. Patients frequently present with nausea, vomiting, abdominal pain, and fatigue subsequently leading to hypovolemic shock. Gastroenteritis and fever are the two most common precipitating events, but other physiological stress such as trauma, surgery, and even dental procedures can trigger adrenal crisis leading to shock. Patients are frequently found with hyponatremia, hyperkalemia, and acute kidney injury. Bolus fluid administration with subsequent maintenance intravenous fluid administration should be implemented as well as initiation of stress dose hydrocortisone once adrenal insufficiency is suspected as a diagnosis. If possible and hemodynamically stable, prompt investigation of adrenal insufficiency should be done with random cortisol and ACTH level. Morning cortisol level should be obtained if possible, for an accurate measurement and ACTH stimulation test is done to establish diagnosis but not at the expense of delaying treatment with hydrocortisone once adrenal insufficiency is suspected as a cause of shock.

Hypovolemic Shock

Hypovolemic shock occurs when there is inadequate organ perfusion secondary to loss of intravascular volume. Due to the loss of volume, there is inadequate perfusion to the organs, which subsequently leads to damage of the organs, triggering inflammatory reactions.[107] Common causes of hypovolemic shocks include acute hemorrhage from trauma, soft tissue injury, generally any condition that would cause loss of volume in the intravascular space.

Cardiogenic Shock

Cardiogenic shock is due to failure of the heart to produce adequate cardiac output. Cardiomyopathic causes of shock include myocardial infarction especially in multi-vessel coronary artery disease, severe right ventricular infarction, acute exacerbation of heart failure in patients with severe underlying dilated cardiomyopathy, stunned myocardium following cardiac arrest, prolonged ischemia or cardiopulmonary bypass, myocardial depression due to advanced septic or neurogenic shock, and myocarditis. Hypertrophic cardiomyopathy can also rarely present with cardiogenic shock.[3] Arrhythmia, both atrial and ventricular, may induce hypotension contributing to state of shock due to decreased output from the arrhythmia. Valvular abnormalities can also cause the heart to decrease cardiac output. Additional causes include severe ventricular septal defects or acute rupture of the intraventricular septum, atrial myxomas, and a ruptured ventricular free wall aneurysm.[1–3,9]

Echocardiography is pivotal in the diagnosis and management of the shock.[108] It is non-invasive and can be rapidly applied. It can supply immediate information to assist in diagnosis and initiation of therapy, while a follow-up advanced study can further refine the diagnosis and provide an in-depth hemodynamic assessment.

Wall motion abnormality, easily seen on bedside echocardiography, can be an early clue to obstructive coronary artery disease. Any assessment of left ventricular contractility needs to take the presence or absence of identifiable segmental wall motion abnormalities into account; if present, urgent revascularization should be considered to enhance prognosis. Wall motion abnormalities, when present, are an independent predictor of cardiovascular events, including myocardial infarction, unstable/stable angina, and congestive heart failure.

A right heart catheter can be helpful for initial diagnosis of shock and for directing subsequent treatments. It can be utilized to monitor hemodynamics such as cardiac output (CO), pulmonary arterial occlusion pressure (PAOP or wedge pressure), pulmonary arterial pressure (PAP), mixed venous oxygen saturation (SvO_2), and stroke volume variation (SVV), to guide fluid management and vasopressor/inotropic support.[100]

In cardiogenic shock caused by acute myocardial infarction, an intra-aortic balloon pump, a mechanical device that increases myocardial oxygen perfusion and indirectly increases cardiac output through afterload reduction, is often utilized to augment systolic blood pressure and assist in perfusing the coronary arteries. However, recent studies have been critical of this device's utilization for lack of survival benefits, and it has been replaced by left ventricular assist devices (LVAD) by most clinicians.[109]

A ventricular assist device (VAD) is an electromechanical device for assisting cardiac circulation. It is utilized to partially or to completely replace the function of a failing heart. More recent studies seem to indicate that placement of LADs may be beneficial and decrease the mortality in patients with severe or refractory cardiogenic shock.[110]

Obstructive Shock

Obstructive shock occurs most commonly due to causes, other than cardiac pump failure, such as right heart infarction, acute pulmonary embolus, cardiac tamponade, or massive pneumothorax.[2]

Acute Right Heart Myocardial Infarction

Acute right heart dysfunction can mimic left ventricular dysfunction resulting in cardiogenic shock. Acute right heart syndrome is associated with myocardial infarction localizing to the right ventricle, massive volume overload, hypoxemic vasoconstriction resulting in acute pulmonary hypertension, and pulmonary embolism (PE) that can lead to shock state in these patients.

Acute Pulmonary Embolus

Diagnostic criteria include dilated right atrium and ventricle, decreased right ventricular contraction, increased pulmonary artery pressures, decreased cardiac output, and intra-cavity emboli. Right ventricle dilatation can be seen in the apical four-chamber view with a right ventricle/left ventricle area ratio > 0.6; gross dilatation is seen with a ratio > 1.0.[111,112]

The McConnell sign is an important sign where there is good apical but poor free wall contraction.[113] However, it can also be found in right ventricular infarction, and its specificity for pulmonary embolism (PE) has been called into question.[114,115] McConnell's sign is a pattern of right ventricular (RV) dysfunction seen on an ECHO where RV akinesia is seen with the apex of the RV sparing. McConnell's sign is highly specific for right heart strain, which can indicate a pathologic condition such as PE (Figure 7-1).

Cardiac Tamponade

An echocardiogram can usually identify a pericardial effusion, except in rare occasions when the fluid is loculated posteriorly. Fluid in the pericardial space is generally easy to differentiate from a pericardial fat pad or a pleural effusion (Figure 7-2).[116] Echocardiographic findings of tamponade include: (1) collapse of right atrium and right ventricle, during relaxation phase or diastole, or collapse of both atria; (2) Inferior vena cava is usually dilated (> 20 mm); (3) mitral peak E-wave velocity > 25%; (4) tricuspid peak E wave velocity drops < 40% in expiration compared to inspiration;

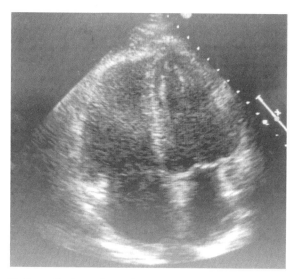

Figure 7-1 • McConnell's sign echocardiogram.

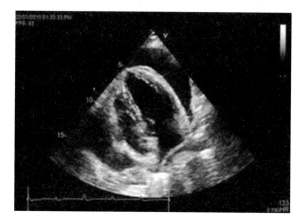

Figure 7-2 • Cardiac tamponade echocardiogram. (Courtesy of Karan Omidvari, MD.)

(5) right and left ventricle outflow tracts with physiologic variations in aorta and pulmonary trunk < 10%; and (6) 10% drop in peak velocity in aorta while increase >10% in right ventricular outflow tract (Figure 7-2).

Dynamic LVOT Obstruction

Dynamic left ventricular outflow obstruction is a rare entity, and its true incidence is unknown. Echo Doppler reveals left ventricular wall hypertrophy, which may alert the clinician to the possibility of hypertrophic obstructive cardiomyopathy and LVOT obstruction.

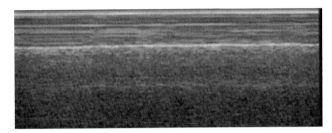

Figure 7-3 • Sea-shore sign. (Courtesy of Karan Omidvari, MD.)

Two-dimensional echo examination reveals close approximation of lateral wall and septum, plus systolic anterior motion of the anterior mitral leaflet. TEE examination often supplements the TTE approach. Color Doppler will reveal turbulent flow through the LVOT with continuous wave Doppler picking up high velocities indicating obstructive and subsequent pulsed-wave Doppler identifying exactly where that obstruction occurs. A classic spectral Doppler pattern is the so-called dagger shaped LVOT flow. Treatment includes re-establishing an adequate intravascular volume, reducing heart rate to enhance diastolic filling time, and ceasing inotropes. Occasionally, LVOT obstruction tokutsubo cardiomyopathy is also described.[117,118]

Tension Pneumothorax

Tension pneumothorax is caused by collapse of the lung creating increased intrathoracic pressure causing vascular collapse and shock. It can easily be demonstrated by lack of seashore sign on the m mode of ultrasound (Figure 7-3) or by lack of lung sliding sign on 2-D mode in association with hemodynamic instability (Figure 7-4).

Acute Pulmonary Embolus

Echocardiography is a very important tool in diagnosis of a shock patient with PE.[111] Diagnostic criteria include dilated right atrium and ventricle, decreased right ventricular contraction, increased pulmonary artery pressures, decreased cardiac output, and intra-cavity emboli. Right ventricle dilatation can be seen in the apical four-chamber view with a right ventricle/left ventricle area ratio > 0.6; gross dilatation is seen with a ratio > 1.0 (Figure 7-5).[119] The McConnell sign is an important sign where there is good apical but poor free wall contraction.[111–113] However, it can also be found in right ventricular infarction, and its specificity for PE has been called into question.[111,112]

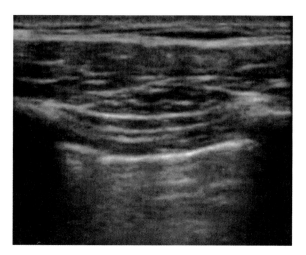

Figure 7-4 • Lung sliding. (Courtesy of Karan Omidvari, MD.)

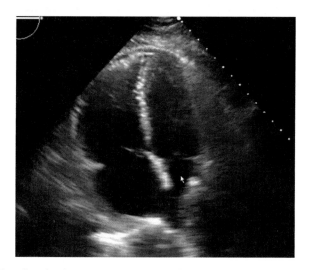

Figure 7-5 • Dilated right ventricle. (Courtesy of Karan Omidvari, MD.)

Hypovolemic Shock

Hemorrhagic shock is a type of hypovolemic shock and is a result of decreased volume from blood loss which can result in shock. There are multiple causes of hemorrhagic shock, of which blunt or penetrating trauma (includes multiple fractures without vessel injury) is the most common, followed by upper (e.g., variceal hemorrhage, peptic ulcer) or lower (e.g., diverticular, arteriovenous malformation) gastrointestinal bleeding.[2] Reduced intravascular volume from fluid loss other than blood can cause

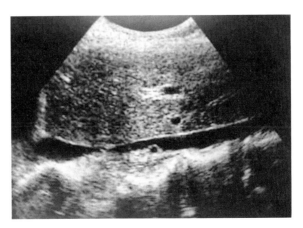

Figure 7-6 • Inferior vena cava compressibility. (Courtesy of Karan Omidvari, MD.)

shock. Volume depletion from loss of sodium and water can occur from diarrhea, vomiting, heat stroke, burns, Steven Johnson syndrome, renal loss, and third space losses.[1–3] Reduced intravascular volume can easily be assessed by bedside ultrasonography if the inferior vena cava can be compressed with the ultrasound probe (Figure 7-6).

Response to fluid resuscitation can be ascertained by several invasive and noninvasive methods with high sensitivity and specificity. Passive leg raising (PLR), pulse pressure variation, systolic pressure variation, stroke volume variation, systolic velocity variation, end-expiratory occlusion technique, echocardiography, and ultrasound can also be used to measure fluid responsiveness (FR).[120]

Passive leg raising (PLR) is accomplished by tilting a patient from a 45-degree semi-recumbent head up position to a 45-degree leg up position. This maneuver can transfer up to 300 mL of blood into the central circulation but avoids compression of the femoral veins. Stroke volume or across either outflow tract is measured before and 1 minute after the PLR. An increment of 10% suggests FR.[121]

A pulse pressure variation of less than 12%, as seen on the arterial waveform, has been shown to be a valid method. Systolic pressure variation is similarly used with the same cut off. The stroke volume variation as determined by cardiac output monitoring. It can also be done by arterial waveform analysis and is equally valid with a similar cut-off value. End-expiratory occlusion is another method. A rise in stroke volume after end-expiration hold for approximately 15 seconds demonstrates fluid responsiveness.[122]

Echocardiography can assess fluid responsiveness by monitoring the left ventricle, aortic outflow, inferior vena cava, and right ventricle. Static measurements and dynamic variables based on heart–lung interactions combine to predict and measure fluid responsiveness and assess response to intravenous fluid resuscitation.[123]

Stroke volume measurement is relatively simple and a good indicator of fluid responsiveness.[123] More than 12% stroke volume variation (SVV) accurately predicts fluid responsiveness with a very high positive predictive value over 14% and less than 10% a high negative predictive value.[123] Variation of 12–14% fall in a gray area, and other causes should be sought.[123]

Recently, it has been shown that even a small fluid challenge (100 mL) can predict FR using variations in aortic velocity time integral (VTI) with TTE.[124]

Point-of-care ultrasound (POC) has been used for many years to measure the diameter and collapsibility of various large vessels including the inferior vena cava, common carotid artery, subclavian vein, internal jugular vein, and femoral vein. It has similarly been utilized to monitor fluid responsiveness and can guide fluid resuscitation in critically ill patients.[125]

Similarly, in ventilated patients, large variations in inferior vena cava (IVC) diameter with intermittent positive pressure ventilation (IPPV) accurately predict FR. A variability of more than 12% identifies responders.[126]

Biorectance is an electrical device based on emission of a high-frequency (50 kHz) and low-amperage (2 mA) alternating electrical current of constant amplitude via a pair of surface electrodes across the left side of the thorax. It can provide noninvasive, continuous bedside hemodynamic measurements such as circulating blood volume and of cardiac index (CI), and stroke volume. Recent studies have suggested that this device can also be utilized to measure FL after a fluid challenge by continuously measuring these parameters.[127,128]

TREATMENT

Hemorrhagic Shock

Blood and blood products are the mainstay of therapy in hemorrhagic shock. Fluid replacement, such as with normal saline, and pressors as a bridge, may be necessary until blood products are available.

Oxygen carriers (OC), such as oxygen hemoglobin-based oxygen carriers (HBOCs) and perfluorocarbons (FPCs), are the most frequent blood substitutes that have been utilized to avoid transfusion of blood products.[129] Hemoglobin-based oxygen carriers (HBOCs) can be derived from two mammalian sources: bovine and human blood, the latter primarily from outdated red blood cell units. Hemoglobin is first separated from the red blood cell stroma through ultrafiltration and purification.[129] Mammalian hemoglobin is chemically modified by polymerization, crosslinking, pyridoxylation, and/or pegylation (addition of polyethylene glycol [PEG] molecules). The pegylation prevents the dissociation of hemoglobin from its native four-chain configuration into its basic alpha-beta dimers.[130] Perfluorocarbons are inert compounds in which fluorine replaces hydrogen atoms. They have a plasma half-life of 12 hours and are stable when refrigerated at 4°C for up to two years.[129]

Nonhemorrhagic Shock

In patients with nonhemorrhagic shock, isotonic or near-isotonic and colloid-containing solutions are the most common solutions used to replace the extracellular fluid deficit. Crystalloid solutions include 0.9 percent saline (with or without dextrose), buffered crystalloids such as lactated Ringer's, Plasma-Lyte, and bicarbonate buffered 0.45 percent saline. Colloid-containing solutions include albumin solution, hyperon-cotic starch, dextran, and gelatin.[131,132] Hyper-oncotic starch solutions are effective but should be avoided since they increase the risk of acute kidney injury, need for renal replacement therapy, and mortality.[133–135]

Distributive Shock

Septic Shock

Stabilizing respiration, establishing venous access, and early administration of fluids and antibiotics are the principals of supportive care for patients with septic shock (Table 7-5).[136]

Shock Secondary to Adrenal Insufficiency

Acute adrenal insufficiency or adrenal crisis describes another condition of shock caused by decreased level of cortisol or inadequate cortisol response to a physiological stress, which can commonly occur in patients with septic shock. Patients frequently present with nausea, vomiting, abdominal pain, and fatigue subsequently leading to hypovolemic shock.[137] Sepsis, trauma, surgery, and even dental procedures can trigger adrenal crisis leading to shock.[128,138] Patients are frequently found with hyponatremia, hyperkalemia, and acute kidney injury. Bolus fluid administration with subsequent maintenance intravenous fluid administration should be implemented as well as initiation of stress dose hydrocortisone once adrenal insufficiency is suspected as a diagnosis. If possible and hemodynamically stable, prompt investigation of adrenal insufficiency should be done with random cortisol and ACTH level. Morning cortisol level should be obtained if possible, for an accurate measurement

Table 7-5	TREATMENT OF SEPSIS SECONDARY BASED ON PATHOLOGY		
	Empiric Treatment	**First Line Treatment**	**Alternative Treatment**
Community Acquired Pneumonia	Ceftriaxone + Azithromycin + Supportive Care	Ceftriaxone + Azithromycin + Supportive Care	Piperacillin-tazobactam (If pseudomonas risk) + Azithromycin + Supportive Care
	+/− Vancomycin (If Methicillin Resistant Staphylococcus Aureus risk)	+/− Vancomycin (If Methicillin Resistant Staphylococcus Aureus risk)	+/− Vancomycin (If Methicillin Resistant Staphylococcus Aureus risk)
Health Care Associated Pneumonia	Vancomycin + Piperacillin-tazobactam + Supportive Care	Piperacillin-tazobactam + Tobramycin + Vancomycin + Supportive Care	Ceftazidime + Tobramycin + Vancomycin + Supportive Care
Urinary Tract Infection	Vancomycin + Piperacillin-tazobactam + Supportive Care	Piperacillin-tazobactam + Supportive Care	Ceftazidime + Vancomycin + Supportive Care
Meningitis	**Patients < 50 years:** Ceftriaxone + Vancomycin	**Patients < 50 years:** Ceftriaxone + Vancomycin	**Penicillin allergies:** Vancomycin + Moxifloxacin + Trimethoprim-sulfamethoxazole
	Patients > 50 years: Ceftriaxone + Vancomycin + Ampicillin	**Patients > 50 years:** Ceftriaxone + Vancomycin + Ampicillin	
Cellulitis	Vancomycin + Piperacillin-tazobactam + Supportive Care	Antibiotics according to culture data + Supportive Care	Antibiotics according to culture data + Supportive Care
Necrotizing Fasciitis	Urgent Surgical Intervention with Vancomycin + Piperacillin-tazobactam + Supportive Care	Urgent Surgical Intervention with Vancomycin + Piperacillin-tazobactam + Supportive Care	Urgent Surgical Intervention with Vancomycin + Piperacillin-tazobactam + Supportive Care
Osteomyelitis	Obtain bone cultures + Vancomycin + Piperacillin-tazobactam + Supportive Care	Bone culture guided antibiotics regimen +/− Surgical debridement with supportive care	Bone culture guided antibiotics regimen +/− Surgical debridement with supportive care

(Continued)

Table 7-5   TREATMENT OF SEPSIS SECONDARY BASED ON PATHOLOGY (*CONTINUED*)

	Empiric Treatment	First Line Treatment	Alternative Treatment
Abscess	Obtain cultures from abscess + Vancomycin + Piperacillin-tazobactam + Surgical Drainage if appropriate + Supportive Care	Obtain cultures from abscess + Vancomycin + Piperacillin-tazobactam + Surgical Drainage if appropriate + Supportive Care	Obtain cultures from abscess + Vancomycin + Piperacillin-tazobactam + Surgical Drainage if appropriate + Supportive Care
Cholecystitis	Piperacillin-tazobactam + Supportive Care	Piperacillin-tazobactam + Supportive Care + Surgical Intervention	Cefepime + Metronidazole + Supportive Care + Surgical Intervention
Cholangitis	Piperacillin-tazobactam + Supportive Care	Piperacillin-tazobactam + Supportive Care + Biliary Drainage OR Surgical Intervention	Cephalosporin OR Ciprofloxacin + Metronidazole + Supportive Care + Biliary Drainage OR Surgical Intervention

and ACTH stimulation test is done to establish diagnosis but not at the expense of delaying treatment with hydrocortisone once adrenal insufficiency is suspected as a cause of shock.[139]

Myxedema Coma

Hypothyroidism is a condition in which your thyroid gland produces insufficient thyroid hormones leading to symptoms such as fatigue, unexplained weight gain, cold sensitivity, bradycardia, hypothermia, and almost all aspects of metabolism. Hypothyroidism can trigger a severe life-threatening form, known as myxedema crisis, which is due to low T3 levels intracellularly leading to shock, respiratory distress, hypothermia, and coma.[140] Patients in suspicion of myxedema crisis treated with thyroid replacement and intravenous fluids. Myxedema crisis is associated with high mortality rate; thus, these patients should be monitored closely in the ICU, intubated for airway protection, and start treatment as soon as possible.[141,142] Treatment includes fluid resuscitation, synthroid, and solu-cortef.

Obstructive Shock

Acute Pulmonary Embolism

The best treatment choice for a patient with PE may be difficult. Each case should be risk stratified to determine the best option. Systemic lysis is indicated for massive PE with or without cardiac arrest. If lysis is contraindicated, surgical embolectomy is the next best choice.[143] Patients in suspicion for PE should be risk stratified with clinical risk scores such as Pulmonary Embolism Severity Index (PESI), Well's Criteria for PE, as well as with biomarkers such as D-Dimer, troponins, and N-terminal pro-brain natriuretic peptide with appropriate imaging studies.[144] Systemic anti-coagulation is a mainstay of treatment for PE, but patients with massive PE with significant hemodynamic instability and pulmonary artery occlusion resulting in right ventricular strain warrant treatment with systemic thrombolysis, catheter-directed thrombolysis (CDT), or surgical embolectomy (SE).[145] Systemic thrombolysis with tissue plasminogen activator (t-PA) significantly increases risk of bleeding as well as increases risk of hemorrhagic strokes.[145] Therefore detailed risk stratification should be performed by an experienced clinician before making the decision to start thrombolysis. Patients with contraindications to t-PA in massive PE or those who fail systemic lysis and develop cardiogenic shock should undergo CDT, which is a catheter that directly introduces t-PA at the occluded site. CDT has been shown to effectively decrease pulmonary artery obstruction, right ventricular diameter, and pulmonary artery systolic pressure without significantly increasing the risk of major hemorrhagic events.[145]

Pericardial Effusion

Pericardial fluid build-up can be incidental, but it can also cause life threatening hemodynamic instability that would require urgent intervention. Large effusions can progress to cardiac tamponade, which is considered an emergency causing decreased compliance of the heart, ventricular interdependence, and decreased left ventricular filling.[146] Treatment for pericardial effusion is ultimately guided by etiology of the effusion, hemodynamic parameters, and size of the effusion.

Primary treatment for cardiac tamponade is pericardiocentesis with intravenous fluids and vasopressors supportive care in order to maintain adequate cardiac output. Pericardiocentesis can be done at the bedside and if needed, rapidly in an emergency. Pericardial window is preferred in patients with recurrent effusions as well as in situations where effusions can reoccur, such as in malignancy.

Patients with pericardial effusion without tamponade features or hemodynamic instability should always be monitored for progression to tamponade. In selective patients, pericardiocentesis should be performed in order to determine the cause of the effusion.[147]

Cardiogenic Shock

Initial approach includes ventilator support if needed, hemodynamic support with inotropic agents or with norepinephrine, and antiplatelet agents such as aspirin. Volume status should be carefully estimated, and volume resuscitation undertaken. Antiplatelet agent is administered as soon as possible and attempts at re-vascularization include angioplasty, stenting, and coronary artery bypass grafting (CABG).

If myocardium oxygen supply is still jeopardized, assist devices such as an intra-aortic balloon pump (IABP), percutaneous heart pump (Impella), ventricular assist device (VAD), and even extracorporeal membrane oxygenation (ECMO) devices can be utilized temporarily and/ or as a bridge to heart transplantation. Surgery to repair injury to damage heart, such as in the case of left ventricular rupture secondary to acute myocardial infarction, may be necessary.

The timing of IABP placement is controversial with IABP-SHOCK II demonstrating that the in-hospital 30-day mortality rate was much improved if the IABP was placed prior to percutaneous coronary intervention (PCI) as opposed to after.[148] However, an earlier registry study had suggested that the mortality was similar whether IABP was placed before or after PCI.[149]

The use of percutaneous heart pump (Impella) has also been controversial. In a 2019 retrospective study, the use of this devise did not demonstrate a 30-day mortality improvement compared to IABPSHOCK trial patients treated with an IABP or medical therapy.[150]

Immediate CABG is the treatment of choice for patients with associated mechanical complications, such as shock. In patients with ST-elevation myocardial infarction (STEMI), revascularization with either PCI or CABG is preferred to fibrinolytic therapy if performed within 120 minutes from initial hospital presentation.[151] For MI with one or two vessel coronary disease, immediate PCI is preferred to CABG. Immediate reperfusion with PCI is preferred to CABG for amenable stenosis or total occlusion of left main coronary, particularly if it is due to thrombotic occlusion. Three vessels coronary artery disease, with or without left main disease, should be considered for immediate CABG.[152] Fibrinolysis is only considered in patients with STEMI only if revascularization is not feasible.[153,154]

▌REFERENCES

1. Dellinger RP, Levy MM, Rhodes A, et al. Surviving Sepsis Campaign: International guidelines for management of severe sepsis and septic shock, 2012. *Intensive Care Med.* 2013;39(2):165-228.
2. Wacker DA, Winters ME. Shock. *Emerg Med Clin North Am.* 2014;32(4):747-758.
3. Kislitsina ON, Rich JD, Wilcox JE, Pham DT, Churyla A, Vorovich EB, Ghafourian K, Yancy CW. Shock - Classification and pathophysiological principles of therapeutics. *Curr Cardiol Rev.* 2019;15(2):102-113.
4. Marik PE, Weinmann M. Optimizing fluid therapy in shock. *Curr Opin Crit Care.* 2019;25(3):246-251.
5. Hardaway RM. Wound shock: A history of its study and treatment by military surgeons. *Mil Med.* 2004 Apr;169(4):265-269.
6. Trunkey DD. History and development of trauma care in the United States. *Clin Orthop Relat Res.* 2000;(374):36-46.
7. Hanigan WC, Sloffer C. Nelson's wound: Treatment of spinal cord injury in 19th and early 20th century military conflicts. *Neurosurg Focus.* 2004;16(1):E4.
8. Kelly PJ. Vietnam, 1968-1969: A place and a year like no other. *Neurosurgery.* 2003;52(4):927-939; discussion 939-943.
9. Kheng CP, Rahman NH. The use of end-tidal carbon dioxide monitoring in patients with hypotension in the emergency department. *Int J Emerg Med.* 2012;5:31.
10. Halacli B, Kaya A, Topeli A. Critically-ill COVID-19 patient. *Turk J Med Sci.* 2020;50(SI-1):585-591.
11. Phua J, Weng L, Ling L, Egi M, Lim CM. Intensive care management of coronavirus disease 2019 (COVID-19): Challenges and recommendations. *Lancet Respir Med.* 2020;10:S2213-2600.
12. Chen X, Liao B, Cheng L, et al. The microbial coinfection in COVID-19. *Appl Microbiol Biotechnol.* 2020;104(18):7777-7785.
13. Arabi YM, Harthi A, Hussein J, et al. Severe neurologic syndrome associated with Middle East respiratory syndrome corona virus (MERS-CoV). *Infection.* 2015;43(4):495-501.
14. The Who MERS-CoV Research Group. State of knowledge and data gaps of Middle East Respiratory Syndrome Coronavirus (MERS-CoV) in humans. *PLoS Curr.* 2013;5.
15. Chow EJ, Doyle JD, Uyeki TM. Influenza virus-related critical illness: Prevention, diagnosis, treatment. *Crit Care.* 2019;23(1):214.
16. Reed C, Chaves SS, Daily Kirley P, et al. Estimating influenza disease burden from population-based surveillance data in the United States. *PLoS One.* 2015;10(3):e0118369.
17. Iuliano AD, Roguski KM, Chang HH, et al. Estimates of global seasonal influenza-associated respiratory mortality: A modelling study. *Lancet.* 2018;391(10127): 1285-1300.
18. Minchole E, Figueredo AL, Omeñaca M, et al. Seasonal influenza A H1N1pdm09 virus and severe outcomes: A reason for broader vaccination in non-elderly, at-risk people. *PLoS One.* 2016;11(11):e0165711.

19. Doyle TM, Matuschak GM, Lechner AJ. Septic shock and nonpulmonary organ dysfunction in pneumonic plague: The role of Yersinia pestis pCD1- vs. pgm-virulence factors. *Crit Care Med.* 2010;38(7):1574-1583.

20. Meregildo-Rodriguez ED, Villegas-Chiroque M. Peste septicémica rápidamente fatal secundaria a peste bubónica primaria inicialmente no diagnosticada: Reporte de caso [Rapidly fatal septicemic plague secondary to undiagnosed primary bubonic plague: case report]. *Rev Peru Med Exp Salud Publica.* 2019;36(3):515-519. Spanish.

21. Sebbane F, Jarrett CO, Gardner D, Long D, Hinnebusch BJ. Role of the Yersinia pestis plasminogen activator in the incidence of distinct septicemic and bubonic forms of flea-borne plague. *Proc Natl Acad Sci U S A.* 2006;103(14):5526-5530.

22. Nelwan EJ. Early detection of plasma leakage in dengue hemorrhagic fever. *Acta Med Indones.* 2018;50(3):183-184.

23. Ranjit S, Kissoon N. Dengue hemorrhagic fever and shock syndromes. *Pediatr Crit Care Med.* 2011;12(1):90-100.

24. Junaid A, Tang H, van Reeuwijk A, et al. Ebola hemorrhagic shock syndrome-on-a-chip. *iScience.* 2020;23(1):100765.

25. Shayan S, Bokaean M, Shahrivar MR, Chinikar S. Crimean-Congo hemorrhagic fever. *Lab Med.* 2015;46(3):180-189.

26. Auwaerter PG, Penn RL. Francisella tularensis (Tularemia). In: Bennet JE, Dolin R, Blaser MJ, eds. *Mandell, Douglas, and Bennett's Principles and Practice of Infectious Diseases.* 9th ed. Philadelphia: Elsevier; 2015:2759.

27. Guha-Sapir D, Hoyois P, Below R. Annual disaster statistical review 2015 [Internet]. Brussels, Belgium: Centre for Research on the Epidemiology of Disasters; 2016 [cited 2017 Oct 5]. 50. Available from http://www.cred.be/sites/default/files/ADSR_2015.pdf.

28. Definitions: emergencies: World Health Organization; Available at http://www.who.int/hac/about/definitions/en/.

29. EM-DAT: The international disaster database [Internet]. Centre for Research on the Epidemiology of Disasters. [cited 2017-10-31]. Available at http://www.emdat.be/.

30. Bell SA, Abir A, Choi H, Cooke C, Iwashyna T. All-cause hospital admissions among older adults after a natural disaster, August 2017. *Ann Emerg Med.* 2018;71(6):746-754.e2.

31. Center for Disease Control and Prevention. Fatal fungal soft-tissue infections after a tornado – Joplin, Missouri, 2011. *MMWR Morb Mortal Wkly Rep.* 2011;60:992.

32. Alvarez E, Stchigel AM, Cano J, et al. Molecular phylogenetic diversity of the emerging, mucoralean fungus *Apophysomyces*: Proposal of three new species. *Rev Iberoam Micol.* 2010;27: 80-89.

33. Kouadio IK, Kamigaki AS, Hammad K, Oshitani H. Infectious disease following natural disasters: Prevention and control measure. *Expert Rev Anti Infect Ther.* 2012;10(1):95-104.

34. Stefanidou M, Athanaselis S, Spiliopoulou C. Health impacts of fire smoke inhalation. *Inhal Toxicol.* 2008;20(8):761-766.

35. Fayard GM. Fatal work injuries involving natural disasters, 1992–2006. *Disaster Med Public Health Prep.* 2009;3(4):201-209.

36. Shusterman D, Kaplan JZ, Canabarro C. Immediate health effects of an urban wildfire. *West J Med.* 1993;158(2):133-138.

37. Pereira BM, Morales W, Cardoso RG, Fiorelli R, Fraga GP, Briggs SM. Lessons learned from a landslide catastrophe in Rio de Janeiro, Brazil. *Am J Disaster Med.* 2013;8(4):253-258.

38. Kennedy IT, Petley DN, Williams R, Murray V. A systematic review of the health impacts of mass Earth movements (landslides). *PLoS Curr.* 2015;7. A recent systematic review analyzing existing studies on mortality and morbidity during landslides, concluding the lack of evidence regarding physical health effects.

39. Baxter PJ, Jenkins S, Seswandhana R, et al. Human survival in volcanic eruptions: thermal injuries in pyroclastic surges, their causes, prognosis and emergency management. *Burns.* 2017;43(5):1051-1069.

40. Bernstein RS, Baxter PJ, Falk H, Ing R, Foster L, Frost F. Immediate public health concerns and actions in volcanic eruptions: lessons from the Mount St. Helens eruptions, May 18-October 18, 1980. *Am J Public Health.* 1986;76(3 Suppl):25-37.

41. Centers for Disease C, Prevention Community needs assessment and morbidity surveillance following an ice storm—Maine, January 1998. *MMWR Morb Mortal Wkly Rep.* 1998;47(17):351-354.

42. Hartling L, Pickett W, Brison RJ. The injury experience observed in two emergency departments in Kingston, Ontario during "ice storm 98." *Can J Public Health Rev Can Sante Publique.* 1999;90(2):95-98.

43. Toloo GS, Yu W, Aitken P, FitzGerald G, Tong S. The impact of heatwaves on emergency department visits in Brisbane, Australia: A time series study. *Crit Care (Lond, Engl).* 2014;18(2):R69.

44. Katsouyanni K, Trichopoulos D, Zavitsanos X, Touloumi G. The 1987 Athens heatwave. *Lancet.* 1988;2(8610):573.

45. Bortolin M, Morelli I, Voskanyan A, Joyce NR, Ciottone GR. Earthquake-related orthopedic injuries in adult population: a systematic review. *Prehosp Disaster Med.* 2017;32(2):201-208.

46. Ramirez M, Peek-Asa C. Epidemiology of traumatic injuries from earthquakes. *Epidemiol Rev.* 2005;27:47-55.

47. Liang NJ, Shih YT, Shih FY, Wu HM, Wang HJ, Shi SF, Liu MY, Wang BB. Disaster epidemiology and medical response in the Chi-Chi earthquake in Taiwan. *Ann Emerg Med.* 2001;38(5):549-555.

48. Llewellyn M. Floods and tsunamis. *Surg Clin N Am.* 2006;86(3):557-578.

49. Jonkman SN, Kelman I. An analysis of the causes and circumstances of flood disaster deaths. *Disasters.* 2005;29(1):75-97.

50. Burton H, Rabito F, Danielson L, Takaro TK. Health effects of flooding in Canada: A 2015 review and description of gaps in research. *Can Water Resour J.* 2016;41(1-2):238-249.

51. Rotheray KR, Aitken P, Goggins WB, Rainer TH, Graham CA. Epidemiology of injuries due to tropical cyclones in Hong Kong: A retrospective observational study. *Injury.* 2012;43(12):2055-2059.

52. Doocy S, Dick A, Daniels A, Kirsch TD. The human impact of tropical cyclones: A historical review of events 1980–2009 and systematic literature review. *PLoS Curr.* 2013;5:16.

53. Mazumdar, S, Mazmdar PG, Kanjilal B, Singh PK. Multiple shocks, coping and welfare consequences: Natural disasters and health shock in the Indian Sundarbans. *PLoS One*. 2014;9(8):e105427.

54. Watson T, Gayer M, Connolly MA. Epidemics after natural disasters. *Emerg Infec Dis*. 2007;13(1):1-5.

55. Vincent JL, De Backer D. Circulatory shock. *N Engl J Med*. 2013;369:1726.

56. Van Sickle C, Schafer K, Grudic GZ, et al. A sensitive shock index for real-time patient assessment during simulated hemorrhage. *Avait Space Environ Med*. 2013;84(9):907-912.

57. Lakhal K, Macq C, Ehrmann S, et al. Noninvasive monitoring of blood pressure in the critically ill: Reliability according to the cuff site (arm, thigh, or ankle). *Crit Care Med*. 2012;40(4):1207-1213.

58. Muntner P, Shimbo D, Carey RM., et al. Measurement of Blood Pressure in Humans: A Scientific Statement in the American Heart Association. *Hypertension*. 2019;73:e35-e66.

59. Williams DJ, Bayliss R, Hinchliffe R. Surgical technique. Intravenous access: Obtaining large-bore access in the shocked patient. *Ann R Coll Surg Engl*. 1997;79(6):466.

60. Reddick AD, Ronald J, Morrison WG. Intravenous fluid resuscitation: Was Poiseuille right? *Emerg Med J*. 2011;28:201.

61. Foëx BA. Discovery of the intraosseous route for fluid administration. *J Accid Emerg Med*. 2000;17:136.

62. Valdes MM. Intraosseous fluid administration in emergencies. *Lancet*. 1977;1:1235.

63. Drozd A, Madziała M. Which vascular access technique should be chosen during hypovolemic shock? *Am J Emerg Med*. 2016;34(9):1886-1887.

64. Cordova CB, Cap AP, Spinella PC. Fresh whole blood transfusion for a combat casualty in austere combat environment. *J Spec Oper Med*. 2014;14:9-12.

65. Hunsaker S, Hillis D. Intraosseous vascular access for alert patients. *Am J Nurs*. 2013;113(11):34-39.

66. Monnet X, Bataille A, Magalhaes E, et al. End-tidal carbon dioxide is better than arterial pressure for predicting volume responsiveness by the passive leg raising test. *Intensive Care Med*. 2013;39(1):93-100.

67. Monnet X, Rienzo M, Osman D, et al. Passive leg raising predicts fluid responsiveness in the critically ill. *Crit Care Med*. 2006;34(5):1402-1407.

68. Préau S, Saulnier F, Dewavrin F, Durocher A, Chagnon JL. Passive leg raising is predictive of fluid responsiveness in spontaneously breathing patients with severe sepsis or acute pancreatitis. *Crit Care Med*. 2010;38(3):819-825.

69. Rapid Review-Evidence Summary: Use of Trendelenburg for Hypotension. McGill University Health Centre: Division of Nursing Research and MUHC Libraries. October 2015.

70. Geerts BF, Bergh LVD, Stijnen T, et al. Comprehensive review: Is it better to use Trendelenberg position or passive leg raising for the initial treatment of hypovolemia? *J Clin Anesth*. 2012;24(8):668-674.

71. Finfer S, Myburgh J, Bellomo R. Intravenous fluid therapy in critically ill adults. *Nat Rev Nephrol*. 2018;14(9):541-557. Erratum in: *Nat Rev Nephrol*. 2018;14(11):717.

72. Hoorn EJ. Intravenous fluids: Balancing solutions. *J Nephrol*. 2017;30(4):485-492. Erratum in: *J Nephrol*. 2020;33(2):387.

73. Goldfarb DS. The normal saline ceremony. *Am J Kidney Dis.* 2010;56(2):A28-A29.

74. Quinlan GJ, Martin GS, Evans TW. Albumin: Biochemical properties and therapeutic potential. *Hepatol Baltim Md.* 2005;41:1211-1219.

75. Casey JD, Brown RM, Semler MW. Resuscitation fluids. *Curr Opin Crit Care.* 2018;24(6):512-518.

76. Pfortmueller CA, Funk G-C, Reiterer C, et al. Normal saline versus a balanced crystalloid for goal-directed perioperative fluid therapy in major abdominal surgery: A double-blind randomised controlled study. *Br J Anaesth.* 2018;120:274-283.

77. Semler MW, Self WH, Wanderer JP, et al. Balanced crystalloids versus saline in critically ill adults. *N Engl J Med.* 2018;378:829-839.

78. Self WH, Semler MW, Wanderer JP, et al. Balanced crystalloids versus saline in noncritically ill adults. *N Engl J Med.* 2018;378:819-828.

79. Jaber S, Paugam C, Futier E, et al. Sodium bicarbonate therapy for patients with severe metabolic acidaemia in the intensive care unit (BICAR-ICU): A multicentre, open-label, randomised controlled, phase 3 trial. *Lancet Lond Engl.* 2018;392:31-40.

80. Finfer S, Bellomo R, Boyce N, et al. A comparison of albumin and saline for fluid resuscitation in the intensive care unit. *N Engl J Med.* 2004;350:2247-2256.

81. Myburgh JA, Finfer S, Bellomo R, et al. Hydroxyethyl starch or saline for fluid resuscitation in intensive care. *N Engl J Med.* 2012;367:1901-1911.

82. Brunkhorst FM, Engel C, Bloos F, et al. Intensive insulin therapy and pentastarch resuscitation in severe sepsis. *N Engl J Med.* 2008;358:125-139.

83. Guidet B, Martinet O, Boulain T, et al. Assessment of hemodynamic efficacy and safety of 6% hydroxyethylstarch 130/0.4 vs. 0.9% NaCl fluid replacement in patients with severe sepsis: The CRYSTMAS study. *Crit Care Lond Engl.* 2012;16:R94.

84. Perner A, Haase N, Guttormsen AB, et al. Hydroxyethyl starch 130/0.42 versus Ringer's acetate in severe sepsis. *N Engl J Med.* 2012;367:124-134.

85. Lewis SR, Pritchard MW, Evans DJ, et al. Colloids versus crystalloids for fluid resuscitation in critically ill people. *Cochrane Database Syst Rev.* 2018; 8:CD000567.

86. Tilton LJ, Eginger KH. Utility of push-dose vasopressors for temporary treatment of hypotension in the emergency department. *J Emerg Nurs.* 2016;42(3): 279-281.

87. Stratton L, Berlin DA, Arbo JE. Vasopressors and inotropes in sepsis. *Emerg Med Clin North Am.* 2017;35(1):75-91.

88. Kislitsina ON, Rich JD, Wilcox JE, Pham DT, et al. Shock - Classification and pathophysiological principles of therapeutics. *Curr Cardiol Rev.* 2019;15(2): 102-113.

89. Manaker S. (2019). Use of vasopressors and inotropes. In: UpToDate, Polly, PE (Ed), Finlay, G (Ed), Use of vasopressors and inotropes. Available at https://www.uptodate.com/contents/use-of-vasopressors-andinotropes?search= vasopressors%20inotropes&source=search_result&selectedTitle=1~150&usage_ type=default&display_rank=1. Updated May July 3, 2020. Accessed May 2021.

90. Overgaard CB, Dzavik V. Inotropes and vasopressors: Review of physiology and clinical use in cardiovascular disease. *Circulation*. 2008;118(10):1047-1056.

91. Bussard RL, Busse LW. Angiotensin II: A new therapeutic option for vasodilatory shock. *Ther Clin Risk Manag*. 2018;14:1287-1298.

92. Huynh N, Kloke J, Gu C, et al. The effect of hypothermia "dose" on vasopressor requirements and outcome after cardiac arrest. *Resuscitation*. 2013;84(2):189-193.

93. Hypothermia after Cardiac Arrest Study Group. Mild therapeutic hypothermia to improve the neurologic outcome after cardiac arrest. *N Engl J Med*. 2002;346(8):549-556.

94. Bernard SA, Gray TW, Buist MD, et al. Treatment of comatose survivors of out-of-hospital cardiac arrest with induced hypothermia. *N Engl J Med*. 2002;346:557-563.

95. Weil MH, Hole DB, Brown EB Jr, Campbell GS, Heath C. Vasopressor agents; Influence of acidosis on cardiac and vascular responsiveness. *Calif Med*. 1958;88(6):437-440.

96. Vidal C, Grassin-Delyle S, Devillier P, et al. Effect of severe acidosis on vasoactive effects of epinephrine and norepinephrine in human distal mammary artery. *J Thorac Cardiovasc Surg* 2014;147(5):1698-1705.

97. Boyd JH, Forbes J, Nakada TA, Walley KR, Russell JA. Fluid resuscitation in septic shock: A positive fluid balance and elevated central venous pressure are associated with increased mortality. *Crit Care Med*. 2011;39:259-265.

98. Murphy CV, Schramm GE, Doherty JA, et al. The importance of fluid management in acute lung injury secondary to septic shock. *Chest*. 2009;136:102-109.

99. Monnet X, Marik PE, Teboul JL. Prediction of fluid responsiveness: An update. *Ann Intensive Care*. 2016;6(1):111.

100. Huygh J, Peeters Y, Bernards J, Malbrain ML. Hemodynamic monitoring in the critically ill: An overview of current cardiac output monitoring methods. *F1000Res*. 2016;5:F1000 Faculty Rev-2855.

101. Bkker J, Gris P, Coffernils M, Kahn RJ, Vincent JL. Serial blood lactate levels can predict the development of multiple organ failure following septic shock. *Am J Surg*. 1996;171(2):221-226.

102. Das JM, Anosike K, Waseem M. Permissive Hypotension in: StatPearls [Internet]. Treasure Island (FL): StatPearls Publishing; 2020 Jan. Available from: https://www.ncbi.nlm.nih.gov/books/NBK430685/. Accessed October 13, 2020.

103. Bickell WH, Wall MJ, Pepe PE, et al. Immediate versus delayed fluid resuscitation for hypotensive patients with penetrating torso injuries. *N Engl J Med*. 1994;331(17):1105-1109.

104. Morrison CA, Carrick MM, Norman MA, et al. Hypotensive resuscitation strategy reduces transfusion requirements and severe postoperative coagulopathy in trauma patients with hemorrhagic shock: Preliminary results of a randomized controlled trial. *J Trauma*. 2011;70(3):652-663.

105. Dinarello CA. Cytokines as mediators in the pathogenesis of septic shock. *Curr Top Microbiol Immunol*. 1996;216:133-165.

106. Chrousos G. The role of stress and the hypothalamic–pituitary–adrenal axis in the pathogenesis of the metabolic syndrome: neuro-endocrine and target tissue-related causes. *Int J Obes*. 2000;24:S50-S55.

107. Standl T, Annecke T, Cascorbi I, Heller AR, Sabashnikov A, Teske W. The nomenclature, definition and distinction of types of shock. *Dtsch Arztebl Int.* 2018;115(45):757-768.

108. McLean AS. Echocardiography in shock management. *Crit Care.* 2016;20:275.

109. Thiele H, Zeymer U, Thelemann N, et al. Intraaortic balloon pump in cardiogenic shock complicating after myocardial infarction: Long-term 6-year outcome of the randomized IABP-Shock II Trial. *Circulation.* 2019;139:395-403.

110. Wang JI, Lu DY, Feldman DN, et al. Outcomes of hospitalizations for cardiogenic shock at left ventricular assist device versus non–left ventricular assist device centers. *J Am Heart Assoc.* 2020;9(23):e017326.

111. Chan CM, Woods C, Shorr AF. The validation and reproducibility of the pulmonary embolism severity index. *J Thromb Haemost.* 2010;8(7):1509-1514.

112. Casazza F, Bongarzoni A, Capozi A, Agostoni O. Regional right ventricular dysfunction in acute pulmonary embolism and right ventricular infarction. *Eur J Echocardiogr.* 2005;6:11-14.

113. McConnell MV, Solomon SD, Rayan ME, et al. Regional right ventricular dysfunction detected by echocardiography in acute pulmonary embolus. *Am J Cardiol.* 1996;78:469-473.

114. Casazza F, Bongarzoni A, Capozi A, Agostoni O. Regional right ventricular dysfunction in acute pulmonary embolism and right ventricular infarction. *Eur J Echocardiogr.* 2005;6:11-14.

115. Tobicki A. Echocardiography diagnosis of pulmonary embolism: A rise and fall of McConnell sign. *Eur J Echocardiogr.* 2005;6:2-3.

116. Ristic AD, Imazio M, Adler Y, et al. Triage strategy for urgent management of cardiac tamponade: A position statement of the European Society of Cardiology Working Group on Myocardial and Pericardial Disease. *Eur Heart J.* 2014;35:2279-2284.

117. Pulido JN, Afessa B, Masaki M, et al. Clinical spectrum, frequency, and significance of myocardial dysfunction in severe sepsis and septic shock. *Mayo Clinic Proc.* 2012:87(7):620-628.

118. Kawaji T, Shiomi H, Morimoto T, et al. Clinical impact of left ventricular outflow tract obstruction in Takotsubo cardiomyopathy. *Circ.* 2015;79(4):839-846.

119. Jardin F, Dubourg O, Bourdarias JP. Echocardiographic pattern of acute cor pulmonale. *Chest.* 1997;111:209-217.

120. Mandeville JC, Colebourn CL. Predicting fluid responsiveness in the critically ill adult. *Br J Intensive Care.* 2013;23:20-26.

121. Cavallaro F, Sandroni CF, Marano C, et al. Review: Diagnostic accuracy of passive leg raising for prediction of fluid responsiveness in adults: Systematic review and meta-analysis of clinical studies. *Intensive Care Med.* 2010; 36(9):1475-83.

122. Monnet X, Marik PE, Teboul JL. Prediction of fluid responsiveness: An update. *Ann Intensive Care.* 2016;6:111.

123. Marik PE, Cavallazzi R, Vasu T, Hirani A. Dynamic changes in arterial waveform derived variables and fluid responsiveness in mechanically ventilated patients: A systematic review of the literature. *Crit Care Med.* 2009;37:2642-2647.

124. Muller L, Toumi M, Bousquet PJ, et al. An increase in aortic blood flow after an infusion of 100 ml colloid over 1 minute Can Predict Fluid Responsiveness: The Mini-Fluid Challenge Study. *Anesthesiology.* 2011;115(3):541-547.

125. Pourmand A, Pyle M, Yamane D, Sumon K, Frasure S. The utility of point-of-care ultrasound in the assessment of volume status in acute and critically ill patient. *World J Emerg Med.* 2019;10(4):232-238.

126. Barbier C, Loubières Y, Schmit C, Hayon J, Ricôme JL, Jardin F, Vieillard-Baron A. Respiratory changes in inferior vena cava diameter are helpful in predicting fluid responsiveness in ventilated septic patients. *Intensive Care Med.* 2004;30(9):1740-1746.

127. Sivakumar S, Lazaridis C. Bioreactance-based noninvasive fluid responsiveness and cardiac output monitoring: A pilot study in patients with aneurysmal subarachnoid hemorrhage and literature review. *Crit Care Res Pract.* 2020;2020:2748181.

128. Jones TW, Houghton D, Cassidy S, MacGowan GA, Trenell MI, Jakovlievic DG. Bioreactance is a reliable method for estimating cardiac output at rest and during exercise. *Br J Anaesth.* 2015;115(3):386-391.

129. Scott MG, Kucik DF, Goodnough LT, Monk TG. Blood substitutes: Evolution and future applications. *Clin Chem.* 1997;43:1724.

130. Natanson C, Kern SJ, Lurie P, et al. Cell-free hemoglobin-based blood substitutes and risk of myocardial infarction and death: A meta-analysis. *JAMA.* 2008;299:2304.

131. Schramko A, Suojaranta-Ylinen R, Kuitunen A, et al. Hydroxyethylstarch and gelatin solutions impair blood coagulation after cardiac surgery: A prospective randomized trial. *Br J Anaesth.* 2010;104:691.

132. Wiedermann CJ. Hydroxyethyl starch—Can the safety problems be ignored? *Wien Klin Wochenschr.* 2004;116:583.

133. Gattas DJ, Dan A, Myburgh J, et al. Fluid resuscitation with 6% hydroxyethyl starch (130/0.4 and 130/0.42) in acutely ill patients: systematic review of effects on mortality and treatment with renal replacement therapy. *Intensive Care Med.* 2013;39:558.

134. Zarychanski R, Abou-Setta AM, Turgeon AF, et al. Association of hydroxyethyl starch administration with mortality and acute kidney injury in critically ill patients requiring volume resuscitation: a systematic review and meta-analysis. *JAMA.* 2013;309:678.

135. Haase N, Wetterslev J, Winkel P, Perner A. Bleeding and risk of death with hydroxyethyl starch in severe sepsis: Post hoc analyses of a randomized clinical trial. *Intensive Care Med.* 2013;39:2126.

136. Howell MD, Davis AM. Management of sepsis and septic shock. *JAMA.* 2017;317:847.

137. Bancos I, Hahner S, Tomlinson J, et al. Diagnosis and management of adrenal insufficiency. *Lancet Diabetes Endocrinol.* 2015;3:216-226.

138. Téblick A, Peeters B, Langouche L, Van den Berghe G. Adrenal function and dysfunction in critically ill patients. *Nat Rev Endocrinol.* 2019;15(7):417-427.

139. Kumar B, Kodliwadmath A, Singh A, Duggal B. Acute adrenal insufficiency as a mysterious cause of shock following percutaneous coronary intervention: A cardiologist's nightmare. *BMJ Case Rep.* 2020;13(3):e233585.

140. Mathew V, Misgar RA, Ghosh S, et al. Myxedema coma: A new look into an old crisis. *J Thyroid Res.* 2011;2011:493462.

141. Ono Y, Ono S, Yasunaga H, et al. Clinical characteristics and outcomes of myxedema coma: Analysis of a national inpatient database in Japan. *J Epidemiol.* 2017;27:117.

142. Mathew V, Misgar RA, Ghosh S, et al. Myxedema coma: A new look into an old crisis. *J Thyroid Res.* 2011;2011:493462.

143. Engelberger RP, Kucher N. Reperfusion treatment for acute pulmonary embolism. *Hamostaseologie.* 2018;38(2):98-105.

144. Howard L. Acute pulmonary embolism. *Clin Med* (Lond). 2019;19(3):243-247. Erratum in: *Clin Med* (Lond). 2019 Jul;19(4):359.

145. Martinez Licha CR, McCurdy CM, Maldonado SM, Lee LS. Current management of acute pulmonary embolism. *Ann Thorac Cardiovasc Surg.* 2020;26(2):65-71.

146. Imazio M, Adler Y. Management of pericardial effusion. *Eur Heart J.* 2013;34(16):1186-1197.

147. Vakamudi S, Ho N, Cremer PC. Pericardial effusions: Causes, diagnosis, and management. *Prog Cardiovasc Dis.* 2017;59(4):380-388.

148. Abdel-Wahab M, Saad M, Kynast J, et al. Comparison of hospital mortality with intra-aortic balloon counterpulsation insertion before versus after primary percutaneous coronary intervention for cardiogenic shock complicating acute myocardial infarction. *Am J Cardiol.* 2010;105:967.

149. Sanborn TA, Sleeper LA, Bates ER, et al. Impact of thrombolysis, intra-aortic balloon pump counterpulsation, and their combination in cardiogenic shock complicating acute myocardial infarction: a report from the SHOCK Trial Registry. Should we emergently revascularize occluded coronaries for cardiogenic shock? *J Am Coll Cardiol.* 2000;36:1123.

150. Schrage B, Ibrahim K, Loehn T, et al. Impella support for acute myocardial infarction complicated by cardiogenic shock. *Circulation.* 2019;139:1249.

151. Ibanez B, James S, Agewall S, et al. 2017 ESC guidelines for the management of acute myocardial infarction in patients presenting with ST-segment elevation: The task force for the management of acute myocardial infarction in patients presenting with ST-segment elevation of the European Society of Cardiology (ESC). *Eur Heart J.* 2018;39:119.

152. Hochman JS. Cardiogenic shock complicating acute myocardial infarction: Expanding the paradigm. *Circulation.* 2003;107:2998.

153. Indications for fibrinolytic therapy in suspected acute myocardial infarction: Collaborative overview of early mortality and major morbidity results from all randomised trials of more than 1000 patients. Fibrinolytic Therapy Trialists' (FTT) Collaborative Group. *Lancet.* 1994;343:311.

154. French JK, Feldman HA, Assmann SF, et al. Influence of thrombolytic therapy, with or without intra-aortic balloon counterpulsation, on 12-month survival in the SHOCK trial. *Am Heart J.* 2003;146:804.

8 ANALGESIA, SEDATION, AND MECHANICAL VENTILATION

Ronaldo C. Go, MD, Ruchi Jain, PharmD,
Jason Steinfeld, BHA, RPT, and Bisma Alam, MD

▍ INTRODUCTION

Mass casualty events (MCEs) are defined as "act[s] of bioterrorism or other public health or medical emergenc[ies]" and constitute national disasters, pandemics or acts of terrorism.[1] The response to these disasters is rapidly becoming a new reality as they continue to overwhelm health care systems. Over the last several decades, the United States has witnessed an increase in these events and as a consequence, hospital and intensive care units (ICUs) around the nation have been urged to develop emergency preparedness protocols. However, there are many challenges that may hinder delivery of standard of care to patients during MCEs, including lack of equipment and supplies and increased demand for resources. Currently, the coronavirus disease 2019 (COVID-19) is the mass casualty event. In this chapter, we aim to summarize potential strategies when mechanical ventilation and pharmaceutical services are limited.

▍ THERAPEUTIC OPTIONS FOR ANALGESIA, SEDATION, AND PARALYSIS IN MECHANICALLY VENTILATED PATIENTS IN THE SETTING OF DRUG SHORTAGES

Pandemics and global sedative shortages have led to a significant increase in demand for analgesics and sedative medications that are essential for the care of critically ill patients.[2-4] This may be attributed to interruption in supply chain, production delays, or increased demand due to higher patient census and acuity.[2] In the case of the COVID-19 pandemic, dramatic increase in patients requiring mechanical ventilation along with analgesics/sedatives to maintain ventilator synchrony and impending exhaustion of these vital agents necessitated exploring safe clinical alternatives.[5] While creating a document providing information on therapeutic alternatives is vital, it is also necessary to develop drug conservation strategies.[2,6] This may be accomplished by performing vigilant inventory tracking, prioritizing supply to the patients who are most likely to benefit and conducting prospective monitoring to limit inappropriate utilization. This is crucial to minimize depletion of the supply on hand.[2,6] The purpose of this section is to provide recommendations for standard and non-standard therapeutic options when faced with medication shortages or limited availability.

General Principles

When faced with shortage situations, it is important to remain mindful of general principles and overarching themes of pharmacotherapy management, as recommended by the Society of Critical Care Medicine's PADIS guidelines.[7] For example, current guidelines recommend analgesia-first or analgosedation (the administration of an analgesic agent before sedative administration) due to the premise that pain is commonly experienced in critically ill patients and is a major reason for agitation.[7] If the absence of pain or discomfort or if analgosedation is inadequate, sedative agents may be required.[7] Non–benzodiazepine-based sedation (e.g., dexmedetomidine or propofol) may be preferred over benzodiazepine-based sedation due to a decrease in duration of mechanical ventilation, ICU length of stay, and frequency of delirium observed in clinical trials.[7] These agents are titrated to the desired clinical effect, guided by validated sedation/analgesia scoring tools (e.g., Richmond Agitation Sedation Scale, Riker Sedation-Agitation Scale, Critical Care Pain Observation Tool) to ensure adequate but not excessive sedation is achieved.[7] During a shortage, clinicians should consider alternative medications from the same class, and if this is not feasible, then an agent from the next tier should be selected. Tables 8-1 to 8-3 provide an overview of both of commonly used and alternative analgesic and sedatives, if shortages of first line medications occur.

Recommended Therapies for Analgesia

In mechanically ventilated patients in the ICU, opioids have become the mainstay of therapy for non-neuropathic pain.[7] They provide analgesia, but they also serve as sedatives at all doses. The three most common agents used are fentanyl, hydromorphone, and morphine. They primarily exert their pharmacological actions through u-receptors, with some also having kappa activity. Advantages include fast onset, ease of titration, provision of patient comfort and reversibility, and hemodynamically

Table 8-1   PROPERTIES AND DOSING OF ANALGESIC MEDICATIONS[5,16]

Opioids	Bolus dose	Intermittent IV Dose	Continuous infusion	Onset (min)	Metabolism	Active Metabolite	Elimination half-life
First-line therapy							
Fentanyl	25–100 mcg	0.35–0.5 mcg/kg every 30–60 min	0.7–10 mcg/kg/hour	1–2	Hepatic	No	2–4 hr
Hydromorphone	0.5–2 mg	0.2–0.6 mg q 1–2 hr	0.5–5 mg/hr	5–15	Hepatic	No	2–3 hr
Second-line therapy							
Morphine	2–10 mg	2–4 mg q 1–2 hr	0.5–30 mg/hr	5–10	Hepatic	Yes	3–4 hr
Ketamine (adjunct to reduce or conserve opioids)	0.1–0.5 mg/kg	0.1–0.5 mg/kg	0.2–1 mg/kg/hr	30–40 seconds	Hepatic	Yes	2–3 hr
Third-line therapy							
Methadone	N/A	2.5–10 IV q 8–12 hr	Not recommended	1–3 days	Hepatic	No	15–60 hr
Remifentanil	1.5 mcg.kg	N/A	0.5–15 mcg/kg/hr	1–3	Blood and tissue esterases	No	3–10 min
Fourth-line therapy							
Sufentanil	N/A	N/A	0.1–1.5 mcg/kg/hr	1–3	Hepatic	No	2–3 hr

Table 8-2   PROPERTIES AND DOSING OF SEDATIVE MEDICATIONS[5,16]

	Bolus dose	Intermittent dose	Continuous infusion	Onset (min)	Metabolism	Active Metabolite	Elimination half-life
First-line therapy							
Dexmedetomidine	1 mcg/kg*	N/A	0.2–1.5 mcg/kg/hr	5–10	Hepatic	No	2–3 hr
Propofol	N/A	N/A	5–50 mcg/kg/min	1–2	Hepatic and extrahepatic	No	3–12 hr; however duration is 3–10 min
Second-line therapy							
lorazepam	1–2 mg	0.5–4 mg every 2–6 hr	1–10 mg/hr	15–20	Hepatic	No	8–15 hr
Midazolam	1–5 mg	0.5–4 mg every 0.5–2 hr	1–10 mg/hr	2–5	Hepatic	Yes	3–11 hr
Ketamine	0.1–0.5 mg/kg	0.1–0.5 mg/kg	0.1–1 mg/kg/hr (light sedation) Doses > 1 mg/kg/hr (deep sedation)[5,14]	30–40 seconds	Hepatic	Yes—norketamine 33% as potent as parent compound	2–3 hr
Third-line therapy							
Phenobarbital	7.5 mg/kg	Sedation: 1–2 mg/kg/day divided every 12 hr Sedation withdrawal: 200 mg followed by 100 mg every 4 hr × 5 doses, 60 mg every 4 hr for 4 doses, and then 60 mg every 8 hr for 3 doses[5]	N/A	5	Hepatic	No	50–120 hr

*Optional due to risk of adverse hemodynamic effects. N/A: not applicable.

Agent	Dose	Time to onset	Half-life	Sedation	EPS	QTC prolongation
Haloperidol	2–10 mg IV q 6 hours	3 to 20 min	18–51 hr	Low	High	High (dose related)
Quetiapine	25–100 mg PO q 12 hours (max 400 mg/day)	20 to 30 min	12 hr	Moderate	Very low	Low
Olanzapine	5–10 mg once daily (max 20 mg daily)	6 hr (peak)	30 hr	Moderate	Low	Low

Table 8-3 ANTIPSYCHOTICS[5,21]

neutral on blood pressure (fentanyl and remifentanil). While all opioids are therapeutically equivalent at equianalgesic doses, the selection of a specific IV opioid agent depends upon pharmacokinetic parameters and adverse effect profile as they vary considerably among agents.

Opioid use is associated with number of side effects and can occur at all dose ranges. The most common side effects are gastrointestinal, respiratory, and central nervous system in nature, occurring in up to 80–90% of patients.[8,9] These may include constipation, dry mouth, nausea, vomiting, respiratory depression, sedation, dizziness, and urinary retention.[8-10] Constipation is commonly experienced by many ICU patients and often requires preemptive use of stool softeners and stimulant cathartics/osmotic agents to improve laxation (Table 8-4).[8] In refractory cases when conventional therapies fail, methylnaltrexone, a peripherally acting mu-receptor antagonist, may be required. It should be avoided in the presence of bowel obstruction because of the risk for intestinal perforation.[11] Respiratory depression is generally dose related and maybe problematic when it is interfering with efforts to wean in mechanically ventilated patients. While naloxone can reverse respiratory depression, it is not recommended after prolonged opioid use because of the risk of precipitating a withdrawal syndrome, including reversal of pain control, tachycardia, pulmonary edema, and hypertension.[8] It is best to withhold further opioids until respiratory rate or ventilation improves.

Tolerance, withdrawal and opioid-induced hyperalgesia can also occur with prolonged use of continuous infusion of opioids.[10,12,13] Other less common reactions include chest wall rigidity (at high doses primarily with fentanyl), histamine release causing urticarial, hypotension, and flushing (primarily with morphine).[14]

Table 8-4	COMMONLY USED MEDICATIONS FOR THE TREATMENT OF CONSTIPATION IN MECHANICALLY VENTILATED PATIENTS			
Type of laxative	**Examples**	**Mechanism of action**	**Dosage**	**Comments**
Stool softeners	Docusate sodium	Reduces the surface tension of the oil-water interface of the stool, allowing incorporation of water and fat into the stools with resultant softening	Usual dose: 100 mg twice daily	Usually combined with a stimulant laxative as a first-line therapy for opioid-induced constipation
Stimulant laxatives	Senna	Increases water and electrolyte secretion by the intestinal mucosa to stimulate peristalsis	Starting dose: 10–15 mL once daily increasing to a maximum of 15 mL twice daily	Usually combined with a stool softener as first-line approach for opioid-induced constipation
	Bisacodyl		Rectal: 10 mg once daily	May cause gastric irritation
Osmotic laxatives	Lactulose	Synthetic disaccharide that is not metabolized by the intestinal enzymes; thus water and electrolytes remain in the intestinal lumen producing an osmotic effect	Starting dose: 15–30 mL (10 to 20 g) daily increasing to a maximum of 20 mL three times daily	Slower onset; it requires 24 to 48 hours to achieve its effect
	Polyethylene glycol	An osmotic agent, polyethylene glycol 3350 causes water retention in the stool; increases stool frequency	17 g once daily and titrate up to maximum of 34 g	• Preferred due to fewer adverse effects • Slower onset; it may require up to 72 hours to produce a bowel movement
	Magnesium citrate	Causes osmotic retention of fluid leading to increased peristaltic activity	195–300 mL single dose	Caution in patients with renal insufficiency

(Continued)

Table 8-4 COMMONLY USED MEDICATIONS FOR THE TREATMENT OF CONSTIPATION IN MECHANICALLY VENTILATED PATIENTS (*CONTINUED*)

Type of laxative	Examples	Mechanism of action	Dosage	Comments
Opioid antagonist (many agents in this class with methylnaltrexone being the most studied)	Methylnaltrexone	Peripheral acting opioid antagonist, thereby inhibiting opioid induced decreased gastrointestinal motility and delay in gastrointestinal transit time	Subq according to weight: • 38 to < 62 kg: 8 mg • 62 to 114 kg: 12 mg • 114 kg: 0.15 mg/kg Maximum: 1 dose/24 hours	• Reserved for refractory cases • Does not induce systemic symptoms of opioid withdrawal • Caution in administering to patients with known or suspected lesions in the intestinal wall (e.g. Ogilvie's syndrome, diverticular disease, infiltrative GI tract malignancies) due to concerns of bowel perforation

Fentanyl is a synthetic opioid and remains the most widely used opioid in the ICU setting due to rapid onset (<1 minute due to greater lipid solubility) and shorter half-life (30 minutes to 2 hours) allowing for easy titration to achieve desired effect. It is 100 times more potent than morphine and lacks histamine-releasing properties. It is largely metabolized in the liver by cytochrome P450 system to norfentanyl, an inactive metabolite, that is then renally excreted. The higher lipophilicity of fentanyl can cause accumulation in the adipose tissue leading to increase in its duration of action. Rapid bolus doses of fentanyl should be administered cautiously as this has been associated with chest-wall rigidity.[14,15] This phenomenon is uncommon but can result in reduced chest wall compliance, making rescue assisted ventilation difficult. It has been primarily described in pediatric patients and following elective procedures. Among adults, it is unlikely to be observed unless bolus doses of 100 mcg are exceeded.[14] The exact mechanism remains poorly understood and appears to be potentiated by both dose and rate of injection administered.

Hydromorphone is a semisynthetic opioid with a relatively longer duration of action (~3 to 4 hr) than fentanyl. It is ~7 times more potent than morphine. It is also less lipophilic than fentanyl resulting in less distribution into the adipose tissue. It is hepatically cleared and does not significantly accumulate in patients with renal failure. For these reasons, hydromorphone may be a reasonable option as a continuous infusion, particularly if fentanyl is unavailable or its use is restricted. The longer duration of action also allows for intermittent dosing strategy.

Morphine is the standard by which other opioids are compared, but the use of morphine as continuous infusion has largely been replaced with fentanyl. Morphine is primarily metabolized in the liver to active metabolites, morphine-3-glucuronide and morphine-6-glucoronide, and these metabolites are eliminated by the kidneys. These metabolites are concerning because they may accumulate in patients with renal dysfunction. Collectively, these properties of relatively slow onset of action, histamine release, and potential for accumulation complicate and limit its utility in mechanically ventilated patients, unless other options are unavailable in shortage scenarios. Despite these shortcomings, it continues to be used for end-of-life for terminally ill patients, pain associated with myocardial infarction, and end of life related dyspnea and discomfort.

Remifentanil is an ultra-short acting mu opioid receptor agonist that possesses potency of one to two times that of fentanyl. It is more commonly employed as an infusion during general anesthesia or monitored anesthesia care. Although, limited data exists for its use for ICU analgesia and sedation, it's appealing due to its ideal pharmacokinetics.[5,16] It has a rapid onset and offset and unlike other opioids is metabolized by plasma esterases into inactive metabolites. This characteristic allows for easy titration without concerns of accumulation or unpredictable drug recovery. On the other hand, it may pose a risk for patients if the infusion is inadvertently interrupted exposing the patient to a loss of analgesia and acute opioid withdrawal.[14] Most of all, its high cost tends to make it prohibitive for more frequent use.

Sufentanil is a phenylpiperidine mu opioid agonist that is approximately 5 to 10 times more potent than fentanyl.[5] Similar to fentanyl, it is highly lipophilic with rapid onset, hepatically metabolized, and lower cost compared to remifentanil.[14] It is also mostly used during induction of general anesthesia.

Methadone is a synthetic opioid with unique characteristics that differentiate it from other opioids. It exerts its activity through binding and activation of mu-receptors as well as antagonizing N-methyl-D-aspartate (NMDA) receptors. It possesses a long duration of action with a half-life that varies from 15 to 60 hours depending on hepatic and CYPs 3A4 and 2B6 enzyme function.[16,17] Due to incomplete tolerance, delayed onset and lack of reliable dose conversions when transitioning from standard opioids, methadone should be initiated at a low dose 5 to 10 mg every 8 to 12 hours, regardless of previous opioid exposure.[5] It should be titrated no more frequently than every 3 to 5 days as methadone concentrations will not reach steady state for a period of 3 to 7 days.[18] A detailed strategy to transition patients from continuous infusion opioids to methadone is provided elsewhere.[17] In clinical practice, it has been employed to facilitate weaning from mechanical ventilation in a patient requiring prolonged or high doses of continuous infusion analgesia. Through this strategy, opioid withdrawal syndrome may be prevented.

Adverse effects such as respiratory depression, QT prolongation, serotonin syndrome, and constipation should be monitored during methadone therapy.[18] Close monitoring for signs of respiratory depression is required as methadone's peak respiratory effects last longer than its peak analgesic effects.[18] Additionally, risk factors for QT prolongation resulting in torsades de pointes include concurrent use with other QT_C prolonging medications, electrolyte imbalances, and presence of structural heart disease. Baseline EKG prior to initiation and with any dose titrations is recommended. Patients receiving methadone should be monitored for signs and symptoms of serotonin syndrome, particularly when used concurrently with other serotonergic medications.

Alternative Routes of Administration

Enteral and/or transdermal agents should be strongly considered to preserve supply of intravenous drugs. This may involve enteral administration of oxycodone or morphine, when possible. Transdermal fentanyl patches are a potential option in hemodynamically stable patients with more stable opioid requirements. However, it should be avoided for the management of acute pain due to 12 to 24 hours delay in onset of action and extent of absorption may be variable and dependent on temperature, permeability, and perfusion to the skin. This strategy should be limited to patients with functioning gastrointestinal tract.[8]

Intermittent or scheduled dosing of medications to facilitate weaning and conserve current supply of the standard agents can also be recommended, when clinically appropriate.[5] Opioids such as hydromorphone or oxycodone allow for intermittent dosing due to their reliably longer duration of action as compared to IV fentanyl.[5]

Recommended Therapies for Sedation

Benzodiazepines including midazolam and lorazepam are two of the most commonly used agents for ICU sedation. They exert their effect through mediating the GABA receptor, thereby providing anxiolysis and anterograde amnesia. They do not significantly cause alteration in blood pressure or heart rate. Benzodiazepine-based continuous sedation is no longer considered first-line therapy given the emerging evidence suggesting that they are associated with prolonged dependence on the ventilator and increased ICU length of stay as compared with propofol or dexmedetomidine.[7] This may be explained by delayed emergence from sedative effects due to prolonged administration, advanced age, and organ dysfunction(s).[16] Additionally, they have an unintended consequence of being associated with increased risk for delirium when administered continuously.[7]

Despite this evidence, benzodiazepines may be appropriate in select patient cases. For example, they may be preferred in patients requiring deep sedation (such as when neuromuscular blockade is used), premedication for procedures, seizures, alcohol withdrawal, and in other scenarios in conjunction with opioid-based analgosedation to sedate patients who are hemodynamically unstable since propofol and dexmedetomidine are commonly associated with hypotension.

When selecting among benzodiazepines, factors influencing decision include onset and duration of action, potency, hepatic dysfunction, renal impairment. Midazolam has a rapid onset of action due to its lipid solubility, which may be useful to control dangerous behaviors quickly. However, with prolonged administration, it may accumulate in the body due to accumulation of an active metabolite. On the other hand, lorazepam has a slower onset of action and is longer-acting, which may be useful for the treatment of alcohol withdrawal. Continuous infusion lorazepam is generally avoided and requires close monitoring for a high anion gap metabolic acidosis, especially in renal failure as a result of diluent, propylene glycol, present in the parenteral formulation.[16] Alternatively, enteral and intermittent use of benzodiazepines should also be considered to minimize intravenous continuous infusion requirements to conserve drug supplies in the setting of ongoing shortage. Furthermore, this strategy may limit the benzodiazepine exposure and accumulation that is more likely to be associated with continuous infusion. Lastly, the routine use of reversal agent flumazenil is not recommended after prolonged infusion because it may precipitate withdrawal symptoms, including seizures.[8] It has a duration of action of approximately 60 minutes, and patients who have received prolonged infusions may become resedated once the effects wear off.

Propofol is an intravenous sedative, hypnotic, and anticonvulsant agent that is most widely used because of its rapid onset and offset of action, ease of titration, and relatively low cost. Thus, when used as a sedative it allows for rapid awakening and helps to differentiate between over-sedation and neurological dysfunction. Like the benzodiazepines, propofol acts on the GABA receptor, although the site of action is different. It is preferred over benzodiazepines because it is associated with shorter time to light sedation and extubation. On the other hand, it has been associated with longer time to extubation when compared with dexmedetomidine, although no difference in mortality or ICU length of stay was reported.[7]

Its utility is limited by its lack of analgesic activity, risk of hypotension and myocardial depression (especially in volume depleted patients), the requirement of mechanical ventilation due to dose dependent respiratory depression, and a rare but potentially fatal condition known as propofol-related infusion syndrome (PRIS). PRIS is characterized by unexplained high anion gap metabolic acidosis, rhabdomyolysis, hyperkalemia, acute kidney injury, arrhythmias, and cardiovascular collapse.[16] Risk factors include prolonged duration of propofol greater than 48 hours, the administration of doses > 80 mcg/kg/minute, and concomitant administration of catecholamines and glucocorticoids.[14] Although the mechanism for PRIS is not well understood, it is thought to be due to mitochondrial dysfunction and impaired fatty acid oxidation. More recent findings suggest PRIS may occur with shorter duration as well.[16] Other complications of propofol include hypertriglyceridemia potentially causing acute pancreatitis. Serum triglycerides should be checked every 3 days and alternative sedative should be considered when triglyceride level exceeds 500 mg/dL.[5] In COVID-19, a higher threshold for triglyceridemia 800 mg/dL has been suggested when considering to withhold infusion.[19] This has been suggested to account for hypertriglyceridemia caused by systemic inflammation secondary to hemophagocytic lymphohistiocytosis.[19] Propofol is a lipid emulsion, so the calorie content must be considered whenever it is administered.

Dexmedetomidine is a central alpha-2 agonist with anxiolytic and opioid sparing properties without depressing the respiratory drive, even in high doses.[20,21] It is roughly eight times more specific and selective than clonidine for the alpha receptors. Dexmedetomidine does not have amnestic property and offers a type of light sedation allowing patients to be sleepy, but interactive, and able to participate in their care.[16] This property may be particularly preferable in patients requiring frequent neurologic assessments. Therefore, it should be avoided in those patients where deep sedation is required.[21] It is often selected in agitated patients who are in the process of weaning from mechanical ventilation, or those with tenuous respiratory function. Furthermore, when compared with benzodiazepine infusions, it has resulted in reduced incidence and duration of delirium.[16] Clinically important bradycardia and hypotension are the most frequent adverse events reports with dexmedetomidine infusion. These effects may be unwanted in patients with hemodynamic instability or those with reduced left ventricular function.

Several studies have also reported success in transitioning patients from dexmedetomidine to enteral clonidine for continued sedation as a strategy to facilitate transfer out of the ICU and reduce the duration of dexmedetomidine infusion.[22] For example, one transition strategy that was utilized in a previous report included initiating enteral clonidine at a dose of 0.2 to 0.3 mg every 6 hours if dexmedetomidine doses were less than 0.7 mcg/kg/hr, body weight less than 100 kg, or older patients.[22] Higher clonidine doses 0.3 mg or more every 6 hours were initiated with dexmedetomidine doses of 0.7 mcg/kg/hr or higher, body weight more than 100 kg, or younger patients. The dexmedetomidine dose was reduced by 25% with each dose of clonidine administered. Clonidine patches should be avoided due to delayed onset of action requiring 3 to 4 days to reach steady state and unpredictable absorption in an ICU patient.

Ketamine is an enantiomeric, rapid-acting, phencyclidine derivative commonly used in anesthesia. Ketamine exerts its activity primarily through nonselective NMDA receptor antagonism [23,24] Additional minor effects are mediated via opioid and GABA blockade, as well as central nervous system anticholinergic pathways.[23,24] Ketamine's notable pharmacokinetic properties include rapid onset of action, elimination half-life of approximately 2–3 hours, lipophilicity with limited protein binding, and hepatic clearance via cytochrome P450-mediated mechanisms. Ketamine has emerged as an attractive option for use in critical care settings due to its ability to provide dose-dependent dissociative effects, akinesia, amnesia, as well as analgesia. Furthermore, it has a favorable hemodynamic profile, preserves respiratory drive, and does not affect gastric motility.[23] For these reasons, it may be a useful addition to analgesics and sedatives in mechanically ventilated patients to promote concomitant analgesic and sedative dose-sparing effects. Recent shortages have also forced many institutions to adopt the use of ketamine as a sedative agent in COVID-19 patients. Despite its theoretical benefit, the current PADIS guidelines recommend low-dose ketamine only as an adjunct to opioid therapy for reducing opioid consumption in post-surgical adults admitted to the ICU based on existing data.[7] Furthermore, prospective clinical trials are lacking to confirm findings that were observed in the retrospective analyses.[24]

Although the standard dosing has yet to be defined, the analgesic effects of ketamine can be seen at lower doses < 0.5 mg/kg/hr while sedative effects may require higher doses > 1 mg/kg/hr.[5] Common adverse effects associated with ketamine use include hypertension, tachycardia, increased secretions, nausea, and vomiting. Emergence reactions are also reported in up to 30% of patients on ketamine and are characterized by psychosis, nightmares, vivid dreams, and hallucinations.[23] This adverse event may be attenuated by administering a benzodiazepine. Concerns about using ketamine in head injured patients have been raised due to its sympathomimetic effects; however, a recent meta-analysis suggests ketamine does not increase intracranial pressure and may not need to be avoided in head injured patients.[23] Overall, ketamine should be reserved as a second- or third-line agent due to its side effect profile, paucity of data, and unfamiliarity with its use.

Phenobarbital, a barbiturate, appears to be an attractive option due to its sedative and hypnotic properties resulting in its off-label use for sedation.[22] Phenobarbital exerts its activity through its action on the gamma aminobutyric acid (GABAA) receptor by prolonging the duration of chloride channel opening whereas benzodiazepines augment the frequency of channel opening.[25] Current PADIS guidelines do not make any recommendations about the use of phenobarbital in their most recent iteration.[7] It is rapidly absorbed following intravenous administration within 5 minutes, peaks at 20 to 30 minutes, and possesses oral bioavailability of greater than 95%.[25] It has a moderate volume of distribution 0.5 to 0.7 L/kg and elimination half-life is 50 to 120 hours, with a median of about 80 hours.[25] This characteristic limits its ability to be rapidly titrated but allows for auto-tapering upon discontinuation. It is metabolized in the liver via CYP2C9 (major) and ~25 to 50% is excreted unchanged in the urine.

Phenobarbital is generally well tolerated. Adverse effects include hypotension and respiratory depression, particularly with high doses. Therapeutic drug monitoring may be considered in certain patients in whom inadequate response is observed, prolonged use, oversedation, or pharmacokinetic variability is anticipated, to achieve serum concentrations of 15–40 mg/L, based on data in patients with epilepsy.[22] Serum concentrations can be obtained at any time during a dosing interval because of its long half-life. Drug interactions with phenobarbital must also be considered as it is a strong inducer of CYP3A and CYP2C enzymes. A delayed attainment of the enzymatic induction has been observed resulting in onset and offset of more than a week with respect to drug-drug interactions.[22]

Antipsychotics

Haloperidol and several second-generation antipsychotics are often considered for patients diagnosed with delirium. They have traditionally not been studied for sedation due to lack of evidence but may be options in the crisis situations (Table 8-3).[5] When considered, they should be used as an adjunctive treatment and avoided in patients that require deep sedation.[5] The lack of respiratory depression makes them potentially attractive alternatives to more conventional sedatives when trying to liberate a patient from mechanical ventilation. These agents block dopamine, serotonin, histamine, a-adrenergic, and muscarinic receptors, resulting in mood stabilizing effects. Though many antipsychotics may help treat agitation, there is limited evidence supporting whether antipsychotics reduce duration of delirium, symptom severity, or other clinically relevant outcomes such as duration of mechanical ventilation or ICU/hospital mortality.[7] Furthermore, there is paucity of data comparing atypical antipsychotics to haloperidol or to one another.[7] Limited evidence suggests they may have similar efficacy when compared to haloperidol in critically-ill patients.[26] Therefore, routine use of antipsychotics is not recommended by the PADIS guidelines for the prevention or treatment of delirium.[7] An off-label use of these agents may be considered through intermittent or scheduled dosing to facilitate extubation in an agitated patient (especially when harmful to oneself or others), but the ongoing need based on clinical response should be addressed regularly.[7] In general, once delirium has been identified, the treatment should focus on identification and correction of the underlying cause. Most commonly used agents in the ICU include haloperidol, quetiapine, and olanzapine.[26]

Haloperidol is most frequently used agent with an onset of activity at 3 to 20 minutes after intravenous administration.[5,21] It does produce a dose-related increase in QT interval; therefore, it should be used cautiously or avoided altogether in patients with a history of heart disease or those receiving other QT-prolonging agents.[8] It should be noted that the optimal dose of haloperidol is not well defined.[8] The newer atypical agents differ from older agents in that they have fewer side effects and may represent reasonable alternatives. Agent specific adverse event profile should also be considered. For example, lower affinity for dopamine receptors may pose a lower risk of extrapyramidal side effects, while their stronger affinity for histamine and alpha-1 receptors leads to more sedation and hypotension observed with quetiapine and olanzapine.[26]

Neuromuscular Blocking Agents

Neuromuscular blocking agents (NMBAs) are part of the pharmacological arsenal used in the management of ARDS. Continuous infusion of cisatracurium, atracurium, vecuronium, or rocuronium can be utilized for patients with severe or refractory hypoxemia, facilitation of mechanical ventilation, and control of patient/ventilator asynchrony (Table 8-5).[27]

Table 8-5   PROPERTIES AND DOSING OF NON-DEPOLARIZING NEUROMUSCULAR BLOCKING AGENTS[28]

	Bolus dose	Intermittent dose	Continuous infusion	Onset (min)	Elimination	Duration (min)
First-line therapy						
Cisatracurium	0.1–0.2 mg/kg	Not applicable	0.5–10 mcg/kg/min	2–3	Hoffman Elimination (RBC esterases)	35–45
Atracurium	0.4–0.5 mg/kg	Not applicable	4–20 mcg/kg/min	3–5	Hoffman Elimination (RBC esterases)	30–40
Second-line therapy						
Rocuronium	0.6–1 mg/kg	50 mg followed by 25 mg given when peripheral nerve stimulation returns	8–12 mcg/kg/min	1–3	33% (renal); ~75% (biliary)	~30
Vecuronium	0.08–0.1 mg/kg	0.1 to 0.2 mg/kg/dose; may be repeated when neuromuscular function returns	0.08 to 0.1 mcg/kg/min	3–5	50% (renal) 35 – 50% (biliary)	45–60

Consideration for intermittent strategy or "as needed" guided use may be prudent to preserve current supply and to minimize long-term adverse effects with their use.[21] The intermittent strategy over continuous infusion is also endorsed by current Surviving Sepsis Campaign COVID-19 guidelines.[28] They recommend initiating with intermittent bolus doses first to test if patient-ventilator dyssynchrony improves before initiating a continuous infusion. If intermittent dosing strategy is inadequate, then a continuous infusion could be considered. Another strategy to conserve supply is the use of train-of-four monitoring when titrating NMBA infusions to ensure the lowest effective dose is being used.

MECHANICAL VENTILATION

Mechanical ventilation is needed for airway protection and hypoxic and/or hypercapnic respiratory failure. High frequency oscillation ventilation, proportional assist ventilation, neurally-adjusted ventilation assist (NAVA), and adaptive support ventilation (ASV) will not be discussed in this chapter.

Volume cycle ventilation (VC) delivers a preset tidal volume.

Synchronized intermittent mechanical ventilation (SIMV) is similar to VC but only a set of breaths are fully supported.

Pressure control ventilation (PCV) is preferred when the plateau pressures > 30. Set ventilator to assist control and match the respiratory rate, FiO_2, PEEP, and I:E ratio to prior VCV settings. Setting the initial inspiratory pressure can be achieved by (1) measuring 75% of the difference of PEAK – PEEP and (2) increasing inspiratory pressure to desired tidal volume.

Pressure regulated volume cycled ventilation (PRVC) is a pressure control with volume assurance. The ventilation adjusts pressure from breath to breath as resistance and compliance changes to meet target volume. Tidal volume, respiratory rate, PEEP, FiO_2, and I:E ratio are set.

Airway pressure release ventilation (APRV) is a modified bilevel allowing spontaneous breath at the upper level pressure and time cycled pressure release. The pressure release allows for improved tidal volume for given change in pressure, but it is short enough so there is no derecruitment. Initial settings would be P_{high} which is $P_{plateau}$, desired P_{mean} + 3 cm H_2O, or desired mean airway pressure; thigh at 4.5–6 seconds, respiratory rate 8–12 breaths per minute, P_{low} at 0 cm H_2O, and T_{low} at 0.5–0.8 seconds. T_{low} is increased if tidal volume is inadequate or increased if too large.[29]

ALTERNATIVES TO TRADITIONAL INVASIVE MECHANICAL VENTILATION

During a crisis surge, tier-based protocols are developed to accommodate the number of patients. Alternatives to traditional mechanical ventilators have been developed including converting BPAP into invasive mechanical ventilation and connecting multiple patients into one ventilator.

V60 to PCV

The Philips Respironics V60 BiPAP can be converted to PCV.[30] On menu tab, go to Mask/Port; select ET/Trach. On exhalation port selection, chose Disposable Exhalation Port (DEP).[30] In Mode Screen, select PCV. On Batch Update of Current Mode Screen, press active batch change. HME Filter and bacterial /viral filter is on the exhalation port.[30] A Ballard is placed between HMEF and ET tube. Delta P (IPAP-EPAP) is used.[30] Heated humidification is not used.

Differential Multi-Ventilation (DMV)

Shortage of mechanical ventilators during the COVID-19 surge prompted "co-ventilation" strategies.[31-38] There are associated challenges unique to co-ventilation. Patients must be paralyzed for complete passive ventilation to prevent dyssynchrony with the ventilator.[36] Ventilator must be set to PCV to individualize the regulation of the tidal volume. There is individualized monitoring of the patient's hemodynamics, flow sensors, and end-tidal CO_2.[36]

Identify Patient Compatibility

Patients are deemed compatible to share DMV if each patient requires (1) > 72 hours need for mechanical ventilation; (2) TV 6–8 ml/kg/PBW; (3) driving pressure 5V16 cm H_2O with an accepted difference of 0–6 cm H_2O; (4) respiratory rate 12–30 breaths per minute; (5) PEEP 5–18 cm H_2O with an accepted difference of up to 5 cm H_2); (6) FiO_2 21–60%; (7) pH ≥ 7.30; (8) both patients have the same respiratory infection status; (9) no severe obstructive lung disease; (10) no contraindication to neuromuscular blockade; and (11) no rapid increase in vasopressor requirements.[37,38]

Setup for DMV

One method to create a DMV involves two regular "wye" breathing circuits, two 'T" connectors, and four heat and moisture exchangers (HME) filters.[37] The T connectors are attached to the inspiratory and expiratory ports, with an HME filter in each expiratory limb.[37,38] At the end of the "wye" circuits, a patient is connected by one HME filter.

Another approach uses two sets of breathing circuits, two HME filters, two antimicrobial filters, two connector cuffs, and two "T" connectors (Figure 8-1).[4] With this approach, the connector cuff is attached to the bottom of the T piece while the antimicrobial filter is connected to one side.[38] Expiratory limbs for both circuits connected to same T piece and the other T piece is connected to both inspiratory limbs. Then the expiratory limbs are connected to the expiratory port on the ventilator and the inspiratory limbs are connected to the inspiratory port on the ventilator.

To individualize ventilator variables, flow restrictors and valves are placed in each circuit.[36] Inline PEEP in expiratory limb causes flow resistance, which is added PEEP to the ventilator PEEP for that patient. Inline

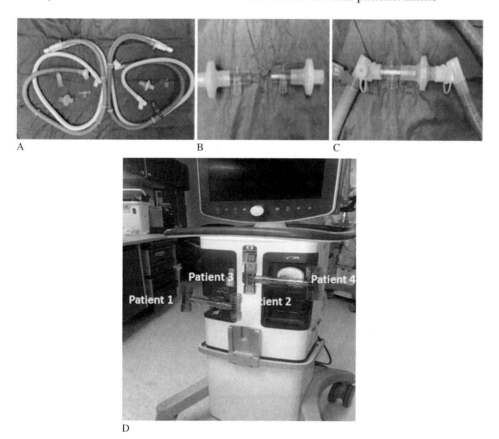

Figure 8-1 • A. Two sets of patient tubing, t-piece, and antimicrobial filters. **B.** T-piece is connected to filter. **C.** Expiratory limb is connected to same T-piece. **D.** Differential multi-ventilation for four patients. (Photos used with permission from Alvin Torres.)

PEEP in the inspiratory limb will limit the PIP from the ventilator into the patient. BVM PEEP can be substituted for inline PEEP.

Initial Settings for Patient on DMV

Note that both patients will require neuromuscular blockade. Train of four (TOF) might not be necessary to minimize entry to the room.[38] Patients should be preoxygenated prior to transfer to DMV. When the patient is still on one patient ventilation, the following baseline parameters are obtained: driving pressure, tidal volume, and respiratory rate. PCV is initiated to match baseline driving pressure, and inspiratory time between 0.6 and 1 seconds to match tidal volume. Respiratory rate, PEEP, and FIO_2 are unchanged. When patient is transferred to DMV, note that driving pressure, PEEP, inspiratory time, and respiratory rate are the same for each patient. The minute volume must be within ± 2 liters/min of baseline of each patient.[38]

Aerosolized Delivery of Medications

Goals of inhaled therapy during mechanical ventilation include assurance of drug delivery, optimization of drug deposition, consistent drug dosing, avoiding inappropriate therapies, achieving reproducible dosing, clinically feasible, safety of inhaled drugs, and controlling costs of aerosolized therapy.[39–42] Plasma levels of drugs were equivalent to lower respiratory tract levels due to lack of oropharyngeal deposition. In COVID-19 patients, pressure meter dosing inhaler (pMDI) may be preferred over nebulizers due to risk of aerosolization.

Pressure Meter Dosing Inhaler

Efficiency of drug delivery via pMDI is dependent on appropriate technique administration. The pMDI must be shaken since failure can decrease respirable dose up to 35%.[43] Actuation at 15 second intervals is similar to actuation at 1 minute intervals.[44] pMDI attached a spacer chamber in the inspiratory limb (32.1% of the dose) improved delivery compared to an elbow adaptor (7.3% of the dose) or when placed at the endotracheal tube (ETT) (29% of the dose).[45] The chamber spacer should be placed 15 cm from the Y piece.[46] Bronchodilator effect of 4 puffs (400 ug) with a pressured meter dosing inhaler (pMDI) is equivalent to 2.5 mg of albuterol nebulizer and increased doses has no additional benefit.[39–42]

Nebulizers

There are three types of nebulizers. Jet nebulizers use compressed air or oxygen to travel across the surface of the liquid medication, causing the

Table 8-6 PRESSURE METER DOSING INHALER VERSUS JET NEBULIZER TECHNIQUE IN INVASIVE MECHANICAL VENTILATION	
pMDI Technique	Jet Nebulizer Technique
1. Suction endotracheal and airway secretions	1. Suction endotracheal and airway secretions
2. Shake pMDI	2. Drug up to 4–6 ml in nebulizer
3. pMDI in space chamber in circuit 15 cm from endotracheal tube	3. Nebulizer attached to inspiratory line 18 cm from Y piece
4. Remove heat and moisture exchange (HME)	4. Turn off flow-by or continuous flow
5. Coordinate actuation with inspiration, 15 seconds in between actuation	5. Gas flow to 6–8 l/min
6. Monitor for adverse effects	6. Tap nebulizer periodically
7. Reconnect HME	7. Remove nebulizer, rinse with sterile water
	8. Reconnect HME

larger particles to travel on the upstream and the smaller particles to leave the nebulizer. This cause additional 6–8 L/min in the ventilator circuit, increasing the tidal volume. Jet nebulizers are affected by residual volume, unlike the ultrasound and vibrating mesh nebulizers. Residual volume (0.1 ml to 2.4 ml) is the amount of remaining medication in the nebulizer after treatment. The greater the residual volume, the less medication that is nebulized. Four to 5 ml is recommended to be filled.[47,48] Jet nebulizers also require a flow of 2 to 8 l/min and must be placed proximal to the humidifier, close to the ventilator[47,48] (Table 8-6).

Aerosolized Medications

In addition to the aerosolized bronchodilators albuterol, levo-albuterol, ipratropium, and inhaled corticosteroids, the following medications can also be aerosolized.[49–68]

Bronchodilators. The role of albuterol, ipratropium, and inhaled corticosteroids in obstructive lung disease such as asthma and COPD are part of standard of care.[69–73] In ALI and ARDS, the beta-agonist lung injury trial (BALTI), a randomized placebo-controlled clinical trial (n = 66) showed that intravenous salbutamol (15 mg/kg/h) compared to placebo had lower lung water at day 7 (9.2 ± 6 vs 13.2 ± 3 ml/kg 95% CI 9.2-8.3 P = 0.038) and lower plateau pressure (23.9 ± 3.8 H_2O vs 29.5 ± 7.2 H_2O P = 0.049).[74] An RCT (N = 282) of albuterol 5 mg every 4 hours for 10 days compared to placebo in ALI did not improve ventilator free days (14.4 vs 16.6 95% CI –4.7 to 0.3 P = 0.087) or rates of death before hospital discharge (23% vs 17.7 % CI – 4.7 to 14.7 P = 0.3).[75] Another RCT

(N = 922) suggested that on demand acetylcysteine with salbutamol was non-inferior to routine administration (every 6 hours until extubation) in ventilator free days, length of stay, and mortality.[76]

Acetylcysteine is a mucolytic. The role of oral acetylcysteine (600 mg PO BID for 12 months) has been investigated in COPD and bronchiectasis for prevention of exacerbations.[77,78] Its role as sole nebulized therapy for mechanically ventilated patients has not been well established.[79,80]

Heparin provides fibrinolytic activation and therefore inhibits coagulation and early inflammatory response.[61–64] It has been investigated for a potential role in inhalation injury associated acute lung injury by preventing fibrin deposition and airway obstruction. A meta-analysis of nine studies (n = 609) suggested mortality in the heparin treatment group was lower (relative risk 0.75) and duration of mechanical ventilation was shorter.[62] Most common regimen is unfractionated heparin (5,000 or 10,000 IU) initiated at 1–4 hours post injury and continued every 4 hours for up to 48 hours.[61] A retrospective study (N = 48) suggested that the use of nebulized heparin with N-acctylcysteine and albuterol contributed to a reduction in duration of mechanical ventilation (P = 0.39).[64]

Hypertonic saline causes an increased osmotic gradient in the bronchial surface, increasing epithelial lining fluid volume and decreasing volume of bronchial epithelial cells.[65] This facilitates mucociliary clearance.[65] This has largely been used in bronchiectasis. The use of the hypertonic saline outside of bronchiectasis has been studied in the pediatric population; although the trials have not shown any benefit.[66–69]

Heliox is an inert gas that has a lower density than air and therefore will decrease frictional resistant with turbulent flow. In non-intubated patients, it enhanced bronchodilator effects of albuterol in asthma, improved acidosis and encephalopathy in COPD, but did not affect overall intubation or mortality rates.[70–72] A small prospective observation study (N = 13) showed that there was a reduction in peak airway pressure (54.1 ± 12.6 cm H_2O vs 47.9 ± 10.8 cm H_2O, P < 0.001) and $PaCO_2$ (64.3 ± 14.9 mm Hg vs 62.3 + 15.1 mm Hg P = 0.01).[73] Another observation cohort (N = 24) using heliox (50:50) for mechanical ventilation in cardiac arrest, showed improved respiratory rate (25 ± 4 versus 23 ± 5) (0.011), minute volume ventilatoin (11.1 ± 1.9 versus 9.9 ± 2.1 L/min) and reducing $PaCO_2$ (5 ± 0.6 versus 4.5 kPa P = 0.011) and peak pressures (21.1 ± 3.3 versus 12.8 ± 3.2 P = 0.024).[74]

Recombinant factor VIIa is a treatment for hemophilia A and B by initiating a clot formation. It has been used as hemostasis for diffuse alveolar hemorrhage when given through bronchoscopy at 50–90 ug/kg or intravenously between 35 and 120 mcg/kg every 2 hours, but higher risk of thrombotic events if given intravenously.[75,76] One case report suggested administration via nebulizer initially with 100 ug/kg and repeated after 20 minutes to obtain hemostasis.[77,78]

Tranexamic acid (TA) is an antifibrinolytic medication to control bleeding in hemophilias and postoperative bleeding. An observation study in pediatric population (n = 19) nebulized tranxexamic acid was given 250–500 mg every 6 hours until hemostasis.[79] In adults, a double blinded randomized controlled trial (N = 47) using nebulized TA 500 mg TID vs placebo showed resolution of hemoptysis within 5 days (96% vs 50%; P < 0.0005), mean hospital length of stay was shorter (5.7 ± 2.5 days vs 7.8 ± 4.6 days P = 0.046), and fewer requiring interventional bronchoscopy or aniogrpahic embolization (0% vs 18.2% P = 0.041).[80]

TROUBLESHOOTING MECHANICAL VENTILATION

Troubleshooting mechanical ventilation requires review of the ventilator pressures, waveforms (Table 8-7), and may require radiographic images. An increased peak pressure without a change in plateau pressure can suggest increased airway resistance endotracheal tube, bronchospasm, or increased secretions. An increased peak and plateau pressure suggest decreased compliance from extrathoracic compression, bronchial intubaion, atelectasis, edema, or pneumothorax. If the difference between peak and plateau > 5 cm H_2O, this can suggest airway resistance.[29]

Driving pressure (DP) is the amount of cyclic deformation imposed on ventilated lung units calculated as plateau pressure – PEEP. Decreasing DP ($\leq$15 cm H_2O is associated with improved outcomes in ARDS).[81]

Ventilator—Induced Lung Injury

Failure to adhere to low tidal volume strategies and peak and plateau pressures < 30 mm Hg can lead to ventilator induced lung injury (VILI). Although there are microscopic VILI, the three main macroscopic VILI are subcutaneous emphysema, pneumomediastinum, and pneumothorax.

Subcutaneous emphysema and pneumomediastinum occurs when and air leaks in between the fascial planes and caused by bronchopleural fistula, asthma, dental extraction, asthma attacks, postoperative and post traumatic bronchopleural fistula, and barotrauma from mechanical ventilation. In mechanical ventilation, strategies to avoid this would be low tidal volumes and plateau pressure (<30 mm H_2O). However the high incidence in COVID-19 despite plateau pressure < 30 mm Hg have suggested another mechanism.[27] Treatment may include lowering or removing PEEP, infraclavicular bore holes, negative pressure VAC therapy,

Table 8-7	DIFFERENT TYPES OF WAVE FORMS AND TREATMENT OPTIONS	
	Description	**Treatment**
Ineffective trigger	• Insensitive trigger setting or untriggered breaths secondary to high intrinsic PEEP or incorrect vent settings	• Apply PEEP • Decrease RR/Vt • Reduce sedation • Increase expiratory time • Decrease trigger threshold
Double trigger	• Inspiratory effort continue even after inspiratory time is finished	• Increase tidal volume • Increase inspiratory time
Auto-trigger	• Inappropriate sensitive trigger thresholds, hiccups, shivering, cardiac oscillations	• Adjust vent settings • Increase sedation
Ineffective flow	• Dip in pressure time curve • Lead to ineffective trigger and auto-PEEP	• Increase flow • Change pattern to deceleration • Change to PCV
Delayed termination	• Expiratory event • Patient's intrinsic timing precedes ventilator's end of inflation • Pressure spike at the end of inspiration on pressure time waveform with rapid decline in inspiration on flow-time waveform • Lead to dynamic hyperinflation, delayed or missed triggers	• Change vent settings
Premature termination	• Expiratory event • Continued inspiration despite termination of ventilator breath • Drop or negative deflection in flow-time, pressure time, and esophageal pressures	• Increase inspiratory time • Remove excessive opioids

and/or chest tube.[82,83] The blow hole technique involves 3 cm incisions down to pectoralis fascia, 2–4 cm below the midclavicular line and packed with moist gauze pads. Note that this was applied in patients not on mechanical ventilation.[83] Another technique, the negative pressure VAC therapy includes anterior wall incisions and application of negative pressure wound therapy devices (Figure 8-2).[82,83]

Tension pneumothorax is a pneumothorax that causes obstructive shock, which can lead to cardiac arrest. It rapidly occurs and sometimes there isn't sufficient time to get a chest radiograph although it is often necessary to confirm the diagnosis. Lung ultrasound can be used with

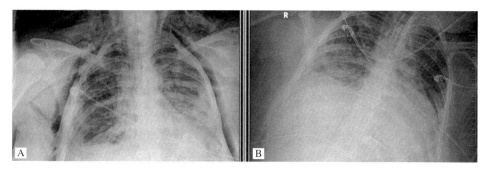

Figure 8-2 • A. Subcutaneous emphysema on PEEP 18. **B.** Subcutaneous emphysema improved on PEEP 0.

finding a lung point or lack of sea shore sign on M mode. However, known fibrotic lung disease might preclude the use of lung ultrasound. Needle decompression is used via 14G needle between the second and third intercostal space at the midclavicular line and if unsuccessful, the fourth and fifth intercostal space at the mid axillary line. This is then followed with tube thoracotomy.

Spontaneous Breathing Trials, Extubation Failure, and Tracheostomy

Spontaneous breathing trials (SBT) are conducted in conjunction with a sedation holiday or spontaneous awakening trial (SAT) when the cause of respiratory failure has improved, no significant metabolic derangements, normalized electrolytes, and no significant need for pressor support. The two most common forms are pressure support (PS) and T-piece and conducted from 30 to 120 minutes. An arterial blood gas may be obtained at the end of the trial to confirm adequate oxygenation and removal of CO_2 or ventilation. An RCT (N = 1153) suggested that a 30 minute trial on PS led to higher successful extubation rates compared to 2 hour T-piece (82.3% versus 74.% Differ 9.2% 95 CI 3.4-13 P = 0.001).[84] A recent meta-analysis of 10 RCT (N = 3165) showed no difference in predictive power of extubation between T-piece and pressure support (PS) (OR = 0.91; 95% CI 0.78-1.07; P = 0.27; I^2 = 79%).[85]

Extubation failure is defined as reintubation within 48 hours, although other literature suggest that it can be up to 1 week.[86-93] Risk factors for extubation failure include age > 65, chronic cardiorespiratory disease, high APACHE II score, pneumonia, cardiogenic cause of respiratory failure, rapid shallow breathing index (F/Vt) >105, positive fluid balance, altered mental status, neurologic patients, PaO_2/FiO_2 < 200, Glasgow Coma Scale < 8, increased secretions, poor cough, and moderate or abundant respiratory secretions.[86] Strategies to prevent or delay reintubation include the use of noninvasive mechanical ventilation and high flow. A metal analysis of 17 randomized control trials (N = 3341) showed that compared to conventional oxygen therapy (COT), NIV reduced re-intubation rate (risk ratio 0.55, 95% CI 0.48-0.91 and short-term mortality RR 9.55, 95% CI 0.48-0.91).[94] In one randomized control trial (N = 604) there was no significant difference between high flow nasal cannula and NIV in median time to reintubation (26.5 [IQR 14–39 hours] vs 21.5 hours [IQR 2–9] [absolute difference −5 hours; 95 CI −34 to 24 hours]).[95] Another randomized control trial (n = 641) suggested benefit of high flow NC with NIV over HFNC alone with reintubation rates 12% versus 20% difference −7.4% [95% CI −13.2% to −1.8%] (P = 0.009).[96]

Tracheostomy is considered for patients requiring prolonged mechanical ventilation to decrease sedation-related delirium, patient comfort, facilitate weaning, decrease ventilator associated pneumonia, tracheal obstruction, and/or laryngeal edema. In the United States, 8–13% of critically ill patients require tracheostomy.[97] Interestingly, at least 1/2 of pre-COVID patients who required tracheostomy do not survive for more than a year, and less than 12% are at home and functionally independent.[98]

Tracheostomy is also an aerosolization risk. In 2003, the SARS outbreak found increased risk for health care workers who did tracheal intubation (OR 6.6 [95% CI 2.3-18.9]), performed tracheostomy (OR 4.2 [1.5–11.5]), placed patients on non-invasive ventilation (OR 3.1 [1.5–11.5]), and manual ventilation before intubation (2.8 [1.3–6.4]).[99]

In the setting of a resource limited crisis or aerosolization risk pandemic such as COVID-19, who, when, and how are important questions that need to be addressed. Adequate personal protective equipment (PPE) must be available, and health care providers with the highest level of expertise with tracheostomy should perform the procedure to decrease operation time and complications. Health workers should enhance PPE such as face shields or powered air-purifying respirators (PAPRs). Studies recommended tracheostomy after 10 days provided that there are signs of clinical improvement.[100,101] The American Academic of Otolaryngology-Head and Neck Surgery recommends tracheostomy of COVID-19 patients around 21 days of mechanical ventilation, partly from a cohort on the SARS outbreak in Hong Kong 2003, suggested little benefit from tracheostomy earlier than 23 days,.[102,103] Viral clearance may be prolonged in critical ill patients, and repeat viral polymerase chain reaction (PCR) may not be available or is not necessarily indicative of infectious potential. One study suggested the PCR can be positive for up to 39 days.[104]

Percutaneous and surgical tracheostomies can be performed, with surgical tracheostomies if the patient has BMI > 30 and small neck or thyroid gland hypertrophy. SARS data also suggested less aerosolization risk to surgical tracheostomies compared to percutaneous tracheostomies.[105,106] However, minimizing the transfer of a patient from the ICU room to the OR might make the percutaneous tracheostomy a more attractive option. Cuffed and nonfenestrated tracheostomy is preferred.

Late tracheostomy (>10 days of mechanical ventilation) may also decrease tracheal stenosis, tracheomalacia, and posterior tracheal wall damage secondary to prolonged over-cuffed intubation, prone position, and repeated intubation and extubation procedures.[107]

Bronchoscopy

The American Association for Bronchology and Interventional Pulmonology (AAABIP) recommends that upper respiratory samples be used to primary diagnosis of COVID-19.[108] Induced sputum is not recommended.[108] If bronchoscopy is performed, it requires a minimum 3 ml of specimen.[108]

REFERENCES

1. Leider JP, DeBruin D, Reynolds N, et al. Ethical guidance for disaster response, specifically around crisis standards of care: A systematic review. *Am J Public Health*. 2017;107:e1-e9.

2. Kanji S, Burry L, Williamson D, Pittman M, et al. Ontario COVID-19 ICU drug task force. Therapeutic alternatives and strategies for drug conservation in the intensive care unit during times of drug shortages: a report of the Ontario COVID-19 ICU Drug Task Force. *Can J Anaesth*. 2020;67:1405-1416.

3. Burry LD, Barletta JF, Williamson D, et al. It takes a village. Contending with drug shortages during disasters. *Chest*. 2020;158:2414-2424.

4. US Food & Drug Administration. FDA drug shortages. Available at www.accessdata.fda.gov/scripts/drugshortages/default.cfm. Accessed November 20, 2020.

5. Ammar MA, Sacha GL, Bass SN, et al. Sedation, analgesia, and paralysis in COVID-19 patients in the setting of drug shortage. *Journal of Intensive Care Medicine*. 2020;1-18.

6. Ahuja T, Merchan C, Arnouk S, et al. COVID-19 pandemic preparedness: A practical guide from clinical pharmacists' perspective. *Am J Health-Syst Pharm*. 2020;77:1510-1515.

7. Devlin JW, Skrobik Y, Gelinas C, et al. Clinical practice guidelines for the prevention and management of pain, agitation/sedation, delirium, immobility, and sleep disruption in adult patients in the ICU. *Crit Care Med*. 2018;46: e825-e873.

8. Jacobi J, Fraser GL, Coursin DB, et al. Clinical practice guidelines for the sustained use of sedatives and analgesics in the critically ill adult. *Crit Care Med*. 2002;30:119-141.

9. Yaksh TL, Wallace MS. Opioids, analgesia, and pain management. In: Brunton LL, Chabner BA, Knollman BC, eds. *Goodman & Gilman's The Pharmacological Basis of Therapeutics*. 12th ed. New York, NY: McGraw-Hill Medical; 2011.

10. Makii JM, Mirski MA, Lewin JJ. Sedation and analgesia in critically ill neurologic patients. *J Pharm Pract*. 2010;23:455-469.

11. Methylnaltrexone [prescribing information] Bridgewater, NJ: Salix Pharmaceuticals LLC; December 2020.

12. Cammarano WB, Pittet JF, Weitz S, et al. Acute withdrawal syndrome related to the administration of analgesic and sedative medications in adult intensive care unit patients. *Crit Care Med*. 1998;26(4):676.

13. Lee M, Silverman SM, Hansen H, et al. A comprehensive review of opioid-induced hyperalgesia. *Pain Physician*. 2011;14(2):145-161.

14. Adams CD, Altshuler J, Barlow BL, et al. Analgesia and sedation strategies in mechanically ventilated adults with COVID-19. *Pharmacotherapy*. 2020;40(12):1180-1191.

15. Roan JP, Bajaj N, Davis FA, et al. Opioids and chest wall rigidity during mechanical ventilation. *Ann Intern Med*. 2018;168:678.

16. Barr J, Fraser GL, Puntillo K, et al. Clinical practice guidelines for the management of pain, agitation, and delirium in adult patients in the intensive care unit. *Crit Care Med*. 2013;41:263-306.

17. Brown R, Kraus C, Fleming M, et al. Methadone: Applied pharmacology and use as adjunctive treatment in chronic pain. *Postgrad Med J*. 2004;80: 654-659.

18. Elefritz JL, Murphy CV, Papadimos TJ, et al. Methadone analgesia in the critically ill. *J Crit Care*. 2016;34:84-88.

19. Devlin JW, O'Neal HR JR, Thomas C, et al. Strategies to optimize ICU liberation (A to F) bundle performance in critically ill adults with coronavirus disease 2019. *Crit Care Expl*. 2020;2:e0139.

20. Panzer O, Moitra V, Sladen RN. Pharmacology of sedative-analgesic agents: Dexmedetomidine, remifentanil, ketamine, volatile anesthetics, and the role of peripheral mu antagonists. *Crit Care Clin*. 2009;25:451-469.

21. Chanques G, Constantin JM, Devlin JW, et al. Analgesia and sedation in patients with ARDS. *Intensive Care Med*. 2020;46(12):2342-2356.

22. Gagnon, DJ, Fontaine GV, Riker RR, et al. Repurposing valproate, enteral clonidine, and phenobarbital for comfort in adult ICU patients: A literature review with practical considerations. *Pharmacotherapy*. 2017;37:1309-1321.

23. Erstad BL, Patanwala AE. Ketamine for analgosedation in critically ill patients. *J Crit Care*. 2016;35:145-149.

24. Hurth KP, Jaworski A, Thomas KB, et al. The reemergence of ketamine for treatment in critically ill adults. *Crit Care Med*. 2020;48:899-911.

25. Phenobarbital sodium injection [prescribing information]. Louisville, KY: Cameron Pharmaceuticals LLC; August 2020.

26. Reznik ME, Slooter AJC. Delirium management in the ICU. *Curr Treat Options Neurol*. 2019;21:59.

27. Warr J, Thiboutot Z, Rose L. Current therapeutic uses, pharmacology, and clinical considerations of neuromuscular blocking agents for critically ill adults. *Ann Pharmacother*. 2011;45(9):1116-1126.

28. Alhazzani W, Moller MH, Arabi YM, et al. Surviving sepsis campaign: Guidelines on the management of critically ill adults with coronavirus disease 2019 (COVID-19). *Intensive Care Med*. 2020;46:854-887.

29. Esteitie R, Go RC, Tabba M. Chapter 12: Mechanical ventilation. In: Go RC, ed. *Critical Care Examination and Board Review*. New York: McGraw Hill; 2019:235-267.

30. Available at: Respironics V60/V60 Plus Ventilator User Manual. http://incenter.medical.philips.com/doclib/enc/11191054/Respironics_V60_Ventilator_User_Manual_(ENG)_-_1047358_M.pdf%3Ffunc%3Ddoc.Fetch%26nodeid%3D11191054. Accessed on October 13, 2020.

31. Available at https://www.differentialmultivent.org. Accessed December 27, 2020.

32. Clarke AL, Stephens AF, Liao S, Byrne TJ, Gregory SD. Coping with COVID-19: Ventilator splitting with differential driving pressures using standard hospital equipment. *Anaesthesia*. 2020;75:872-880.

33. Bunting L, Roy S, Pinson H, et al. A novel inline PEEP valve design for differential multi-ventilation. *Am J Emerg Med*. 2020;38(10):2045-2048.

34. Roy S, Bunting L, Stahl S, Textor D. Inline positive end-expiratory pressure valves: The essential component of individualized split. *Crit Care Explor*. 2020;2(9):e0198.

35. Levin MA, Shah A, Shah R, et al. Differential ventilation using flow control valves as a potential bridge to full ventilatory support during the COVID-19 crisis: From bench to bedside. *Anesthesiology*. 2020;133:892-904.

36. de Jongh FHC, de Vries HJ, Warnaar RSP, et al. Ventilating two patients with one ventilator: Technical setup and laboratory testing. *ERJ Open Res*. 2020;6(2):00256-2020.

37. Tonnetti T, Zanella A, Pizzilli G, et al. One ventilator for two patients: Feasibility and considerations of a last resort solution in case of equipment shortage. *Thorax*. 2020;75:517-519.

38. Beitler JR, Kallet R, Kacmarek R, et al. Columbia University Vagelos College of Physicians & Surgeons – New York-Presbyterian Hospital – Ventilator sharing protocol: Dual-patient ventilation with a single mechanical ventilator for use during critical ventilator shortages – version 4, March 27, 2020. Available at http://www.gnyha.org/wp-content/uploads/2020/03/Ventilator-Sharing-Protocol-Dual-Patient-Ventilation-with-a-Single-Mechanical-Ventilator-for-Use-during-Critical-Ventilator-Shortages.pdf. Accessed on October 15, 2020.

39. Dhand R. How should aerosols be delivered during invasive mechanical ventilation? *Respiratory Care*. October 2018;62(10):1343-1367.

40. Dhand R, Duarte AG, Jubran A, Jenne JW, Fink JB, Fahey PJ, Tobin MJ. Dose-response to bronchodilator delivered by metereddose inhaler in ventilator-supported patients. *Am J Respir Crit Care Med*. 1996;154(2 Pt1):388-393.

41. Duarte AG, Momii K, Bidani A. Bronchodilator therapy with metered-dose inhaler and spacer versus nebulizer in mechanically ventilated patients: comparison of magnitude and duration of response. *Respir Care*. 2000;45(7):817-823.

42. Manthous CA, Hall JB, Schmidt GA, Wood LD. Metered-dose inhaler versus nebulized albuterol in mechanically ventilated patients. *Am Rev Respir Dis*. 1993;148(6 Pt 1):1567-1570.

43. Everard ML, Devadason SG, Summers QA, Le Soue¨f PN. Factors affecting total and "respirable" dose delivered by a salbutamol metered dose inhaler. *Thorax*. 1995;50(7):746-749.

44. Fink JB, Dhand R, Duarte AG, Jenne JW, Tobin MJ. Aerosol delivery from a metered-dose inhaler during mechanical ventilation. An in-vitro model. *Am J Respir Crit Care Med*. 1996;154(2Pt1):382-387.

45. Rau JL, Harwood RJ, Groff JL. Evaluation of a reservoir device for metered-dose bronchodilator delivery to intubated adults. An in vitro study. *Chest*. 1992;102(3):924-930.

46. Ari A, Areabi H, Fink JB. Evaluation of aerosol generator devices at 3 locations in humidified and non-humidified circuits during adult mechanical ventilation. *Respir Care*. 2010;55(7):837-844.

47. Rau JL. Design principles of liquid nebulization devices currently in use. *Respir Care*. 2002;47(11):1257-1275; discussion 1275-1278.

48. Kallet RH. Adjunct therapies during mechanical ventilation: airway clearance techniques, therapeutic aerosols, and gases. *Respir Care*. 2013;58(6):1053-1073.

49. Nair S, Thomas E, Pearson SB, Henry MT. A randomized controlled trial to assess the optimal dose and effect of nebulized albuterol in acute exacerbations of COPD. *Chest*. 2005;128(1):48-54.

50. Truitt T, Witko J, Halpern M. Levalbuterol compared to racemic albuterol: Efficacy and outcomes in patients hospitalized with COPD or asthma. *Chest*. 2003;123(1):128-135.

51. Global Strategy for Asthma Management and Prevent. Available at https://ginasthma.org/. Accessed Dececember 24, 2020.

52. Global Initiative for Chronic Obstructive Lung Disease. Available at https://gold-copd.org/wp-content/uploads/2020/11/GOLD-REPORT-2021-v1.1-25Nov20_WMV.pdf. Accessed December 24, 2020.

53. May CS, Palmer KN. Effect of aerosol ipratropium bromide (SCH 1000) on sputum viscosity and volume in chronic bronchitis. *Br J Clin Pharmacol*. 1977;4(4):491-492.

54. Perkins GD, McAuley DF, Thickett DR, Gao F. The beta-agonist lung injury trial (BALTI): A randomized placebo-controlled clinical trial. *Am J Respir Crit Care Med*. 2006;173(3):281-287.

55. National Heart, Lung, and Blood Institute Acute Respiratory Distress Syndrome (ARDS) Clinical Trials Network, Matthay MA, Brower RG, et al. Randomized, placebo-controlled clinical trial of an aerosolized β_2-agonist for treatment of acute lung injury. *Am J Respir Crit Care Med*. 2011;184(5):561-568.

56. van Meenen DMP, van der Hoeven SM, Binnekade JM, et al. Effect of on-demand vs routine nebulization of acetylcysteine with salbutamol on ventilator-free days in intensive care unit patients receiving invasive ventilation: A randomized clinical trial. *JAMA*. 2018;319(10):993-1001.

57. Qi Q, Ailiyaer Y, Liu R, et al. Effect of N-acetylcysteine on exacerbations of bronchiectasis (BENE): A randomized controlled trial. *Respir Res*. 2019;20(1):73.

58. Zheng JP, Wen FQ, Bai CX, et al. Twice daily N-acetylcysteine 600 mg for exacerbations of chronic obstructive pulmonary disease (PANTHEON): A randomised, double-blind placebo-controlled trial. *Lancet Respir Med.* 2014;2(3):187-194.

59. Han DW, Ji W, Lee JC, Song SY, Choi CM. Efficacy of nebulized acetylcysteine for relieving symptoms and reducing usage of expectorants in patients with radiation pneumonitis. *Thorac Cancer.* 2019;10(2):243-248.

60. Masoompour SM, Anushiravani A, Tafaroj Norouz A. Evaluation of the effect of nebulized N-acetylcysteine on respiratory secretions in mechanically ventilated patients: Randomized clinical trial. *Iran J Med Sci.* 2015;40(4):309-315.

61. Miller Ac, ELamin E, Suffredini AF. MD1 inhaled anticoagulation regimens for the treatment of smoke inhalation–associated acute lung injury. *Crit Care Med.* 2014;42(2):413-419.

62. Lan X, Huang Z, Tan Z, Huang Z, Wang D, Huang Y. Nebulized heparin for inhalation injury in burn patients: A systematic review and meta-analysis. *Burns Trauma.* 2020;8:tkaa015.

63. Juschten J, Tuinman PR, Juffermans NP, Dixon B, Levi M, Schultz MJ. Nebulized anticoagulants in lung injury in critically ill patients-an updated systematic review of preclinical and clinical studies. *Ann Transl Med.* 2017;5(22):444.

64. McGinn KA, Weigartz K, Lintner A, Scalese MJ, Kahn SA. Nebulized heparin with N-acetylcysteine and albuterol reduces duration of mechanical ventilation in patients with inhalation injury. *J Pharm Pract.* 2019 Apr;32(2):163-166.

65. Carro LM, Martinez-Garcia MA. Nebulized hypertonic saline in noncystic fibrosis bronchiectasis: A comprehensive review. *Ther Adv Respir Dis.* 2018;13: 1-15.

66. Everard ML, Hind D, Ugonna K, et al. SABRE: A multicentre randomised control trial of nebulised hypertonic saline in infants hospitalised with acute bronchiolitis. *Thorax.* 2014;69(12):1105-1112.

67. Angoulvant F, Bellêttre X, Milcent K, et al. Effect of nebulized hypertonic saline treatment in emergency departments on the hospitalization rate for acute bronchiolitis: A randomized clinical trial. *JAMA Pediatr.* 2017;171(8):e171333.

68. Teunissen J, Hochs AH, Vaessen-Verberne A. The effect of 3% and 6% hypertonic saline in viral bronchiolitis: A randomised controlled trial. *Eur Respir J.* 2014;44(4):913-21.

69. Flores P, Mendes AL, Neto AS. A randomized trial of nebulized 3% hypertonic saline with salbutamol in the treatment of acute bronchiolitis in hospitalized infants. *Pediatr Pulmonol.* 2016;51(4):418-425.

70. El-Khatib MF, Jamaleddine G, Kanj N, et al. Effect of heliox- and air-driven nebulized bronchodilator therapy on lung function of patients with asthma. *Lung.* 2014;192(3):377-383.

71. Maggiore SM, Richard JC, Abroug F, et al. A multicenter, randomized trial of noninvasive ventilation with helium-oxygen mixture in exacerbations of chronic obstructive lung disease. *Crit Care Med.* 2010;38(1):145-151.

72. Jolliet P, Ouanes-Besbes L, Abroug F, et al. A multicenter randomized trial assessing the efficacy of helium/oxygen in severe exacerbations of chronic obstructive pulmonary disease. *Am J Respir Crit Care Med.* 2017;195(7):871-880.

73. Leatherman JW, Romero RS, Shapiro RS. Lack of benefit of heliox during mechanical ventilation of subjects with severe air-flow obstruction. *Respir Care.* 2018;63(4):375-379.

74. Beurskens CJ, Brevoord D, Lagrand WK, et al. Heliox improves carbon dioxide removal during lung protective mechanical ventilation. *Crit Care Res Pract.* 2014;2014:954814.

75. Pathak V, Kuhn J, Gabriel D, Barrow J, Jennette JC, Henke DC. Use of activated factor VII in patients with diffuse alveolar hemorrhage: A 10 years institutional experience. *Lung.* 2015;193(3):375-379.

76. Baker MS, Diab KJ, Carlos WG, Mathur P. Intrapulmonary recombinant factor VII as an effective treatment for diffuse alveolar hemorrhage: A case series. *J Bronchology Interv Pulmonol.* 2016;23(3):255-258.

77. Esper RC, Estrada IE, de la Torre León T, Gutiérrez AO, López JA. Treatment of diffuse alveolar hemorrhage secondary to lupus erythematosus with recombinant activated factor VII administered with a jet nebulizer. *J Intensive Care.* 2014;2(1):47.

78. Hoffman M, Monroe MDIII. The action of high-dose factor VIIa in a cell-based model hemostasis. *Dis Mon.* 2003;49:1-7.

79. O'Neil ER, Schmees LR, Resendiz K, Justino H, Anders MM. Inhaled tranexamic acid as a novel treatment for pulmonary hemorrhage in critically ill pediatric patients: An observational study. *Crit Care Explor.* 2020;2(1):e0075.

80. Wand O, Guber E, Guber A, Epstein Shochet G, Israeli-Shani L, Shitrit D. Inhaled tranexamic acid for hemoptysis treatment: A randomized controlled trial. *Chest.* 2018 Dec;154(6):1379-1384.

81. Bugedo G, Retamal J, Bruhn A. Driving pressure: A marker of severity, safety limit or goal of mechanical venitlation? *Crit Care.* 2017;21(199):1-7.

82. Taylor BC, McGowan S. Use of closed incision negative pressure therapy for massive subcutaneous emphysema. *Cureus.* 2020;12(3):e7399.

83. Herlan DB, Landreneau RJ, Ferson PF. Massive spontaneous subcutaneous emphysema. acute management with infraclavicular blow holes. *CHEST.* 1992;102(2):503-505.

84. Subirà C, Hernández G, Vázquez A, et al. Effect of pressure support vs T-piece ventilation strategies during spontaneous breathing trials on successful extubation among patients receiving mechanical ventilation: A randomized clinical trial [published correction appears in JAMA. 2019 Aug 20;322(7):696]. *JAMA.* 2019;321(22):2175-2182.

85. Li Y, Li H, Zhang D. Comparison of T-piece and pressure support ventilation as spontaneous breathing trials in critically ill patients: A systematic review and meta-analysis. *Crit Care.* 2020;24(1):67.

86. Thille AW, Richard JCM, Brochard L. The decision to extubate in the intensive care unit. *Am J Respir Crit Care Med.* 2013;187(12):1294-1302.

87. Esteban A, Alía I, Gordo F, et al.; The Spanish Lung Failure Collaborative Group. Extubation outcome after spontaneous breathing trials with T-tube or pressure support ventilation. *Am J Respir Crit Care Med.* 1997;156:459-465.

88. Esteban A, Alía I, Tobin MJ, et al. Spanish Lung Failure Collaborative Group. Effect of spontaneous breathing trial duration on outcome of attempts to

discontinue mechanical ventilation. *Am J Respir Crit Care Med.* 1999;159:512-518.

89. Vallverdú I, Calaf N, Subirana M, Net A, Benito S, Mancebo J. Clinical characteristics, respiratory functional parameters, and outcome of a two-hour T-piece trial in patients weaning from mechanical ventilation. *Am J Respir Crit Care Med.* 1998;158:1855-1862.

90. Epstein SK, Ciubotaru RL, Wong JB. Effect of failed extubation on the outcome of mechanical ventilation. *Chest.* 1997;112:186-192.

91. Epstein SK, Ciubotaru RL. Independent effects of etiology of failure and time to reintubation on outcome for patients failing extubation. *Am J Respir Crit Care Med.* 1998;158:489-493.

92. Frutos-Vivar F, Ferguson ND, Esteban A, et al. Risk factors for extubation failure in patients following a successful spontaneous breathing trial. *Chest.* 2006;130:1664-1671.

93. Demling RH, Read T, Lind LJ, Flanagan HL. Incidence and morbidity of extubation failure in surgical intensive care patients. *Crit Care Med.* 1988;16:573-577.

94. Zhou X, Yao S, Dong P,Chen B, Xu Z, Wang H. Preventive use of respiratory support after scheduled extubation in critically ill medical patients – A network meta-analysis of randomized controlled trials. *Critical Care.* 2020;24:370.

95. Hernández G, Vaquero C, Colinas L, et al. Effect of postextubation high-flow nasal cannula vs noninvasive ventilation on reintubation and postextubation respiratory failure in high-risk patients: A randomized clinical trial. *JAMA.* 2016;316(15):1565-1574.

96. Thille AW, Muller G, Gacouin A, et al. Effect of postextubation high-flow nasal oxygen with noninvasive ventilation vs high-flow nasal oxygen alone on reintubation among patients at high risk of extubation failure: A randomized clinical trial. *JAMA.* 2019;322(15):1465-1475.

97. Mehta AB, Syeda SN, Bajpayee L, Cooke CR, Walkey AJ, Wiener RS. Trends in tracheostomy for mechanically ventilated patients in the United States. *Am J Respir Crit Care Med.* 2015;192:446-454.

98. Vargas M, Sutherasan Y, Brunetti I, et al. Mortality and long-term quality of life after percutaneous tracheotomy in intensive care unit: A prospective observational study. *Minerva Anestesiol.* 2018;84:1024-1031.

99. Tran K, Cimon K, Severn M, Pessoa-Silva CL, Conly J. Aerosol generating procedures and risk of transmission of acute respiratory infections to healthcare workers: A systematic review. *PLoS One.* 2012;7:e35797.

100. Takhar A, Surda P, Ahmad I, et al. Timing of tracheostomy for prolonged respiratory wean in critically ill coronavirus disease 2019 patients: A machine learning approach. *Crit Care Explor.* 2020;2(11):e0279.

101. McGrath BA, Brenner MJ, Warrillow SJ, et al. Tracheostomy in the COVID-19 era: Global and multidisciplinary guidance. *Lancet Respir Med.* 2020;8(7):717-725.

102. Leung GM, Hedley AJ, Ho LM, et al. The epidemiology of severe acute respiratory syndrome in the 2003 Hong Kong epidemic: An analysis of all 1755 patients. *Ann Intern Med.* 2004;141(9):662-673.

103. Parker NP, Schiff BA, Friz MA, et al. Tracheotomy recommendations during the COVID-19 pandemic. Available at https://www.entnet.org/

content/tracheotomy-recommen dations-during-covid-19-pandemic. Updated April 2,2020. Accessed December 21, 2020.

104. Chen C, Gao G, Xu Y, et al. SARS-CoV-2-positive sputum and feces after conversion of pharyngeal samples in patients with COVID-19. *Ann Intern Med.* 2020;172(12):832-834.

105. Tien HC, Chughtai T, Jogeklar A, Cooper AB, Brenneman F. Elective and emergency surgery in patients with severe acute respiratory syndrome (SARS). *Can J Surg.* 2005;48:71-74.

106. Chee VW, Khoo ML, Lee SF, Lai YC, Chin NM. Infection control measures for operative procedures in severe acute respiratory syndrome-related patients. *Anesthesiology.* 2004;100:1394-1398.

107. Mattioli F, Fermi M, Ghirelli M, et al. Tracheostomy in the COVID-19 pandemic. *Eur Arch Otorhinolaryngol.* 2020;277(7):2133-2135.

108. Wahidi MM, Lamb C, Murgu S, et al. American Association for Bronchology and Interventional Pulmonology (AABIP) statement on the use of bronchoscopy and respiratory specimen collection in patients with suspected or confirmed COVID-19 infection. *J Bronchology Interv Pulmonol.* 2020;27(4):e52-e54.

ENDOCRINOLOGIC ISSUES DURING CRISIS

9

Shruti Pandiri, MD, Anne Marie Van Hoven, MD, and Colette M. Knight, MD

▌ INTRODUCTION

The endocrine system is a major network that integrates metabolic and hormonal signals in the human body. It encompasses a large system of organs including the pituitary gland, thyroid, adrenal gland, reproductive organs, pancreas, and bone.[1] Any environmental changes or perturbations are likely to have long-lasting effects on multiple endocrine axes.[2] Pandemics or other types of crises often result in stressful events that affect normal endocrine signaling, resulting in alterations in baseline endocrine function or exacerbation of pre-existing conditions. Further, some events are impactful enough to fundamentally change the approach to the practice of endocrinology and can alter usual clinical practices and guidelines. We are currently experiencing such a shift as we progress through the coronavirus disease 2019 (COVID-19) pandemic, which has caused greater than 110 million infections worldwide and > 2.4 million deaths. The viral infection is caused by the severe acute respiratory syndrome coronavirus 2 (SARS-CoV-2). Acute COVID-19 viral infection has been shown to have significant effects on multiple endocrine organs and systems, some of which are short-lived but others that can persist for a long time (see Table 9-1). Recent viral pandemics such as severe acute respiratory syndrome (SARS) in 2003 and middle east respiratory syndrome (MERS) in 2012 were associated with pituitary dysfunction, adrenal insufficiency, impaired glycemic control associated with lability in glycemic excursions, and increased insulin resistance.[3-6] Of significant interest is the mechanism by which newly discovered pathogens like SARS CoV-2 may choose to utilize metabolic pathways such as the renin angiotensin-aldosterone system (RAAS) and the angiotensin converting enzyme-2 (ACE-2) receptor more specifically as the entry point of infection to cells. This pathway has significant importance as it is readily activated in multiple endocrine systems. Given the consequences of these burgeoning pandemics on the metabolic milieu, it seems plausible that a deliberate and structured

Table 9-1 EFFECT OF COVID-19 ON ENDOCRINE ORGANS		
Endocrine Organ	**Mechanism**	**Clinical Presentation**
Pituitary	Cell edema and necrosis Inflammatory markers mediated injury Immune mediated injury	Hypophysitis
Thyroid	Destruction of follicular cells Decreased type 1 deiodinase activity Hypothalamic dysfunction	Subacute thyroiditis Euthyroid-sick syndrome Hypothyroidism
Adrenal	Adrenal necrosis Adrenal vasculitis Adrenal infiltration	Hypocortisolism
Pancreatic Islet	Islet cell damage Inflammation Acute pancreatitis	Hyperglycemia
Gonads	Destruction of seminiferous tubules Orchitis	Male hypogonadism Subfertility

approach to the identification and management of endocrine and metabolic disorders is essential to adaptation during times of crisis. Here we will present a general overview on how crises may affect the manifestation of endocrine disorders. More specifically, we will review how the current COVID-19 pandemic has affected the endocrine pathways and axes, the current information and the current knowledge that has been gained, and insights on how to better prepare for emerging crises.

HYPOTHALAMUS PITUITARY ADRENAL AXIS

In general, the stress response is mediated primarily by the corticotrophin-releasing hormone (CRH) and locus coeruleus-norepinephrine (LC-NE) sympathetic system in a synergistic way. This pathway is often activated by inflammatory factors and cytokines, which stimulate the release of ACTH from the anterior pituitary, which then drives the production and secretion of cortisol from the adrenal gland. Ultimately this activated pathway has a negative feedback on ACTH signaling, which ultimately dampens the stress response by inhibiting the inflammatory cascade.[7,8]

Although the exact mechanism is still unclear, it has been deduced that COVID-19 can affect the hypothalamic-pituitary axis. Angiotensin converting enzyme-2 (ACE2), which is present in multiple human organs, has been identified as the possible route of cellular entry for COVID-19.[9] The hypothalamus and pituitary gland are known to express ACE2, thus making it a target for COVID-19.[10] Garg and colleagues proposed three different mechanisms of how COVID-19 can affect the hypothalamic-pituitary axis. The first mechanism is explained by direct injury to the cells resulting in cell edema and necrosis. Second is indirect injury mediated by inflammatory markers such as interleukin-1, interleukin-6, and tumor necrosis factor-alpha. Third is immune mediated, resulting in hypophysitis.[11]

Given that the genetic similarity between SARS-CoV-2 and SARS-CoV is 79.5%, inferences can be made from studies of patients affected by SARS-CoV in 2003.[12] Leow and colleagues evaluated 61 survivors of SARS-CoV for hormonal abnormalities three months after recovery for up to one year. Of the 61 survivors, 39.3% had hypocortisolism.[13] They finally concluded that SARS-CoV causes reversible hypophysitis or direct hypothalamic injury, leading to abnormalities of the hypothalamic-pituitary adrenal axis and hypothalamic-pituitary thyroid axis.[13] This type of cortisol deficiency has been described in other disorders such as chronic fatigue syndrome, post-traumatic stress disorder, and primary fibromyalgia syndrome.[13–15] Tan and colleagues demonstrated that patients with COVID-19 had a marked stress response and had much higher levels of serum cortisol when compared to people without COVID-19. They also found that elevated serum cortisol concentrations were associated with higher rates of mortality.[16]

In contrast, Alzahrani and colleagues found that patients with COVID-19 had low ACTH and low serum cortisol levels, suggestive of central adrenal insufficiency. They measured ACTH, morning serum cortisol level, and dehydroepiandrosterone sulfate levels during the first two days of admission in 28 patients with COVID-19 infection. Their findings demonstrated that patients with COVID-19 had impaired adrenocortical response.[17]

▌HYPOTHALAMUS PITUITARY THYROID AXIS

Critical Illness and Thyroid Disorders

Critical illness and stress are often associated with alterations in thyroid function.[18] The most common disorder is the euthyroid-sick syndrome (decreased thyroid function tests associated with a non-thyroidal illness) that is associated with decreased thyroid stimulating hormone (TSH), thyroxine (T4) and triiodothyronine (T3), and elevated reverse T3 (rT3).[19,20] The euthyroid sick syndrome involves both peripheral and central axis disturbance. The initial phase is due to decrease in thyroid hormone binding and activation of thyroid deiodinases. However, prolonged illness is associated with hypothalamic dysfunction resulting in impaired secretion of thyroid releasing hormone (TRH).[21,22] There is a growing school of thought that the syndrome could represent both a protective response and a maladaptive response. Several studies have revealed that low levels of thyroid hormone is a predictor of poor outcome and increased mortality in the critically ill patients.[23,24]

COVID-19 and Thyroid Function

The emergence of the COVID-19 pandemic has once again brought the concerns of thyroid hormone perturbations during acute illness to the forefront. Persons with acute COVID-19 infections have been shown to have a variety of thyroid disorders including subacute thyroiditis and hypothyroidism, which are either caused or exacerbated by the viral infection. Various mechanisms have been proposed for thyroid dysfunction in patients with COVID-19. These include secondary hypothyroidism due to disruption of the hypothalamus-pituitary-thyroid axis, autoimmune thyroiditis and thyrotoxicosis due to release of inflammatory markers, and subacute thyroiditis.[25–29] The presence of ACE-2 receptors in thyroid follicular cells has been described as a possible source of viral entry into the thyroid gland resulting in subacute thyroiditis.[28]

Leow and colleagues found that some survivors had thyroid dysfunction, which was attributed to either hypophysitis or thyroiditis leading to abnormal function.[13]

Recent reports have compared thyroid function in patients with COVID-19 to those without the disease and found that TSH, Total T4, and Total T3 were lower in patients with COVID-19.[30,31]

A retrospective study done in Italy evaluated thyroid function in 287 patients hospitalized for COVID-19. Of these patients, 20.2% were found to have thyrotoxicosis. The authors hypothesized that thyrotoxicosis was a result of destructive thyroiditis as it resolved spontaneously and had negative TRAb. They also found an association between thyrotoxicosis and circulating levels of interleukin-6, suggesting that the thyroid gland is likely affected by the inflammatory markers associated with COVID-19 infection.[16] However, it is important to note that in many of the studies reporting thyroid hormone alterations in persons with COVID-19, most of the affected patients are euthyroid.[26]

To date there are no specific guidelines on when testing is indicated for thyroid disorders for persons with critical illness. In this case it is best to monitor the clinical presentation and check thyroid function tests when there are objective symptoms and signs for thyroid disorder.[30,32]

The current evidence suggests that most patients with COVID-19 infection remain euthyroid, but the most common thyroid abnormality is the euthyroid sick syndrome followed by a subacute thyroiditis that is mediated by an acute inflammatory process that results in destruction of follicular cells, which may result in increased extrusion of thyroid hormone.[30,32,33] Most of the alterations in thyroid function are transient and should improve during the convalescent period. Whether preexisting autoimmune thyroid disorder increases the risk of developing a thyroid disorder during COVID-19 infection is unknown. Treatment of a developing thyroid condition should be approached cautiously as several studies have shown that there is a high likelihood of recovery. For those patients already on thyroid therapy, they should be continued with close monitoring to assess if there is a need for dose adjustment of the treatment.[32]

HYPOTHALAMUS PITUITARY REPRODUCTIVE AXIS

The expression of ACE2 in spermatogonia and Leydig and Sertoli cells makes testes vulnerable to COVID-19 infection.[34] This was described in a case report of a young man with COVID-19 infection who presented with orchitis.[21,35] A study published in 2006 examined testes of six patients that died from SARS infection. After reviewing the findings from the study, the authors concluded that orchitis is a complication of SARS.[36] Postmortem examination of testes in COVID-19 patients showed seminiferous tubular injury, reduced Leydig cells, and lymphocytic inflammation. These findings are suggestive of significant testicular damage.[37] Li and colleagues examined semen samples of 38 patients affected by COVID-19. The results of semen analysis showed that 15.8% were positive for COVID-19.[38]

Another retrospective study performed in China compared reproductive function in men affected with COVID-19 infection and healthy men. The authors noted that the serum testosterone level did not vary significantly among the two groups, but they did find an elevated serum luteinizing hormone level and significant decrease in serum testosterone to luteinizing hormone ratio in those affected by COVID-19. They concluded that these findings were most likely due to possible damage to the Leydig cells. Men with COVID-19 infection were also found to have an elevated serum prolactin level.[39]

ACE2 receptors are less predominant in the female reproductive system compared to the male reproductive system.[24,25] It has been noted that COVID-19 may affect the hypothalamic-pituitary-gonadal axis resulting in lower levels of serum estrogen and progesterone.[40,41]

Thus, in viral pandemics there seems to be a dichotomy where men are disproportionately affected compared to women.

DIABETES AND CRITICAL ILLNESS

Diabetes Management and the Critically Ill Patient

As recently as 20 years ago, there was no data that glycemic control in the critically ill patient was necessary. Considered a compensatory reaction to illness, treatment of hyperglycemia was difficult based on the SQ insulins available and the resources required for intravenous insulin. In November 2001, a landmark article was published in the *New England Journal of Medicine*. The article, by lead author Greet Van den Berghe at the University of Leuven, Belgium, showed that glycemic control in mechanically ventilated surgical patients on early enteral nutrition improved ICU and in-hospital survival.[42] The goal for glycemic control was an unprecedented range of 80–110mg/dl. In addition, this approach reduced blood stream infections, acute renal failure requiring dialysis, red cell transfusions, and critical illness polyneuropathy. As with many landmark articles, the medical community spent the better part of the next decade trying to refute or reproduce these findings and did not succeed. The data became more confusing and the conclusions hotly debated by the decreased risk of some outcomes and yet the increased mortality risk associated with hypoglycemia. In 2009, the NICE-SUGAR investigators published the data delineating what has become the goalpost for glycemic control in the ICU. The inpatient goal of 140–180mg/dl was shown to be associated with less mortality than the tighter range of 81–108mg/dl. The medical community settled on this range as a middle of the road approach where the patient was not put in danger of hypoglycemia but the sugars were not allowed to elevate into the 200 and 300s with no intervention.

While the goal may be largely agreed upon, the mechanism whereby acute illness increases blood glucose in still unknown. On an outpatient basis, hyperglycemia can be the harbinger of infection or inflammation. Patients with no history of diabetes often have hyperglycemia in the setting of steroid use or myocardial infarction or sepsis. This so-called stress hyperglycemia has been felt, although perhaps not proven, to bely a predisposition to the development of diabetes. Patients with stress hyperglycemia may be at increased risk to develop diabetes later in life in the same way that those women with gestational diabetes (the stress being pregnancy) have a much higher risk of developing subsequent diabetes than does the general population. Kar and colleagues showed that in 40 patients that had hyperglycemia during critical illness hyperglycemia, less than a 1/3 of patients had normal oral glucose tolerance tests at 3 months and 12 months post ICU stay.[43] Other investigators have looked into this, but the data is limited by different definitions of stress hyperglycemia versus diabetes and heterogeneity of the patient populations. A meta-analysis of four studies by Abdelhamid and colleagues showed that the odd ratio for development of diabetes in a population with stress hyperglycemia was 3.48.[44] It seems a reasonable conclusion, therefore, that patients with stress hyperglycemia should be screened for diabetes down the road.

COVID-19 and Diabetes Management

COVID-19 has brought on challenges with regard to diabetes and glycemic control unlike any we have seen. What is the mechanism of hyperglycemia in COVID-19? Is it the same problem of critical illness hyperglycemia simply made worse by the use of high dose steroids, or is there damage to the pancreas by the virus itself? Further complicating the issue is the use of enteral nutrition in these patients, which further escalates insulin resistance. One argument for pancreatic damage from the virus stems from the anecdotal increased incidence of diabetic ketoacidosis (DKA) in these patients upon presentation to the hospital. One Chinese study reported pancreatic injury assessed by elevations of plasma amylase and lipase in 17% of their patients with COVID-19. Regardless of the etiology, glycemic control in COVID-19 has proven exceptionally difficult given the severity of illness, the significant degree of hyperglycemia seen, the use of steroids and tube feeds, and the balance of exposure and treatment required from frequent blood glucose monitoring.

The COVID-19 pandemic has propelled a review of the current protocols and treatment paradigms that are used for treatment of hyperglycemia emergencies and inpatient hyperglycemia.[45] Is it really necessary in light of the exposure risk and need to preserve personal protective equipment (PPE) to utilize an insulin infusion with the requisite q1 hour fingerstick monitoring in patients with COVID-19 and DKA? It has been well studied whether intravenous insulin is required for patients with diabetic emergencies, particularly DKA. Several studies have looked at IV insulin with q1 hour finger sticks versus SQ insulin with q2 hour finger sticks, and both approaches have been shown to be acceptable.[46–50] The problem with these studies in the setting of COVID-19 is that these were all patients with uncomplicated DKA. These were not acutely ill patients with tenuous clinical pictures and therefore labile insulin requirements. These data, while perhaps promising in trying to defer ICU admission purely for an insulin infusion in a patient who is otherwise healthy and low risk, do not apply to our COVID-19 patient population. Because of this, COVID-19 patients in DKA still need the resource intensive insulin infusion with q1 hour fingerstick monitoring until the acidosis is cleared.

It is said that adversity breeds innovation, so perhaps it is time to bring to the forefront those technologies that have been previously unused in the inpatient setting. Continuous glucose monitors can be applied to the patient and the data transmitted to a remote device. This is a technology utilized by parents of small children with type 1 diabetes so they can always be aware of their blood glucose. This would enable less fingerstick testing and therefore less exposure and less utilization of PPE by nurses and patient care techs. The accuracy of these devices in the acute setting, with intensity of blood glucose changes in clinically tenuous patients, is potentially the limitation here. In measuring an interstitial rather than a blood glucose, these devices are not as accurate when the blood glucose is changing rapidly and consistently lag about 10 minutes behind blood glucose changes. It would need to be studied further whether this 10 minute lag is clinically significant in the acutely ill.

CONCLUSION

The endocrine system with its vast interaction with neural and metabolic pathways is highly susceptible to changes during times of stress or crisis. The endocrine system is robust and has multiple innate responses that foster rapid adaptation to stress, inflammation, or immune modulation. In times of crisis, the presentation of endocrine conditions can be variable, and at times it is difficult to identify a single unifying clinical presentation or the best mode of treatment. As such, critical care providers have to remain dogged in their clinical diagnostic skills and acumen. In the acute setting, strict attention to detail is imperative, but for many patients long-term follow-up will be required.

REFERENCES

1. Golden SH, Robinson KA, Saldanha I, Anton B, Landenson PW. Prevalence and incidence of endocrine and metabolic disorders in the United States: A comprehensive review. *J Clin Endocrinol Metab*. 2009;94(6):1853-1878.

2. Manibusan MK, Touart LW. A comprehensive review of regulatory test methods for endocrine adverse health effects. *Crit Rev Toxicol*. 2017;47(6):433-481.

3. Badawi A, Ryoo SG. Prevalence of comorbidities in the Middle East respiratory syndrome coronavirus (MERS-CoV): A systematic review and meta-analysis. *Int J Infect Dis*. 2016;49:129-133.

4. Chatterjee S, Ghosh R, Biswas P, et al. COVID-19: The endocrine opportunity in a pandemic. *Minerva Endocrinol*. 2020;45(3):204-227.

5. Somasundaram NP, Ranathunga I, Ratnasamy V, et al. The impact of SARS-Cov-2 virus infection on the endocrine system. *JES*. 2020;4(8):bvaa082. doi: 10.1210/jendso/bvaa082.

6. Yang JK, Feng Y, Yuan MY, et al. Plasma glucose levels and diabetes are independent predictors for mortality and morbidity in patients with SARS. *Diabet Med*. 2006;23(6):623-8.

7. O'Connor TM, O'Halloran DJ, Shanahan F. The stress response and the hypothalamic-pituitary-adrenal axis: From molecule to melancholia. *Qjm*. 2000;93(6):323-333.

8. Tsigos C, Kyrou I, Kassi E, et al. Stress: Endocrine physiology and pathophysiology. ed. A.B. Feinglod KR, Boyce A, et al. [Updated 2020 Oct 17], *Endotext*. 67.

9. Hamming I, Timens W, Bulthuis MLC, Lely AT, Navis GJ, van Goor H. Tissue distribution of ACE2 protein, the functional receptor for SARS coronavirus. A first step in understanding SARS pathogenesis. *J Pathol*. 2004;203(2):631-637.

10. Pal R, Banerjee M. COVID-19 and the endocrine system: Exploring the unexplored. *J Endocrinol Invest*. 2020;43(7):1027-1031.

11. Garg MK, Gopalakrishnan M, Yadav P, Misra S. Endocrine involvement in COVID-19: Mechanisms, clinical features, and implications for care. *Indian J Endocrinol Metab*. 2020;24(5):381-386.

12. Wu A, Peng Y, Huang B, et al. Genome composition and divergence of the novel coronavirus (2019-nCoV) originating in China. *Cell Host Microbe*. 2020;27(3):325-328.

13. Leow MKS, Kwek DSK, Ng AWK, Ong KC, Kaw GJL, L LSU. Hypocortisolism in survivors of severe acute respiratory syndrome (SARS). *Clin Endocrinol (Oxf)*. 2005;63(2):197-202.

14. Demitrack MA, Dale JK, Straus SE, et al. Evidence for impaired activation of the hypothalamic-pituitary-adrenal axis in patients with chronic fatigue syndrome. *J Clin Endocrinol Metab*. 1991;73(6):1224-1234.

15. Yehuda R. Hypothalamic–pituitary–adrenal alterations in PTSD: Are they relevant to understanding cortisol alterations in cancer? *Brain Behav Immun*. 2003;17(1):73-83.

16. Tan T, Khoo B, Mills EG, et al. Association between high serum total cortisol concentrations and mortality from COVID-19. *Lancet Diabetes Endocrinol*. 2020;8(8):659-660.

17. Alzahrani AS, Mukhtar N, Aljomaiah A, et al. The impact of Covid-19 viral infection on the hypothalamic-pituitary-adrenal axis. *Endocr Pract*. 2020:S1530-891X(20)48393-4.

18. Adler SM, Wartofsky L. The nonthyroidal illness syndrome. *Endocrinol Metab Clin North Am*. 2007;36(3):657-672.

19. Economidou F, Douka E, Tzanela M, Nanas S, Kotanidou A. Thyroid function during critical illness. *Hormones (Athens)*. 2011;10(2):117-124.

20. Van den Berghe G. Non-thyroidal illness in the ICU: a syndrome with different faces. *Thyroid*. 2014;24(10):1456-1465.

21. Bello G, Ceaichisciuc I, Silva S, Antonelli M. The role of thyroid dysfunction in the critically ill: A review of the literature. *Minerva Anestesiol*. 2010;76(11):919-928.

22. Mebis L, Van den Berghe G. Thyroid axis function and dysfunction in critical illness. *Best Pract Res Clin*. 2011;25(5):745-757.

23. Gutch M, Kumar S, Gupta K. Prognostic value of thyroid profile in critical care condition. *Indian J Endocrinol Metab*. 2018;22(3):387-391.

24. Wang F, Pan W, Wang H, Wang S, Pan S, Ge J. Relationship between thyroid function and ICU mortality: A prospective observation study. *Critical Care*. 2012;16(1):11.

25. Kothandaraman N, Rengaraj A, Xue B, et al. COVID-19 endocrinopathy with hindsight from SARS. *Am J Physiol Endocrinol Metab*. 2021;320(1):E139-e150.

26. Lania A, Sandri MT, Cellini M, Mirani M, Lavezzi E, Mazziotti G. Thyrotoxicosis in patients with COVID-19: The THYRCOV study. *Eur J Endocrinol*. 2020;183(4):381-387.

27. Muller I, Cannavaro D, Dazzi D, et al. SARS-CoV-2-related atypical thyroiditis. *Lancet Diabetes Endocrinol*. 2020;8(9):739-741.

28. Rotondi M, Coperchini F, Ricci G, et al. Detection of SARS-COV-2 receptor ACE-2 mRNA in thyroid cells: A clue for COVID-19-related subacute thyroiditis. *J Endocrinol Invest*. 2020:1-6.

29. Wang W, Su X, Ding Y, et al. Thyroid Function Abnormalities in COVID-19 Patients. *Front Endocrinol (Lausanne)*. 2021;11:623792.

30. Khoo B, Tan T, Clarke SA, et al. Thyroid function before, during, and after COVID-19. *J Clin Endocrinol Metab*. 2020;106(2):e803-e811.

31. Lui DTW, Lee CH, Chow WS, et al. Thyroid Dysfunction in Relation to Immune Profile, Disease Status, and Outcome in 191 Patients with COVID-19. *J Clin Endocrinol Metab*. 2021;106(2):e926-e935. doi: 10.1210/clinem/dgaa813.

32. Caron P. Thyroid disorders and SARS-CoV-2 infection: From pathophysiological mechanism to patient management. *Annales d'endocrinologie*. 2020;81(5): 507-510.

33. Brancatella A, Ricci D, Cappellani D, et al. Is subacute thyroiditis an underestimated manifestation of SARS-CoV-2 infection? Insights from a case series. *J Clin Endocrinol Metab*. 2020;105(10):e3742-e3746.

34. Wang Z, Xu X. scRNA-seq profiling of human testes reveals the presence of the ACE2 receptor, a target for SARS-CoV-2 infection in spermatogonia, Leydig and Sertoli cells. *Cells*. 2020;9(4).

35. La Marca A, Busani S, Donno V, Guaraldi G, Ligabue G, Girardis M. Testicular pain as an unusual presentation of COVID-19: A brief review of SARS-CoV-2 and the testis. *Reprod Biomed Online*. 2020;41(5):903-906.

36. Xu J, Qi L, Chi X et al. Orchitis: a complication of severe acute respiratory syndrome (SARS). *Biol Reprod*. 2006;74(2):410-416. doi: 10.1095/biolreprod.

37. Yang M, Chen S, Huang, et al. Pathological findings in the testes of COVID-19 patients: Clinical implications. *Eur Urol Focus*. 2020;6(5):1124-1129.

38. Li D, Jin M, Bao P, Zhao W, Zhang S. Clinical characteristics and results of semen tests among men with coronavirus disease 2019. *JAMA Network Open*. 2020;3(5):e208292-e208292.

39. Ma L, Xie W, Li D, et al. Effect of SARS-CoV-2 infection upon male gonadal function: A single center-based study. medRxiv. 2020:2020.03.21.20037267.

40. Madjunkov M, Dviri M, Librach C. A comprehensive review of the impact of COVID-19 on human reproductive biology, assisted reproduction care and pregnancy: A Canadian perspective. *J Ovarian Res*. 2020;13(1):140.

41. Mauvais-Jarvis F, Klein SL, Levin ER. Estradiol, progesterone, immunomodulation, and COVID-19 outcomes. *Endocrinology*. 2020;161(9).

42. Van den Berghe G, Wouters P, Weekers F, et al. Intensive insulin therapy in critically ill patients. *N Engl J Med*. 2001;345(19):1359-1367.

43. Kar P, Plummer MP, Abdelhamid YA, et al. Incident diabetes in survivors of critical illness and mechanisms underlying persistent glucose intolerance: A prospective cohort study. *Crit Care Med*. 2019;47(2):e103-e111.

44. Ali Abdelhamid Y, Kar P, Finnis ME, et al. Stress hyperglycaemia in critically ill patients and the subsequent risk of diabetes: A systematic review and meta-analysis. *Crit Care*. 2016;20(1):301.

45. Korytkowski M, Antinori-Lent K, Drincic A, et al. A pragmatic approach to inpatient diabetes management during the COVID-19 pandemic. *J Clin Endocrinol Metab*. 2020;105(9):dgaa342. doi: 10.1210/clinem/dgaa342.

46. Gianchandani R, Esfandiari NH, Ang L, et al. Managing hyperglycemia in the COVID-19 inflammatory storm. *Diabetes*. 2020;69(10):2048-2053.

47. Umpierrez GE, Cuervo R, Karabell A, Latif K, Freire AX, Kitabchi AE. Treatment of diabetic ketoacidosis with subcutaneous insulin aspart. *Diabetes Care*. 2004;27(8):1873-1878.

48. Umpierrez GE, Latif K, Stoever J, et al. Efficacy of subcutaneous insulin lispro versus continuous intravenous regular insulin for the treatment of patients with diabetic ketoacidosis. *Am J Med*. 2004;117(5):291-296.

49. Zhou K, Al-Jaghbeer MJ, Lansang MC. Hyperglycemia management in hospitalized patients with COVID-19. *Cleve Clin J Med*. 2020.

50. Zhu L, She ZG, Cheng X, et al. Association of blood glucose control and outcomes in patients with COVID-19 and pre-existing Type 2 diabetes. *Cell Metabolism*. 2020;31(6):1068-1077.e3.

10 STRATEGIES IN ACUTE RESPIRATORY DISTRESS SYNDROME

Anjan Devaraj, MD and Michael McBrine, MD

INTRODUCTION

Acute respiratory distress syndrome (ARDS) is a distinct type of respiratory failure that manifests as acute, diffuse lung inflammation that causes hypoxemia and is associated with high mortality. Early recognition of the syndrome and the prompt use of appropriate ventilator and adjunct strategies to manage the disease is essential in reducing critical care morbidity and mortality. This chapter will cover how ARDS is a common cause of hypoxemia in the critically ill patient and will go over strategies for the early diagnosis of the disease. Later, the chapter will also go over strategies to manage and help these patients recover, including the key tenets of mechanical ventilatory support and the indications for noninvasive ventilatory support. Finally, adjunct strategies to help clinicians struggling with refractory hypoxemia will be reviewed, including the use of recruitment maneuvers, open lung ventilation, paralysis, proning, and extracorporeal membrane oxygenation (ECMO), among other modalities.

DEFINITION AND CAUSES OF HYPOXEMIA

Hypoxemia is defined as low levels of oxygen in the blood; more specifically, it is frequently defined as a level of partial pressure of oxygen that is less than 60 mm Hg in arterial blood. This cutoff is physiologically significant as there is rapid dissociation of oxygen from hemoglobin below this value that ultimately leads to a significantly reduced oxygen carrying capacity.[1] In the critical care unit, ARDS is always high on the differential for a patient with acute hypoxemia.

Hypoxemia is divided into five distinct etiologies: decreased inspired levels of oxygen, hypoventilation, impaired diffusion, ventilation perfusion mismatch, and right to left shunt. Clinically, both a low level of inspired oxygen and hypoventilation can be excluded in the critical care unit due the clinician controlling a patient's minute ventilation and fraction of inspired oxygen with a ventilator. Impaired diffusion is also rarely a cause of hypoxemia in the mechanically ventilated patient due to oxygen being a perfusion and not diffusion limited gas. As a result, most causes of hypoxemia in critically ill patients are due to ventilation perfusion mismatch and shunt (Figure 10-1).

ARDS causes hypoxemia by causing alveolar filling from a diffuse inflammatory process, resulting in ventilation perfusion mismatch and shunt as described below.

PATHOGENESIS, DEFINITION, AND EPIDEMIOLOGY OF ARDS

The hypoxemia driven by ARDS is caused by the leaking of protein rich fluid from lung capillaries into their adjacent alveoli, a process driven by the inflammatory response to the original inciting event. The increase of fluid and inflammation in the alveoli and interstitial space in turn decreases the ability of oxygen to move from the alveoli to the capillaries, thereby causing hypoxemia.

The process where ARDS develops has been classified into three distinct stages, which may overlap[2]

1. An exudative phase, termed diffuse alveolar damage, where the epithelium of the alveoli are disrupted and neutrophils infiltrate

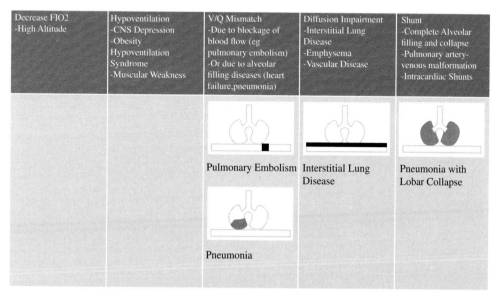

Figure 10-1 • Schematic showing causes of hypoxemia. (Adapted from Glenny, RW. Teaching ventilation/perfusion relationships in the lung. *Advances in Physiology Education*. 2008;32(3):192-195.)

the interstitium and alveoli in response to some insult causing lung inflammation

2. A proliferative phase, where after initial inflammation there is deposition of interstitial and alveolar collagen occurring alongside a decrease of the initial burst of neutrophils

3. A fibrotic phase, characterized by residual diffuse alveolar fibrosis and scarring in patients with prolonged (> 2 weeks) ARDS.

Since any disease process that can cause lung inflammation can lead to ARDS, it has a wide breadth of etiologies. Etiologies of ARDS are typically divided into direct (injuring lung) versus indirect (extrapulmonary injury causes), though ultimately both direct and indirect causes of ARDS lead to lung inflammation (Table 10-1).

Definition and History of ARDS

ARDS was first described in a case series in 1967 where 12 patients were noted to have hypoxemia and bilateral opacities on chest x-rays in the context of preceding traumas or infections.[3] At this time, it was called adult respiratory distress syndrome to distinguish it from respiratory distress syndrome in infants.

While the 1967 case series allowed for a rough idea of what ARDS was, it wasn't until 1988 when a more specific set of criteria were proposed to define the disease.[4] This definition used a lung injury score that graded lung injury from 0–4 in four different categories: radiographic opacities,

Table 10-1 DIRECT VS INDIRECT CAUSES OF ARDS	
Direct vs Indirect Injury in ARDS	
Direct	Indirect
Aspiration Pneumonitis	Sepsis
Pneumonia	Trauma
Pulmonic Contusion	Blood Transfusions
Toxic Inhalation	Pancreatitis
Near Drowning	Drug Overdose
Reperfusion Injury (e.g. Lung Transplant)	Adverse Medication Effects

Source: Adapted from Spadaro S, Park M, Turrini C, et al. Biomarkers for acute respiratory distress syndrome and prospects for personalised medicine. *Journal of Inflammation.* 2019;16(1):1.

degree of hypoxemia, amount of positive end expiratory pressure (PEEP) required to ventilate the patient, and respiratory system compliance. An average score of 2.5 or higher diagnosed ARDS. The main drawback of this definition was that it didn't exclude cardiogenic edema, as it assumed clinicians would do so automatically. However, it was the first time the notion of a P/F ratio (ratio of PO_2, the partial pressure of oxygen in a patient's arterial blood, divided by FIO_2, the fraction of oxygen in inspired air delivered to the patient) would be used for the disease, recognizing that the degree of respiratory support given needed to be accounted for to determine the degree of patient's hypoxemia.

In 1994, an American-European Consensus Conference (AECC) published a new de-facto definition of ARDS which defined it as an acute syndrome with bilateral infiltrates on chest radiography, hypoxemia with a P/F ratio < 200, and exclusion of cardiac failure by clinical exam or a pulmonary artery occlusion pressure of 18 mm Hg or less.[5] This definition also formally recognized there was a spectrum of disease severity, designating patients with the aforementioned criteria but a P/F ratio of < 300 as having acute lung injury (ALI), and those with a P/F ratio less than 200 of having ARDS. However, the 1994 definition still neglected to account for the use of PEEP in determining the severity of hypoxemia. Given this criticism and others, in 2012 the Berlin Definition of ARDS was introduced, which acts as the current definition of the disease.

The Berlin Definition of ARDS is a clinical entity whereupon within one week of a known precipitant, a patient has (a) new or worsening respiratory symptoms, (b) bilateral opacities on chest imaging that are not fully explained by cardiac failure of fluid overload, and (c) hypoxia defined as a P/F ratio less than 300, all while being maintained on positive pressure ventilation (either via an endotracheal or tracheostomy tube or through noninvasive means) with a minimum PEEP of 5 cm H_2O[6] (Table 10-2). This definition also stratified ARDS into mild (P/F < 300), moderate (P/F < 200), or severe (P/F < 100) categories. Ultimately, since the current definition of ARDS represents the hypoxic manifestation of lung injury caused by several different mechanisms, strategies to identify, manage, and treat the condition are essential for any clinician delivering critical care.

Epidemiology of ARDS

Given the relatively broad definition of ARDS and the inherent difficulty in its diagnosis, it is difficult to elucidate the exact incidence of the disease. The reported incidence of ARDS has ranged from 75 per 100,000 population per the National Heart and Lung Task force in the USA[7] to as low as

Table 10-2 BERLIN DEFINITION OF ARDS	
Criteria	**Definition**
Timing	Within 1 week of precipitant
Chest Imaging	Bilateral Opacities not explained by lobar collapse
Origin of Edema	Respiratory Failure not fully explained by cardiac failure or fluid overload
Oxygenation	
Mild	200 mm Hg ≤ Arterial P/F ≤ 300 mm Hg with PEEP or CPAP ≥ 5
Moderate	100 mm Hg ≤ Arterial P/F ≤ 200 mm Hg with PEEP or CPAP ≥ 5
Severe	Arterial P/F ≤ 100 mm Hg with PEEP or CPAP ≥ 5

PEEP, positive end expiratory pressure; CPAP, continuous positive airway pressure.

Source: Adapted from Ranieri VM, Rubenfeld GD, Thompson BT, et al. Acute respiratory distress syndrome: The Berlin Definition. *J Am Med Assoc* 2012;307(23):2526–2533.

1.5 per 100,000 in Europe.[8] The incidence of ALI has been estimated to be 78.9 cases per 100,000 person-years. The discordance between these numbers reflects the difficulty in clinicians defining and identifying the disease, and as such these numbers likely under-represent the prevalence of the syndrome.

NONINVASIVE SUPPORT IN ARDS

Indications and Use in Practice

Due to the degree of hypoxemia seen in ARDS, all patients are typically treated with what we will term noninvasive support or invasive ventilation. Noninvasive support includes but is not limited to the use of high flow nasal cannula (HFNC) and noninvasive ventilation (NIV, commonly used as continuous positive airway pressure and/or bilevel), whereas invasive ventilation indicates the use of an advanced airway (endotracheal tube or tracheostomy tube) with the addition of mechanical ventilation.

Most clinicians suggest the use of invasive mechanical ventilation for moderate to severe ARDS (defined as a P/F ratio < 200) and not noninvasive modalities. This recommendation is driven in part by data that suggest increased mortality with NIV in this patient population.[9] If NIV is utilized in mild ARDS (defined as P/F ratio less than 300, but greater than 200), the decision to transition to invasive ventilation should be made quickly (within 30–60 minutes) if (a) the patient's oxygenation is not improving on noninvasive support and (b) if further deoxygenation is expected given the patient's clinical trajectory. This approach is driven by data showing increased mortality in the delay of intubation while using HFNC.[10] Otherwise, in mild ARDS, the decision to intubate should still be based on other indications for intubation, such as the patient failing to maintain adequate spontaneous minute ventilation or risk of patency or protection of the patient's airway.

It can be difficult to recognize mild ARDS, as the epidemiology data presented earlier suggests. Further confounding the problem is that not all of these patients are on positive pressure ventilation to begin with, and not all of them have available blood gases at the time of assessment. From a practical standpoint one should consider ARDS on the differential (and recognize the prompt need for either noninvasive support or mechanical ventilation) in any patient utilizing NIV with an expiratory positive airway pressure (EPAP) or a continuous positive airway pressure (CPAP) at 5 cm H_2O or lower, or any patient whose oxygenation saturation (SpO_2) cannot be kept greater than 90% with either 6 liters of nasal cannula, 10 liters or greater with a venturi face mask, or 10 liters or greater with a non-rebreather face mask (whichever oxygen delivery device is available).

When choosing between HFNC or NIV in the setting of mild ARDS, the data is not entirely clear. Among patients with hypoxemic respiratory failure, HFNC lessened mortality and intubation rates compared to noninvasive ventilation or standard oxygen therapy.[11] However, this study was not specific to ARDS patients and was not sufficiently powered. The data does suggest that HFNC is inferior to NIV in patients whose primary process includes hypercapneic acidosis from COPD and acute cardiogenic pulmonary edema.[12,13] However, by virtue of the definition of ARDS being a hypoxemic, not hypercapnic process, driven by a non-cardiogenic etiology, HFNC may be a reasonable alternative to NIV in patients with mild ARDS.

Noninvasive Support in COVID-19

As the data emerges from the recent COVID-19 pandemic, there are recommendations from the Society of Critical Care Medicine advocating for the use of HFNC over NIV. These recommendations are based on the aforementioned studies analyzing HFNC and acute hypoxemic respiratory failure, as well as an article in July 2020 that noted a few small size, low powered studies which showed improved outcomes in COVID-19 patients treated with HFNC over standard oxygen therapy.[14] Of note, there is also a debate about the risk of aerosolization of infectious particles with HFNC, but it is generally thought that this risk is low when flow rates are kept below 40 liters.[15] Early in the pandemic, some providers initially recommended prompt intubation for patients even with mild ARDS, largely prompted by fears of increased risk of aerosolization of the virus and risking infection in health care workers. As of yet, sufficient high quality studies have not been performed to support this practice pattern.

▌ INTUBATION AND MECHANICAL VENTILATION

Indications

Given the rapid disease progression and severe hypoxemia seen in ARDS, most patients are ultimately managed on a ventilator with an endotracheal or tracheostomy tube.

The key principle behind ventilator use in ARDS is to minimize both ventilator induced lung injury and patient self-induced lung damage. This strategy aims to compensate for the physiologic decrease in lung compliance that is seen with ARDS. The goal as such is to ventilate the lungs utilizing low tidal volumes, 4–6 cc/kg, to minimize the damage from barotrauma. At the same time, clinicians aim to utilize PEEP to prevent damage from atelectrauma and allow the lungs time to recover from the proliferative and exudative phase of ARDS, and prevent progression to the fibrotic phase.[16] This strategy targeting a low tidal volume, which is defined as 6 ml/kg of predicted body weight, or PBW, and aiming for a plateau pressure less than 30 is one that was famously described in 2000.[17]

Initial Settings

After intubating a patient for moderate to severe ARDS, initial ventilator settings should be set with the PEEP at 8 cm H_2O and FIO_2 at 100%, and the tidal volume set at 6 ml/kg of predicted body weight (PBW). We recommend starting with a volume-limited mode to easily control tidal volume. The calculations for PBW can be found in the Table 10-3.

The above settings come from the ARDS network low tidal volume study trial,[17] which showed benefit from low tidal volume ventilation. This study also solidified prior beliefs that a targeted low plateau pressure (less

Table 10-3 INITIAL VENTILATOR SETTINGS

Initial ventilator settings

Calculate predicted body weight (PBW)

Male =	$50 + 2.3$ [height (inches) $- 60$] **OR**
	$50 + 0.91$ [height (cm) $- 152.4$]
Female	$45.5 + 2.3$ [height (inches) $- 60$] **OR**
=	$45.5 + 0.91$ [height (cm) $- 152.4$]

Set mode to volume assist-control

Set initial tidal volume to 6 ml/kg **PBW**

Set initial ventilator rate ≤35 breaths/min to match baseline minute ventilation

Source: Adapted from The Acute Respiratory Distress Syndrome Network, et al. Ventilation with
   lower tidal volumes as compared with traditional tidal volumes for acute lung injury and the acute
   respiratory distress syndrome. *N Engl J Med.* 2000;342:1301–1308.

than 30) would also be beneficial. The plateau pressure itself can be measured by performing an inspiratory pause on the ventilator, which causes the machine to give the patient a breath and hold it. During this pause, airway pressure and alveolar pressure equalize, and this value can be used as a surrogate for the degree of barotrauma the alveoli are experiencing.

From a practical standpoint, the initial ventilator settings calculated from the table correspond to 275 ml, 350 ml, and 425 ml for a 5 foot, 5 foot 6 inches, and 6 foot woman, respectively, as well as 300, 375, and 450 for a 5 foot, 5 foot 6, and 6 foot man, respectively. The respiratory rate should be set at a range of 14–22 to approximate the patient's prior minute ventilation.

Titrating Settings

After initial intubation and ventilation, settings should be rapidly titrated to the patient's degree of hypoxemia and acidosis. With regards to the PEEP and FiO_2 settings, further titration, with a goal PaO_2 between 55 and 80 mm Hg,[18] can be performed in accordance with the Table 10-4 from the ARDSNET study.[17]

Despite subsequent studies showing no difference between high or low PEEP strategies in ARDS patients,[19] clinicians err on the higher side of PEEP so as to maximize alveolar recruitment and minimize atelectasis.

Table 10-4 TITRATING OXYGEN AND PEEP IN VENTILATED PATIENTS							
Arterial oxygenation and PEEP							
Oxygenation goal: PaO_2 55 to 80 mmHg or SpO_2 88 to 95 percent							
Use these FiO_2/PEEP combinations to achieve oxygenation goal:							
FiO_2	0.3	0.4	0.5	0.6	0.7	0.8	0.9	1.0
PEEP	5	5 to 8	8 to 10	10	10 to 14	14	14 to 18	18 to 24
PEEP should be applied starting with the minimum value for a given FiO_2.							

Source: Adapted from The Acute Respiratory Distress Syndrome Network, et al. Ventilation with lower tidal volumes as compared with traditional tidal volumes for acute lung injury and the acute respiratory distress syndrome. *N Engl J Med.* 2000;342:1301–1308.

While not statistically significant, those studies on respiratory mechanics in ARDS showed a trend toward increased PEEP usage leading to lower mortality.[19]

The tidal volume should be kept to 6 ml/kg PBW, while also trying to keep the patient's plateau pressure less than 30 cm H_2O. Lastly, clinicians can have reasonable flexibility with changing the patient's respiratory rate, but typically aim for a respiratory rate of less than 35, and try to lower the respiratory rate to a number where auto-peep (breath stacking) is minimized or not seen but the patient's pH is kept > 7.25 (Table 10-5). In addition, it is important to try to keep the patient sedated sufficiently to prevent patient-ventilator dyssynchrony as it has been shown to increase ventilator length of use and morbidity[20] but not too deeply to impair readiness testing as described in the weaning section.

The above titrating principles are based on data showing decreased mortality in the ARDSNET study by focusing on reducing barotrauma and ventilator induced lung damage at high plateau pressures.

Driving Pressure

While all of the above data suggests that lung protective ventilator strategies (low tidal volumes, plateau < 30, higher PEEP) lead to better patient outcomes, optimizing the exact tidal volume and PEEP for an individual patient remains challenging. Some authors have suggested that one way to approach individual optimization is to look at the alveolar pressure changes that occur with ventilation as opposed to the maximal alveolar pressure (which is reflected by the plateau pressure). Perhaps large

Table 10-5 TIDAL VOLUME ADJUSTMENT IN VENTILATED PATIENTS
Subsequent tidal volume adjustment
Plateau pressure goal: Pplat ≤30 cm H_2O
Check inspiratory plateau pressure with 0.5 second inspiratory pause at least every four hours and after each change in PEEP or tidal volume.
If Pplat >30 cm H_2O, decrease tidal volume in 1 mL/kg PBW steps to 5 or if necessary to 4 mL/kg PBW.
If Pplat <25 cm H_2O and tidal volume <6 mL/kg, increase tidal volume by 1 mL/kg PBW until Pplat >25 cm H_2O or tidal volume = 6 mL/kg.
If breath stacking (autoPEEP) or severe dyspnea occurs, tidal volume may be increased to 7 or 8 mL/kg PBW if Pplat remains ≤30 cm H_2O.

Source: Adapted from The Acute Respiratory Distress Syndrome Network, et al. Ventilation with lower tidal volumes as compared with traditional tidal volumes for acute lung injury and the acute respiratory distress syndrome. *N Engl J Med.* 2000;342:1301–1308.

changes in alveolar pressure, or the driving pressure (symbolized as the delta in pressure, or Δ P), that occur during each breath are responsible for ventilator induced lung injury.[21] Δ P can be calculated as the Plateau pressure – PEEP or tidal volume / lung compliance. A 2015 study[21] found that the driving pressure was most predictive of an increased 60-day survival. Practically, Δ P can be thought of as a number that describes the relationship between a specified tidal volume set on the ventilator and the inherent lung volume available to receive the breath at the beginning of inspiration.[21] A lower number suggests a more compliant lung that does not experience a large change in alveolar pressure with a given breath. Other authors have suggested that maintaining a driving pressure < 14 leads to better outcomes.[22] It follows that titration of a patient's tidal volume and PEEP targeting a lower driving pressure may lead to a better outcome for that individual patient than following a static plateau pressure or a PEEP chart. Physiologically, driving pressure is still fundamentally about optimizing ventilator settings to prevent ventilator induced lung injury while maximizing compliance of the lung, but further studies need to validate the findings described above.

Weaning Settings and Extubation

Similar to other patients with respiratory failure, we prefer weaning patients with ARDS from mechanical ventilation with daily spontaneous breathing trials (SBTs). This process, called readiness testing, starts when a patient's oxygenation has improved so that they require a PEEP of 8 cm H_2O or less and their FIO_2 requirement is 50% or less while still maintaining a $PaO_2 > 55$. In addition, patients should be taking spontaneous breaths, have a pH >7.25, and should be hemodynamically stable. Given the newer data showing improved outcomes and successes at extubation with pressure support ventilation (PSV) over T-piece (no pressure support given),[23] new guidelines[24] have been created advocating for the use of PSV over T-piece. Once on PSV, a patient passes a trial if they avoid the following within 120 minutes:[25]

- Respiratory rate fewer than 8 or more than 35 per minute for 5 minutes or longer
- Hypoxemia ($SpO_2 < 88\%$ for $\geq$ 5 minutes)
- Abrupt change in mental status
- Acute cardiac arrhythmia
- Two or more of the following: tachycardia, bradycardia, accessory muscle use, sweating, or visible dyspnea

If a patient passes the trial, one may move forward with extubation. If patients have risk factors that place them at high risk for reintubation and there are no resource limitations, extubating to HFNC or NIV should be considered. While not conclusive, there is data supporting this approach.[26]

ADJUNCT VENTILATOR STRATEGIES IN REFRACTORY HYPOXEMIA IN ARDS

Refractory Hypoxemia

Even with the evidence-based approach described above in managing patients with ARDS on ventilators, it is not uncommon to have refractory hypoxemia, defined as ongoing hypoxemia with a P/F ratio < 150 despite low volume mechanical ventilation. Likewise, patients may have significant ventilator dyssynchrony with low tidal volumes and high respiratory rates. Here we will describe adjunct therapies that can be utilized in these scenarios and the evidence supporting their use.

Changing Modes of Ventilation

If a patient continues to have significant dyssynchrony or if there is difficult in keeping the plateau pressure < 30 cm/H_2O, switching to a pressure limited mode of ventilation may be helpful. Pressure limited modes are the most well studied in comparison to volume control modes in ARDS.

In some studies, pressure limited modes are associated with lower peak airway pressures, increased synchrony, and more homogeneous gas distribution when compared to volume control modes.[27] This mode is best utilized in patients with little variation in their compliance in order to target and maintain a low targeted tidal volume.

While there are other modes of ventilation, including pressure-regulated volume control, airway pressure release ventilation, and neurally adjusted ventilator assist, there is limited data about their efficacy in ARDS and their use may be best employed at centers that are familiar with these modes. Ultimately, if a trial of an alternate mode of ventilation is employed, close monitoring over the next few hours after the change is essential in order to measure changes in gas exchange, airway pressures, and synchrony.

Recruitment Maneuvers

Another ventilator strategy involves the use of a recruitment maneuver: a short burst of a high level of PEEP to prevent atelectrauma and to open up closed non-gas exchanging alveoli. Recruitment maneuvers can be performed individually or as the first step of open lung ventilation (see below). When performed individually, high levels of PEEP (35 cm H_2O) are applied for 40 seconds before reverting back to the patient's prior PEEP. There have been individual trials showing a mortality benefit with this approach, but a meta-analysis in 2017 failed to confirm this finding.[28] Nevertheless, it is a reasonable salvage therapy given its ease of use and minimal adverse effects provided excessive PEEP and duration are limited.[29]

Open Lung Ventilation

Open lung ventilation (OLV) is another strategy that can be attempted in refractory hypoxemic patients. It employs the use of a recruitment maneuver to recruit non-gas exchanging alveoli, and couples it with subsequent titration of PEEP to maintain the patency of alveoli and minimize atelectasis. The data behind this strategy is conflicting, and a 2017 meta-analysis showed improved mortality with this technique.[30] However the largest international RCT using open lung ventilation, also published in 2017, showed possible harm.[31] There is not a well-established protocol for OLV as a result of the discordant data. Many institutions perform a recruitment maneuver with a PEEP approximating 35 cm H_2O, then drop the PEEP to 30 cm H_2O for 2 minutes, then 25 cm H_2O for 2 minutes. Subsequently, decremental decreases in the PEEP by 2 cm H_2O increments for 2 minutes each until the SpO_2 drops by 2% or more or until the PEEP is 2 cm H_2O above the prior PEEP. This new PEEP level is maintained if the peak pressures are kept to less than 45 cm H_2O and the plateau pressures are less than 30 H_2O, and there is overall improved oxygenation in the patient. Otherwise we return back to the prior PEEP.

ADJUNCT NON-VENTILATOR STRATEGIES

As discussed earlier in the chapter, utilizing lung protective ventilator strategies (low tidal volumes, plateau < 30, higher PEEP) is the core principle in the management of patients with ARDS. However, there are other therapies utilized in the ICU that merit discussion in the evidence-based care of ARDS patients.

Proning

In ARDS, the hypoxemia present is driven by both shunt physiology and by v/q mismatch. This physiology is at times exacerbated by the supine position. When supine, the dorsal alveoli are atelectatic and filled with protein rich fluid in part due to the hydrostatic forces associated with this position. These dorsal alveoli are not well ventilated, but are being perfused, and hypoxemia results. In contrast, the more ventral alveoli are often over-distended as a result of positive pressure breaths being redirected away from those dorsal atelectatic regions. However, these ventral units are less well perfused than the dorsal units. The physiologic processes occurring dorsally and ventrally lead to significant V/Q mismatch as the best perfused regions of the lung (dorsal) receive the least ventilation while the over ventilated regions (ventral) receive less perfusion.

However, prone positioning helps ameliorate these regional differences, thus making ventilation more homogeneous. When prone, the previously dependent lung continues to receive the majority of the blood flow as alveoli reopen (recruitment) as a result of both PEEP and decreased transpulmonary pressure. In contrast, the newly dependent lung continues to receive the minority of the blood flow as alveoli begin to collapse. This improvement in ventilation/perfusion that is seen with proning can last well after a return to the supine position, as the data below suggests. Furthermore, the overdistention and ventilator induced barotrauma these previously ventral alveoli experienced has also decreased due to prone positioning.[32]

Given the physiology behind this maneuver, it is not surprising that numerous studies showed an improvement in oxygenation with proning in ARDS.[33] However, it was not until PROSEVA[32] was published in 2013 that a mortality benefit was shown. In this study, they enrolled 466 patients with ARDS, with a P/F < 150 within 33 hours of intubation. The major difference in this trial was the marked increase in time spent prone when compared to previous studies (at least 16 hours). The end result of the study was a significant reduction in the 90-day mortality (24 versus 41 percent). In addition, the patients enrolled in the proning arm of the study needed fewer rescue modalities like ECMO or iNO.

In 2019, a meta-analysis of 25 studies also concluded that there was a lower 28-day mortality when proning was utilized for patients with moderate to severe ARDS.[34] Given all of the above, the recommendation to use proning is consistent with guidelines from the American Thoracic Society, European Society of Intensive Care Medicine, and Society of Critical Care Medicine.[35] Contraindications do exist and include increased intracranial pressure, trauma, and spinal instability among others. In addition, complications including pressure ulcers, nerve compression, and dislodgement of tubes and IVs can be seen.

Given the robust data mentioned above demonstrating a mortality benefit, proning was an expert WHO recommendation for COVID-19 patients with severe hypoxemic respiratory failure.[36] In addition, self proning has been recommended for the hypoxemic but non-intubated patient based on several small studies that showed an improvement in oxygenation.[37] There is insufficient data as of yet to know if proning helps to avoid intubation.

Extracorporeal Membrane Oxygenation

Extracorporeal membrane oxygenation (ECMO) is a mechanical circulatory support device that has been used for acute respiratory failure since the 1970s, and in some cases, as a bridge to lung transplant. While venous-arterial (VA) ECMO can be used for both hemodynamic support and for hypoxemia/hypercapnia, venous-venous, or V-V ECMO, has been primarily reserved for those patients who are persistently hypoxemic (P/F < 70) despite conventional therapeutic strategies. The CESAR trial[38] from 2009 enrolled 180 patients in the United Kingdom who had severe hypoxemic respiratory failure. These patients were transferred to ECMO centers in the United Kingdom, and those in the intervention arm had increased survival without disability at six months (63% versus 47%). This trial was criticized for the heterogeneity in ventilator strategies employed and the fact that many of the patients in the intervention arm were never actually started on ECMO. This study suggested that those individuals with severe respiratory failure did better at an ECMO center.

The EOLIA trial from 2018[39] enrolled 249 patients with severe ARDS (defined as a P/F ratio < 50 for > 3 hours or P/F < 80 for > 6 hours) and assigned them to an intervention of early V-V ECMO versus conventional lung protective ventilator strategies. This study was stopped early, and there ultimately was not a statistically significant improvement in 60-day mortality. However, the ECMO arm of the study did have improved oxygenation, less renal failure, and fewer ischemic strokes. In addition, survival was highest in those patients who were randomized to ECMO early (within 2 days). Limitations of this study included the high amount of severely hypoxemic patients who crossed over into the ECMO arm of the study and the much greater utilization of prone positioning (known to improve mortality) in the placebo arm of the study.

A meta-analysis from 2019[40] combined the data from both EOLIA and CESAR and from three other observational studies to conclude that there was evidence to support an improved 60-day mortality rate (34% versus 47%) with ECMO utilization. This study did note that there was a moderate risk of major bleeding associated with ECMO and that this technique was best utilized in centers that are comfortable with ECMO.

Finally, in relation to the recent COVID-19 epidemic, numerous case series have emerged from various centers regarding their experiences, but disease specific recommendations have not been forthcoming at this point. The WHO released guidelines[36] that suggested the utilization of the EOLIA hypoxemia criteria (P/F ratio < 50 for > 3 hours or P/F ratio < 80 for > 6 hours) as a reason to consider an ECMO referral in centers with the applicable expertise.

Neuromuscular Blockade

Neuromuscular blocking agents (NMBAs) block transmission of neurologic signals at the neuromuscular junction and induce paralysis of skeletal muscles. The most commonly used class of NBMAs in the critically ill are the nondepolarizing NMBAs which competitively inhibit the activation of the acetylcholine receptor either by blocking binding or preventing a transformational change. While these medicines have been used widely in critically ill patients, the data supporting their use has always been sparse. The literature has shown an improvement in oxygenation with their use[41] but also shown evidence of harm.[42] Consensus guidelines have been created,[43] though written as weak recommendations based on the evidence available, paralytics remain commonly used. While NBMAs do not have sedative, amnestic, or analgesic properties, they can be used for refractory hypoxemia, shivering in the setting of hypothermia, ventilator asynchrony, and in the setting of increased abdominal pressures or intracranial pressures. With the advent of lung protective ventilator strategies, breath stacking, a form of dyssynchrony, has become a prominent phenomenon in ICUs. Many ARDS patients want larger tidal volumes than we administer and work against the ventilator to accomplish this goal.

The ACURASYS[44] trial published in 2010 intriguingly showed an improvement in the adjusted 90-day survival rate when cisatracurium was utilized for 48 hours soon after the initiation of mechanical ventilation in ARDS patients. The study patients all had a P/F ratios less than 150 and were also managed with conventional lung protective ventilation strategies. Importantly, this study did not encounter an increase in adverse outcomes, specifically muscle weakness. One theory about the perceived efficacy in this study was that paralytics ameliorated the breath stacking and those non-lung protective volumes that occurred during breath stacking.

However, given the lack of research comparing the effects of paralytics with deep sedation versus a lighter sedation strategy, the Reevaluation of Systemic Early Neuromuscular Blockade (ROSE)[45] trial was undertaken. This trial also enrolled patients with ARDS and a P/F < 150 who had been intubated for less than 48 hours and again utilized cisatracurium. Notably, this study used lighter sedation in their control arm and used higher levels of PEEP (average of 12) uniformly throughout the study. At 90 days, there was no difference in the mortality between their treatment and control arm.[45]

Based on the data available, there still is a role for paralytics in certain patients with ARDS, particularly those with ventilator dyssynchrony. However, its use for all patients with ARDS and a P/F < 150 is not supported by the currently available data.

Inhaled Vasodilators

Inhaled vasodilators, particularly inhaled nitric oxide, have been utilized in ICUs for severe ARDS for the past 40 years. In principle, these medications are inhaled into well oxygenated airways, then traverse into the local pulmonary vascular system and cause vasodilation. The result is an increase in perfusion to well ventilated alveoli (away from poorly ventilated alveoli) and an improvement in oxygenation. While principally sound, this theory has not been shown to consistently deliver on its promise. Studies have described patients whose gas exchange does not improve with the administration of iNO and noted that specific factors like high baseline pulmonary vascular resistance, responsiveness to positive end-expiratory pressure (PEEP), and the absence of sepsis or septic shock may predict responsiveness to iNO.[46]

Given the somewhat contradictory findings above, and the complexity of the pulmonary vascular system, it is not surprising that multiple meta-analyses have failed to show a mortality benefit. The Cochrane review in 2016 included 16 papers with over 1,300 participants and did not show any mortality benefit.[47] This study also noted that there was a significant transient increase in oxygenation at 24 hours that occurred at the expense of more acute renal failure.

Inhaled prostaglandins, epoprostenol for example, have also been studied in severe ARDS. Similar to iNO, the data suggests it improves oxygenation in severe ARDS but does not affect mortality.[48] These drugs may be preferable to iNO given they do not need a sophisticated delivery mechanism like iNO. However, during the recent COVID epidemic, they have been less preferable than inhaled iNO due to the frequency with which the ventilator circuit needs to be disconnected. With epoprostenol, the filter at the expiratory port of the ventilator circuit needs to be changed more frequently than when using iNO. When the circuit is disrupted, there is potential increased aerosolization and increased risk of transmission.

Fluid Management

Despite many years of research, determining an optimal fluid strategy remains challenging when trying to apply the available data to a specific patient. Previous best practices like the pulmonary artery catheter have fallen by the wayside as our knowledge has evolved. The surviving sepsis campaign has made expert based recommendations involving fluid resuscitation, but only a minority of ARDS patients have underlying infection as an etiology of their disease. In addition, in the early phase of ARDS, when increased capillary permeability is present, excessive administration of fluid increases vascular hydrostatic forces and increases pulmonary edema.

The bulk of the fluid strategy in managing ARDS patients stems from a 2006 article that compared a conservative fluid strategy versus a more liberal strategy.[49] One thousand patients were randomized to either a liberal strategy which targeted a central venous pressure (CVP) of 10 to 14 mm Hg or a pulmonary artery occlusion pressure (PAOP) of 14 to 18 mm Hg. In this liberal fluid group, the patients were ultimately positive 6,992 mL over the course of a week, or roughly a liter a day. The conservative fluid group targeted a CVP < 4 mm Hg or a pulmonary artery occlusion pressure (PAOP) < 8 mm Hg. This group was roughly net even in their fluid balance (exactly negative 136 mL) over the course of the week. While there was not a mortality benefit with a conservative fluid strategy, those patients had evidence of improved oxygenation and more ventilator free days than those patients in the liberal group. Given the above, from a practical standpoint, targeting a close to even (to sometimes negative) fluid balance in ARDS patients is preferred after initial resuscitation attempts have concluded.

Glucocorticoids

Similar to vasodilators, studies looking at the impact of glucocorticoids on ARDS outcomes have been ongoing for almost 40 years. Given the antifibrotic and anti-inflammatory properties of glucocorticoids, they have been an attractive potential therapy in ARDS due to the underlying physiology outlined earlier in the chapter. However, the data available has never conclusively shown a benefit[50] and in fact, many of the studies were conducted before the advent of the ARDSnet trials referenced earlier.

Recently, a trial was published that examined the effects of dexamethasone in patients with moderate to severe ARDS[50] whose primary outcome was the number of ventilator free days. This study showed a statistically significant increase in ventilator free days in the dexamethasone group when administered at 20 mg daily for 5 days, followed by 10 mg daily for 5 days. In addition, the authors found a decrease in the 60-day all-cause mortality without an increase in adverse events.

When considering the use of corticosteroids in ARDS patients, it is also important to consider the other potential indications like pneumonia, septic shock, and more recently, COVID-19 when choosing a dose. While the data supporting these other indications is beyond the scope of this chapter, the well-read physician will be cognizant of these other indications.

CONCLUSION

ARDS is a life-threatening cause of hypoxemia in the critically ill patients, and early recognition of this syndrome is crucial for any clinician working in the critical care unit. Rapid identification of patients progressing to ARDS with the use of the Berlin Criteria and P/F ratio is critical, and prompt and judicious use of mechanical ventilator support to preserve lung function and minimize inflammatory mediated damage is essential. The key concept of lung protective ventilation via low tidal volumes is essential in minimizing mortality among these critically ill patients. Adjunct strategies and therapies, such as OLV, recruitment maneuvers, and the use of diuretics, paralytics, proning, and ECMO can also be utilized in the attempt to minimize mortality and complications related to mechanical ventilation. While ARDS remains a cause of high mortality in the ICU, knowledge of the approaches outlined above will give any clinician the best tools to care for their patients.

▌ REFERENCES

1. Barcroft J, Roberts F. The dissociation curve of haemoglobin. *J Physiol.* 1909;39(2):143.
2. Tomashefski J Jr. Pulmonary pathology of the adult respiratory distress syndrome. *Clin Chest Med.* 1990;11(4):593.
3. Ashbaugh D, Bigelow DB, Petty T, Levine B. Acute respiratory distress in adults. *The Lancet.* 1967;290(7511):319-323.
4. Murray JF, Matthay MA, Luce JM, Flick MR. An expanded definition of the adult respiratory distress syndrome. *Am Rev Respir Dis.* 1988;138(3):720-723.
5. Bernard GR, Artigas A, Brigham KL, et al. Report of the American-European Consensus conference on acute respiratory distress syndrome: Definitions, mechanisms, relevant outcomes, and clinical trial coordination. *J Crit Care.* 1994;9(1):72-81.
6. Ferguson ND, Fan E, Camporota L, et al. The Berlin definition of ARDS: An expanded rationale, justification, and supplementary material. *Intensive Care Med.* 2012;38(10):1573-1582.
7. Lewandowski K, Lewandowski M. Epidemiology of ARDS. *Minerva Anestesiol.* 2006;72(6):473-477.
8. Villar J, Slutsky AS. The incidence of the adult respiratory distress syndrome. *Am J Respir Crit Care Med.* 1989;140(3):814-816.
9. Bellani G, Laffey JG, Pham T, et al. Noninvasive ventilation of patients with acute respiratory distress syndrome. Insights from the LUNG SAFE study. *Am J Respir Crit Care Med.* 2017;195(1):67-77.
10. Kang BJ, Koh Y, Lim C-M, et al. Failure of high-flow nasal cannula therapy may delay intubation and increase mortality. *Intensive Care Med.* 2015;41(4):623-632.
11. Frat J-P, Thille AW, Mercat A, et al. High-flow oxygen through nasal cannula in acute hypoxemic respiratory failure. *N Engl J Med.* 2015;372(23):2185-2196.
12. Osadnik CR, Tee VS, Carson-Chahhoud KV, Picot J, Wedzicha JA, Smith BJ. Non-invasive ventilation for the management of acute hypercapnic respiratory failure due to exacerbation of chronic obstructive pulmonary disease. *Cochrane Database Syst Rev.* 2017;7(7):CD004104.
13. Vital FM, Ladeira MT, Atallah ÁN. Non-invasive positive pressure ventilation (CPAP or bilevel NPPV) for cardiogenic pulmonary oedema. *Cochrane Database Syst Rev.* 2013;(5):CD005351.
14. Rochwerg B, Solo K, Darzi A, Chen G, Khamis AM. Update Alert: Ventilation techniques and risk for transmission of coronavirus disease, including COVID-19. *Ann Intern Med.* 2020;173(6):W122.
15. Leonard S, Atwood CW, Walsh BK, et al. Preliminary findings on control of dispersion of aerosols and droplets during high-velocity nasal insufflation therapy

using a simple surgical mask: Implications for the high-flow nasal cannula. *Chest.* 2020;158(3):1046-1049.

16. Mauri T, Lazzeri M, Bellani G, Zanella A, Grasselli G. Respiratory mechanics to understand ARDS and guide mechanical ventilation. *Physiol Meas.* 2017;38(12):R280.

17. Network ARDS. Ventilation with lower tidal volumes as compared with traditional tidal volumes for acute lung injury and the acute respiratory distress syndrome. *N Engl J Med.* 2000;342(18):1301-1308.

18. Mortelliti MP, Manning HL. Acute respiratory distress syndrome. *Am Fam Physician.* 2002;65(9):1823.

19. National Heart L, Network BIACT. Higher versus lower positive end-expiratory pressures in patients with the acute respiratory distress syndrome. *N Engl J Med.* 2004;351(4):327-336.

20. De Wit M, Miller KB, Green DA, Ostman HE, Gennings C, Epstein SK. Ineffective triggering predicts increased duration of mechanical ventilation. *Crit Care Med.* 2009;37(10):2740-2745.

21. Amato MB, Meade MO, Slutsky AS, et al. Driving pressure and survival in the acute respiratory distress syndrome. *N Engl J Med.* 2015;372(8):747-755.

22. Bellani G, Laffey JG, Pham T, et al. Epidemiology, patterns of care, and mortality for patients with acute respiratory distress syndrome in intensive care units in 50 countries. *JAMA.* 2016;315(8):788-800.

23. Subirà C, Hernández G, Vázquez A, et al. Effect of pressure support vs T-piece ventilation strategies during spontaneous breathing trials on successful extubation among patients receiving mechanical ventilation: a randomized clinical trial. *JAMA.* 2019;321(22):2175-2182.

24. Schmidt GA, Girard TD, Kress JP, et al. Official executive summary of an American Thoracic Society/American College of Chest Physicians clinical practice guideline: Liberation from mechanical ventilation in critically ill adults. *Am J Respir Crit Care Med.* 2017;195(1):115-119.

25. Girard TD, Kress JP, Fuchs BD, et al. Efficacy and safety of a paired sedation and ventilator weaning protocol for mechanically ventilated patients in intensive care (Awakening and Breathing Controlled trial): A randomised controlled trial. *Lancet.* 2008;371(9607):126-134.

26. Hernández G, Vaquero C, González P, et al. Effect of postextubation high-flow nasal cannula vs conventional oxygen therapy on reintubation in low-risk patients: A randomized clinical trial. *JAMA.* 2016;315(13):1354-1361.

27. Prella M, Domenighetti G. Effects of short-term pressure-controlled ventilation on gas exchange, airway pressures, and gas distribution in patients with acute lung injury/ARDS: Comparison with volume-controlled ventilation. *Chest.* 2002;122(4):1382-1388.

28. Goligher EC, Hodgson CL, Adhikari NK, et al. Lung recruitment maneuvers for adult patients with acute respiratory distress syndrome. A systematic review and meta-analysis. *Ann Am Thorac Soc.* 2017;14(Supplement 4):S304-S311.

29. Fan E, Wilcox ME, Brower RG, et al. Recruitment maneuvers for acute lung injury: A systematic review. *Am J Respir Crit Care Med.* 2008;178(11):1156-1163.

30. Lu J, Wang X, Chen M, et al. An open lung strategy in the management of acute respiratory distress syndrome: A systematic review and meta-analysis. *Shock*. 2017;48(1):43-53.

31. Cavalcanti AB, Suzumura ÉA, Laranjeira LN, et al. Effect of lung recruitment and titrated positive end-expiratory pressure (PEEP) vs low PEEP on mortality in patients with acute respiratory distress syndrome: a randomized clinical trial. *JAMA*. 2017;318(14):1335-1345.

32. Guérin C, Reignier J, Richard JC, et al. Prone positioning in severe acute respiratory distress syndrome. *N Engl J Med*. 2013;368(23):2159-2168.

33. Jolliet P, Bulpa P, Chevrolet JC. Effects of the prone position on gas exchange and hemodynamics in severe acute respiratory distress syndrome. *Crit Care Med*. 1998;26(12):1977-1985.

34. Aoyama H, Uchida K, Aoyama K, et al. Assessment of therapeutic interventions and lung protective ventilation in patients with moderate to severe acute respiratory distress syndrome: A systematic review and network meta-analysis. *JAMA Network Open*. 2019;2(7):e198116.

35. Fan E, Del Sorbo L, Goligher EC, et al. American Thoracic Society, European Society of Intensive Care Medicine, and Society of Critical Care Medicine. An official American Thoracic Society/European Society of Intensive Care Medicine/Society of Critical Care Medicine clinical practice guideline: Mechanical ventilation in adult patients with acute respiratory distress syndrome. *Am J Respir Crit Care Med*. 2017;195(9):1253-1263.

36. World Health Organization. Clinical management of COVID-19: Interim guidance, 27 May 2020. World Health Organization; 2020.

37. Coppo A, Bellani G, Winterton D, et al. Feasibility and physiological effects of prone positioning in non-intubated patients with acute respiratory failure due to COVID-19 (PRON-COVID): A prospective cohort study. *Lancet Respir Med*. 2020;8(8):765-774.

38. Peek GJ, Mugford M, Tiruvoipati R, et al. Efficacy and economic assessment of conventional ventilatory support versus extracorporeal membrane oxygenation for severe adult respiratory failure (CESAR): A multicentre randomised controlled trial. *Lancet*. 2009;374(9698):1351-1363.

39. Combes A, Hajage D, Capellier G, et al. Extracorporeal membrane oxygenation for severe acute respiratory distress syndrome. *N Engl J Med*. 2018;378(21):1965-1975.

40. Munshi L, Walkey A, Goligher E, et al. Venovenous extracorporeal membrane oxygenation for acute respiratory distress syndrome: a systematic review and meta-analysis. *Lancet Respir Med*. 2019;7(2):163-172.

41. Gainnier M, Roch A, Forel JM, et al. Effect of neuromuscular blocking agents on gas exchange in patients presenting with acute respiratory distress syndrome. *Crit Care Med*. 2004;32(1):113-119.

42. Watling SM, Dasta JF. Prolonged paralysis in intensive care unit patients after the use of neuromuscular blocking agents: A review of the literature. *Crit Care Med*. 1994;22(5):884-893.

43. Murray MJ, DeBlock HF, Erstad BL, et al. Clinical practice guidelines for sustained neuromuscular blockade in the adult critically ill patient: 2016 update--executive summary. *Am J Health-Syst Pharm.* 2017;74(2):76-78.

44. Papazian L, Forel JM, Gacouin A, et al. Neuromuscular blockers in early acute respiratory distress syndrome. *N Engl J Med.* 2010;363(12):1107-1116.

45. Moss M, Huang DT, Brower RG, et al. Early neuromuscular blockade in the acute respiratory distress syndrome. *N Engl J Med.* 2019;380(21):1997-2008.

46. Puybasset L, Rouby JJ, Mourgeon E, et al. Factors influencing cardiopulmonary effects of inhaled nitric oxide in acute respiratory failure. *Am J Respir Crit Care Med.* 1995;152(1):318-328.

47. Afshari Arash, Brok J, Møller AM, et al. Inhaled nitric oxide for acute respiratory distress syndrome (ARDS) and acute lung injury in children and adults. *Cochrane Database Syst Rev.* 2010;7:CD002787.

48. Fuller BM, Mohr NM, Skrupky L, et al. The use of inhaled prostaglandins in patients with ARDS: A systematic review and meta-analysis. *Chest.* 2015;147(6):1510-1522.

49. Wiedemann HP, Wheeler AP, Bernard GR, et al. Comparison of two fluid-management strategies in acute lung injury. *N Engl J Med.* 2006;354(24):2564-2575.

50. Villar J, Ferrando C, Martínez D, et al. Dexamethasone treatment for the acute respiratory distress syndrome: A multicentre, randomised controlled trial. *Lancet Respir Med.* 2020;8(3):267-276.

11 ACUTE KIDNEY INJURY AND RENAL REPLACEMENT THERAPY

Renu D. Muttana, MD

INTRODUCTION

Acute kidney injury (AKI) is a decline in renal function commonly seen in critically ill patients. During times of crisis, detection and treatment of AKI has become more complicated.

AKI

AKI has been associated with poor patient outcomes.[1,2] Intrinsic risk factors include advanced age starting from 65 to 75 years of age, comorbid conditions including preexisting chronic kidney disease, diabetes mellitus, proteinuria, heart disease, chronic obstructive pulmonary disease, chronic liver disease, and peripheral vascular disease.[1] The extrinsic or modifiable factors include sepsis, cardiac and vascular surgery, administration of iodinated contrast, traumas, burn injuries, medication and drug toxicities, and / or hypovolemia.[1,2]

The criteria for detection and staging of AKI continue to evolve. It involves changes with glomerular filtration through changes with serum creatinine and urine output. In 2004, the Acute Dialysis Quality Initiative (ADQI) introduced the Risk, Injury, Failure, Loss of kidney function, End stage renal disease classification (RIFLE).[3] The Acute Kidney Injury Network (AKIN) proposed their classification in 2007.[4] In 2012, with both validated initiatives possessing strengths and limitations, the Kidney Disease Improving Global Outcome (KDIGO) work group integrated the RIFLE and AKIN classifications to standardize the definition and severity of AKI.[5] The KDIGO criteria was set forth to provide a single definition for purposes of clinical practice, research, and public health initiatives (Table 11-1).[1]

Despite all of this, only functional kidney impairment is being classified. The need for biomarkers to assess AKI risk stratification, diagnosis early kidney stress and subclinical acute kidney injury may allow for

Table 11-1 STAGING OF AKI		
Stage	**Serum Creatinine**	**Urine Output**
1	1.5–1.9 times baseline OR ≥ 0.3 mg/dl (≥ 26.5 mmol/l) increase	< 0.5 ml/kg/h for 6–12 hours
2	2.0–2.9 times baseline	< 0.5 ml/kg/h for ≥ 12 hors

3	3.0 times baseline
	OR
	Increase in serum creatinine to $\geq$
	   4.0 mg/dl (≥ 353.6 mmol/l)
	OR
	Initiation of renal replacement therapy
	OR
	In patients < 18 years, decrease in
	   eGFR to < 35 ml/min per 1.73 m^2
		< 0.3 ml/kg/h for ≥ 24
		   hours
		OR
		Anuria for ≥ 12 hours

development of possible preventative and treatment options for AKI. Acute kidney stress referring to the pre-injury phase can possibly be identified through the expression of cell cycle arrest biomarkers.[6] Subclinical AKI is an awareness of injury occurring before alterations in glomerular filtration. Promising serum and urinary biomarkers under investigation include neutrophil gelatinase-associated lipocalin (NGAL), cystatin-C (Cys-c), kidney injury molecule-1 (KIM-1), interleukin-18 (IL-18), fatty acid binding proteins (FABPs), tissue inhibitor of metalloproteinases 2 (TIMP -2), insulin-like growth factor binding protein 7(IGFBP7), and endogenous ouabain (EO).[7] The clinical utility of these biomarkers remains undetermined.

Renal functional reserve (RFR) is a concept of the kidney having the ability to increase the glomerular filtration rate (GFR) in response to physiological and pathological stressors. Serum creatinine levels do not begin to rise until after significant amount of the GFR is already lost and kidney damage has taken place. The ability to test the RFR of the kidney may provide insight to subclinical kidney disease, parenchymal loss due to injury, and potentially fibrosis.[8] This parallels the use of an exercise stress test for cardiac function. Areas of testing may be directed toward glomerular and tubular kidney function. Glomerular functional reserve testing is not routinely utilized in clinical practice at this time, while tubular functional reserve testing in AKI has adopted to use of furosemide.[8] The furosemide stress test (FST), developed by Chawla and colleagues in 2013, is an assessment of tubular function with predictive capacity to identify patients with severe and progressive AKI.[9] In this study, Lasix was administered at 1–1.5 mg/kg to critically ill patients with KDIGO Stage 1 and 2 AKI. Urine output was assessed at 2 hours with a cutoff of 200 ml to predict progression to KDIGO Stage 3 within 14 days. A preliminary study revealed that FST outperformed biochemical biomarkers for prediction of progression to AKI, need for RRT, and inpatient mortality.[10]

EPIDEMIOLOGY

Recognition of AKI has increased with the development and acceptance of diagnostic criteria such as RIFLE, AKIN, and KDIGO. In studies done from 2006 to 2015, incidence of AKI ranged from 19.2% to 74.5%.[11] A review of large cohort studies from 2004–2012 using the KDIGO criteria, revealed a world incidence of 1 in 5 adults and 1 in 3 children experiencing AKI during an episode of hospitalization.[12] The Acute Kidney Injury – Epidemiological Prospective Investigation (AKI – EPI) was an international cross-sectional study that identified 57.3% of patients had AKI in the first week of ICU admission using the KDIGO criteria.[13] Worsening severity of AKI was associated with increased mortality.[13] Renal replacement therapy (RRT) is utilized in 10–15% of critically ill patients.[14] The population incidence of AKI patients requiring RRT has been rapidly rising by 10% per year in an analysis from 2000 to 2009.[15] AKI occurred in 24% of trauma patients admitted to the ICU, of which 10% required RRT.[16] AKI was found in 38% of burn patients admitted to the ICU with 12% requiring RRT.[17] Long-term outcome of AKI requiring RRT was found to have a twenty eight fold risk of progressive CKD Stage 4 or 5 and two fold increased risk of death.[18]

ETIOLOGY

The pathophysiology of AKI remains unclear. Proposed renal pathophysiology for AKI includes global renal hypoperfusion, hypoxia, dysregulation of inflammatory response, direct toxin injury, tubular epithelial cell death, and/or acute tubular necrosis (ATN).[19–22] Common causes precipitating AKI in critically ill patients include sepsis, shock, surgery, trauma, acute liver failure, and exposure to nephrotoxins.

Treatment of rhabdomyolysis remains the rapid initiation of intravenous fluids and treatment of underlying injury. Life threatening electrolyte abnormalities such as hyperkalemia may require RRT. The accessibility of appropriate treatments poses a challenge in injuries sustained in the battlefield or disaster affected areas.

In burns and inhalation injury, AKI-related risk factors include older age, chronic hypertension, diabetes mellitus, high total body surface area (TBSA) percent burnt, high abbreviated burn severity index (ABSI) score, inhalation injury, rhabdomyolysis, surgery, high acute physiology and chronic health evaluation (APACHE II) score, high sequential organ function assessment (SOFA) score, sepsis, and mechanical ventilation.[17] Development of AKI is multifactorial and a part of multiorgan failure. Initial treatment to support hemodynamic stability is fluid resuscitation. Mortality rates in these patients are several-fold higher compared to other critically ill patients.[23]

Intra-abdominal hypertension (IAH) and abdominal compartment syndrome (ACS) are observed in medical and surgical critically ill patients possibly leading to AKI. Intra-abdominal pressure (IAP) measurements are obtained by the transduction of bladder pressures. IAH is defined as a sustained or repeated increased intra-abdominal pressure $\geq$ 12 mm Hg. ACS is defined as sustained or repeated increased intra-abdominal pressure $\geq$ 20 mm Hg with new organ dysfunction.[24] An observational study showed IAP can predict the occurrence of AKI in patients who underwent abdominal surgeries.[25] The pathophysiology causing the decrease in glomerular filtration is suspected to be renal hypoperfusion due to reduced arterial blood inflow and venous blood outflow along with the increase in renal parenchymal pressures.[26] Surgical intervention was initially mainstay treatment for IAH and ACS. Patients with ACS may require decompressive laparotomy. With more awareness and recognition of IAH and ACS, early nonsurgical interventions may be helpful in preventing organ dysfunction, including AKI. These strategies focus on improving abdominal wall compliance, evacuating and decompressing the gastrointestinal tract, draining fluid collections, correcting positive fluid balance, and minimizing capillary leak.[24]

NONDIALYTIC MANAGEMENT

Identification of high-risk patients for developing AKI may allow for earlier diagnosis and implementation of preventive strategies. Attempts to achieve hemodynamic stability can be through the use of fluid administration and vasoactive medications. Isotonic crystalloid solution, such as 0.9% sodium chloride, was the mainstay treatment for critically ill patients. However, the high chloride concentration posed concern to switch to balanced crystalloid solution due to being more physiologically consistent with the content of plasma. In 2018, a large study found fewer major adverse kidney events by 30 days in the balanced crystalloid group therefore shifting support for the use of solutions such as lactated ringer's or Plasma-Lyte solutions instead of 0.9% sodium chloride.[27] However, a meta-analysis review in 2019, which included this study, concluded that the use of balanced crystalloids compared to 0.9% normal saline did not improve rates of mortality, AKI, or use of RRT.[28] The avoidance of nephrotoxic agents and appropriate medication dosing is proposed to prevent the development and/or worsening of AKI.

AKI related complications include electrolyte abnormalities, acid-base disturbances, and fluid/volume status. In non-life-threatening scenarios not requiring RRT, medical management may be utilized.

Measures to correct hyperkalemia focus on causing an intracellular potassium shift and excretion. This shift is promoted by the use of insulin, bicarbonate, and/or beta-adrenergic agonists. Intravenous dextrose is given to prevent hypoglycemia with insulin administration. In attempts to excrete potassium, diuretics and/or potassium binders may be utilized. Loop diuretics are often used for renal potassium excretion. Medications such as sodium polystyrene sulfonate, sodium zirconium cyclosilicate, or patiromer are used for gastrointestinal excretion. Intravenous calcium administration is necessary in life threatening hyperkalemia for cardiac stability.

The benefit of bicarbonate administration for the treatment of metabolic acidosis in the critically ill patient remains controversial. A clinical trial in the *Lancet* from 2018 investigated intravenous sodium bicarbonate administration in ICU patients with severe acidemia. The primary outcome of death from any cause by day 28 and the presence of at least one organ failure at day 7 was not affected by sodium bicarbonate administration.[29] Another study in 2018 enrolled septic patients with metabolic acidosis and administered sodium bicarbonate. This study proposed no association with improved outcome for the patients who received sodium bicarbonate therapy but was associated with improved survival in patients with AKI Stage 2 or 3 and severe acidosis.[30] Sodium bicarbonate therapy presents complications of hypokalemia, hypocalcemia, hypernatremia, extracellular volume overload, and hypercapnia causing deleterious effects in patients with respiratory acidosis.

Fluid overload is a complication in the critically ill patient with AKI leading to increased mortality. The fluid management in these patients is a balance between treatment of underlying processes, maintaining hemodynamic stability, and preventing AKI while avoiding the complications of fluid overload. The judicious adaptation of strategies to assess a patient's volume status and recognize fluid overload may be helpful to guide intravenous fluid therapy in critically ill patients. Some strategies include accurate documentation of intake and output, knowledgeable interpretation of brain natriuretic peptide values, and use of diagnostic imaging. These imaging tools include chest radiographs, thoracic ultrasound, and ultrasound of inferior vena cava diameter.[31] Diuretic therapy is the mainstay treatment for non-life-threatening fluid overload. However, the use of diuretic therapy is accompanied by electrolyte abnormalities requiring regular lab monitoring and electrolyte replacement when indicated.

DIALYTIC THERAPY

RRT can be initiated in life threatening complications or refractory to conservative management. The RRT modalities available for renal support include peritoneal dialysis and extracorporeal treatments such as intermittent hemodialysis (IHD), continuous renal replacement therapy (CRRT), and prolonged intermittent renal replacement therapy (PIRRT) also referred to as extended daily dialysis. Different machines and dialysis solutions are required depending on the modality being utilized. Despite the similar indications for RRT, each modality has specific advantages and barriers to treatment dependent on the patient's clinical state as well as the situational capabilities where the treatment is being administered.

Indications for immediate RRT include severe hyperkalemia, metabolic acidosis, pulmonary edema, and/or complications due to uremia (uremic pericarditis, pleuritis, encephalopathy or coagulopathy.[1] The optimal timing to initiate RRT in the critically ill patient with AKI without these complications remains yet to be determined. A meta-analysis done by the Cochrane Database of Systematic Review in 2018 reviewed five randomized control trials with a total of 1,084 participants. These studies compared outcomes in early start RRT versus standard start RRT using continuous renal replacement therapy (CRRT) and/or intermittent hemodialysis (IHD). The review reported the lack of high quality of evidence to support early initiation of RRT with the possibility of increased risk of adverse events.[32] An updated meta-analysis in 2020 reviewed 18 RCTs from 1997 to 2018, involving 2,856 patients, investigating the timing of RRT in critically ill patients with AKI. This review revealed no benefit in early RRT support for patients with critically ill or community acquired AKI.[33] In July 2020, the STARRT-AKI (Standard versus Accelerated Initiation of Renal Replacement Therapy with Acute Kidney Injury) trial presented accelerated initiation of RRT in the critically ill patient with AKI was not associated with lower risk of death at 90 days as compared to standard initiation of therapy.[34] The relative criteria investigated for initiating renal replacement therapy have included KDIGO AKI Stage 2 or 3 paying attention to changes in serum creatinine and urine output, monitoring biomarkers, levels of blood urea, response failure to diuretics treatments as seen in the FST.[34-36]

Extracorporeal Renal Replacement Therapies

Extracorporeal RRT circulates the patient's blood through an extracorporeal circuit involving a purification device (filter or dialyzer) and then returns the "purified" blood to the patient. Access to a patient's circulation is obtained from the sterile insertion of an uncuffed, non-tunneled, double lumen central venous catheter into a large vein such as internal jugular veins, femoral veins, or subclavian veins. KDIGO recommendations are for ultrasound guided insertion of catheters to increase probability of success and reduce risk of complications. Also recommended is to obtain a chest radiograph after catheter insertion for placement confirmation and assessing for possible procedural complications.[1] A functioning vascular access is essential for the adequacy of extracorporeal RRT. In the dialyzer, the patient's blood and dialysis solution interact via a semipermeable membrane to allow for the diffusion of solutes and ultrafiltration or convection of water.

Intermittent hemodialysis (IHD) was the first extracorporeal RRT available in the intensive care unit. A human HD apparatus was developed in the 1940s with widespread use of IHD for the treatment of AKI by the 1950s. The high efficiency of IHD is advantageous for patients requiring fast solute removal such as severe hyperkalemia in crush injuries. Administering RRT with IHD, especially in the critically ill patient, is limited by hemodynamic instability. Refractory intradialytic hypotension complicates IHD treatments and may result in the early termination of treatments.

With its introduction in the 1980s, continuous renal replacement therapy (CRRT) soon became the preferred RRT modality in the critically ill patient. CRRT therapies include continuous hemodialysis, continuous hemofiltration, and continuous hemodiafiltration. CRRT allows for hemodynamic stability, correction of electrolyte and acid-base imbalances, continuous control of volume status, and reduced risk of cerebral edema.

Prolonged intermittent renal replacement therapies (PIRRT) are the "hybrid" of RRT. These modalities are sustained low-efficiency dialysis

(SLED) for solute removal and sustained low-efficiency ultrafiltration (SCUF) for fluid removal. SLED and SCUF generally run over the course of 8–12 hours per day but may be variable. The machines allow for slower solute and/or water removal compared to IHD, therefore maintaining hemodynamic stability.

Peritoneal Dialysis

Peritoneal dialysis (PD) is the renal replacement modality utilizing the peritoneal cavity and membrane to achieve diffusion and osmosis for solute and fluid removal, respectively. The dialysis solution, usually a glucose containing fluid, is instilled, via catheter, into the peritoneal cavity. Here the solution comes in contact with the blood via the peritoneal membrane housing peritoneal capillaries to move solute and water. Aside from these anatomical components, factors affecting the dialysis and fluid removal are the prescription of volume of solution instilled (dwell volume), how often the solution is exchanged (dwell time), and the type of solution instilled.

PD was first introduced in the 1920s initially for the treatment of uremia in humans. Early investigations utilized intermittent PD for treatment of uremia and eventually hyperkalemia and fluid overload. Intermittent PD was complicated by access issues, fluid leakage, and peritonitis. The introduction of the Tenckhoff catheter in the 1960s and continuous ambulatory PD in the 1970s changed the landscape for utilization of PD, however, evolving mostly in the setting of treatment for end stage renal disease (ESRD).

Treatment of AKI in critically ill patients requiring dialytic therapies was overshadowed by development and availability of extracorporeal therapies such as continuous renal replacement therapies and intermittent hemodialysis. The International Society for Peritoneal Dialysis (ISPD) issued guidelines in 2020 in support of the use of PD in AKI in adults.[37] The supporting evidence for such guidelines was presented in a 2017 Cochrane review that concluded insufficient evidence exists to determine a difference between PD and extracorporeal therapies in terms of all-cause mortality or kidney function recovery in the treatment of AKI. However, this determination came along with the recommendation for further, larger randomized controlled studies to support the efficacy of PD in AKI.[38] A randomized control trial of 125 patients at a well experienced PD unit in Saudi Arabia found that patients who started on tidal volume PD had better outcomes of mortality, infection rates, duration of requiring RRT, renal recovery, and ICU length of stay compared to those receiving CVVHDF.[39] This is a promising study in support of acute start

PD in the critically ill patient with AKI; however, the results need to be reproducible in more widespread clinical settings. In 2018, a prospective study compared the respiratory mechanics of AKI patients requiring PD and HD while on invasive mechanical ventilation. Their evaluation of 37 patients of continuous PD and 94 patients on HD revealed no difference in the improvement in these patients pre- and post-dialysis.[40]

In acute PD, most PD catheters may be placed at the bedside under local anesthesia by appropriately trained staff. Recommendations from the ISPD are to utilize the flexible, fenestrated, and tunneled Tenckhoff catheter versus the non-tunneled rigid catheter. These characteristics allow for Tenckhoff catheters to remain in place if long term RRT is required and have less complications such as leakage of dialysate, inadequate drainage, intrabdominal bleeding, and peritonitis, compared to rigid catheters.[41] Due to increased risk of peritonitis, rigid PD catheters are recommended to be replaced every 3–5 days if they are used for acute RRT with PD.[42] Improvised options for PD access in situations of limited resources included placement of sterile nasogastric tubes, suprapubic catheters, intercostal drainage tubes, hemodialysis catheters, and percutaneous cavity drainage catheters.[43]

PD modalities include continuous ambulatory PD (CAPD) and automated PD (APD). CAPD is the manual exchange of dialysate into and out of the peritoneal cavity taking advantage of gravity. APD utilizes hydraulic pumps in the "cycler" machine to cycle the dialysate solution through the peritoneal cavity. APD is more widely used in the treatment of AKI; however, there is a dependency on the availability of cyclers and trained staff. Therefore, in a resource limited setting, CAPD may be the preferred method. CAPD is dependent upon manual fluid exchanges and does not require a cycler machine. In extreme environments with no electricity, patients are able to undergo RRT via CAPD. The appropriate and effective PD prescription dosing for patients with AKI remains unclear. Alterations in dwell volume, dwell time, number of exchanges, and dialysate solutions are likely required to approach a clinically effective PD prescription for each individual patient.

▌CHOICE OF RENAL REPLACEMENT THERAPY MODALITY

The choice of RRT modality in the critically ill patient is dependent on several factors, including clinical appropriateness and infrastructure availability. A patient's hemodynamic stability, RRT indication, ability to obtain a functioning dialysis access, availability of equipment, and staff experience with the modalities are all considerations in deciding upon the appropriate RRT. All modalities offer advantages and barriers for patients requiring RRT and need to be considered in the decision-making process (Table 11-2). The answer to which is the "best" modality for the critically ill patient with AKI remains the source of much debate. A review of 17 RCT and observational studies from 2004 to 2014 comparing extended daily dialysis with CRRT showed similar mortality outcomes in the RCTs but lower mortality rate in observational studies.[44] A cohort study including 232 patients receiving either SLED or CRRT revealed similar 30-day mortality and short-term renal recovery in both groups.[45] There is a lack of RCTs to support which RRT modality is better suited for the critically ill patient. A multicenter observational study on RRT in the critically ill burn patient revealed earlier and higher dose CRRT modality was preferred in most centers.[46] In the intensive care unit, the choice of RRT is often based on the patient's clinical condition, equipment/machine accessibility, availability of trained staff, resources, and cost. In situations requiring a high demand for RRT and strained resources, staff, and equipment, all available modalities of RRT should and can be utilized to treat critically ill patients. Such were the experiences with the COVID-19 pandemic, where institutions were forced to rely on all RRT modalities.[47]

▌RENAL REPLACEMENT THERAPY IN CRISIS

Renal replacement therapies are dependent on resource availability. These resources include staff, machines, and supplies. These resources can and have been strained during periods of high demand for RRT as being seen during disasters such as earthquakes and the COVID-19 pandemic. The International Society of Nephrology (ISN) established the Renal Disaster Relief Task Force (RDRTF) after the 1988 Spitak earthquake in Armenia to address to overwhelming need for RRT in crush syndromes and rhabdomyolysis occurring in these devastated areas. In the 1999 earthquake in Marmara, Turkey, the quick intervention of RDRTF and Medecins Sans Frontieres (MSF) to identify patients at high risk for AKI, transport patients, provide trained staff, supply equipment, and provide RRT aided in the treatment of hundreds of crush syndrome patients.[48] The RDRTF continued to intervene in other earthquake disasters around the globe. In these situations, IHD presented as the preferred RRT due to advantages of rapid clearance of potassium, ability to treat several patients per day on the same machine, and minimal need for anticoagulation. However, the need for a water supply presents an obstacle to treatment with IHD in these devastated areas.[49] Innovative and conservative strategies to provide RRT were implemented worldwide to address the rapidly growing

Table 11-2 POTENTIAL ADVANTAGES AND CHALLENGES OF RRT MODALITIES[1,45]		
Type of RRT Modality	Advantages	Challenges
CRRT	• Hemodynamic stability due to slower and controlled fluid and solute removal • Preferred RRT for patients with brain injury	• Need for established infrastructure • Staff training required • Immobilization of patient • Need for continuous anticoagulation • Slower rate of toxin and solute clearance • Potential higher costs
IHD	• Rapid toxin and low molecular weight substances removal • Allows time for other diagnostic or therapeutic procedures • Potential lower costs compared to CRRT • Decreased anticoagulation exposure	• Hemodynamic instability • Need for established infrastructure • Complex staff training required • Need for adequate water supply
SLED / SCUF	• Hemodynamic stability • Decreased anticoagulation exposure	• Slower rate of solute and toxin removal • Need for established infrastructure • Complex staff training • Need for adequate water supply
PD	• No coagulopathy complications related to access and system clotting • No systemic anticoagulation required • No need for vascular assess	• Inability to set fluid removal rate and/or volume • Fluid removal can only be assessed at end of cycle • Inexperienced centers/staff may lead to delays in initiating treatment • Need for specialized trained staff for PD access placement

(Continued)

Table 11-2 POTENTIAL ADVANTAGES AND CHALLENGES OF RRT MODALITIES[1,45] (CONTINUED)		
Type of RRT Modality	**Advantages**	**Challenges**
	• Minimal blood loss • Hemodynamic stability • Less induced inflammatory state • Technically simple staff training required • Less and minimal infrastructure required • No need for electricity or water supply to perform therapy • Can limit staff exposure in isolation settings • Potential lower cost	• Concern for protein loss • Requires intact peritoneal cavity • Risk of peritonitis • High glucose exposure from dialysate solutions

need for RRT in COVID-19 patients. A New York City institution deeply impacted by COVID-19 devised a multifaceted approach to meet the growing need for RRT. Strategies included lengthening periods of "sharing" CRRT machines to decrease filter utilization, decreasing CRRT dialysate rates to conserve dialysate solutions, training extended staff to perform CRRT, utilizing IHD for patients on low dose vasopressor support, treating with ultrafiltration only therapies to conserve dialysate solutions, communication with vendors to secure supplies, and coordinating within the institution's network to allocate staff, supplies, and resources where most needed.[50]

With the longstanding history of PD, we have seen its usefulness in situations of war, natural disasters, and resource limited settings. During earthquakes and hurricanes, ESRD patients can continue with RRT due to it not requiring electricity for CAPD, large equipment, a water supply, and/or need for transportation to HD units.[43] The increasing RRT needs in patients infected with SARS-CoV-2 created strain on dialysis resources.

Another New York City institution found some relief by implementing acute PD for COVID-19 patients with AKI.[51] PD can offer a potential relief along with possible advantages. PD training is relatively simple and can be easily learned by staff. PD cycler machines for APD can be set up for a 24-hour period and therefore limiting infection transmission risk and less personal protective equipment (PPE) usage. In settings where cycler machines are not available or unable to be used (i.e., no electricity), CAPD or manual exchanges may be performed to perform RRT. PD theoretically would have minimal issues with hypercoagulable patients, as seen in patients with COVID-19 compared to other RRT given that no vascular access is required for the therapy. The dialysate solutions for PD are prepared commercially. In resource limited settings, the availability of dialysate solutions may become a barrier to treatment. PD solution is able to be locally prepared using more readily available intravenous fluids with caution to sterility of the solution.[43,52] In disaster situations resulting in crush injury induced AKI, PD may not be the preferred RRT due to the hypercatabolic state of these patients and need for fast solute removal from complications of hyperkalemia; however, in dire situations it may be the only option.

CONCLUSION

AKI is a major complication in the critically ill patient. Preventative and early detection measures are key to decreasing the incidences of AKI in these patients. Hopefully more inclusive diagnostic criteria and the clinical utilization of chemical biomarkers will lead to promising results in decreasing AKI in intensive care units. With the progression to severe stages of AKI, complications of AKI can be treated with medical management and RRT, if available, can be initiated in refractory cases. The RRT modality chosen will rely on a multitude of factors from the patient's clinical status to the available infrastructure. In situations compromising the usual standard of care measures to provide lifesaving treatments, the innovative and collaborative strategies are necessary to continue to provide care for these critically ill patients.

Despite this knowledge of AKI and the availability of options with RRT modalities, the prognosis for these critically ill patients continues to remain poor. Therefore, continued curiosity for research and exploration into renal pathophysiology, early detection markers, and directed renal therapies aimed at the improvement of these outcomes is greatly welcomed.

REFERENCES

1. KDIGO AKIWG: Kidney Disease: Improving Global Outcomes (KDIGO). Clinical practice guideline for acute kidney injury. *Kidney Int Suppl.* 2012;2:1-141.

2. Chawla LS, Abell L, Mazhari R, et al. Identifying critically ill patients at high risk for developing acute renal failure: A pilot study. *Kidney Int.* 2005;68: 2274-2280.

3. Bellomo R, Ronco C, Kellum JA, et al. Palevsky P and the ADQI workgroup. Acute renal failure—definition, outcome measures, animal models, fluid therapy and information technology needs: The Second International Consensus Conference of the Acute Dialysis Quality Initiative (ADQI) Group. *Crit Care.* 2004;8:R204.

4. Mehta RL, Kellum JA, Shah SV, et al. Acute Kidney Injury Network: Report of an initiative to improve outcomes in acute kidney injury. *Crit Care.* 2007;11:R31.

5. Lopes JA, Jorge S. The RIFLE and AKIN classifications for acute kidney injury: A critical and comprehensive review. *Clin Kidney J.* 2013;6:8-14.

6. Katz N, Ronco C. Acute kidney stress—A useful term based on evolution in the understanding of acute kidney injury. *Crit Care.* 2016;20:23.

7. Pozzoli S, Simonini M, Manunta P. Predicting acute kidney injury: Current status and future challenges. *J Nephrol.* 2018;31(2):209-223.

8. Chawla LS, Ronco C. Renal stress testing in the assessment of kidney disease. *Kidney Int Rep.* 2016;1(1):57-63.

9. Chawla LS, Davison DL, Brasha-Mitchell E, et al. Development and standardization of a furosemide stress test to predict the severity of acute kidney injury. *Crit Care.* 2013;17(5):R207.

10. Brasha-Mitchell E, et al. Furosemide stress test and biomarkers for the prediction of AKI severity. *J Am Soc Nephrol.* 2015;26(8):2023-2031.

11. Bellomo R, Ronco C, Mehta RL, et al. Acute kidney injury in the ICU: From injury to recovery: reports from the 5th Paris International Conference. *Ann Intensive Care.* 2017;7(1):49.

12. Susantitaphong P, Cruz DN, Cerda J, et al. World incidence of AKI: A meta-analysis [published correction appears in *Clin J Am Soc Nephrol.* 2014;9(6):1148]. *Clin J Am Soc Nephrol.* 2013;8(9):1482-1493.

13. Hoste EA, Bagshaw SM, Bellomo R, et al. Epidemiology of acute kidney injury in critically ill patients: the multinational AKI-EPI study. *Intensive Care Med.* 2015;41(8):1411-1423.

14. Pickkers P, Ostermann M, Joannidis M, et al. The intensive care medicine agenda on acute kidney injury. *Intensive Care Med.* 2017;43(9):1198-1209.

15. Hsu RK, McCulloch CE, Dudley RA, Lo LJ, Hsu CY. Temporal changes in incidence of dialysis-requiring AKI. *J Am Soc Nephrol.* 2013;24(1):37-42.

16. Søvik S, Isachsen MS, Nordhuus KM, et al. Acute kidney injury in trauma patients admitted to the ICU: A systematic review and meta-analysis. *Intensive Care Med.* 2019;45(4):407-419.

17. Folkestad T, Brurberg KG, Nordhuus KM, et al. Acute kidney injury in burn patients admitted to the intensive care unit: A systematic review and meta-analysis. *Crit Care*. 2020;24(1):2.

18. Lo LJ, Go AS, Chertow GM, et al. Dialysis-requiring acute renal failure increases the risk of progressive chronic kidney disease. *Kidney Int*. 2009;76(8):893-899.

19. Peerapornratana S, Manrique-Caballero CL, Gómez H, Kellum JA. Acute kidney injury from sepsis: Current concepts, epidemiology, pathophysiology, prevention and treatment. *Kidney Int*. 2019;96(5):1083-1099.

20. Poston JT, Koyner JL. Sepsis associated acute kidney injury. *BMJ*. 2019;364:k4891.

21. Eriksson M, Brattström O, Mårtensson J, Larsson E, Oldner A. Acute kidney injury following severe trauma: Risk factors and long-term outcome. *J Trauma Acute Care Surg*. 2015;79(3):407-412.

22. Assanangkornchai N, Akaraborworn O, Kongkamol C, Kaewsaengrueang K. Characteristics of creatine kinase elevation in trauma patients and predictors of acute kidney injury. *J Acute Med*. 2017;7(2):54-60.

23. Brusselaers N, Monstrey S, Colpaert K, Decruyenaere J, Blot SI, Hoste EA. Outcome of acute kidney injury in severe burns: A systematic review and meta-analysis. *Intensive Care Med*. 2010;36(6):915-925.

24. Mohmand H, Goldfarb S. Renal dysfunction associated with intra-abdominal hypertension and the abdominal compartment syndrome. *J Am Soc Nephrol*. 2011;22(4):615-621.

25. Demarchi AC, de Almeida CT, Ponce D, et al. Intra-abdominal pressure as a predictor of acute kidney injury in postoperative abdominal surgery. *Ren Fail*. 2014;36(4):557-561.

26. Villa G, Samoni S, De Rosa S, Ronco C. The pathophysiological hypothesis of kidney damage during intra-abdominal hypertension. *Front Physiol*. 2016;7:55.

27. Semler MW, Self WH, Wanderer JP, et al. Balanced crystalloids versus saline in critically ill adults. *N Engl J Med*. 2018;378(9):829-839.

28. Liu C, Lu G, Wang D, et al. Balanced crystalloids versus normal saline for fluid resuscitation in critically ill patients: A systematic review and meta-analysis with trial sequential analysis. *Am J Emerg Med*. 2019;37(11):2072-2078.

29. Jaber S, Paugam C, Futier E, et al. Sodium bicarbonate therapy for patients with severe metabolic acidaemia in the intensive care unit (BICAR-ICU): A multicentre, open-label, randomised controlled, phase 3 trial [published correction appears in *Lancet*. 2018;392(10163):2440]. *Lancet*. 2018;392(10141):31-40.

30. Zhang Z, Zhu C, Mo L, Hong Y. Effectiveness of sodium bicarbonate infusion on mortality in septic patients with metabolic acidosis. *Intensive Care Med*. 2018;44(11):1888-1895.

31. Claure-Del Granado R, Mehta RL. Fluid overload in the ICU: Evaluation and management. *BMC Nephrol*. 2016;17(1):109.

32. Fayad AII, Buamscha DG, Ciapponi A. Timing of renal replacement therapy initiation for acute kidney injury. *Cochrane Database Syst Rev*. 2018; 12(12):CD010612.

33. Zhang L, Chen D, Tang X, Li P, Zhang Y, Tao Y. Timing of initiation of renal replacement therapy in acute kidney injury: An updated meta-analysis of randomized controlled trials. *Ren Fail*. 2020;42(1):77-88.

34. STARRT-AKI Investigators; Canadian Critical Care Trials Group; Australian and New Zealand Intensive Care Society Clinical Trials Group. Timing of initiation of renal-replacement therapy in acute kidney injury [published correction appears in *N Engl J Med*. 2020 Jul 15]. *N Engl J Med*. 2020;383(3):240-251.

35. Klein SJ, Brandtner AK, Lehner GF, et al. Biomarkers for prediction of renal replacement therapy in acute kidney injury: A systematic review and meta-analysis. *Intensive Care Med*. 2018;44(3):323-336.

36. Lumlertgul N, Peerapornratana S, Trakarnvanich T, et al. Early versus standard initiation of renal replacement therapy in furosemide stress test non-responsive acute kidney injury patients (the FST trial). *Crit Care*. 2018;22(1):101.

37. Cullis B, Al-Hwiesh A, Kilonzo K, et al. ISPD guidelines for peritoneal dialysis in acute kidney injury: 2020 update (adults). *Perit Dial Int*. 2021;41(1):15-31.

38. Liu L, Zhang L, Liu GJ, Fu P. Peritoneal dialysis for acute kidney injury. *Cochrane Database Syst Rev*. 2017;12(12):CD011457.

39. Al-Hwiesh, A, Abdul-Rahman, I, Finkelstein, F, et al. Acute kidney injury in critically ill patients: A prospective randomized study of tidal peritoneal dialysis versus continuous renal replacement therapy. *Ther Apher Dial*. 2018;22(4):371–379.

40. Almeida CP, Balbi AL, Ponce, D. Effect of peritoneal dialysis vs. haemodialysis on respiratory mechanics in acute kidney injury patients. *Clin Exp Nephrol*. 2018;22:1420–1426.

41. Wong SN, Geary DF. Comparison of temporary and permanent catheters for acute peritoneal dialysis. *Arch Dis Child*. 1988;63(7):827-831.

42. Daugirdas JT, Blake PG, Ing TS, eds. *Handbook of Dialysis*. 5th ed. Philadelphia, PA: Lippincott Williams & Wilkins; 2014:453.

43. Gorbatkin C, Finkelstein FO, Kazancioglu RT. Peritoneal dialysis during active war. *Semin Nephrol*. 2020;40(4):375-385.

44. Zhang L, Yang J, Eastwood GM, Zhu G, Tanaka A, Bellomo R. Extended daily dialysis versus continuous renal replacement therapy for acute kidney injury: A meta-analysis. *Am J Kidney Dis*. 2015;66(2):322-330.

45. Kitchlu A, Adhikari N, Burns KE, et al. Outcomes of sustained low efficiency dialysis versus continuous renal replacement therapy in critically ill adults with acute kidney injury: A cohort study. *BMC Nephrol*. 2015;16:127.

46. Chung KK, Coates EC, Hickerson WL, et al. Renal replacement therapy in severe burns: A multicenter observational study. *J Burn Care Res*. 2018;39(6):1017-1021.

47. Fisher R, Clarke J, Al-Arfi K, et al. Provision of acute renal replacement therapy, using three separate modalities, in critically ill patients during the COVID-19 pandemic. An after action review from a UK tertiary critical care centre [published online ahead of print, 2020 Dec 28]. *J Crit Care*. 2020;62:190-196.

48. Vanholder R, Sever MS, De Smet M, Erek E, Lameire N. Intervention of the Renal Disaster Relief Task Force in the 1999 Marmara, Turkey earthquake. *Kidney Int*. 2001;59(2):783-791.

49. Gibney RT, Sever MS, Vanholder RC. Disaster nephrology: Crush injury and beyond. *Kidney Int*. 2014;85(5):1049-1057.

50. Division of Nephrology, Columbia University Vagelos College of Physicians. Disaster response to the COVID-19 pandemic for patients with kidney disease in New York City. *J Am Soc Nephrol*. 2020;31(7):1371-1379.

51. El Shamy O, Patel N, Abdelbaset MH, et al. Acute start peritoneal dialysis during the COVID-19 pandemic: Outcomes and experiences. *J Am Soc Nephrol*. 2020;31(8):1680-1682.

52. Ponce D, Balbi A. Acute kidney injury: Risk factors and management challenges in developing countries. *Int J Nephrol Renovasc Dis*. 2016;9:193-200.

TRANSPLANTATION 12

Ella Illuzzi, ANP and John Oropello, MD

▌ INTRODUCTION

Solid organ transplantation (SOT) of kidney, liver, pancreas, intestine, heart, and lung is one of the biggest advances in medicine and has become a life-saving treatment for end-stage organ diseases. One particular peril to organ transplantation is the risk of emerging infectious diseases. Over the last several decades, infectious respiratory diseases such as severe acute respiratory syndrome coronavirus (SARS-CoV), influenza A/H1N1, and more recently SARS-CoV-2, the virus that causes COVID-19, have threatened the general public and have challenged the transplantation community.[1]

Some of these emerging diseases have been limited to specific geographic areas, and transplantation centers have been able to adapt and proceed with transplantation safely and efficiently. However, COVID-19, a novel, rapidly growing, highly contagious virus, has forced drastic changes in medical practice within a short period of time. It has greatly impacted transplantation centers throughout the United States and worldwide, while increasing pressure on intensive care units (ICU) who faced a surge of COVID-inflicted critical illness.

▌ EPIDEMIOLOGY

COVID-19 was first identified as the source of a cluster of pneumonia cases in Wuhan, China.[2] It spread rapidly throughout China, followed by increasing cases throughout the world and by March 2020 the World Health Organization (WHO) declared an international pandemic. As of October 2020, nearly 34 million cases and over 1 million deaths have been reported worldwide.[3]

The COVID-19 virus is particularly transmissible. The most common modes of transmission are through respiratory droplets during close-range contact with an asymptomatic or symptomatic carrier and to a lesser degree, contact transmission.[4,5] Airborne transmission is less likely, but raises potential risk during aerosol-generating procedures such as endotracheal intubation, open suctioning, and bronchoscopy.[6] The virus has also been detected in stool, ocular secretions, and semen, but their role in transmission remains unknown.[7]

The general population lacks immunity and is at risk for acquiring the novel coronavirus. The average incubation period for COVID-19 is approximately 5 days[8] and around 97.5% of individuals who develop symptoms usually do so within 11.5 days.[9] The most common symptoms among hospitalized individuals were fever, dry cough, shortness of breath, fatigue, nausea/vomiting, diarrhea, and myalgia.[10] The spectrum of symptoms vary from mild febrile illness to severe illness, including acute respiratory distress syndrome (ARDS), acute kidney injury, and multi-organ failure. Older age and medical conditions such as diabetes, cardiovascular disease, chronic pulmonary disease, chronic kidney disease, chronic liver disease, malignancy, obesity, and recipients of solid organ transplants are associated with increased risk for severe COVID 19 illness.[11]

▌TRANSPLANT CANDIDATES

At this time, there are over 100,000 individuals in need of a lifesaving organ transplant on the United Organ Network for Organ Sharing (UNOS) waitlist.[12] With the COVID-19 pandemic, transplantation centers faced many new challenges. These new challenges were related to organ procurement, screening policy of donor and recipient, risk of transmission to recipient or health care workers, decision to proceed with or postpone transplantation, and resources availability.[1,13–15] In light of the multiple, aforementioned challenges, many transplant centers have decided to curtail and some even suspend their transplant activity. As of April 11, 2020, there was a 51.1% decline in donor organ transplantations throughout the United States and 90 6% in France.[16] Figure 12-1 shows the trend between the increase in COVID-19 infections and a substantial decline in overall SOT procedures in the United States and France.[16]

There are no evidence-based guidelines on proceeding with or postponing organ transplantation during a pandemic and each transplant center varies in their practices with the support of transplant societies' recommendations and guidance. It is imperative that transplant centers continually assess disease prevalence in their area and balance medical resources and availability against the need to continue organ transplantation.[17] In addition, ensure resources such as available ICU beds, ventilators, blood products, or other medical resources if complications occur.

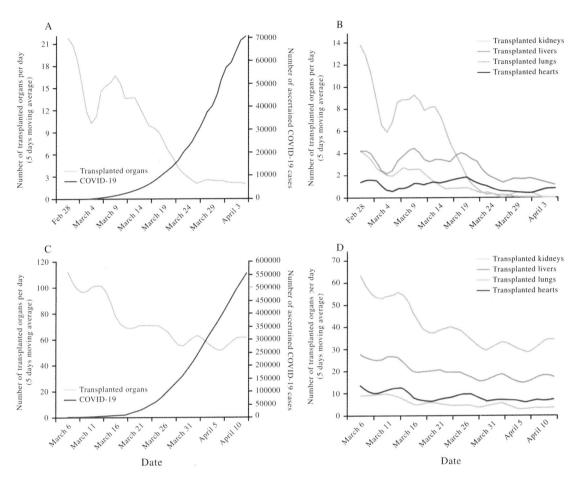

Figure 12-1 • Trends in COVID-19 in France and the United States and recovery of organs and solid-organ transplantation procedures from deceased donors. **(A, C)** Number of COVID-19 diagnoses and number of solid organs recovered for transplantation over time in France **(A)** and the United States **(C)**. **(B, D)** Total number of transplants from deceased donors, with separate trend lines for kidney, liver, heart, and lung, over time in France **(B)** and the United States **(D)**. (From Loupy A, Aubert O, Reese PP, Bayer F, Jacquelinet C. Organ procurement and transplantation during COVID-19 pandemic. *Lancet*. 2020;395:e95-e96.)

If the virus is rampant in a certain area, this increases the potential risk of nosocomial transmission to a recipient or to health care workers. A transplant center, under certain circumstances, may decide to proceed with deceased donor transplantation, but temporarily suspend elective living donor or non-urgent deceased donor transplantation.[1]

The decision to continue transplantation should be taken cautiously and case by case with special considerations based on disease progression. Furthermore, a decrease in donor organ availability is expected related to limitations on institutional resources and the evolving data on the risk of donor-derived disease transmission.[14] Transplant centers may have to prioritize individuals awaiting transplantation who are most likely to die without an organ offer and delay those who can wait longer.

Transplant candidates are considered to be at greater risk of severe infection due to their higher rate of underlying medical conditions.[11] A virus such as COVID-19 can pose a threat to the patient's transplant eligibility, jeopardizing their chances for a life-saving organ. General recommendations for COVID-19 prevention by the CDC have been made to limit in-person medical visits, ensure personnel protective equipment (PPE) is being correctly utilized, clean and disinfect areas visited by persons under investigation (PUI) or confirmed COVID-19, and monitor health care workers for signs or symptoms of illness.[18,19] Furthermore, each transplantation center should develop their own outpatient policy tailored to their patient population and needs. The continuation of medical management and maintenance for end-stage organ disease is essential. However, the need for non-urgent procedures and scheduled routine visits should be evaluated. Telemedicine including virtual visits, phone calls, text messaging, and emailing should be utilized, and laboratory testing should be performed locally. If an outpatient appointment is warranted, implement a COVID-19 screening questionnaire prior to the visit. Lastly, ensure patients have enough refills for medications and if possible, make use of pharmacy delivery services. The main priority of transplant candidates should always be to avoid infection. Therefore, it is imperative to emphasize prevention including, but not limited to, wearing a mask, social distancing, frequent hand washing, and adhering to travel restrictions.

There is limited information on waitlisted candidates infected with or exposed to COVID-19, and it remains unclear if individuals with active or recent infection can be safely transplanted. However, it is anticipated that individuals undergoing transplantation with active infection result in poor outcomes.[17] Given the lack of definitive treatment, candidates with active COVID-19 infection should be deferred for transplantation until clinically improved and the virus is undetectable.[20] It is suggested to screen all potential recipients with an organ offer for COVID-19 symptoms prior to admission and if confirmed recent SARS-CoV-2 positive, candidates may be considered for transplantation 14–21 days after symptoms resolve and 1 or 2 negative SARS-CoV-2 diagnostics tests.[14] This recommendation is encouraged in order to avoid potential complications post-transplantation as well as exposure to the health care team or other transplant recipients.

TRANSPLANT RECIPIENTS

There has been a significant concern regarding the outcome of COVID-19-infected transplant recipients. They are also considered a vulnerable group, who are at risk for infection due to underlying medical conditions, transplant-related cytopenias, frequent contact with the health care system, and required immunosuppression post-transplantation.[21] It has been reported that transplant recipients who become infected with COVID-19 are at higher risk for severe disease and poorer outcomes than the general population.[22] Furthermore, there is a concern that post-transplantation immunosuppression may result in poor virologic control leading to increasing severity of disease and prolonged viral shedding.[22] However, the effects of immunosuppression on the novel coronavirus are not well established.

Some data suggests that immunosuppression may have a desirable effect and be protective against the excessive pro-inflammatory response of the virus.[23] In a large, multicenter study of 482 SOT recipients with COVID-19 infection (66% were kidney or kidney/pancreas, 15.1% were liver, 11.8% were heart, and 6.2% were lung), the 28-day mortality rate was 20.5% and older age, higher rates of underlying medical comorbidities, and radiographic chest abnormalities on presentation were directly related to mortality, but transplant-related type and intensity of immunosuppression were not.[24] Of the hospitalized recipients with COVID-19 infection, 39% required ICU care and 31% required mechanical ventilation.

Considering the novelty of the virus, there is no clear guidance on the medical management and therapeutic approach for transplant recipients with COVID-19 infection. Although there is limited data, it is recommended to treat transplant recipients with the same management guidelines as non-transplant patients.[21] Table 12-1 provides guidelines for the adult treatment of SARS-CoV-2 (COVID-19) used by the Mount Sinai Hospital.[25]

However, special considerations should be taken when treating COVID-19 in SOT recipients. This includes providing an optimal immunosuppression regimen and monitoring for potential drug-drug interactions and adverse effects of treatment.[21] To date, there are no guidelines for adjusting immunosuppression in transplant recipients with COVID-19 infection. It is suggested that modifications to immunosuppression should be individualized based on disease severity, the specific immunosuppressant agents, time from organ transplantation, and risk of graft rejection.[22]

The American Association for the Study of Liver Diseases (AASLD) recommends lowering the overall level of immunosuppression, specifically reducing the anti-metabolite dosage and closely monitoring calcineurin

Table 12-1 MOUNT SINAI HEALTH SYSTEM ADULT TREATMENT GUIDELINES FOR COVID-19[25]		
Illness Severity	**Therapy Options**	**Considerations**
Not Hospitalized or Asymptomatic	Supportive care	
Mild Illness Hospitalized (>94% on room air) and NOT requiring supplemental oxygen	Supportive care	Initiation of corticosteroids is not recommended.
Moderate Illness SpO$_2$ ≤ 94% on RA or requiring low-flow nasal cannula	Supportive care **Consider:** • **Anticoagulation** • **Dexamethasone** • **Remdesivir EUA** • **Convalescent plasma or SARS-CoV-2 specific antibody therapy**	**Anticoagulation**—per hospital protocol **Dexamethasone 6 mg IV/PO once daily for up to 10 days**. Patients with symptom duration of < 7 days have not demonstrated benefit from dexamethasone. Dexamethasone should not be continued after discharge unless patient has a history of being on chronic steroid therapy. **Remdesivir EUA-** On May 1, 2020, the FDA issued an EUA for the use of remdesivir in hospitalized patients. Remdesivir is not recommended in patients with an eGFR < 30 mL/min or with an ALT/AST > 5 times with upper limit of normal. Health care providers must document in the medical record that the patient/caregiver has been given information consistent with the "Fact Sheet for Patients and Parents/Caregivers" and have been informed that remdesivir is not FDA-approved but its use is authorized under an EUA. Initiation of EUA remdesivir requires approval by each institution's designated multidisciplinary approval committee. **Convalescent plasma**—On August 23, 2020, the FDA issue an EUA for the use of convalescent plasma in hospitalized patients.

(Continued)

Table 12-1 MOUNT SINAI HEALTH SYSTEM ADULT TREATMENT GUIDELINES FOR COVID-19[25] (*CONTINUED*)		
Illness Severity	**Therapy Options**	**Considerations**
Severe Illness **Patient requiring** non-rebreather, high flow nasal cannula, or non-invasive ventilation (i.e., BiPAP)	Supportive care **Recommend:** • **Anticoagulation** • **Dexamethasone** • **Remdesivir EUA** • **Convalescent plasma or SARS-CoV-2 specific antibody therapy**	See above.
Critical Illness **Patient requiring** mechanical ventilation and/ or extracorporeal membrane oxygenation (ECMO)	Supportive care **Consider** • **Anticoagulation** • **Dexamethasone**	Evaluation for the appropriateness of remdesivir and/or convalescent plasma will be on a case-by-case basis. Currently, data demonstrating benefit of either therapy are lacking in these populations. *Infectious disease (ID) consult is strongly recommended for the use of remdesivir and convalescent plasma therapy.

inhibitor levels.[14] However, precaution should be taken when reducing or discontinuing immunosuppression in transplant patients; this can potentially lead to graft rejection, flare in certain autoimmune liver diseases, and adrenal insufficiency.[14] Clinicians managing transplant recipients with COVID-19 should consult a transplant specialist prior to adjusting immunosuppression. It is also recommended that transplant recipients without COVID-19 infections continue immunosuppressive agents with no anticipatory adjustments.[14]

Strict infection prevention is essential to keeping transplant recipients from acquiring this life-threatening virus. Pertaining to hospitalized transplant recipients without COVID-19 infection, designate a separate ICU and ward isolated from patients under investigation for COVID-19 infection or with confirmed COVID-19 infection. Limit the number of team members and personnel permitted to enter patient rooms. In addition, implement a strict visitor policy to minimize risk of transmission from visitors.

Outpatient office visits and adhering to the same precautions described in the previous section of this chapter are critical. Additionally, the use of virtual physical therapy and educational sessions are encouraged. Educate patients to use an electronic medical app to record and trend vital signs and their current state of health. Table 12-2 illustrates COVID-19 prevention strategies for routine or follow up outpatient visits.

▌ CARE IN THE ICU

Severe cases of COVID-19 may be associated with ARDS, septic shock, cardiac dysfunction, thromboembolic disease, cytokine storm, and exacerbation of underlying medical conditions.[21] Patients that have acquired severe COVID-19 infection are usually critically ill and require ICU care. As previously mentioned, transplant candidates and recipients are at greater risk for severe illness due to COVID-19 and may ultimately require admission to the ICU. Transplant candidates are in end-stage organ failure and a virus such as COVID-19 can cause additional complications and rapid decompensation of their underlying disease. Moreover, transplant recipients with COVID-19 infection are equally susceptible to critical illness due to their underlying medical comorbidities and immunocompromised state. Therefore, high-quality ICU care is essential to the outcomes of this vulnerable population of patients.

Critically ill patients with COVID-19 may require vasopressor support, ventilatory support, renal replacement therapy, and certain pharmacologic interventions. The Surviving Sepsis Campaign (SSC) issued *Guidelines on the Management of Critically Adults with Coronavirus Disease 2019 (COVID-19)* in March 2020, which offers expert advice to clinicians caring for these critically ill patients.[26] The National Institute of Health (NIH) developed a summary of these recommendations for the care of critically ill patients with COVID-19.[21] Table 12-3 summarizes the management of critically ill patients with COVID-19.[21]

Table 12-2 PREVENTION OF COVID-19 OUTPATIENT STRATEGY	
TELEMEDICINE	**ELECTRONIC MEDICAL APP**
• Virtual visit • Phone call • Text messaging • Email • Virtual educational classes • Virtual physical therapy	• Vital signs • General clinical status • Screening for COVID-19 signs and symptoms

Table 12-3 CARE OF CRITICALLY ILL PATIENTS WITH COVID-19[21]

Summary Recommendations

Hemodynamic Support:
- The Panel recommends norepinephrine as the first-choice vasopressor (AII).
- For adults with COVID-19 and refractory septic shock who are not receiving corticosteroids to treat their COVID-19, the Panel recommends using low-dose corticosteroid therapy ("shock-reversal") over no corticosteroid therapy (BII).

Ventilatory Support:
- For adults with COVID-19 and acute hypoxemic respiratory failure despite conventional oxygen therapy, the Panel recommends high-flow nasal cannula (HFNC) oxygen over noninvasive positive pressure ventilation (NIPPV) (BI).
- In the absence of an indication for endotracheal intubation, the Panel recommends a closely monitored trial of NIPPV for adults with COVID-19 and acute hypoxemic respiratory failure for whom HFNC is not available (BIII).
- For adults with COVID-19 who are receiving supplemental oxygen, the Panel recommends close monitoring for worsening respiratory status and that intubation, if it becomes necessary, be performed by an experienced practitioner in a controlled setting (AII).
- For patients with persistent hypoxemia despite increasing supplemental oxygen requirements in whom endotracheal intubation is not otherwise indicated, the Panel recommends considering a trial of awake prone positioning to improve oxygenation (CIII).
- The Panel recommends against using awake prone positioning as a rescue therapy for refractory hypoxemia to avoid intubation in patients who otherwise require intubation and mechanical ventilation (AIII).
- For mechanically ventilated adults with COVID-19 and acute respiratory distress syndrome (ARDS), the Panel recommends using low tidal volume (VT) ventilation (VT 4–8 mL/kg of predicted body weight) over higher tidal volumes (VT >8 mL/kg) (AI).
- For mechanically ventilated adults with COVID-19 and refractory hypoxemia despite optimized ventilation, the Panel recommends prone ventilation for 12 to 16 hours per day over no prone ventilation (BII).
- For mechanically ventilated adults with COVID-19, severe ARDS, and hypoxemia despite optimized ventilation and other rescue strategies, the Panel recommends using an inhaled pulmonary vasodilator as a rescue therapy; if no rapid improvement in oxygenation is observed, the treatment should be tapered off (CIII).
- There are insufficient data to recommend either for or against the routine use of extracorporeal membrane oxygenation (ECMO) for patients with COVID-19 and refractory hypoxemia.

Acute Kidney Injury and Renal Replacement Therapy:
- For critically ill patients with COVID-19 who have acute kidney injury and who develop indications for renal replacement therapy, the Panel recommends continuous renal replacement therapy (CRRT), if available (BIII).
- If CRRT is not available or not possible due to limited resources, the Panel recommends prolonged intermittent renal replacement therapy rather than intermittent hemodialysis (BIII).

Rating of Recommendations: A = Strong; B = Moderate; C = Optional

Rating of Evidence: I = One or more randomized trials with clinical outcomes and/or validated laboratory endpoints; II = One or more well-designed, nonrandomized trials or observational cohort studies; III = Expert opinion

▌ TO TRANSPLANT OR NOT TO TRANSPLANT

In April 2020, the Center for Medicare and Medicaid Services (CMS) recommended limiting all nonessential elective surgeries and procedures, which excluded transplant surgery and categorized transplant surgery as Tier 3b, "do not postpone."[27] CMS advised if surgery is required to save a life, manage severe illness, or avoid further complications from an underlying medical condition it should not be delayed.

There have been a plethora of issues and debates regarding transplantation during a pandemic. Resource availability, associated care, and ethical considerations are important factors in whether or not to continue transplantation. Each center should be responsible in developing specific policies and protocols based on their local situation with the guidance of transplant societies. Such policies and protocols should include measures to protect the health care team, pre-transplant management, organ donation, organ transplantation, and follow-up care. Transplant societies such as American Society of Transplant Surgeons (ASTS), the American Society of Transplantation (AST), The Transplant Society (TTS), the International Society for Heart and Lung Transplantation (ISHLT), and Association of Organ Procurement Organizations (AOPO) play an important role and should provide transplant centers with their expert advice and continuous support during this rapidly evolving pandemic.

The COVID-19 pandemic will continue to threaten the general public as well as the transplant community until a definitive treatment and vaccine is available. There is limited data on the impact of the pandemic on individuals awaiting and those who have undergone transplantation. Therefore, it is essential for transplant centers, clinicians, and patients to make informed decisions and take the proper precautions to ensure safety throughout this challenging time. Transplant centers must stay apprised of emerging and evolving information on this new disease, be adaptable to the changes, and individualized decision making to continue the quality of the life-improving and life-saving practice of transplantation.

▌ REFERENCES

1. Kumar D, Manuel O, Natori Y. COVID-19: A global transplant perspective on successfully navigating a pandemic. *Am J Transplant*. 2020;20:1773-1779.
2. Zhu N, Zhang D, Wang W, et al. A novel coronavirus from patients with pneumonia in China, is 2019. *N Engl J Med*. 2020;382:727-733.

3. WHO. Coronavirus disease (COVID-19) situation reports. https://covid19.who. int. Updated October 1, 2020. Accessed October 1, 2020.

4. Chu DK, Akl EA, Duda S, et al. COVID-19 Systemic Urgent Review Group Effort (SURGE) studying authors. Physical distancing, face masks, and eye protection to prevent person-to-person transmission of SARS-CoV-2 and COVID-19: A systematic review and meta-analysis. *Lancet*. 2020;395:1973-1987.

5. Wiersinga WJ, Rhodes A, Cheng AC, Peacock SJ, Prescott HC. Pathophysiology, transmission, diagnosis, and treatment of coronavirus disease 2019 (COVID-19). *JAMA*. 2020;324(8):782-793.

6. WHO. Modes of transmission of virus causing COVID-19: Implications for IPC precaution recommendations: Scientific brief. https://apps.who.int/iris/handle/10665/331601. Published March 27, 2020. Accessed October 1, 2020.

7. Patel KP, Vunnam SR, Patel PA, et al. Transmission of SARS-CoV-2: An update of current literature. *Eur J Clin Microbiol Infec Dis*. 2020;39(11):2005-2011.

8. Cheng HY, Jian SW, Liu DP, et al. Contact tracing assessment of COVID-19 transmission dynamics in Taiwan and risk at different exposure periods before and after symptom onset. *JAMA Intern Med*. 2020;180(9):1156-1163.

9. Lauer SA, Grant KH, Bi Q, et al. The incubation of coronavirus disease 2019 (COVID-19) from publicly reported confirmed cases: Estimation and application. *Ann Intern Med*. 2020;172(9):577-582.

10. Guan WJ, Ni ZY, Hu Y, et al. Clinical characteristics of coronavirus disease 2019 in China. *N Engl J Med*. 2020;382:1708-1720.

11. Centers for Disease Control and Prevention. Evidence used to update the list of underlying medical conditions that increase a person's risk of severe illness from COVID-19. https://www.cdc.gov/coronavirus/2019-ncov/need-extra-precautions/people-with-medical-conditions.html. Updated October 6, 2020. Accessed October 6, 2020.

12. United Organ Network for Organ Sharing. Transplant trends. https://unos.org/data/transplant-trends/. Updated October 1, 2020. Accessed October 1, 2020.

13. Zhang H, Dai H, Xie X, et al. Solid organ transplantation during the COVID-19 pandemic. *Frontiers in Immunology*. 2020;11:1392.

14. American Association for the Study of Liver Diseases. Clinical Insights for hepatology and liver transplant providers during the COVID-19 pandemic. https://www.aasld.org/sites/default/files/2020-06/AASLD-COVID19-ExpertPanelConsensusStatement-June252520-v2-FINAL.pdf. Published June 25, 2020. Accessed October 1, 2020.

15. Galvan NN, Moreno NF, Garza JE, et al. Donor and transplant candidate selection for solid organ transplantation during the COVID-19 pandemic. *Am J Transplant*. 2020.

16. Loupy A, Aubert O, Reese PP, Bayer F, Jacquelinet C. Organ procurement and transplantation during COVID-19 pandemic. *Lancet*. 2020;395:e95-e96.

17. American Society of Transplantation. 2019-nCoV (Coronavirus): FAQs for organ transplantation. https://www.myast.org/sites/default/files/COVID19%20FAQ%20Tx%20Centers%206.18.2020.pdf. Updated June 18, 2020. Accessed October 6, 2020.

18. Centers for Disease Control and Prevention. Healthcare facilities: Managing operations during the COVID-19 pandemic. https://www.cdc.gov/coronavirus/2019-ncov/hcp/guidance-hcf.html. Published June 28, 2020. Accessed October 6, 2020.

19. Centers for Disease Control and Prevention. Cleaning and disinfecting your facility. https://www.cdc.gov/coronavirus/2019-ncov/community/disinfecting-building-facility.html. Published June 29, 2020. Accessed October 6, 2020.

20. The Transplant Society. Guidance on coronavirus disease 2019 (COVID-19) for transplant clinicians. https://tts.org/26-tid/tid-resources/749-tis-covid-test. 2020. Updated July 14, 2020. Accessed October 6, 2020.

21. COVID-19 Treatment Guidelines Panel. Coronavirus disease 2019 (COVID-19) treatment guidelines. National Institutes of Health. https://www.covid19treatmentguidelines.nih.gov/. Published October 13, 2020. Accessed October 13, 2020.

22. Pereira MR, Mohan S, Cohen DJ, et al. COVID-19 in solid organ transplant recipients: Initial report from the US epicenter. *Am J Transplant.* 2020;20(7):1800-1808.

23. Kates OS, Fisher CF, Stankiewicz-Karita HC, et al. Earliest cases of coronavirus disease 2019 (COVID 19) identified in solid organ transplant recipients in the United States. *Am J Transplant.* 2020;20:1885-1890.

24. Kates OS, Haydel BM, Florman SS. Coronavirus disease 2019 in solid organ transplant: A multicenter cohort study. *Clin Infect Dis.* 2020 Aug 7:ciaa1097. Online ahead of print.

25. Mount Sinai Hospital. Mount Sinai Health System adult treatment guidelines for SARS-CoV-2 infection (COVID-19). https://www.mountsinai.org/files/MSHealth/Assets/HS/About/Coronavirus/MSHS-Treatment-Guidelines-COVID.pdf. Updated September 27, 2020. Accessed October 30, 2020.

26. Alhazzani, W, Moller MH, Arabi YM, et al. Surviving Sepsis Campaign: Guidelines on the management of critically ill adults with coronavirus disease 2019 (COVID-19). *Crit Care Med.* 2020;46(5):854-867.

27. Centers for Medicare and Medicaid Services. Non-emergent, elective medical services, and treatment recommendations. https://www.cms.gov/files/document/cms-non-emergent-elective-medical-recommendations.pdf. Published April 7, 2020. Accessed October 13, 2020.

EXTRACORPOREAL MEMBRANE OXYGENATION USE DURING CRISIS IN CRITICAL CARE 13

Samantha K. Brenner, MD, MPH

▌ INTRODUCTION

Extracorporeal membrane oxygenation (ECMO) is a resource-intensive rescue strategy, which is powered by a centrifugal pump and serves as a mechanical circulatory support (MCS) device. The two most common indications are either life-threatening pulmonary or cardiac failure or some combination of the two. ECMO can be used in the field as a temporizing measure providing supportive care, if the right team and equipment are available for placement and a safe transfer plan to an ECMO-capable center is readily available. Importantly, ECMO serves as a temporizing measure awaiting either organ recovery or a more permanent device or surgery, such as organ transplant. Effective use of ECMO requires a specialized team of providers to monitor both the patient and the circuit. A team approach reduces ECMO complication rates, which are predominantly renal failure and coagulation disorders—both bleeding and clotting.

Depending on the indication, different configurations of ECMO can be used. For example, in cases of out-of-hospital cardiac arrest, venoarterial (VA) ECMO has been used successfully. In the context of acute and severe respiratory failure, venovenous (VV) ECMO has been employed in the treatment of trauma, burning, and drowning victims, as well as epidemic diseases such as 2009 H1N1 influenza, Middle East Respiratory Syndrome (MERS), and the SARS-CoV-2 pandemic.

This chapter summarizes the technological evolutions in ECMO, its common configurations and indications, as well as covering common complications. At the close of the chapter, considerations for disaster preparedness and crisis applications of ECMO are discussed.

▍OVERVIEW OF THE EVOLUTION OF ECMO TECHNOLOGY

ECMO was developed to serve as a cardiopulmonary bypass circuit for use outside of the confines of the operating room for longer durations of supportive care. In 1953, almost 20 years after the case that inspired the idea, Gibbon successfully used the first external perfusion and oxygenation support to perform the first successful heart operation.[1] In 1972, Hill and colleagues described a case of a thoracic trauma patient who developed refractory respiratory distress post-thoracic surgery. His treatment team took the unprecedented step of using peripheral cannulation to support him for 75 hours.[2]

ECMO has continued to evolve since that time, both in technological advancements and in its applications.[3,4] For example, the initial pumps used for ECMO were constructed of roller pumps with silicon oxygenators and had higher complication rates than the new hollow-fiber polymethylpentene oxygenators and centrifugal pumps.[5–8] Using polymethylpentene instead of silicone in the oxygenators reduces platelet consumption and decreases resistance to blood flow.[6] These oxygenators are less prone to damage and last longer, as a result of the nonmicroporous consistency of these fibers. Ultimately, liquid, which causes oxygenator failure, is less likely to diffuse across than previous oxygenators.[7] In addition, the new pumps consist of polycarbonate housing with a magnetically-rotated impeller, which decreases sheer stress on the blood cells.[7] Finally, the connecting PVC tubing is now either coated in heparin-based or synthetic anticoagulants, which decreases thrombosis rates.[5,7,9] Improvements in cannulation strategies have facilitated extubation and ambulation for patients requiring prolonged ECMO runs.[10–13]

Collectively, these technological advances have made ECMO cheaper and simpler, but still necessitate a team approach for best outcomes. The improvements in ease of use, decreased complication rates, and trends toward improved survival rates have resulted in increased use of ECMO over time. Concomitantly, the applications and indications for ECMO have continued to be expanded.[14–16] The evolution and use of ECMO has not been linear over time. Randomized controlled trials of VV ECMO in particular have been plagued by an inability to demonstrate its efficacy. In the 1990s, Morris and colleagues were unable to demonstrate a statistical difference between ECMO and conventional therapy.[17] Ten years later, the Conventional ventilation or ECMO for Severe Adult Respiratory failure (CESAR) trial's unfortunate trial design foiled the conclusions when the researchers unwittingly conducted randomization on transfer to an ECMO center instead of measuring the effects of administration of ECMO itself.[18] In 2018, the ECMO to Rescue Lung Injury in Severe ARDS (EOLIA) trial was poised to measure the effectiveness of VV ECMO in ARDS, but the institutional review board stopped the trial early, as ECMO appeared to be too effective for the trial to ethically continue. Unfortunately, in the final analysis, they had recruited too few patients to meet their power calculations and intention-to-treat analysis failed find a significant difference.[19] Due to the lack of definitive evidence and difficulty in carrying out randomized controlled trials in this field, ECMO has experienced fits and starts in popularity. Furthermore, ECMO has consistently been found to increase the costs of providing care to patients.[18]

Based on cumulative registry data from the Extracorporeal Life Support Organization (ELSO), as of 2015, ECMO has most commonly been used in neonates (53%), with adult cases constituting only 23% of over 65,000 cases. By 2017, ELSO was reporting over 87,000 cases, most of which were respiratory and a growing number, 8%, were for extracorporeal cardiopulmonary resuscitation (ECPR).[1,20]

CIRCUIT COMPONENTS AND COMMON CONFIGURATIONS

ECMO is an external (hence, extracorporeal) pump that provides several primary functions: blood oxygenation, carbon dioxide removal, and/or cardiac output. These feats are accomplished using a centrifugal pump to drain blood from the patient's venous system through a large-bore cannula, then through a membrane oxygenation system, which simultaneously extracts carbon dioxide via fresh gas flow.[20] The hollow polymethylpentine fibers inside the oxygenator are semipermeable and have gas flow through them. Gas exchange occurs because the blood flows around the hollow fibers.[7] The sweep gas circulates through the oxygenator and is controlled by the blender, which assists in the combination of ambient air with oxygen gas.[7] The oxygenated, carbon dioxide-depleted blood is then returned to the circulatory system again through a large-bore cannula.[21] When ECMO is being placed, consideration must be given to adequate cannula sizing for the expected amount of flow required (3–4 mL/kg/min), while also seeking to minimize complications from large-bore vascular access.[5,22] If available, an ultrasound is recommended to calculate the size of the vessel and ensure the chosen cannula is less than two-thirds the size of the vessel or 1-3F sizes smaller than the vessel.[23]

The general components of the ECMO circuits are available from different manufactures and are as follows (see Figure 13-1):[5,20]

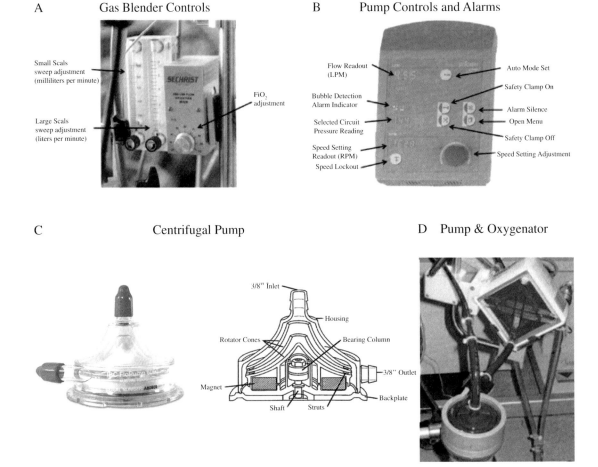

Figure 13-1 • ECMO Components. **A** shows the gas blender controls to control both the rate of carbon dioxide removal as well as increase the fraction of inspired oxygen, as needed. **B** is an example of a console, and the types of indicators and alarms usually available. **C** shows a centrifugal pump as well as a schematic. **D** depicts the oxygenator on the upper right corner, which is connected to a pump like the one shown in **C** The blood is flowing from the patient to the pump and then to the oxygenator before returning to the patient. (Parts A and B used, with permission, from Keebler ME, Haddad EV, Choi CW, et al. Venoarterial extracorporeal membrane oxygenation in cardiogenic shock. *JACC Heart Fail*. 2018;6(6):503-516. Part C from *Some Introduction of ECMO Centrifugal Pump Magnet*. https://www.magnet-sdm.com/2020/03/13/introduction-ecmo-centrifugal-pump-magnet/. Copyright © 2020 SDM Magnetics Co., Ltd. Part D used, with permission, from MacLaren G, Combes A, Bartlett RH. Contemporary extracorporeal membrane oxygenation for adult respiratory failure: Life support in the new era. *Intensive Care Med*. 2012;38:210-220.)

- One or more large bore cannula(s)
- PVC connection tubing
- Pump

- Oxygenator
- Blender
- Console (controls and alarms)

Each ECMO circuit needs to be configured based on its indication for use. The nomenclature describes the circuitry employed. For example, for cardiac failure, veno-arterial (VA) should be used. For respiratory failure, veno-venous (VV) cannulations are most commonly used. VA ECMO is used when there is combined respiratory and cardiac failure. By convention, the first letter denotes the source of deoxygenated blood coming from the body to the pump, and the second letter (and, if applicable, the third letter) describe(s) the return site of the oxygenated blood running from the pump back to the body.

For cases of respiratory failure in which VV ECMO is being used, the cannulation tends to follow one of two formations: either two catheters with one femoral and one internal jugular, or one double-lumen catheter placed in the right internal jugular vein. Both configurations are shown in Figure 13-2. As illustrated in Figure 13-2, the solitary double-lumen catheter, named a Wang-Zwische (after its inventors) or more commonly Avalon catheter, acts as a catheter within a catheter: blood is removed from ports in both the superior and inferior vena cavae of the outer catheter and retuned to the right atrium using the internal catheter.[24] The placement of these single catheters with a double lumen requires transesophageal echography or fluoroscopy to ensure that the catheter flow is directed toward the tricuspid valve to maximize oxygenated blood return and decrease mixing.[24] The advantage of this single catheter configuration is decreased vascular complications, recirculation, and increased mobility for patients.[5]

When VA ECMO cannulation is under consideration for cardiogenic shock, there are two conventional configurations that are predominantly in use: central or peripheral cannulation, both of which are depicted in Figure 13-3.[20] Central cannulation refers to right atrial drainage and return of oxygenated blood directly into the ascending aorta.[1] Peripheral cannulation most commonly is accomplished with two femoral cannulas, one arterial and one venous. However, more recently, to increase mobility, peripheral cannulation is sometimes performed in the upper extremities, not just femoral.[20] In cases of combined cardiogenic shock and pulmonary failure, veno-arterio-venous is more commonly used as it provides a third cannula that returns oxygenated blood to the right heart at the level of the tricuspid valve to prevent Harlequin or North/South syndrome. In other words, adequate cerebral oxygenation is ensured, by providing oxygenated blood directly to the venous system.[20]

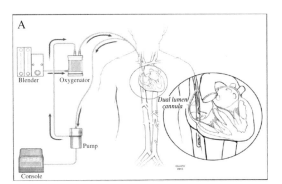

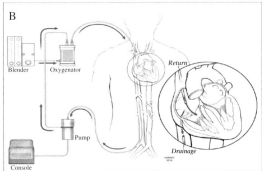

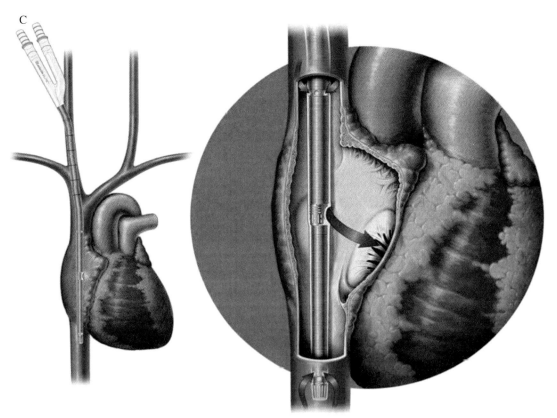

Figure 13-2 • Typical VV ECMO Cannulation Configurations. **A** is a schematic of a single catheter with a dual lumen veno-venous ECMO configuration. **B** delineates the blood flow in a femoral VV ECMO cannulation in which there is a venous femoral drain limb and a right atrial return limb. Alternatively, bilateral femoral venous cannulation is also an option (not shown). **C** Close up of VV ECMO single cannula shows access through the right internal jugular vein. The external cannula has several drain ports that flow to the drain line with a single internal return port aimed to the tricuspid valve. (Parts A and B used, with permission, from Sen A, Callisen HE, Alwardt CM, et al. Adult venovenous extracorporeal membrane oxygenation for severe respiratory failure: Current status and future perspectives. *Ann Card Anaesth.* 2016;19(1):97-111. https://www.annals.in/text.asp?2016/19/1/97/173027. The device in Part C is indicated for extracorporeal life support procedures due to respiratory failure. Reprinted with permission, Getinge, Wayne, New Jersey.)

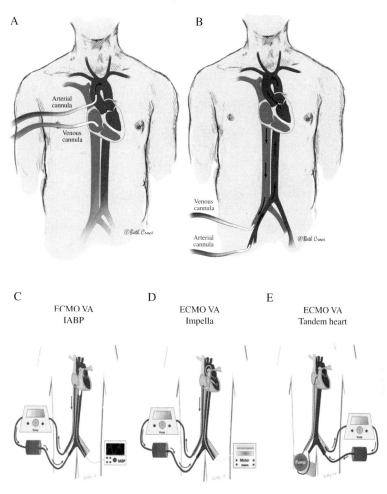

Figure 13-3 • Common VA ECMO Configurations. **A** shows central veno-arterial ECMO cannulation right atrial drain limb and left atrial return limb. **B** shows peripheral veno-arterial ECMO cannulation with a femoral venous drain line and a femoral arterial return limb. Alternative peripheral VA ECMO configurations include axillary or carotid arterial return limbs (not shown). **C, D,** and **E** show VA ECMO configurations with other mechanical devices for cardiac unloading, balloon pump, impella, and Tandem heart, respectively. (Parts A and B used, with permission, from Marasco SF, Lukas G, McDonald M, McMillan J, Ihle B. Review of ECMO (extra corporeal membrane oxygenation) support in critically ill adult patients. *Heart Lung Circ*. 2008;17S:S41-S47. Parts C-E used, with permission, from Brasseur A, Scolletta S, Lorusso R, Taccone FS. Hybrid extracorporeal membrane oxygenation. *J Thorac Dis*. 2018;10(4):S707-S715; Nancy International Ltd, subsidiary AME Publishing Company, conveyed through Copyright Clearance Center, Inc.)

VA ECMO alone can sometimes cause increased cardiac strain and over-distention as a result of increased aortic afterload associated with the return limb. This cardiac strain can prove antithetical to cardiac recovery. Therefore, ensuring ventricular unloading can sometimes be essential in the setting of VA ECMO for cardiogenic shock patients depending on their hemodynamics. Increasingly, VA ECMO is now being combined with other MCS devices to improve ventricular unloading (Figure 13-3):

- VA ECMO + intraortic pulsatile balloon pump (IABP)[25,26]
- VA ECMO + left ventricular Impella device (Abiomed Inc., USA), aka: ECpella[3,26]
- VA ECMO + Tandem Heart pump (Cardiac Assist, Inc., Pittsburgh, PA, USA)[26]

Table 13-1 shows the pros and cons of these configurations. These configurations also have the advantage of facilitating ECMO weaning if cardiac function is slow to recover.[3,4,26] Although data is sparse, there are other hybrid VA ECMO configurations with increasing numbers of ECMO drainage limbs that are also being reported in the literature. The configurations are theoretically designed to improve venous drainage, optimize systemic hemodynamics, improve oxygenation, decrease LV work and dilation, and reduce pulmonary edema.[26]

▌INDICATIONS FOR USE

Clinicians should consider the use of VA ECMO for cardiogenic shock, whereas patients with respiratory failure should be considered for VV ECMO. In cases where both cardiac and pulmonary failure are present, VA ECMO should be considered, particularly because VV ECMO is contraindicated in cases of right ventricular (RV) failure.[1]

VA ECMO

For the purposes of VA ECMO consideration, cardiogenic shock should be defined as systolic blood pressure of less than 90 mm Hg or 30 mm Hg less than basal in hypertensive patients for greater than 30 minutes, with use of vasopressors or inotropes to keep systolic blood pressure greater than 90 mm Hg, despite adequate intravascular volume, and a cardiac index of less than 2.2 L/min/m^2.[1,27] Table 13-2 shows the common indications for VA ECMO, i.e. common etiologies of cardiogenic shock amenable to recovery.

Ideally, clinicians should strive to obtain the patient's hemodynamic measurements by Swan-Ganz catheter prior to mechanical support placement, as well as an echocardiogram to rule out immediately reversible or treatable conditions such as tamponade or pulmonary embolism.[27] However, in an acute crisis situation such as during a cardiac arrest, a

Table 13-1 ADVANTAGES AND DRAWBACKS OF HYBRID VA ECMO CONFIGURATIONS[26]

Configuration	Pros	Cons
VA ECMO + IABP	• LV unloading • Increased coronary perfusion	• Possible decrease in cerebral blood flow • Not shown in metanalysis to provide mortality benefit
VA ECMA + Impella = ECpella	• LV unloading • Shown in several propensity- or case-matched studies to show improved survival over VA ECMO alone	• Increased hemolysis risk
VA ECMO + Tandem-Heart	• LV unloading	• Not well-studied, efficacy unknown/unproven

Note: The purpose of hybrid VA ECMO configurations with other MCS devices is protection against worsening LV failure through LV venting. See Figure 13-3 for visualizations of each configuration.

ECpella = VA ECMO with LV impella vent; IABP = intraortic pulsatile balloon pump; LV = left ventricle.

Swan-Ganz catheter may not be readily available or logistically feasible. Instead, VA ECMO can be placed as a salvage maneuver to stabilize the patient.[28]

VV ECMO

VV ECMO should be considered for cases of refractory respiratory failure, either hypoxemic or hypercarbic.[7] Specifically, reversible or treatable disease processes that cause acute respiratory distress syndrome (ARDS) are common indications including viral or bacterial pneumonias, and trauma patients. Other conditions include patients with severe air leak syndromes, primary graft failure in lung transplant patients, or patients pre-transplant.[21] Additionally, VV ECMO can also be employed in rare cases of complex airway management or pulmonary hemorrhage/massive hemoptysis.[1,7] In general, VV ECMO should be considered when patient

Table 13-2 COMMON INDICATIONS FOR VA ECMO[21,48]

Clinical Condition	Common Clinical Context
Post-cardiotomy	Unable to come off of cardiopulmonary bypass following cardiac surgery
Post-heart transplant	In the setting of primary graft failure
Decompensated cardiomyopathy	Known long-standing cardiomyopathy as a temporizing bridge to durable implantable device or transplant, particularly if: • Biventricular failure is noted (i.e., CI < 2.2 L/min/m^2, RAP ≥ 15 mm Hg, RAP:PCWP > 0.8, PAPi < 1.85) • Increasingly instability as measured by rising lactate (> 5mg/dL) or higher pressor or inotropic requirements despite initial stabilization efforts
Myocarditis	Fulminant, decompensated
Acute coronary syndrome[27,49]	Complicated by cardiogenic shock, particularly if there is: • Cardiac arrest • Hypoxemia (PaO$_2$/FiO$_2$ ratio < 80 on PEEP ≥ 10) • Persistent VT (storm) • Biventricular failure (i.e., CI < 2.2 L/min/m^2, RAP ≥ 15 mm Hg, PCWP ≥ 18, PAPi < 1.0) particularly if Lactate > 5 mg/dL
Toxic or metabolic cardiac depression	Profound, persistent cardiac depression due to: • Drug overdose • Sepsis • Severe hypothermia (< 28°C) with cardiac instability[20]
Witnessed in-hospital cardiac arrest (E-CPR)[76,104]	Usually in the context of a well-developed E-CPR program in which the ECMO team is deployed for every cardiac arrest, and cannulas are placed early during the arrest if the patient is not recovering.
Refractory ventricular arrhythmias[20]	Such as VT storm

CI= cardiac index; FiO$_2$ = fraction of inspired oxygen; iNO = inhaled nitric oxide; PaO$_2$/FiO$_2$ = partial pressure of oxygen to fraction of inspired oxygen ratio; PAPi = pulmonary arterial pulsatility index; PCWP = pulmonary capillary wedge pressure; RAP = right atrial pressure; VT= ventricular tachycardia.

mortality is predicted to be greater than 80%, despite optimal use of less invasive strategies.[5]

Optimization of mechanical support care prior to VV ECMO can be seen in the treatment algorithm in Figure 13-4. Since no formal consensus on VV ECMO indications exist, Figure 13-4 has been adapted from previous expert opinions.[29–32] The general contours of the approach are to maximize pre-ECMO mechanical ventilation oxygenation and ventilation through rescue therapies, which if they fail, should prompt the consideration of ECMO in patients without contraindications (Table 13-3). It should be noted that while guidelines and best practices exist for VV ECMO initiation, clinical consideration should be given not only to absolute cutoff values but also to the rate of clinical demise.[5] Furthermore, in terms of pre-ECMO mechanical ventilation optimization, Grasso and colleagues have suggested that measurement of transesophageal pressure with an esophageal manometer may be the most specific means of determining the optimal PEEP and obviate the need for ECMO in some cases. Using the measured transpulmonary pressure, instead of using plateau pressure as a surrogate, leads to a more nuanced PEEP titration to target a transpulmonary pressure of 25 cm H_2O. Although this approach is based in physiological reasoning, trial data demonstrating the efficacy of this approach remain lacking.[33]

▌PATIENT SELECTION

Patient selection is paramount. Similar to other advanced medical treatment tools, unfortunately, ECMO can sustain life in the absence of a reasonable probability of meaningful recovery. Therefore, one of the central considerations for ECMO placement is the likelihood of organ recovery. Hemodynamically or physiologically devastating, but temporary and reversible, single organ failure patients are the best candidates for this form of MCS device, as opposed to patients with acute multisystem organ failure.[5,21,34] Furthermore, because end-organ failure predicts poor survival, early re-perfusion and oxygenation with ECMO prior to multisystem end-organ damage is the standard. In other words, late initiation of ECMO can render the treatment medically futile.[20,35] In light of this, many ECMO guidelines now have specific time-based parameters for when ECMO use is most appropriate.[32] This understanding is important in crisis situations. Specifically, it is likely best to create mobile teams to deploy ECMO in the field and transport patients to safety, if the treatment is going to be effective.[20]

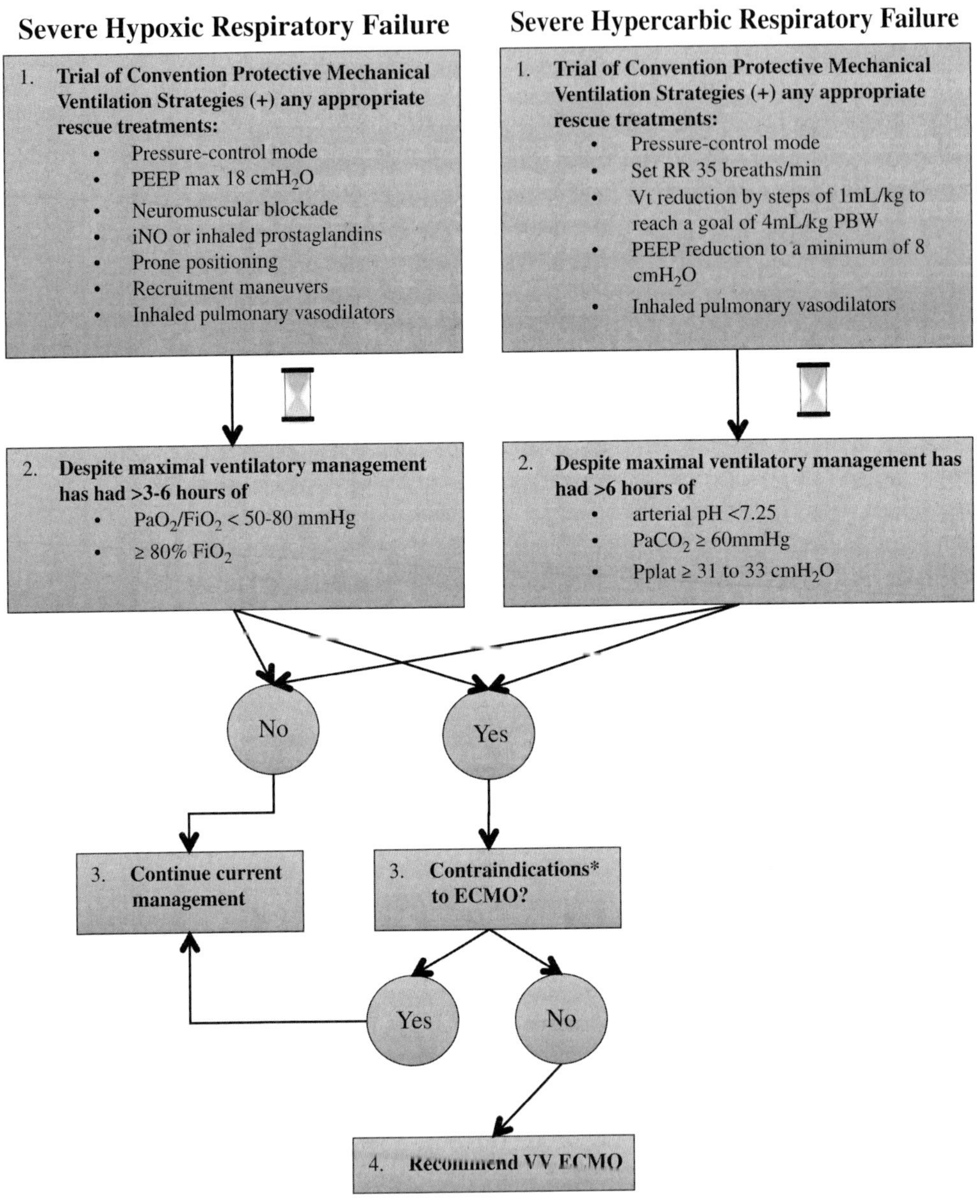

Severe Hypoxic Respiratory Failure

1. **Trial of Convention Protective Mechanical Ventilation Strategies (+) any appropriate rescue treatments:**
   - Pressure-control mode
   - PEEP max 18 cmH$_2$O
   - Neuromuscular blockade
   - iNO or inhaled prostaglandins
   - Prone positioning
   - Recruitment maneuvers
   - Inhaled pulmonary vasodilators

2. **Despite maximal ventilatory management has had >3-6 hours of**
   - PaO$_2$/FiO$_2$ < 50-80 mmHg
   - ≥ 80% FiO$_2$

Severe Hypercarbic Respiratory Failure

1. **Trial of Convention Protective Mechanical Ventilation Strategies (+) any appropriate rescue treatments:**
   - Pressure-control mode
   - Set RR 35 breaths/min
   - Vt reduction by steps of 1mL/kg to reach a goal of 4mL/kg PBW
   - PEEP reduction to a minimum of 8 cmH$_2$O
   - Inhaled pulmonary vasodilators

2. **Despite maximal ventilatory management has had >6 hours of**
   - arterial pH <7.25
   - PaCO$_2$ ≥ 60mmHg
   - Pplat ≥ 31 to 33 cmH$_2$O

No   Yes

3. **Continue current management**

3. **Contraindications* to ECMO?**

Yes   No

4. **Recommend VV ECMO**

Figure 13-4 • Algorithm for VV ECMO Consideration in Severe Hypoxic or Hypercapnic Respiratory Failure.[5,18,19,29,30,32,34]
*Contraindications to ECMO can be found in Table 13-4. FiO$_2$ = fraction of inspired oxygen; IBW = ideal body weight; iNO = inhaled nitric oxide; PaCO$_2$ = arterial partial pressure of carbon dioxide; PaO$_2$/FiO$_2$ = partial pressure of oxygen to fraction of inspired oxygen ratio; PEEP = positive end-expiratory pressure; Pplat = plateau pressure; RR = respiratory rate; Vt = tidal volume.

Table 13-3 COMMON RELATIVE CONTRAINDICATIONS TO ECMO	
Clinical Parameter	**Specific Considerations**
Acute multisystem organ failure	Excluding, of course, cardiac or respiratory failure, which are the indications for ECMO
Mechanical ventilation > 7 days	Specifically pertains to VV ECMO
Advanced age	≥ 65 years
Chronic organ failure	Examples: • Advanced chronic obstructive pulmonary disease (particularly, if not a lung transplant candidate) • Interstitial lung disease (particularly, if not a lung transplant candidate) • Liver cirrhosis • End-stage renal failure • End-stage cardiomyopathy patients who are neither heart transplant nor durable ventricular assist device candidates
Clinical frailty scale score	≥ 3
Malignancy with a poor or uncertain prognosis	Specifically: • Disseminated malignancy • Hematologic malignancy • Those patients actively undergoing chemotherapy •
Immunocompromised patients	Examples: • Solid organ transplantation patients (lung and heart transplants being notable possible exceptions) • HIV/AIDS • Graft vs host disease
Prior neurological dysfunction	Examples: • Dementia[48] • Prior stroke • Seizure disorder • Prior neurotrauma • Prior intracranial hemorrhage

(Continued)

Table 13-3 COMMON RELATIVE CONTRAINDICATIONS TO ECMO (*CONTINUED*)	
Clinical Parameter	**Specific Considerations**
Clinical Prediction Scores predicting < 50% survival	• **RESP** score ≤ −1 for VV ECMO[40,105] (see Table 13-5) • **SAVE** Score ≤ 0 for VA ECMO[44] (see Table 13-4)
Contraindications to anticoagulation	

Note: No consensus surrounds absolute contraindications to ECMO, therefore clinical teams must work together to examine each case and determine ECMO candidacy.

RESP = Respiratory ECMO Survival Prediction; SAVE = Survival after veno-artial ECMO.

Survival and Quality of Life

In all comers, survival to hospital discharge for VV ECMO and VA ECMO is similar, around 50%.[15,20,36,37] Unfortunately, 3- and 6-month survival can be significantly lower.[20,38] However, survival rates differ significantly based on indication and on age, with older patients having lower survival rates regardless of whether VV or VA ECMO is employed.[21] Quality of life for survivors of ECMO are worse than age-matched healthy controls but about equal or sometimes better than age-matched patients living with chronic diseases.[20,39]

VV ECMO Patient Selection

In the case of VV ECMO, patients who receive ECMO for asthma exacerbations tend to fare better,[40] as do patients with viral and bacterial pneumonias.[15] Patients receiving VV ECMO for traumas or burns may have worse survival.[15] Likewise, as described above, patients with multisystem organ failure do worse than those with single organ failure.[15] Higher pre-ECMO lung compliance,[30] along with having been on mechanical ventilation for longer than 7–10 days, is also associated with worse survival.[15,30,35,41] The Respiratory ECMO Survival Prediction (RESP) score was validated on over 3,000 patients and can be used pre-implantation of VV ECMO to predict survival rate (Table 13-5).[40]

VA ECMO Patient Selection

When considering VA ECMO placement, indication plays a significant role in predicting survival as well. For example, reversible causes of myocardial injury, such as myocarditis,[42] have better survival than post-cardiotomy[43] or acute myocardial injury.[20] The lowest survival rates are seen with ECPR.[20] Women and patients with higher body mass index fare worse on VA ECMO.[20] Similar to VV ECMO, time on mechanical ventilation prior to VA ECMO placement is associated with worse outcomes, but time in the case of VA ECMO is measured in hours instead of days. Similar to VV ECMO, a large group of almost 4,000 patients was used to develop the Survival After Veno-arterial ECMO score (SAVE), which can be reviewed in Table 13-4.[44]

Relative Contraindications

Appropriate patient selection for ECMO is critical. There is still no consensus on what the absolute contraindications to ECMO might be. To further confuse matters, different authors site differing lists of absolute contraindications. Therefore, Table 13-3 details a broad list of clinical conditions for which strong bias against using ECMO should be considered.[5,31] However, each institution should develop its own clinical guidelines to assist in this complex decision-making process.

▌ ECMO MANAGEMENT

In general, ECMO management is centered on the principles of mechanical support to facilitate organ rest and recovery. Therefore, maintaining physiologic homeostasis is at the forefront of the management goals. A detailed list of physiologic goals is provided in Table 13-6. Broadly speaking, clinicians should strive to restore and maintain normal organ function, acid-base balance, negative fluid balance, and neurologic status.[20] Enteral nutrition should be initiated within 48–72 hours when feasible.[7,32] Diuresis and fluid removal, while important for weaning, are best accomplished at a rate that allows for physiologic accommodation to prevent suctioning around the inflow cannula that causes "chatter." Other less common causes of "chatter" include coughing, cannula malposition, and kinking or obstructive shock such as cardiac tamponade or pneumothorax.[7] For further reference, ELSO also provides a comprehensive set of guidelines and resources for the management of ECMO.[45]

A team of specialized ECMO clinicians is needed to coordinate management of ECMO cases, as more data is showing this model is likely to improve outcomes,[46,47] and most importantly, provides the critical coordination of care needed for these complex patients.[20] As part of the multidisciplinary approach, early mobilization should be initiated whenever possible.[32]

Table 13-4 VA ECMO SURVIVAL PREDICTION SCORE: SAVE SCORE	
Parameter	**Score**
Diagnosis	
Myocarditits	3
Refractory VT/VF	2
Graft failure post-heart or lung transplant	3
Congenital heart disease	-3
Other diagnosis	0
Age (yrs)	
18 to 38	7
39 to 52	4
53 to 62	3
≥ 63	0
Weight (kg)	
≤ 65	1
65–89	2
≥ 90	0
Acute pre-ECMO organ failure (include all that apply)	
Liver failure[a]	−3
Central nervous system dysfunction[b]	−3
Renal failure[c]	−3
Chronic kidney disease (eGR < 60 mL/min/1.73 m^2) for $\geq$ 3 months	−6
Duration of mechanical ventilation pre-ECMO (hours)	
≤ 10	0
11 to 29	−2
≥ 30	−4

Table 13-4 VA ECMO SURVIVAL PREDICTION SCORE: SAVE SCORE (*CONTINUED*)

Parameter	Score
Peak inspiratory pressure ≤ 20 cm H_2O	3
Pre-ECMO cardiac arrest	–2
Diastolic blood pressure before ECMO ≥ 40 mm Hg	3
Pulse pressure before ECMO ≥ 20 mm Hg	–2
HCO_3 before ECMO ≤15 mmol/L	–3
Constant value to add to all calculations	–6
Total Score	**–35 to 17**

Hospital Survival by Risk Class	Risk Class	Survival
> 5	I	75%
1 to 5	II	58%
–4 to 0	III	42%
–9 to –5	IV	30%
≤ –10	V	18%

Note: The SAVE score can be calculated prior to placement of VA ECMO to assist in determining the patient's likelihood of survival based on co-morbidities and prior clinical course. An online calculator is available at www.save-score.com. It is not a substitute for clinical judgment and as the list of relative contraindications suggest, it is not comprehensive in considering all factors that may result in poor outcomes on VA ECMO.

[a]Liver failure defined as bilirubin ≥33 μmol/L or elevation of serum aminotransferases (ALT or AST) >70 UI/L.

[b]Central nervous system dysfunction includes any patient with neurotrauma, stroke, encephalopathy, intracranial hemorrhage, or seizure.

[c]Renal dysfunction is defined as acute renal insufficiency, Cr >1.5 mg/dL.

Source: Reproduced, with permission, from Schmidt M, Burrell A, Roberts L, et al. Predicting survival after ECMO for refractory cardiogenic shock: The survival after veno-arterial-ECMO (SAVE)-score. *Eur Heart J.* 2015;36(33):2246-2256. Copyright © 2015, Oxford University Press.[44]

Besides the physiologic considerations of the patient, there are other mechanical considerations to maintain the ECMO circuitry. For example, the circuit tubing, oxygenator, and pump must be visually inspected at minimum daily, but preferably every 8–12 hours, to ensure thrombosis

Table 13-5 VV ECMO SURVIVAL PREDICTION SCORE: RESP SCORE	
Parameter	Score
Age, yr	
18 to 49	0
50 to 59	−2
≥ 60	−3
Immunocompromised status[a]	−2
Mechanical ventilation prior to initiation of ECMO	
< 48 hours	3
48 hours to 7 days	1
> 7 days	0
Acute respiratory diagnosis group (select only one)	
Viral pneumonia	3
Bacterial pneumonia	3
Asthma	11
Trauma and burn	3
Aspiration pneumonitis	5
Other acute respiratory diagnosis	1
Non-respiratory or chronic respiratory diagnosis	0
Central nervous system dysfunction[b]	−7
Acute associated (nonpulmonary infection)	−3
Neuromuscular blockade agents before ECMO	1
Nitric oxide use before ECMO	−1
Bicarbonate infusion or IV bolus prior to ECMO	−2
Cardiac arrest before ECMO	−2
$PaCO_2$, mm Hg	
< 75	0

Table 13-5 VV ECMO SURVIVAL PREDICTION SCORE: RESP SCORE (*CONTINUED*)

Parameter	Score
≥ 75	–1
Peak inspiratory pressure, cm H_2O	
< 42	0
≥ 42	–1
Total Score	**–22 to 15**

Hospital Survival by Risk Class	Risk Class	Survival
≥ 6	I	92%
3 to 5	II	76%
–1 to 2	III	57%
–5 to –2	IV	33%
≤ –6	V	18%

Note: The RESP score can be calculated prior to placement of VV ECMO to assist in determining the patient's likelihood of survival based on co-morbidities and prior clinical course. An online calculator is available at www.respscore.com. It is not a substitute for clinical judgment and as the list of relative contraindications suggest, it is not comprehensive in considering all factors that may result in poor outcomes on VV ECMO.

[a]Immunocompromised is defined as hematological malignancies, solid tumor, solid organ transplantation, human immunodeficiency virus, and cirrhosis.

[b]Central nervous system dysfunction includes any patient with neurotrauma, stroke, encephalopathy, intracranial hemorrhage, or seizure.

Source: Adapted with permission of the American Thoracic Society. Copyright © 2021 American Thoracic Society. All rights reserved. Schmidt M, Bailey M, Sheldrake J, et al. Predicting survival after extracorporeal membrane oxygenation for severe acute respiratory failure. The Respiratory Extracorporeal Membrane Oxygenation Survival Prediction (RESP) score. *Am J Respir Crit Care Med*. 2014;189(11):1374-1382. The American Journal of Respiratory and Critical Care Medicine is an official journal of the American Thoracic Society. Readers are encouraged to read the entire article for the correct context at https://www.atsjournals.org/doi/full/10.1164/rccm.201311-2023OC. The authors, editors, and The American Thoracic Society are not responsible for errors or omissions in adaptations.[40]

is not developing (see Figure 13-5). Regular physical examination of the patient should be performed to ensure the cannulas are not bleeding or moving. Routine x-ray monitoring can be used to ensure the cannulas remain in good position.[5]

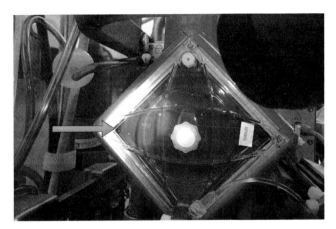

Figure 13-5 • VV ECMO Oxygenator Thrombosis. Arrow points to the thrombus seen at the corner of the oxygenator.

The console and blender allow clinicians to adjust the ECMO circuit according to the patient's physiologic needs. Instead of using a ventilator, hypoxemia can be treated using the ECMO circuit either by using the blender to increase the FiO_2 or by using the console to increase the rate of flow on the ECMO. Likewise, hypercarbia should be managed by using the blender to increase the ECMO fresh gas flow, also known as the sweep, instead of increasing ventilator parameters.[21] In difficult to manage cases, neuromuscular blockade can also be added to assist in reaching the physiologically acceptable goals as described in Table 13-6.[5]

VA ECMO Management Considerations

In VA ECMO cases, the goal is to minimize inotrope usage, while still maintaining enough cardiac contractility to ensure left ventricular emptying.[21] As mentioned previously, ideally, a Swan-Ganz catheter should be placed prior to VA ECMO cannulation. However, if ECMO was placed emergently, once the patient is stabilized, the Swan-Ganz catheter should be placed to assist in routine monitoring, to gauge hemodynamic changes, and to facilitate the weaning process. Assessing cardiac hemodynamics is also essential as VA ECMO displaces the blood from the venous circulation to the arterial circulation creating higher left ventricular afterload and decreasing both right and left ventricular preload.[48] The Swan-Ganz catheter should be used to determine whether or not the left ventricle is demonstrating evidence of pressure overload, requiring venting (if not already vented, see Table 13-1 and Figure 13-3) as well as to determine

Table 13-6 GENERAL MANAGEMENT PRINCIPLES[5,20,45,55]

Clinical Parameter Goals	Recommended Indications
Circuit flow	50–100 mL/kg/min
Mean arterial pressure	> 60 mm Hg
Patient weight	Attempt to achieve patient's dry weight
Anticoagulation	Activated partial thromboplasin time 1.2–1.8 times above normal
Hemoglobin	Normal, or 8–9 g/dL if SaO_2 > 85%
Platelets (in non-bleeding patients)	> 20×10^9/L
Platelets (for bleeding patients)	$50–100 \times 10^9$/L
D-dimer	Abrupt increases may signal impending oxygenator failure
Plasma-free hemoglobin	< 0.5–1.0 g/L
	If not at goal, consider re-evaluating anticoagulation, cannula position, pump speed, and long-term viability of pump.

VV ECMO SPECIAL CONSIDERATIONS[5,7,21]

SaO_2	≥ 80%
PaO_2	≥ 60%
$PaCO_2$	Within normal limits
Inspiratory pressure	< 25 cm H_2O
Plateau pressure	< 30 cm H_2O
Tidal volume	< 4 mL/kg ideal body weight
PEEP	10–18 cm H_2O
Respiratory rate	10–12 breaths/min

$PaCO_2$ = partial pressure of carbon dioxide; SaO_2 = oxygen saturation.

right-sided hemodynamics and assess whether or not biventricular failure is present, to assist in management and weaning plan.[27,49]

Maintaining adequate cerebral oxygenation in peripheral VA ECMO cannulation is a point of particular concern. Oxygenated blood from the

VA ECMO circuit meets the variably oxygenated blood flow from the heart somewhere in the aorta. Depending on the flow from each, cardiac versus ECMO, and the degree of oxygenation from the lungs, patients on VA ECMO can suffer from deoxygenated blood reaching the brain instead of the ECMO-circuit oxygenated blood. If undiagnosed, these patients develop cyanosis (hence, the name Harlequin syndrome), and, if untreated, they go on to develop negative cerebral outcomes.[20] Therefore, a *right* radial arterial cannulation is the preferred site for monitoring and ensuring adequate cerebral perfusion, as the right radial artery shares a blood supply most similar to the cerebral blood supply. Oximetry of the right upper extremity, either ear lobe, or central nervous system oxygenation monitoring systems are alternative and adjunctive forms of monitoring when arterial access is a challenge.[21]

VV ECMO Management Considerations

VV ECMO management is different, as lung-rest is the goal, not cardiac support. For VV ECMO cases, protecting the lungs is accomplished by minimizing any iatrogenic baro-, atelect-, or volu-trauma, through protective ventilatory settings.[21,50] Specifically, the FiO_2 on the ECMO should be turned up so that the FiO_2 on the ventilator can reach a goal of $\leq$ 60%.[30] If the ability to draw blood samples post-oxygenator has been provided for in the configuration of the circuit, the PO_2 should be $\geq$ 200 mm Hg. Mechanical ventilation settings should be set to ensure peak inspiratory pressure of $\leq$ 30 cm H_2O and arterial $PaO_2 \geq$ 60% or pulse oximetry readings of $\geq$ 80%.[7,30] Baro- and volu-trauma can be limited by reducing tidal volumes < 4 mL/kg of ideal body weight, decreasing peak inspiratory pressures 20–25 cm H_2O, and decreasing set respiratory rate.[51] Atelectrauma can be decreased by using a higher level of positive end-expiratory pressure (PEEP), such as 10–18 cm H_2O; however, studies conflict as to the mortality benefits or harm of PEEP levels.[7,30,52]

In a VV ECMO circuit with two cannulas, depending on the relative positioning of those cannulas, recirculation can occur in the setting of increasing the pump flow. This creates a shunt phenomenon, which paradoxically worsens hypoxia. Sampling blood oxygenation from both inflow and outflow cannulas can aid in making the diagnosis.[7] Given the fluctuations over time of native lung and cardiac function, juxtaposed with the different available cannulation configurations, understanding the meaning of changes in PaO_2 while on VV ECMO can be extremely complex. An excellent summary and series of case examples are provided in Bartlett's physiologic review of VV ECMO, which is useful for understanding these principles.[22]

▌ ECMO WEANING

VA ECMO Weaning

There are several indications of cardiac recovery including increasing blood pressure or lower levels of inotropes and vasopressors, increasing or return of pulsatility on arterial pressure waveform ($\geq$ 30 mm Hg), improving PaO_2 specifically, in a *right* radial arterial line.[20,21] Furthermore, it is advisable that the CVP $\leq$ 15 mm Hg indicating that the patient is adequately diuresed, and a pulmonary arterial pulsatility index (PAPi) of $\geq$ 1.5 to ensure adequate right ventricular recovery. Institutional guidelines vary considerably on the specifics of timing and amount, but the commonly accepted test for assessing native cardiac function is to decrease the ECMO flows in a step-wise fashion, so as not to create large hemodynamic variations for the newly recovering heart.[20] A measure of physiologic function should be assessed during this weaning procedure. This can be a visual assessment with echocardiogram or a calculation using the Fick equation and mixed venous saturation.[20] This weaning process is recommended to be performed in the setting of therapeutic anticoagulation, as the flows will need to be decreased to rates that are increasingly thrombogenic.[21,45] Figure 13-6 shows a suggested weaning algorithm.

VV ECMO Weaning

Signs of and conditions consistent with lung recovery in patients on VV ECMO include improvements in the chest x-ray (as demonstrated by clearing/decreased consolidations), improving white blood cell counts, weaning of vasopressors, decreased lactate, and net negative fluid balance.[7] The weaning of VV ECMO is not flow dependent; however, weaning down the flows can help ensure decreased hemodynamic disturbances once the ECMO is in fact removed.[7] Most importantly, the blender should be used to decrease the sweep fresh gas flow through the ECMO circuit to low levels, e.g., < 30% FiO2 and sweep of < 2 L/min.[5] Some centers perform what is known as a Cilley test, in which the FiO_2 on the ventilator is turned to 100% while the FiO_2 on ECMO is 21%; if the O_2 saturation goes to 100%, it is considered a positive test, and VV ECMO is considered weanable.[7] Alternatively, more commonly, the VV ECMO circuit can be weaned off if the patient can be adequately oxygenated and ventilated with moderate ventilator settings such as those listed below:[5,21,45]

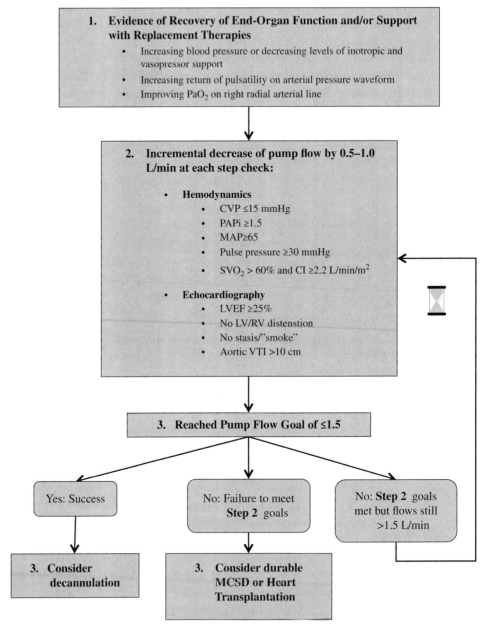

Figure 13-6 • VA ECMO Weaning Algorithm. This suggested weaning algorithm should only be attempted when signs of hemodynamic stability and cardiac recovery are evident. CI= cardiac index; FiO_2 = fraction of inspired oxygen; LV = left ventricle; LVEF = left ventricular ejection fraction; MAP = mean arterial pressure; MCSD = mechanical circulatory support device; PaO_2 = arterial partial pressure of oxygen; PAPi = pulmonary arterial pulsatility index; RV = right ventricle; SVO_2 = mixed venous oxygen saturation; VTI = velocity-time integral. (Used, with permission, from Keebler ME, Haddad EV, Choi CW, et al. Venoarterial extracorporeal membrane oxygenation in cardiogenic shock. *JACC Heart Fail.* 2018;6(6):503-516.)

- Tidal volume ~6 mL/kg ideal body weight
- Respiratory rate < 25 breaths/min
- FiO_2 < 0.6
- PEEP < 15 cm H_2O
- Plateau pressure < 30 cm H_2O

COMPLICATIONS

Complication rates of ECMO are monitored by international organizations, such as the Extracorporeal Life Support Organization (ELSO), which tracks cases and complications in participating ECMO centers.[36,53] The ELSO registry report from 2004 reports that for patients receiving ECMO for either cardiac or respiratory failure, the most common mechanical failures are as follows:[36]

- Oxygenator failure (16–18%)
- Cannula positioning problems (7–11%)
- Pump malfunction (2–4%)

On the patient-level, cumulative data from the ELSO registry, starting in 1988 and going through 2004, reported that in adults the most common complications were surgical site bleeding (22–32%), followed by cannula site bleeding (12–13%), and hemolysis (5–8%).[36] By contrast, data from a meta-analysis conducted with over 1,700 ECMO cases identified the three most frequent patient-level complications from the newer ECMO circuits as renal failure requiring renal replacement therapy (52%), bacterial pneumonia (33%), and bleeding (29%).[37]

Coagulopathy and Hemorrhagic Complications

Prior to the technological advances in circuitry components, thrombosis was one of the most common complications seen with ECMO.[5,54] For example, in a large review of hematologic complications in ESLO registry patients from 1986 to 2013, Murphy and colleagues found high rates of oxygenator clots, systemic thrombosis, and cannula site bleeding.[5] The pathophysiology of increased thrombosis in ECMO is thought to be secondary to blood-device interactions, namely blood interacting with non-endothelial surfaces causing an inflammatory and prothombotic response, specifically, thrombin generation leading to clot formation both in the ECMO circuit and in the patient's microcirculation.[7,55] Therefore, in spite of the improvements in circuitry, ECMO still poses a thrombotic risk, so anticoagulation of patients on an ECMO circuit is advised.[5] There are ways to minimize the thrombotic risk above anticoagulation alone and risk factors to avoid when possible:[55]

- Immediate post-operative state
- Open surgical field with air-blood interface
- Complex ECMO circuitry, e.g.:
  - high circuit tubing volumes and therefore, high non-endothelial surface areas
  - high number of connection sites (creates turbulent flow)

Conversely, another facet of the same immunological inflammatory response is that ECMO can also result in the consumption and dilution of clotting factors, and therefore, bleeding is also a common complication in patients with these large bore cannulas.[21] Commonly, these consumptive processes can lead to platelet dysfunction, thrombocytopenia, disseminated intravascular coagulation, hyperfibinolysis, or acquired von Willebrand syndrome due to high shear stress.[1,55] The rate of bleeding on ECMO is estimated to be somewhere between 10 and 35%, but remains difficult to measure due to differing definitions among studies.[37,56] Data from a systemic review by Auborn and colleagues suggests that it is specifically patients with elevated activated partial thromboplastin times who were more likely to bleed while on ECMO. This finding suggests that some significant proportion of bleeding events while on ECMO may actually be iatrogenic. Further confirmatory studies are required, but it does suggest that some proportion of bleeding events may be preventable through careful monitoring and administration of anticoagulation.[56] Hemolysis is a less common cause of dropping hemoglobin in ECMO patients. Monitoring routine plasma-free hemoglobin levels ($> 10\%$ = concerning) assists in making the diagnosis, indicating that the circuit configuration requires repair. The most common sites of bleeding are surgical site bleeding (19%), cannula site bleeding (17%), pulmonary hemorrhage (8%), gastrointestinal hemorrhage (5%), and intracranial hemorrhage (4%).[57]

Renal Complications

Patients requiring ECMO frequently have their course complicated by acute kidney injury (AKI) necessitating renal replacement therapy (RRT). Ultrafiltration can be directly spliced into the ECMO circuit, via an in-line hemofilter or by incorporating a continuous renal replacement machine into the ECMO circuit.[58] The potential advantages of these types of in-line configurations are decreasing the number of patient vascular access sites, which is theorized to decrease the incidence of competing blood flow, maintain venous access sites for other uses, and decrease the number of infectious, thrombotic and bleeding complications associated with temporary hemodialysis catheters.[20,55] However, it is important to note, that these in-line connections increase the complexity of the circuit, which poses a theoretical thrombotic risk in and of itself.[55,58] The incidence of AKI requires RRT ranges from about 50–60% in adult ECMO cases.[37,38] While in-hospital survival is similar to patients who do not require RRT while on ECMO, 3-month survival appears to be worse for patients who do require RRT.[38] Perhaps due to this increased long-term mortality, studies have found that patients who start RRT while on ECMO are unlikely to go on to develop long-standing end-stage renal disease, requiring life-long hemodialysis.[58]

Neurological Complications

A broad range of neurologic complications have been reported with ECMO including acute ischemic stroke (5%), intracranial hemorrhage (2–4%), seizures (1–2%), subclinical cognitive impairment, and peripheral neuropathy.[20,39,59,60] The incidence of some of these complications have not been well-studied or reported, making it difficult to assess their frequency. Of all of the bleeding complications seen with ECMO, intracranial hemorrhage (ICH) remains a rare, but important, complication. ICH carries an elevated relative risk of mortality of 1.19–4.43 when compared to non-ICH ECMO patients,[59,60] as well as significantly increased length of stay and higher rates of discharge to a long-term care facility.[59]

Infectious Complications

Based on data from the ELSO registry, of the over 2,000 adult patients studied, secondary infections while on ECMO occur in about 21% of cases,[61] which is lower than the 33% reported in recent metanalysis.[37] In adults, *Candida species*, *Pseudomonas aeruginosa*, and *Staphylococcus aureus* are the most common causative agents.[61] Treatment of infections should follow normal protocols based on available culture data and known hospital biome and bacterial and fungal resistance patterns.[7] However, detection of infection can sometimes be more challenging if temperature regulation is being employed; other clinical signs of infection such as chest x-rays and white blood cell counts have to be relied on more heavily in the context of ECMO. Current data suggests that secondary infections while on ECMO are correlated with increased duration of ECMO support required as well as increased mortality.[61]

Circuit-Specific Complications

Local peripheral cannulation site complications most commonly include leg ischemia, which remains a preventable complication (10–30%).[20,23,37]

This complication is easily preventable with ultrasound-guided cannula placement to ensure proper sizing along with the addition of limb-perfusion catheter if a larger than ideal cannula is clinically deemed necessary to ensure sufficient perfusion or drainage by the cannulas.[23] Other circuit-component-specific complications are also seen with ECMO, such as systemic gas embolism, dislodgement of ECMO cannulas resulting in hemorrhage, upper body hypoxia due to inadequate retrograde oxygenation (more common in VA ECMO), pump failure, and oxygenator failure requiring replacement.[48] Coupled with daily visual inspection, daily d-dimer levels can be helpful to monitor over time as a sharp increase in d-dimer without other clinical reason can signal an impending oxygenator failure.[55] Unlike oxygenator thrombosis and failure, pump failure cannot be determined by visual inspection; instead, clinicians should listen for a noisy pump or look for signs of intravascular hemolysis and/or hemoglobinuria.[55]

Drug Removal

In vitro studies have demonstrated that the polyvinylchloride (PVC) tubing used in ECMO circuitry seems to be responsible for a significant proportion of drug adsorption. Likely lipophilic medications, such as antimicrobials and sedative agents, are most susceptible to this phenomenon, regardless of priming fluid used.[20,62-64] Based on further in vitro investigations, it appears that the new surface modified coatings used in the newer circuits are, in part, contributing to the drug adsorption phenomenon.[65] This makes monitoring drug levels, particularly for anti-infective agents, crucial to ensuring effective dosing.[20]

▌ CRISIS STANDARD OF CARE: SPECIAL CONSIDERATIONS

There are certain indications for ECMO that are more likely to arise in wartime situations, natural disasters, terrorist attacks, or other times of crises such as global pandemic infections.[66] What follows is a more in-depth discussion of each of the scenarios and indications for ECMO, which warrant further consideration.

ECPR

As mentioned previously, ECMO is being increasingly used for ECPR, despite poor outcomes.[61] One extremely helpful tool during a cardiac arrest, if available, is to obtain a point-of-care echocardiogram, which will allow the clinician to rule out both pulmonary embolism and cardiac tamponade as treatable, reversible causes of the arrest.[23] The correct timing of initiation of ECMO to perform ECPR remains debated and under study. There exists a tension between waiting too long to initiate ECMO and loose valuable perfusion time versus initiating a treatment that carries risk and is ultimately unnecessary if the patient would have developed return of spontaneous circulation (ROSC) on their own.[23] Another distinction, which is particularly relevant for fieldwork (outside of a hospital setting) and (in-hospital) crisis situations, is the distinction between witnessed in-hospital arrests and out-of-hospital arrests.

However, it is important to note, whereas ECMO is generally used as a salvage therapy with patients who are unlikely to survive, ECPR still represents the least likely to survive group even among ECMO patients. Furthermore, just like ECMO for other indications, but to an even greater extent, ECPR requires a team approach to CPR and a complicated on-call system to ensure that trained clinicians are available at any time.[67] In fact, the ECPR studies on ECMO often note that the time of day of in-hospital cardiac arrests is heavily weighted toward the evenings. As such, on-call staff and supplies have to be ready for use at any moment.[67–69]

ECPR Initiation Criteria

One option, if available, is to use end-tidal $CO_2 < 10$ mm Hg after 20 minutes of CPR. Others have suggested using a time cutoff, for example, after $\geq$ 10–30 minutes of conventional CPR without ROSC should prompt ECMO in eligible cases.[70–73] One of the challenges of a time-based criteria is that even for institutions in which 10 minutes is the criteria, cannulation is not instantaneous upon determining candidacy and actual cannulations at those institutions can still take up to 60 minutes of CPR to accomplish.[72] However, if after 60 minutes of conventional CPR, ECMO cannulation is attempted, survival rates are reported to be very low.[72] An alternative criterion for initiation of ECPR is cardiac standstill found on a sub-xyphoid window with point-of-care ultrasound during CPR pulse checks. Cardiac standstill for >10 minutes is 90% sensitive and 100% specific for non-ROSC. Therefore, some have alternatively proposed using the finding of cardiac standstill after two cycles of CPR, then ECMO can be considered assuming no contraindications to ECMO are present (Table 13-3), and the underlying causes of the arrest are thought to be reversible.[23]

In-Hospital Arrests

An important question is neurologic status post-ECPR with some centers reporting the Glasgow-Pittsburgh Cerebral Performance (CPC) categories 1–2 (good neurologic function) in all or almost all survivors,[70,72,74,75] and other centers reporting low (e.g., 28%) rates of good neurologic function.[71] Consistently, patients who received ECPR, a cardiac cause of cardiac arrest, are reported to have higher survival rates.[71,74] In-hospital survival rates from ECPR range from 30–50%.[71,72,74–76] While randomized trials have not been conducted in this area, propensity-score and matching studies have been conducted finding ECPR to have lower mortality rates than conventional CPR,[71,76] and a higher percentage of favorable neurological outcomes.[76] However, not all propensity matched studies have found a survival benefit, which has left the implementation of ECPR extremely variable among institutions, particularly because it is an extremely resource-intensive program to implement.[73]

Out-of-Hospital Arrests

Out-of-hospital arrests are a more heterogeneous entity and difficult to study systematically. Interestingly, one study conducted in Japan suggests that for these un-witnessed arrests, sometimes with unknown downtime, increased pupillary diameter even by 1 mm on arrival to the emergency department may be predictive of poor neurological outcomes if ECPR is indicated.[77] Therefore, ideally, patients who suffer out-of-hospital cardiac arrests may be eligible for ECPR if:[67,69,77]

- no contraindications to ECMO (Table 13-3)
- witnessed cardiac arrest
- conventional CPR was initiated within the first 5–15 minutes of the arrest
- pupils are equal and reactive and not dilated

One study from Paris, France, details the launching of a mobile ECPR program for a trained team of intensivists or emergency medicine physicians and nurses to arrive to the site of the arrest within 10 minutes of arrest and cannulated eligible patients in the field to decrease low blood flow states and poor perfusion during patient transport to the hospital.[67] ECPR for out of hospital arrests appears to improve survival compared to matched controls when exclusion criteria are applied, but data conflicts as to whether or not ECPR improves the percentage of patients who have a good CPC score on discharge.[77,78] If no strict exclusion criteria to the out-of-hospital ECPR are applied, then there is no difference in mortality in matched controls, which suggests the importance of patient selection to determine eligibility for ECPR.[79] ECPR for out-of-hospital cardiac arrests is reported to be around 15–40%.[68,69,77]

Traumas, Drowning, and Burns

Trauma and burn patients are known to develop a severe inflammatory response, which can affect the lungs. In those cases, VV ECMO has been employed to support patients through their respiratory illness.[2] The survival data in this patient population is mixed. It appears that because trauma victims tend to be younger than other adult patients who develop infectious causes of respiratory failure, those patients may do better.[80] However, trauma patients who do receive ECMO appear to have higher survival rates than historical controls even if those survival rates may sometimes be lower than that of patients receiving VV ECMO for other indications.[81,82] One study has suggested that in the trauma population, as with VV ECMO more generally, early cannulation, defined in this case as within 5 days of mechanical ventilation, has improved outcomes.[82] Based on survey data of trauma surgeons, use of ECMO in trauma patients remains limited in part secondary to availability of ECMO as well as clinicians' disinclination to utilize it as a tool for organ support.[83]

Victims of drowning are often hypothermic and can suffer from respiratory failure and cardiac arrest, and VA ECMO has been trialed in these cases. While individual case reports have touted successes,[84] a case series out of France suggests that in adults, these cases have poor outcomes.[85]

2009 H1N1 Influenza Pandemic

Since 2009 when the H1N1 influenza epidemic spread around the world, the viral pneumonia and subsequent ARDS that took hold in some patients was sometimes treated with VV ECMO. In fact, there is some evidence that new ECMO centers were established because of and during this pandemic, some of which are still not part of the ELSO registry.[86] A series of studies was published looking at the efficacy of VV ECMO in improving survival rates in this disease. The highest level of evidence was a randomized control trial called the CESAR trial; however, unfortunately, the way the randomization was performed, the trial ended up being a study measuring the effects of transfer to an ECMO-capable center. It was found that there is, in fact, a mortality benefit to being treated at ECMO-capable tertiary or quaternary care centers.[18] In response to these criticisms of the CESAR trial, some of the same researchers used UK registry data to track patients who referred for ECMO to tertiary care hospitals but did not receive ECMO and found that those patients who did not receive ECMO had similar mortality rates to those patients who were not referred for ECMO.[87] Therefore, the question of whether or not ECMO has a mortality benefit in H1N1 has been relegated to propensity matching and case-control studies. A metanalysis by Zangrillo and colleagues concluded that VV ECMO for H1N1 influenza does, in fact, reduce mortality compared to mechanical ventilation alone to about 28%.[88] These findings suggest that VV ECMO in influenza has a better prognosis than VV ECMO for all comers. Controlled studies published since then or not included in the metanalysis have demonstrated similar findings, or have demonstrated that the ECMO cohort was consistently sicker than the non-ECMO cohort, while having a similar mortality rate.[89–91] However, given the lack of randomized evidence, the debate continues to rage on in the critical care community as to the efficacy of ECMO in viral pneumonias and ARDS more generally.[92,93]

Other Infections

A small case series has been published about avian influenza A (H7N9), which noted there were some successful cases, but had no control group for comparison. In the case of the coronarviurs (MERS-CoV) causing Middle East respiratory syndrome (MERS), 17 patients received ECMO while 18 controls did not, and it was found that the ECMO patients had a higher survival rate. However, with such small numbers and no corroborating studies, conclusions are difficult to draw.[94]

SARS-CoV-2 Pandemic

Unfortunately, the novel coronavirus (SARS-CoV-2) causing coronavirus disease 2019 (COVID-19) has engendered a global pandemic infecting patients in countries all over the world and creating in its wake no shortage of cases of severe respiratory illness, and all too often, death. At the time of this writing, limited large-scale trials are available, but will likely be forthcoming. Early in the pandemic, the virus was contained in China and other Far Eastern countries. Metanalyses from these countries early in our collective global experience with the disease suggested that ECMO was not helpful and had a higher than usual mortality rate in COVID-19 when compared with other viral pneumonias.[95,96] A few months later, two case series from Europe and the United States, with 32 patients and 11 patients, respectively, showed promising outcomes with ECMO but were published so early as to have not enough follow up time to be conclusive regarding mortality rates of the use VV ECMO in COVID-19.[97,98] More recently, another two cases series, both from single centers in the United States, show very promising outcomes with ECMO in COVID-19 (close to 100% survival).[99,100] However, these findings are not consistent with ELSO's current reporting of outcomes with COVID-19, which is reporting about ~50% of patients surviving to hospital discharge.[45] Therefore, the question remains open, pending further data as the efficacy of VV ECMO for the viral pandemic caused by SARS-CoV-2.

ETHICAL AND RESOURCE CONSIDERATIONS WITH ECMO

Capacity Overload and Resource Allocation Strategies

Recent pandemics in the last two decades have called into question the allocation strategy of first-come-first serve that is typically applied during normal medical resource allocation (i.e., in the absence of expected shortages).[32,66] There are ethical models beyond the scope of this chapter, which can be applied to come up with resource allocation strategies.[66] However, resource allocation planning is essential particularly because many countries operate their hospitals already at extremely high capacities, which means meeting the resource needs of seasonal surges like influenza or epidemic surges like COVID-19 extremely challenging.[66] Specifically, mistakenly using a limited resource like ECMO early in a pandemic on poor candidates can put considerable strain on a health care system, especially given that patients usually have a longer hospital course when ECMO is employed, and withdrawal of care can be legally challenging.[101] Instead, clinicians should discuss *a priori* the possibility of limiting ECMO support to those with better expected outcomes and shorter ECMO runs.[102] This is especially important for ECMO, as in the same way that ECMO provides organ rest and support, it can also prolong the inevitable process of dying, if clinicians do not apply its use wisely.

Expert opinions have suggested that prior to a pandemic or crisis situation, ECMO teams should prepare in advance as much as possible. Table 13-7 shows some preparatory steps that have been recommended to ensure the medical team is ready to meet the needs and challenges of resource strains associated with providing ECMO in a crisis situation.[86] There are three general categories of preparation: physical plan, staffing, and ethical considerations. Often overlooked is the importance of a quality assurance or research team dedicated to ensuring that there is institutional accountability and learning on the part of the whole team from the crisis.[32,66]

Withdrawal of Care

Researchers and clinicians continue to debate the ethics of ECMO. Particularly, a significant areas of debate asks: Should there be an arbitrary or specific time limit on the duration that a patient may be allowed to receive ECMO support?[5,103] In practice, most institutions give patients on

Table 13-7 PREPARING TO PROVIDE ECMO IN A CRISIS SITUATION[32,86,102,106]	
Action Item	**Description**
Establish a chain of command	In addition, consider creating clinical processes and guidelines for dealing with a high-demand of ECMO utilization
Inventory management plan	Make a careful inventory of: • supplies available • supplies that are missing/need to be stocked up on Decide who will be managing and keeping track of inventory during the crisis, reordering needed supplies, etc.
Resource management plan	• Predict the average length of ECMO utilization per patient to determine the number of patients that can be served at any given time or over a given time period; this gives realistic institutional expectations of the capacitance of the ECMO team. • Consider the systemic situations in which ECMO use might not be employed in order to save all available resources for less-resource/personnel-intensive strategies. • Consider preferential ECMO support to those patients who are most likely to have historically better outcomes and shorter expected ECMO support.
Tiered ECMO selection criteria	Consider tiered indications for ECMO based on definitions of the current capacity limitations of the system. • Develop institutional definitions for: • conventional capacity • saturated capacity or extended capacity (beyond the normal number of beds) • overwhelmed capacity • Selective indication criteria during times when capacitance is stretched thin, but not saturated or overwhelmed • Restrictive indication criteria during system saturation • ECMO no longer offered if system is overwhelmed and circuits or staff are unavailable, possible triage or referral system to other hospitals in selected cases

Table 13-7 PREPARING TO PROVIDE ECMO IN A CRISIS SITUATION[32,86,102,106] (CONTINUED)

Action Item	Description
Create teams	Consider creating teams with different areas of expertise, consider carefully how many teams you will need of each kind to fill the expected needs, and if relevant the expected staff attrition incurred by the crisis: • insertion teams: physician(s), ± physician extenders, nurses, and perfusionists • management teams: physician(s), ± physician extenders, nurses, nursing aids, and ECMO specialist or perfusionist(s) • specialist teams: physicians who can be content-area specialists in areas of common complications with ECMO, such as infectious disease, renal, hematological, and palliative care specialists • ethics team: consideration to be given to how to allocate resources, particularly in terms of initiating ECMO in questionable cases and also, importantly, if circuits are limited and patients are not faring well on ECMO • quality assurance team: review outcomes in real time to provide feedback to clinical teams as well as provide research support, if applicable
Simulation drills	Time allowing
Infection control measures	If preparing for an infectious disease epidemic, develop infection control guidelines specific for ECMO patients, as relevant.
Other staff safety measures	Any other relevant considerations, such as teams being deployed into war zones, will need to take significantly greater staff safety considerations into account.
Outside hospital transport	• Determine if your crisis response will be limited to in-hospital patients or those coming from other facilities. • Determine also if you will have a mobile insertion team, other than the one located on-site. • Consider creating a network of hospitals to which you can safely transfer ECMO patients to if your hospital becomes overwhelmed. • Create logistical processes for transfer (i.e., is the receiving or transferring team to travel with the patient)

ECMO about 2–3 weeks on circuit before considerations of withdrawal are discussed, unless the patient's survivability comes into question before that time.[5] Case reports demonstrate patients have survived ECMO even after longer runs; however, the rarity and practicality of that phenomenon seem to suggest that extremely long ECMO runs are impractical and perhaps prolonging death instead of prolonging life, given the poor quality of life for many on this level of hemodynamic and respiratory support.[7] Withdrawal of care should be considered on a case-by-case basis by the medical team. If efforts are considered futile, a high likelihood of poor quality of survival is evident, or there is progressive multisystem organ failure despite maximal medical therapies then goals of care discussions should be initiated with family.[32] Regardless of crisis circumstances or routine medical care, every effort should be made to include the families, and when possible, the patients in these difficult decisions. Understandably, shared decision making remains much more challenging to accomplish in crisis and pandemic situations.[86]

▌ CONCLUSION

ECMO is a versatile MCS device that can be employed as a rescue strategy in the setting of an emergent, life-threatening pulmonary or cardiac failure. ECMO remains resource intensive and expensive with frequent common complications. ECMO requires a specialized treatment team focused on implementing sound management practices to promote good patient outcomes and ensure patient safety. ECMO is feasible to perform in the field and in crisis situations, but requires a specialized, highly trained team to do so, and an extraction and hospital transfer plan to be used effectively. Since ECMO is supportive care awaiting organ recovery, clinicians should be prepared for the drawback of longer, more costly hospital courses, with the potential advantage of improved clinical outcomes in carefully selected patients.

▌ REFERENCES

1. Makdisi G, Wang I. Extra Corporeal Membrane Oxygenation (ECMO) review of a lifesaving technology. *J Thorac Dis.* 2015;7(7):E166-E176.
2. Hill DJ, O'Brien TG, Murray JJ, et al. Prolonged extracorporeal oxygenation for acute post-traumatic respiratory failure (shock-lung syndrome). *N Engl J Med.* 1972;286(12):629-634.
3. Patel SM, Lipinski J, Al-Kindi SG, et al. Simultaneous venoarterial extracorporeal membrane oxygenation and percutaneous left ventricular decompression

therapy with impella is associated with improved outcomes in refractory cardiogenic shock. *ASAIO J.* 2019;65(1):21-28.

4. Sayer GT, Baker JN, Parks KA. Heart rescue: The role of mechanical circulatory support in the management of severe refractory cardiogenic shock. *Curr Opin Crit Care.* 2012;18(5):409-416.

5. MacLaren G, Combes A, Bartlett RH. Contemporary extracorporeal membrane oxygenation for adult respiratory failure: Life support in the new era. *Intensive Care Med.* 2012;38:210-220.

6. Peek GJ, Killer HM, Reeves R, Sosnowski AW, Firmin RK. Early experience with a polymethyl pentene oxygenator for adult extracorporeal life support. *ASAIO J.* 2002;48(5):480-482.

7. Sen A, Callisen HE, Alwardt CM, et al. Adult venovenous extracorporeal membrane oxygenation for severe respiratory failure: Current status and future perspectives. *Ann Card Anaesth.* 2016;19(1):97-111.

8. Khoshbin E, Roberts N, Harvey C, et al. Poly-methyl pentene oxygenators have improved gas exchange capability and reduced transfusion requirements in adult extracorporeal membrane oxygenation. *ASAIO J.* 2005;51(3):281-287.

9. Videm V, Svennevig JL, Fosse E, et al. Reduced complement activation with heparin-coated oxygenator and tubings in coronary bypass operations. *J Thorac Cardiovasc Surg.* 1992;103(4):806-813.

10. Langer T, Santini A, Bottino N, et al. "Awake" extracorporeal membrane oxygenation (ECMO): Pathophysiology, technical considerations, and clinical pioneering. *Crit Care.* 2016;20(1):1-10.

11. Langer T, Vecchi V, Belenkiy SM, et al. Extracorporeal gas exchange and spontaneous breathing for the treatment of acute respiratory distress syndrome: An alternative to mechanical ventilation? *Crit Care Med.* 2014;42(3):211-220.

12. Schechter MA, Ganapathi AM, Englum BR, et al. Spontaneously breathing extracorporeal membrane oxygenation support provides the optimal bridge to lung transplantation. *Transplantation.* 2016;100(12):2699-2704.

13. Abrams D, Javidfar J, Farrand E, et al. Early mobilization of patients receiving extracorporeal membrane oxygenation: A retrospective cohort study. *Crit Care.* 2014;18(1):1-9.

14. Sauer CM, Yuh DD, Bonde P. Extracorporeal membrane oxygenation use has increased by 433% in adults in the United States from 2006 to 2011. *ASAIO J.* 2015;61(1):31-36.

15. Nehra D, Goldstein AM, Doody DP, Ryan DP, Chang Y, Masiakos PT. Extracorporeal membrane oxygenation for nonneonatal acute respiratory failure: The Massachusetts General Hospital Experience from 1990 to 2008. *Arch Surg.* 2009;144(5):427-432.

16. Karagiannidis C, Brodie D, Strassmann S, et al. Extracorporeal membrane oxygenation: Evolving epidemiology and mortality. *Intensive Care Med.* 2016;42(5):889-896.

17. Morris AH, Wallace CJ, Menlovet RL, et al. Randomized clinical trial of pressure-controlled inverse ratio ventilation and extracorporeal CO2 removal for adult respiratory distress syndrome. *Am J Respir Crit Care Med.* 1994;149:295-305.

18. Peek GJ, Mugford M, Tiruvoipati R, et al. Efficacy and economic assessment of conventional ventilatory support versus extracorporeal membrane oxygenation for severe adult respiratory failure (CESAR): A multicentre randomised controlled trial. *Lancet.* 2009;374(9698):1351-1363.

19. Combes A, Hajage D, Capellier G, et al. Extracorporeal membrane oxygenation for severe acute respiratory distress syndrome. *N Engl J Med.* 2018;378(21):1965-1975.

20. Keebler ME, Haddad EV, Choi CW, et al. Venoarterial extracorporeal membrane oxygenation in cardiogenic shock. *JACC Heart Fail.* 2018;6(6):503-516.

21. Marasco SF, Lukas G, McDonald M, McMillan J, Ihle B. Review of ECMO (extra corporeal membrane oxygenation) support in critically ill adult patients. *Heart Lung Circ.* 2008;17S:S41-S47.

22. Bartlett RH. Physiology of gas exchange during ECMO for respiratory failure. *J Intensive Care Med.* 2017;32(4):243-248.

23. Zhang Z. Echocardiography for patients undergoing extracorporeal cardiopulmonary resuscitation: A primer for intensive care physicians. *J Intensive Care.* 2017;5(1):1-9.

24. Wang D, Zhou X, Liu X, Sidor B, Lynch J, Zwischenberger JB. Wang-Zwische double lumen cannula—toward a percutaneous and ambulatory paracorporeal artificial lung. *ASAIO J.* 2008;54(6):606-611.

25. Annamalai SK, Buiten L, Esposito ML, et al. Acute hemodynamic effects of intra-aortic balloon counterpulsation pumps in advanced heart failure. *J Card Fail.* 2017;23(8):606-614.

26. Brasseur A, Scolletta S, Lorusso R, Taccone FS. Hybrid extracorporeal membrane oxygenation. *J Thorac Dis.* 2018;10(4):S707-S715.

27. Cove ME, MacLaren G. Clinical review: Mechanical circulatory support for cardiogenic shock complicating acute myocardial infarction. *Crit Care.* 2010;14(5):235.

28. Basir MB, Schreiber T, Dixon S, et al. Feasibility of early mechanical circulatory support in acute myocardial infarction complicated by cardiogenic shock: The Detroit cardiogenic shock initiative. *Catheter Cardiovasc Interv.* 2018;91(3):454-461.

29. Zhang Z, Gu WJ, Chen K, Ni H. Mechanical ventilation during extracorporeal membrane oxygenation in patients with acute severe respiratory failure. *Can Respir J.* 2017;2017:1783857.

30. Wu MY, Huang CC, Wu TI, Wang CL, Lin PJ. Venovenous extracorporeal membrane oxygenation for acute respiratory distress syndrome in adults prognostic factors for outcomes. *Med (United States).* 2016;95(8):1-9.

31. Zochios V, Brodie D, Charlesworth M, Parhar KK. Delivering extracorporeal membrane oxygenation for patients with COVID-19: What, who, when and how? *Anaesthesia.* 2020;75(8):997-1001.

32. Shekar K, Badulak J, Peek G, et al. Extracorporeal Life Support Organization (ELSO) coronavirus disease 2019 interim guidelines: A consensus document from an international group of interdisciplinary extracorporeal membrane oxygenation providers. *ASAIO J.* 2020;66(7):707-721.

33. Grasso S, Terragni P, Birocco A, et al. ECMO criteria for influenza A (H1N1)-associated ARDS: Role of transpulmonary pressure. *Intensive Care Med.* 2012;38(3):395-403.

34. Zochios V, Brodie D, Parhar KK. Towards precision delivery of ECMO in COVID-19 cardiorespiratory failure. *ASAIO J.* 2020;66(7):731-733.

35. Patroniti N, Zangrillo A, Pappalardo F, et al. The Italian ECMO network experience during the 2009 influenza A(H1N1) pandemic: Preparation for severe respiratory emergency outbreaks. *Intensive Care Med.* 2011;37(9):1447-1457.

36. Conrad SA, Rycus PT, Dalton H. Extracorporeal life support registry report 2004. *ASAIO J.* 2005;51(1):4-10.

37. Zangrillo A, Landoni G, Biondi-Zoccai G, et al. A meta-analysis of complications and mortality of extracorporeal membrane oxygenation. *Crit Care Resusc.* 2013;15(3):172-178.

38. Kielstein JT, Heiden AM, Beutel G, et al. Renal function and survival in 200 patients undergoing ECMO therapy. *Nephrol Dial Transplant.* 2013;28(1):86-90.

39. Mehta A, Ibsen LM. Neurologic complications and neurodevelopmental outcome with extracorporeal life support. *World J Crit Care Med.* 2013;2(4):40.

40. Schmidt M, Bailey M, Sheldrake J, et al. Predicting survival after extracorporeal membrane oxygenation for severe acute respiratory failure: The Respiratory Extracorporeal Membrane Oxygenation Survival Prediction (RESP) score. *Am J Respir Crit Care Med.* 2014;189(11):1374-1382.

41. Kanji HD, McCallum J, Norena M, et al. Early veno-venous extracorporeal membrane oxygenation is associated with lower mortality in patients who have severe hypoxemic respiratory failure: A retrospective multicenter cohort study. *J Crit Care.* 2016;33(2016):169-173.

42. Cheng R, Hachamovitch R, Kittleson M, et al. Clinical outcomes in fulminant myocarditis requiring extracorporeal membrane oxygenation: A weighted meta-analysis of 170 patients. *J Card Fail.* 2014;20(6):400-406.

43. Biancari F, Dalén M, Perrotti A, et al. Venoarterial extracorporeal membrane oxygenation after coronary artery bypass grafting: Results of a multicenter study. *Int J Cardiol.* 2017;241:109-114.

44. Schmidt M, Burrell A, Roberts L, et al. Predicting survival after ECMO for refractory cardiogenic shock: The survival after veno-arterial-ECMO (SAVE)-score. *Eur Heart J.* 2015;36(33):2246-2256.

45. Extracorporeal Life Support Organization (ELSO) Guidelines. https://www.elso.org/Resources/Guidelines.aspx. Accessed June 16, 2020.

46. Dalia AA, Ortoleva J, Fiedler A, Villavicencio M, Shelton K, Cudemus GD. Extracorporeal membrane oxygenation is a team sport: Institutional survival benefits of a formalized ECMO team. *J Cardiothorac Vasc Anesth.* 2019;33(4):902-907.

47. Tehrani BN, Truesdell AG, Sherwood MW, et al. Standardized team-based care for cardiogenic shock. *J Am Coll Cardiol.* 2019;73(13):1659-1669.

48. Kapur NK, Jumean MF. Defining the role for percutaneous mechanical circulatory support devices for medically refractory heart failure. *Curr Heart Fail Rep.* 2013;10(2):177-184.

49. Esposito M, Bader Y, Pedicini R, Breton C, Mullin A, Kapur NK. The role of acute circulatory support in ST-segment elevation myocardial infarction complicated by cardiogenic shock. *Indian Heart J*. 2017;69:668-674.

50. Schmidt M, Stewart C, Bailey M, et al. Mechanical ventilation management during extracorporeal membrane oxygenation for acute respiratory distress syndrome: A retrospective international multicenter study. *Crit Care Med*. 2015;43(3):654-664.

51. Ranieri VM, Terragni PP, Del Sorbo L, et al. Tidal volume lower than 6 ml/kg enhances lung protection: Role of extracorporeal carbon dioxide removal. *Anesthesiology*. 2009;111(4):826-835.

52. Modrykamien AM, Hernandez OO, Im Y, et al. Mechanical ventilation in patients with the acute respiratory distress syndrome and treated with extracorporeal membrane oxygenation: Impact on hospital and 30 day postdischarge survival. *ASAIO J*. 2016;62(5):607-612.

53. Bartlett RH. Extracorporeal Life Support Registry Report 1995. *ASAIO J*. 1997;43(1):104-107.

54. Thomas J, Kostousov V, Teruya J. Bleeding and thrombotic complications in the use of extracorporeal membrane oxygenation. *Semin Thromb Hemost*. 2018;44(1):20-29.

55. Murphy DA, Hockings LE, Andrews RK, et al. Extracorporeal membrane oxygenation-hemostatic complications. *Transfus Med Rev*. 2015;29(2):90-101.

56. Aubron C, DePuydt J, Belon F, et al. Predictive factors of bleeding events in adults undergoing extracorporeal membrane oxygenation. *Ann Intensive Care*. 2016;6(1).

57. Brodie D, Bacchetta M. Extracorporeal membrane oxygenation for ARDS in adults. *N Engl J Med*. 2011;365(20):1905-1914.

58. Askenazi DJ, Selewski DT, Paden ML, et al. Renal replacement therapy in critically ill patients receiving extracorporeal membrane oxygenation. *Clin J Am Soc Nephrol*. 2012;7(8):1328-1336.

59. Nasr DM, Rabinstein AA. Neurologic complications of extracorporeal membrane oxygenation. *J Clin Neurol*. 2015;11(4):383-389.

60. Fletcher-Sandersjöö A, Thelin EP, Bartek J, et al. Incidence, outcome, and predictors of intracranial hemorrhage in adult patients on extracorporeal membrane oxygenation: A systematic and narrative review. *Front Neurol*. 2018;9(JUL):1-10.

61. Bizzarro MJ, Conrad SA, Kaufman DA, Rycus P. Infections acquired during extracorporeal membrane oxygenation in neonates, children, and adults. *Pediatr Crit Care Med*. 2011;12(3):277-281.

62. Preston TJ, Hodge AB, Riley JB, Leib-Sargel C, Nicol KK. In vitro drug adsorption and plasma free hemoglobin levels associated with hollow fiber oxygenators in the extracorporeal life support (ECLS) circuit. *J Extra Corpor Technol*. 2007;39(4):234-237.

63. Mehta NM, Halwick DR, Dodson BL, Thompson JE, Arnold JH. Potential drug sequestration during extracorporeal membrane oxygenation: Results from an ex vivo experiment. *Intensive Care Med*. 2007;33(6):1018-1024.

64. Shekar K, Fraser JF, Smith MT, Roberts JA. Pharmacokinetic changes in patients receiving extracorporeal membrane oxygenation. *J Crit Care*. 2012;27(6):741.e9-741.e18.

65. Preston TJ, Ratliff TM, Gomez D, et al. Modified surface coatings and their effect on drug adsorption within the extracorporeal life support circuit. *J Extra Corpor Technol*. 2010;42(3):199-202.

66. DeLaney E, Smith MJ, Harvey BT, et al. Extracorporeal life support for pandemic influenza: The role of extracorporeal membrane oxygenation in pandemic management. *J Extra Corpor Technol*. 2010;42(4):268-280.

67. Lamhaut L, Jouffroy R, Soldan M, et al. Safety and feasibility of prehospital extra corporeal life support implementation by non-surgeons for out-of-hospital refractory cardiac arrest. *Resuscitation*. 2013;84:1525-1529.

68. Wang C-H, Chou N-K, Becker LB, et al. Improved outcome of extracorporeal cardiopulmonary resuscitation for out-of-hospital cardiac arrest – A comparison with that for extracorporeal rescue for in-hospital cardiac arrest. *Resuscitation*. 2014;85:1219-1224.

69. Johnson NJ, Acker M, Hsu CH, et al. Extracorporeal life support as rescue strategy for out-of-hospital and emergency department cardiac arrest. *Resuscitation*. 2014;85:1527-1532.

70. Bednarczyk JM, White CW, Ducas RA, et al. Resuscitative extracorporeal membrane oxygenation for in hospital cardiac arrest: A Canadian observational experience. *Resuscitation*. 2014;85:1713-1719.

71. Shin TG, Choi J-H, Joon Jo I, et al. Extracorporeal cardiopulmonary resuscitation in patients with inhospital cardiac arrest: A comparison with conventional cardiopulmonary resuscitation. *Crit Care Med*. 2011;39(1):1-7.

72. Chen Y-SS, Chao A, Yu H-YY, et al. Analysis and results of prolonged resuscitation in cardiac arrest patients rescued by extracorporeal membrane oxygenation. *J Am Coll Cardiol*. 2003;41(2):197-203.

73. Lin J-W, Wang M-J, Yu H-Y, et al. Comparing the survival between extracorporeal rescue and conventional resuscitation in adult in-hospital cardiac arrests: Propensity analysis of three-year data. *Resuscitation*. 2010;81:796-803.

74. Chen JS, Ko WJ, Yu HY, et al. Analysis of the outcome for patients experiencing myocardial infarction and cardiopulmonary resuscitation refractory to conventional therapies necessitating extracorporeal life support rescue. *Crit Care Med*. 2006;34(4):950-957.

75. Chen Y-S, Yu H-Y, Huang S-C, et al. Extracorporeal membrane oxygenation support can extend the duration of cardiopulmonary resuscitation. *Crit Care Med*. 2008;36:2529-2535.

76. Chen Y-S, Lin J-W, Yu H-Y, et al. Cardiopulmonary resuscitation with assisted extracorporeal life-support versus conventional cardiopulmonary resuscitation in adults with in-hospital cardiac arrest: An observational study and propensity analysis. *Lancet*. 2008;372(16).

77. Maekawa K, Tanno K, Hase M, Mori K, Asai Y. Extracorporeal cardiopulmonary resuscitation for patients with out-of-hospital cardiac arrest of cardiac

origin: A propensity-matched study and predictor analysis. *Crit Care Med.* 2013;41(5):1186-1196.

78. Sakamoto T, Morimura N, Nagao K, et al. Extracorporeal cardiopulmonary resuscitation versus conventional cardiopulmonary resuscitation in adults with out-of-hospital cardiac arrest: A prospective observational study. *Resuscitation.* 2014;85:762-768.

79. Choi DS, Kim T, Ro YS, et al. Extracorporeal life support and survival after out-of-hospital cardiac arrest in a nationwide registry: A propensity score-matched analysis. *Resuscitation.* 2016;99(2016):26-32.

80. Chang CH, Chen HC, Caffrey JL, et al. Survival analysis after extracorporeal membrane oxygenation in critically ill adults. *Circulation.* 2016;133(24):2423-2433.

81. Bosarge PL, Raff LA, McGwin G, et al. Early initiation of extracorporeal membrane oxygenation improves survival in adult trauma patients with severe adult respiratory distress syndrome. *J Trauma Acute Care Surg.* 2016;81(2):236-241.

82. Michaels AJ, Schriener RJ, Kolla S, et al. Extracorporeal life support in pulmonary failure after trauma. *J Trauma - Inj Infect Crit Care.* 1999;46(4):638-645.

83. Raff L, Kerby JD, Reiff D, et al. Use of extracorporeal membranous oxygenation in the management of refractory trauma-related severe acute respiratory distress syndrome: A national survey of the Eastern Association for the Surgery of Trauma. *Trauma Surg Acute Care Open.* 2019;4(1):1-5.

84. Wang CH, Chou CC, Ko WJ, Lee YC. Rescue a drowning patient by prolonged extracorporeal membrane oxygenation support for 117 days. *Am J Emerg Med.* 2010;28(6):750.e5-750.e7.

85. Champigneulle B, Bellenfant-Zegdi F, Follin A, et al. Extracorporeal life support (ECLS) for refractory cardiac arrest after drowning: An 11-year experience. *Resuscitation.* 2015;88:126-131.

86. Ramanathan K, Antognini D, Combes A, et al. Planning and provision of ECMO services for severe ARDS during the COVID-19 pandemic and other outbreaks of emerging infectious diseases. *Lancet Respir Med.* 2020;8(5):518-526.

87. Noah MA, Peek GJ, Finney SJ, et al. Referral to an extracorporeal membrane oxygenation center and mortality among patients with severe 2009 influenza A(H1N1). *JAMA.* 2011;306(15):1659-1668.

88. Zangrillo A, Biondi-Zoccai G, Landoni G, et al. Extracorporeal membrane oxygenation (ECMO) in patients with H1N1 influenza infection: A systematic review and meta-analysis including 8 studies and 266 patients receiving ECMO. *Crit Care.* 2013;17(1):1-8.

89. Weber-Carstens S, Goldmann A, Quintel M, et al. Extracorporeal lung support in H1N1 provoked acute respiratory failure: The experience of the German ARDS Network. *Dtsch Arztebl Int.* 2013;110(33-34):543-550.

90. Pham T, Combes A, Roze H, et al. Extracorporeal membrane oxygenation for pandemic influenza a(H1N1)-induced acute respiratory distress syndrome a cohort study and propensity-matched analysis. *Am J Respir Crit Care Med.* 2013;187(3):276-285.

91. Aokage T, Palmér K, Ichiba S, Takeda S. Extracorporeal membrane oxygenation for acute respiratory distress syndrome. *J Intensive Care.* 2015;3(1):1-8.

92. Morris AH, Hirshberg E, Miller RR, Statler KD, Hite RD. Counterpoint: Efficacy of extracorporeal membrane oxygenation in 2009 influenza A(H1N1): Sufficient evidence? *Chest*. 2010;138(4):1-4.

93. Park PK, Dalton HJ, Bartlett RH, et al. Point: Efficacy of extracorporeal membrane oxygenation in 2009 influenza A(H1N1): Sufficient evidence? *Chest*. 2010;138(4):776-778.

94. Alshahrani MS, Sindi A, Alshamsi F, et al. Extracorporeal membrane oxygenation for severe Middle East respiratory syndrome coronavirus. *Ann Intensive Care*. 2018;8(1).

95. Henry BM, Lippi G. Poor survival with extracorporeal membrane oxygenation in acute respiratory distress syndrome (ARDS) due to coronavirus disease 2019 (COVID-19): Pooled analysis of early reports Brandon. *J Crit Care*. 2020;58:27-28.

96. Ñamendys-Silva SA. ECMO for ARDS due to COVID-19. *Heart Lung*. 2020; 49(4):348-349.

97. Jacobs JP, Stammers AH, St Louis J, et al. Extracorporeal membrane oxygenation in the treatment of severe pulmonary and cardiac compromise in COVID-19: Experience with 32 patients. *ASAIO J*. 2020;66(7):722-730.

98. Sultan I, Habertheuer A, Usman AA, et al. The role of extracorporeal life support for patients with COVID-19: Preliminary results from a statewide experience. *J Card Surg*. Published online 2020:1-4

99. Mustafa AK, Alexander PJ, Joshi DJ, et al. Extracorporeal membrane oxygenation for patients with COVID-19 in severe respiratory failure. *JAMA Surg*. Published online 2020:E1-E3.

100. Kon ZN, Smith DE, Chang SH, et al. Extracorporeal membrane oxygenation support in severe COVID-19. *Ann Thorac Surg*. 2021;111(2):537-543.

101. Maclaren G, Fisher D, Brodie D. Preparing for the most critically ill patients with COVID-19: The potential role of extracorporeal membrane oxygenation. *JAMA-J Am Med Assoc*. 2020;323(13):1245-1246.

102. Prekker ME, Brunsvold ME, Bohman JK, et al. Regional planning for extracorporeal membrane oxygenation allocation during coronavirus disease 2019. *Chest*. 2020;158(2):603-607.

103. Lindén V, Palmér K, Reinhard J, et al. High survival in adult patients with acute respiratory distress syndrome treated by extracorporeal membrane oxygenation, minimal sedation, and pressure supported ventilation. *Intensive Care Med*. 2000;26(11):1630-1637.

104. Avalli L, Maggioni E, Formica F, et al. Favourable survival of in-hospital compared to out-of-hospital refractory cardiac arrest patients treated with extracorporeal membrane oxygenation: An Italian tertiary care centre experience. *Resuscitation*. 2011;83:579-583.

105. Brunet J, Valette X, Buklas D, et al. Predicting survival after extracorporeal membrane oxygenation for ARDS: An external validation of RESP and PRESERVE scores. *Respir Care*. 2017;62(7):912-919.

106. Lindén V, Palmér K, Reinhard J, et al. Inter-hospital transportation of patients with severe acute respiratory failure on extracorporeal membrane oxygenation - National and international experience. *Intensive Care Med*. 2001;27(10):1643-1648.

14 POST CRITICAL CARE IN THE GERIATRIC POPULATION

Laurie G. Jacobs, MD, FACP, AGSF and Robert A. Zorowitz, MD, MBA, FACP, AGSF, CMD

▌ INTRODUCTION

Older adults are particularly vulnerable in a disaster or a pandemic. This increase in risk is multifactorial, and includes intrinsic factors such as underlying physiologic alterations associated with aging, a diminished physiologic reserve, visual and hearing impairment, impaired mobility, and frailty, a clinical phenotype associated with a reduced ability to overcome stressors. Other factors impacting older adults are extrinsic and include the need for prescription medications, inadequate social supports and social isolation, food insecurity and low economic status, all of which are associated with an increased risk of morbidity in older adults during a disaster or pandemic.[1] Triage, care, and rehabilitation of older adult victims of disasters or pandemics must consider these issues in developing care plans.

Half of the deaths from Hurricane Katrina were in adults age 75 and older,[2] and an estimated 95% of those who died after the Great East Japan earthquake in March 2011 were above age 60.[3] The risk of severe illness and mortality from the recent COVID-19 pandemic has disproportionately afflicted older adults. In 2019, it was estimated that more than 703 million persons were aged 65 or older, 1 in 11 of the world's population. By 2050, it is expected that 1 in 6 will be aged 65 or greater. Older adults comprise an increasingly larger proportion with increasing longevity, particularly in industrialized nations. This is particularly true in higher income nations across North America, Europe, and East Asia; however, the population is aging most rapidly in Eastern and South-Eastern Asia, Latin America, and the Caribbean.[4]

Older adults are often defined by age thresholds. Commonly, age 65 to 74 years defines the "young-old," 75 to 84 years, the "old-old," and 85+ years, the "oldest-old." Women currently predominate in the oldest categories although this gap is narrowing. These definitions may be useful to categorize phenomena seen at different decades of life, while understanding that heterogeneity in physiology and functional ability is greatest during these years of life.

During a disaster or pandemic, older adults may be among the first to be affected. They have greater social and environmental susceptibility to the effects of a disaster and significant barriers to their ability to seek help and medical care. Older adults requiring acute medical care may have an atypical presentation of injury, disease, response to medications or treatment, and unanticipated complications causing delayed recovery and increased mortality. Intrinsic and acquired physiologic changes of aging, concurrent conditions, complex clinical decision-making, frailty, and disability all contribute to the challenges in providing medical care for older adults during a disaster or pandemic, the topic of this chapter.

▌ HEALTH CARE RESOURCE ALLOCATION DURING DISASTERS

Disasters and pandemics require specific and extensive health care resources such as medications, equipment, critical care beds, and treatments. When the supply falls below that required to provide care for a population, or the cost rises above what a society can provide, discussions about allocation and rationing of resources arise. The elderly are often the focus. Potential risks, benefits, and actual and opportunity costs of an intervention or resource, such as the availability of intensive care unit (ICU) beds or ventilators in the most recent COVID-19 pandemic, are weighed, although defining criteria for an individual or a population is challenging. Rationing may occur at a national or local level depending on the circumstances.

Often expensive resources in short supply, such as ICU beds, are provided to individuals with a longer predicted life expectancy. Older adults may be most vulnerable in this analysis; however, age alone should not be used as the defining parameter. Rationing should be based upon objective information as well as patients' wishes. That said, patients' wishes regarding resuscitation and critical care may or may not be known at the time of triage. The principle of distributive justice is that allocation of health care resources should be to those who benefit the most. Intensive care physicians in Italy during the COVID-19 pandemic were first faced with these difficult choices. The American Geriatrics Society[5] has outlined principles, aimed at helping to develop strategies for allocating resources equitably when they are in short supply (Table 14-1A).

Table 14-1A AMERICAN GERIATRICS SOCIETY PRINCIPLES REGARDING ALLOCATION OF HEALTH CARE RESOURCES

- Age should never be used as a means for categorically excluding someone from what is ordinarily the standard of care, nor should age "cut-offs" be used in allocation strategies.
- When assessing comorbidities, the disparate impact of social determinants of health including culture, ethnicity, socioeconomic status, and other factors should be considered.
- Multifactor resource allocation strategies that equally weigh in-hospital survival and severe comorbidities contributing to short-term. (Strategies for making allocation decisions should primarily—and equally—weigh how severe comorbidities and survival in hospital might contribute to the short-term risk for death.)
- To avoid biased resource allocation strategies, criteria such as "life-years saved" and "long-term predicted life expectancy" should not be used because they disadvantage older adults.
- Triage committees and officers who have no direct clinical role in the care of the patients being considered for allocation of limited resources should be familiar with resources available.
- Institutions should develop resource allocation strategies that are transparent, applied uniformly, and developed with forethought and input from the multiple disciplines.
- Widespread and carefully considered advance care planning discussions are of paramount importance in achieving ethical care decisions based on the individual's values, preferences, and goals.

Table 14-1B PRINCIPLES OF HOSPITAL PRESCRIBING FOR OLDER ADULTS

- Avoid prescribing for symptoms before a diagnosis is made.
- Avoid prescribing for symptoms of adverse effects of another agent.
- Consider whether medication is necessary and if nonpharmacologic approaches exist.
- Identify the goals of treatment and treatment targets.
- Consider life expectancy and the time required to achieve therapeutic benefit.
- Consider route of administration, dosing intervals, time, and cost if equivalency exists.
- Avoid starting two new medications simultaneously.
- Ensure whether dosing is appropriate for renal function and lean body mass.
- Anticipate and observe for well-known adverse effects.
- Consider deprescribing nonessential medications, supplements, herbs, and drugs given as prophylaxis in the ICU or as needed (prn).
- Evaluate for drug-drug, drug-food, and drug-disease interactions.

HOSPITAL CARE OF OLDER ADULTS

Goals of Care

Determining goals of care during a disaster, whether an earthquake, war, or global pandemic, may not always be easy or convenient. Nevertheless, understanding and honoring patients' preferences remains paramount. When the prevalence of severe illness or injury outstrips available resources, therapeutic choices may be limited. It is doubly difficult when a relatively new disease lacks adequate prognostic models as clinicians experienced with the COVID-19 pandemic.[6] This introduces significant uncertainty into predictive models and complicates the clinician's ability to communicate potential outcomes with the patient.

Goals of care may be defined as "the overarching aims of medical care for a patient that are informed by patients' underlying values and priorities, established within the existing clinical context, and used to guide decisions about the use of or limitation(s) on specific medical interventions."[7] Although age may be a factor in estimating prognosis, age should never be the sole factor under consideration. Establishing the clinical context requires informing the patient of the prognosis and potential disease trajectories. Evidence-based communication approaches, such as the Serious Illness Conversation method,[8] allow clinicians to align clinical treatments and recommendations with patients' values,[9] while acknowledging clinical uncertainty.

Transitioning Older Adults from the ICU

Older adults may be admitted to an ICU during a disaster or pandemic for critical illness defined as impairment in one or more vital organs such that there is a high probability of imminent or life-threatening deterioration in the patients' condition. Triage decisions often require frequent reassessment. Older patients admitted to the ICU are reassessed at least daily for continuing benefit, although discharge criteria are often unclear and inconsistent. A decision to transition a complex high acuity patient, who no longer requires critical care (due to improved condition or a lack of continuing benefit), to a medical or surgical floor requires planning to ensure stability and to prevent return to the ICU. Issues to be addressed include: (1) treatment and medication reconciliation and reordering, (2) reassessment of advance directives, (3) safety within the setting of reduced monitoring, and (4) communication regarding handoffs in care and continuing clinical issues. Continuing consultation, initially by intensivists, is often ideal to a successful transition.

Delirium

Delirium is an acute disorder of attention and cognition, commonly due to an acute illness, post-surgical complication, or a complication of hospitalization. Disproportionately occurring in the elderly, delirium may lead to increased functional impairment, loss of independence, increased morbidity and mortality, and institutionalization.[10] Delirium is potentially preventable, but is often underdiagnosed and its manifestations overlooked.[11]

Delirium may be referred to as an "acute confusional state" or "acute brain failure." It is the most common neuropsychiatric syndrome occurring in acute care, with a prevalence ranging from 10% on general medicine wards to as high as 85% in critical care units.[12] During a disaster or pandemic, the significance of delirium cannot be overstated. It may occur at any point and with any provocation. During the COVID-19 pandemic, delirium was recognized as a presenting sign of infection, sometimes the only presenting sign, with other signs and symptoms following within a few days.[13] Delirium may complicate the ICU or post-operative course, and is associated with an increase in length of stay and mortality. Delirium must be taken as seriously as other systemic complications attributed to a pandemic or other disaster.

Delirium is characterized by an acute onset with a fluctuating course, inattention, impaired consciousness, and cognitive impairment which involves disorientation, memory impairment, or alteration in language. The differential diagnosis of delirium includes major depressive disorder, dementia, and psychotic disorders (Table 14-2).

There are a variety of instruments to evaluate patients for delirium. The most useful tools incorporate a broad range of domains and can be employed for both diagnosis and determination of severity. The most common are the *Confusion Assessment Method* (CAM, CAM-S),[14] the *Delirium Rating Scale* (DRS),[15] and the *Memorial Delirium Assessment Scale*,[16] all of which may be used for both diagnosis and severity. The CAM involves assessment of four domains: (1) acute change in mental status with a fluctuating course, (2) inattention, (3) disorganized thinking, and (4) altered level of consciousness. The diagnosis requires both features (1) and (2) and either (3) or (4). Although designed for the ICU, the CAM-ICU does not measure severity, and the CAM-ICU-7,[17] while designed to measure severity, does not have as broad domain coverage as other instruments and has not been as extensively studied. Selection of an instrument should be based on the time required to perform the assessment, the training required, and the setting.

Table 14-2 DIFFERENTIAL DIAGNOSIS OF DELIRIUM[35,36]				
Sign	Delirium	Dementia	Depression	Psychosis
Acute onset	+	-	-	+
Fluctuating symptoms	+	-	-	-
Inattention	+	±	±	±
Altered consciousness	+	-	-	-
Disorganized thinking	+	±	-	+
Altered psychomotor activity	+	±	+	+

± *indicates that feature may be present*

Risk factors for delirium include predisposing and precipitating factors. Predisposing factors include pre-existing dementia, multiple medications, visual or hearing impairment, multiple comorbid conditions, depression, immobilization, history of cerebrovascular disease, alcohol abuse, and advanced age, among others. The more predisposing factors that are present, the fewer precipitating factors are necessary to cause delirium. Although surgical procedures are the leading precipitating factor, almost any acute insult may cause delirium in a vulnerable patient. Adverse medication effects, fluid and electrolyte disorders, hypoxemia, renal failure, heart failure, and infections are among the triggers that may result in delirium.

Due to the multifactorial causality, prevention of delirium in hospitalized patients requires a multidimensional approach. *The Elder Life Program,*[18] for example, targets six known risk factors in hospitalized elderly patients, including cognitive impairment, sleep deprivation, immobilization, vision impairment, hearing impairment, and dehydration. By minimizing unnecessary medications and applying non-pharmacological interventions, study patients demonstrated significantly fewer episodes of delirium, delirium days, and, interestingly, fewer falls. This was systematized and packaged as the *Hospital Elder Life Program* (HELP),[19] which has been validated in numerous subsequent studies.

In addition to managing the underlying causative condition, care of delirium requires addressing as many predisposing factors as possible. The clinician should assess for potentially reversible risk factors and address those that may be correctable. Environmental factors, such as excessive lighting or noise, should be avoided. Behavioral symptoms can be addressed with nonpharmacologic approaches such as using a sitter, music, and touch; for example, neuroleptics should be avoided. If absolutely necessary, high-potency antipsychotic agents are preferred (off-label), targeted to treatment of specific behaviors, and discontinued as soon as possible. Studies have shown that proactive, multifactorial interventions and consultation by a geriatrician for older adults at risk for delirium in the ICU or hospital may reduce the incidence, severity, and duration of delirium.[20]

Although delirium may resolve within days or weeks following resolution of the acute precipitating condition, it may also cause long-term cognitive and functional impairment. ICU-associated delirium is more frequently associated with long-term cognitive impairment, functional decline, and death. While prevention is key, immediate recognition of delirium and early intervention is critical to effective treatment.

Prevention of Thrombosis

Prevention of thrombosis in high-risk hospitalized patients is the standard of care. Thrombosis risk is higher in older adults than in other age groups. Virchow's triad—stasis, immobility, and hypercoagulability—identify risk factors, which are highly prevalent in trauma or infectious pandemics. COVID-19 infection is associated with a heightened risk for venous and arterial thromboses; stroke, myocardial infarction, and venous thromboembolic disease is observed more frequently than would be expected. Markedly high d-dimer levels are associated with high thrombotic risk from stasis, excessive inflammation, endothelial dysfunction, and platelet activation. A "cytokine storm" is associated with progression of hypoxemia in respiratory infections, often accompanied by SIRS (systemic inflammatory response syndrome), increasing thrombotic risk.

Anticoagulant and/or mechanical prophylaxis is recommended during hospitalization and following discharge for some patients who have not regained mobility or have a continuing high risk, such long bone fractures, for example. Selection of anticoagulants and dosing should follow clinical guidelines with attention to drug interactions and monitoring of platelets and hemoglobin, despite an increased risk of anticoagulant-associated bleeding risk in older adults, as their thrombotic risk is also elevated. Venous filters, removable or not, provide short term prevention for embolization of lower extremity thromboses, but increase the long-term risks of the post-thrombotic syndrome, particularly in older adults.

Falls and Restraints

Falls occurring in hospitalized older adults are not uncommon adverse events and may cause injury and disability. There are many contributing causes. Patients may attempt to get out of bed alone, with an intravenous line attached, in low light, and may misjudge their strength and mobility. Others fall due to manifestations of illness, trauma, or treatment, such as hypotension. Patients may become hypoxic after removing supplemental oxygen trying to get up and become confused. A standardized approach to fall prevention includes use of a "Fall Risk Prediction Tool" to identify risk factors such as a history of falls, use of an assistive device for ambulation, polypharmacy, delirium, dementia, sensory impairment, low body mass, muscle weakness, and other contributing factors. These tools identify patients requiring closer monitoring and should trigger patient education and awareness. All falls should be followed by a clinical assessment to determine reversible or modifiable contributors and extrinsic or environmental hazards. By addressing, reducing, or eliminating as many contributing factors as possible, the clinician may reduce the probability of a future injurious fall.

During an infectious pandemic, compliance with infection control measures, such as the time required for staff to don personal protective equipment before they can assist a patient, stresses already existing staff demands. Staff availability may also be reduced. Interventions may include reducing sedatives, increasing lighting, moving a bed lower to the ground, using video monitoring, and putting the call button and personal items within reach.

Restraints are intended to prevent patients from falling and from harming themselves but have been found to be ineffective. They inhibit patients' autonomy and dignity, and can cause further harm. Physical restraints, such as vests, gloves, wrist and ankle ties, as well as bedrails, have not been shown to be effective in reducing falls or injuries for adults in acute care hospitals, thus are discouraged and often highly regulated. Bedside alarms, including pressure mats, infrared movement detectors, cord-activated alarms, and wearable devices, used to alert staff when patients attempt to leave the bed or a chair, also have not been effective. They may be considered restraints and can contribute to agitation. Chemical restraints, including sedating medications such as benzodiazepines or antipsychotic agents are given to prevent agitation and inadvertent removal of lines and tubes, may be used in the ICU setting, but may result in significant adverse effects and are strongly discouraged by regulations. Sitters, staff members who remain at the bedside to assist a patient at risk for falls move about, are effective but expensive. Many hospitals employ video surveillance by staff for several rooms of patients to try to reduce the cost of sitters but provide oversight and staff availability. Frequent rounding is also used to identify and assist patients who wish to move from the bed.

Prevention of Pressure Injuries

Pressure injuries, previously referred to as pressure ulcers or bedsores, are a potentially avoidable adverse consequence of immobility and have been termed "skin failure." They are associated with pain, infection, a diminished quality of life, increased health care utilization, and even death. Although pressure injuries may develop in anyone, older adults have an age-associated loss of subcutaneous tissue, in addition to other risks such as immobility, diminished sensory input or consciousness, urinary or fecal incontinence, impaired nutrition, and acute illness. Pressure ulcer incidence is often reportable; their prevalence is a marker of hospital quality. Prevention, surveillance, and treatment of pressure injuries must be undertaken by all members of the interdisciplinary team, including physicians.

Prevention strategies include standardized risk assessment using tools such as the Braden Scale[21] coupled with attention to preventative skin care, nutrition, frequent repositioning, and support surfaces that reduce the interface tissue pressure and duration, limit shear and friction forces, reduce contact with moisture, and provide accessibility for patient care. Mattresses selected for prevention and treatment include foam alternatives or pressure-relieving overlays (static or dynamic); the benefit of alternating pressure pads, gel, water, sheepskin, and air mattress overlays is unclear. Wheelchair cushions (foam, gel, air) are important. "Donut" or "waffle" cushions should be avoided. Patients require surveillance of skin surfaces such as the back of the head, sacrum, and heels at hospital admission and at least daily thereafter, with standardized documentation of observed ulcer size, location, stage, any drainage, and description of the ulcer bed.

During the COVID-19 pandemic, prone positioning has been used as a postural intervention to improve pulmonary function, thus oxygenation levels, for patients who are alert and breathing independently, as well as for those who are sedated and supported by mechanical ventilation.

Pressure injuries have been found on the face and body in prone patients. Positioning devices, repositioning, creams, and dressing are recommended for prevention and to decrease facial skin breakdown.[22]

Treatment of pressure injuries is subject to the old adage, "you can put anything you like on a pressure ulcer except the patient." Dressing choices are determined by the cause of the wound (pressure, shear, moisture, and friction), the characteristics (size, stage, drainage, and presence of devitalized tissue), and the need to reduce bacterial infection, absorb fluid, prevent skin maceration, prevent pain on changes, and provide a moist and vital microenvironment for cellular proliferation and ingrowth. They include transparent films, foams, hydrocolloids, petroleum-based nonadherent materials, alginate, hydrogel, and gauze soaked in saline.

Diagnosis of osteomyelitis in the setting of a pressure ulcer is a common problem. Fever may not always be present. The physical examination is not helpful. Laboratory tests are nonspecific and may demonstrate an elevated leukocyte count or erythrocyte sedimentation rate greater than 100. Cultures of wounds usually reflect colonization; blood cultures may identify the organism. Findings on plain radiographs, such as periosteal elevation, cortical disruption, medullary involvement, and osteolysis, occur too late for intervention. Magnetic resonance imaging and PET-CT (positron emission and computerized tomography) scans, although sensitive and specific, are expensive and often impractical. A bone biopsy for culture and pathology is the gold standard.

Nutrition

Protein-calorie undernutrition can be found in about half of hospitalized older adults, but is pervasive in those who receive ICU care and have high caloric requirements due to fever, inflammation, and the work of breathing. Weight loss due to catabolic demand ensues and is associated with poor outcomes regarding survival and function. Measurement is often affected by edema and underlying conditions and is not useful. Weight gain may not indicate weight recovery. Older adults may have anorexia and/or be unable to consume sufficient calories. Efforts to provide nutrition include oral, enteral and parenteral, total, or supplemental, and are discussed elsewhere in this volume. Hospitalized older adults who are able to eat independently may simply need assistance opening packaging and feeding, which may be overlooked. Observation of older adults consuming meals after a transition from the ICU is important to identify swallowing problems, cough, and aspiration, which, in addition to compounding respiratory issues, poses an infection control risk for others.

Infection Control, Secretions, Incontinence, and Lines

The risk of aerosolization and transmission of COVID-19 can increase during respiratory care, aspiration, intubation, as well as during personal care of patients. The risk for viral respiratory transmission is influenced by aerosol or droplet properties, indoor airflow, virus-specific factors, and host-specific factors.[23] Efforts to prevent aerosolization should be pursued alongside the use of personal protective equipment including masks, respirators, goggles, gowns, and gloves.

The risk of transmitting infection due to contact with mucosal surfaces, secretions, and bodily fluids during patient care and via fomites is exacerbated in a pandemic, but has always existed. Older adults may be at higher risk for *Clostridium difficile* infection, MRSA (Methicillin-resistant *staphylococcus aureus*), and other drug-resistant organisms, due to prior colonization, congregate living, and increased prior use of antibiotics.

Urinary incontinence must be managed without the use of indwelling bladder catheters as much as possible as catheter use is a well-known risk for the development of bladder infections, another adverse quality metric measured in hospitals. Frequent toileting using a schedule or careful use and disposal of diapers is necessary. Bowel incontinence or diarrhea is more problematic, and external collection devices may need to be employed.

Similarly, extended use of peripheral and central intravenous catheters may lead to hematogenous infection and is a marker of quality. During a pandemic, as always, attention to sterile insertion of lines with documentation of the time and date is important.

Disability, Deconditioning, and Physical Therapy

Immobility in the ICU and on hospital wards rapidly leads to neuromuscular weakness, wasting, and functional disability. Older adults may have diminished muscular reserve and premorbid disabilities. Early mobility rehabilitation in the ICU has been found to shorten ICU stay, reduce delirium and mortality, and increase muscle strength at ICU transfer and ability to ambulate at hospital discharge.[24] These programs require significant physical, occupational, and respiratory staff resources and may not be feasible everywhere.

Continued physical therapy aimed at bed mobility, transfers, bathing, dressing, and walking, along with occupational therapy to enable activities of daily living such as dressing, eating, and toileting, is essential for older adults to maximize their function following trauma or infection associated with ICU and hospital care. No recommendations regarding a specific type or amount of physical therapy required for benefit can be made as this depends upon the status of an individual. The extent to which these services are provided depends upon the health system and financing, and may also be subject to rationing in a disaster.

MEDICATION MANAGEMENT IN HOSPITALIZED OLDER ADULTS

Principles of Prescribing for Hospitalized Older Adults

Physiologic changes associated with aging which influence medication prescribing are listed in Table 14-3. Pharmacodynamic changes with aging are not well described; however, several important findings include a decline in sensitivity to beta blockers at the receptor level and an increase in response to opioids and benzodiazepines, regardless of the pharmacokinetic changes.

Medication prescribing for hospitalized older adults may be complex (Table 14-1B). Polypharmacy, often defined as the regular use of five or more medications, may result from the treatment of several co-existing conditions, or from a panoply of medications prescribed for one condition, such as heart failure. During a disaster or pandemic, emergency admissions of older adults may not have included the critical step of medication reconciliation to assess chronic prescribed and "over-the-counter" agents, herbs and supplements, their dosing, and indications. Medication reconciliation should occur as early as possible during a hospital or ICU admission and be repeated following ICU transfer, prior to hospital discharge and as part of any transition in care.

Optimizing Prescribing During a Disaster or Pandemic

Medication management during a disaster[25] requires parsimony as shortages of drugs may occur due to manufacturing and/or supply chain issues. A listing of essential medications and therapeutic alternatives should be developed. Strategies to limit their use should be identified. Nursing time for drug administration may also be limited by staffing shortages or the need to redeploy existing staff. When possible, changes to less frequent dosing of medications may assist. Although this may be achieved by using long-acting formulations, their absorption may be less predictable, reducing the utility of this option. Alternative agents or less frequent dosing may be possible. Eliminating unnecessary medications and streamlining the medication regimen or "deprescribing" may not only reduce the risk of adverse drug reactions and drug-drug interactions, but will also reduce

Table 14-3 PHARMACOKINETIC CHANGES OF AGING INFLUENCING PRESCRIBING		
Parameter	**Alteration**	**Implication for Care**
Absorption	Rarely affected	Achlorhydria (innate or medication-induced) may impair iron absorption.
		Drug-drug or drug-food interactions can modify absorption.
Distribution	Increase in tissue fat: water	Increased volume of distribution, increasing the half-life of fat-soluble drugs such as benzodiazepines.
	Illness-induced decline in plasma proteins	Increased nonprotein-bound active drug such as phenytoin.
Metabolism	Decline in hepatic mass and blood flow may slow metabolism	
	Selected metabolic functions (phase I) may decline, e.g., CYP2C19	
Elimination	Age-related decline in glomerular filtration, may be estimated by the Cockcroft-Gault equation: Creatinine Clearance = $\dfrac{(140 - \text{age})(\text{weight in kg})(0.85 \text{ if female})}{72(\text{stable serum creatinine in mg/dL})}$ The Modification of Diet in Renal Disease (MDRD) estimate has not been validated in adults > 85 years old.	Accumulation of water-soluble drugs such as dabigatran, which may increase risk for bleeding.

the time nurses spend distributing medications,[26] allowing for more bed-side care.

Changes in how agents are administered or the timing of administration may be needed. For example, an assessment of whether oral or intravenous administration saves staff time may be important. Changes in drug monitoring may be required or precipitate a change in drug selection. For example, INR (international normalized ratio) tests for monitoring warfarin may be unreliable due to co-morbid illness, and alternative direct oral anticoagulants may be used instead.

Finally, medication changes may be needed for infection control reasons, including reducing the use of short acting insulins and thereby the need for frequent blood glucose monitoring. Medications given by inhalation or nebulizers may be restricted to prevent aerosolization of infectious agents.

Clinical Trials and Off-label Prescribing

Clinical research is critical during a pandemic or disaster to describe clinical phenomena and evaluate new interventions and treatments. During the COVID-19 pandemic, several challenges for clinical trial research have arisen.[27] New methods with attention to infection control for study staff during the COVID-19 pandemic use non-face-to-face electronic and video methodologies for consent and evaluations. To support rapid evaluation of treatments, some investigators have allowed alterations in protocols for enrollment and retention, potentially affecting statistical power or results. In addition, competing protocols may jeopardize sufficient and timely enrollment. Insufficient collaboration in data collection and analysis across sites has occurred despite common electronic medical record platforms.

"Off-label" medications that have U.S. Food and Drug Administration (FDA) approval for a different indication have been widely abused by some physicians in their zeal to offer some treatment, and lack of understanding of the FDA process to ensure safety was seen for medications such as hydroxychloroquine, which potentially caused harm. Off-label use of new agents, with the FDA approval, were rapidly evaluated for a response sufficient to embark upon a clinical trial. The pressure for rapid results may lead to analysis prior to sufficient enrollment or to studies without adequate controls.

All of these issues impact older adults who may not present as ideal candidates for trials but may represent the majority of individuals impacted by a disaster or pandemic, are more subject to harm due to intrinsic and comorbid conditions, and may be more challenging in the consent procedures due to sensory and cognitive impairments. The FDA is committed to enrollment of older adults in clinical trials.[28] The World Health Organization in 2016 released the "Guidance for Managing Ethical Issues in Infectious Disease,"[29] which states that research conducted during an outbreak should be designed and implemented with other public health interventions and protect the safety of participants.

MANAGEMENT OF COMMON SYMPTOMS IN HOSPITALIZED OLDER ADULTS

The clinical management of pain, insomnia, anxiety and agitation (see section on delirium), dyspnea, and constipation in older adults bear special mention due to their frequency in hospitalized patients during a disaster or pandemic and special considerations required for older adults.

Pain

Pain in the context of a disaster or pandemic is usually acute due to injury and noxious stimuli, but has the potential to become chronic or persistent (defined as greater than six months duration). In addition, a prior chronic pain syndrome may exist. The perception of acute pain may be blunted or present in an altered way such as a behavioral disturbance, insomnia, or a depressed mood. Somatic pain (e.g., fractures or surgery), visceral pain (e.g., gastrointestinal or urologic pathology), or neuropathic pain are seen in victims of a disaster. The assessment includes location, duration, quality, radiation, and provocative factors. Pharmacological treatments have several caveats for older adults (Table 14-4). Nonpharmacologic treatments for pain may be used independently or together with medication. The patient may benefit from consultation with a palliative care or pain specialist.

Insomnia

Insomnia is a common complaint in older adults in general, and in hospitalized patients in particular. Changes in sleep associated with aging, the environment, and comorbid conditions often lead to difficulty falling asleep, an increase in awakenings, and difficulty returning to sleep. Nonpharmacologic interventions are less useful for hospitalized patients.

All sedative hypnotics are associated with an increased incidence of falls and delirium in older adults and should be used with caution. Older individuals admitted to the hospital may take sedative hypnotic agents chronically, including benzodiazepines, which are habit form-ing and associated with withdrawal syndrome similar to chronic alcohol use. Awareness and management is critical to prevent withdrawal, and a very slow taper may be required. Chronic use of benzodiazepines is to be avoided in older adults. The use of first-generation antihistamines such as diphenhydramine is also strongly discouraged in older adults as these agents are sedating and have associated anticholinergic effects causing constipation, urinary retention, tachycardia, and delirium.

Medications that can be prescribed for insomnia include the short-acting agents eszopiclone, zaleplon, and zolpidem, but these may have adverse effects similar to benzodiazepines. Melatonin or ramelteon, a melatonin agonist, may be effective. The antidepressants mirtazapine and trazodone are often used off-label for their sedating effect in older adults with agitation and confusion.

Constipation

Constipation is common but may be underdiagnosed in older hospitalized patients due to dehydration, minimal oral intake, medications (anticho-linergics, opioids, calcium channel blockers, etc.), lack of exercise, elec-trolyte, and medical disorders. Constipation in older adults may present as abdominal discomfort or diarrhea occurring around an impaction. Treatment aims at increasing stool bulk and transit time. Both outpa-tient and hospital management include increased hydration, bulk agents (psyllium, methylcellulose, and others) and stimulants (senna and bisaco-dyl), nonabsorbable substances (lactulose, PEG3350, magnesium salts), or occasionally, lubiprostone, a secretory agent. In the hospital setting, enemas and dis-impaction may be required.

Hyperglycemia and Hypoglycemia

Hyperglycemia and hypoglycemia in older adults in the hospital setting is common due to the high prevalence of type II diabetes. The American Diabetes Association (ADA) Standards of Medical Care in Diabetes, released in 2019, recommends treatment to achieve glucose levels between 140 and 180 mg/dL (7.8–10 mmol/L) for both critical and non-critical hospitalized patients to improve outcomes associated with uncontrolled hyperglycemia while minimizing the risk of hypoglycemia.[30] Glycemic control is influenced by many factors, including infection, steroid ther-apy, stress, and nutrition. Often this requires insulin therapy regardless of the prior medication regime, although the occurrence of hypoglycemia is

Table 14-4 PAIN PHARMACOTHERAPY IN OLDER ADULTS		
Medication Class, Drug	**Pain type**	**Prescribing for Older Adults**
Acetaminophen	Mild-moderate somatic or visceral	Reduced daily dose if liver dysfunction. May be compounded with opiates.
NSAIDs (ibuprofen, naproxen, indomethacin)	Mild-moderate somatic, visceral, or neuropathic	Renal dysfunction, hypertension, bleeding, edema, and exacerbation of heart failure may occur. Chronic use should be accompanied by GI prophylaxis.
Steroids (methylprednisolone, prednisone, dexamethasone)	All	Short term use only. Same warnings as with NSAIDS. May cause delirium, insomnia, hyperglycemia, reduced wound healing, lowered resistance to infection.
Anticonvulsants (gabapentin, pregabalin)	Neuropathic indications	Delirium, sedation, dizziness, edema may occur. Many interactions. Should not be used as a primary agent.
Antidepressants (nortriptyline, desipramine [TCAs], duloxetine, venlafaxine [SNRIs])	Neuropathic pain	All may have anticholinergic effects (constipation, urinary retention, confusion); TCAs may cause hypotension and cardiac rhythm effects. Renal function may limit SNRI use. SNRIs have other adverse effects. Venlafaxine may increase blood pressure as tapered.

(Continued)

Table 14-4 PAIN PHARMACOTHERAPY IN OLDER ADULTS (*CONTINUED*)		
Medication Class, Drug	**Pain type**	**Prescribing for Older Adults**
Opioids (tramadol, hydrocodone, oxycodone, fentanyl transdermal, etc.)	Moderate to severe pain of all types	Increased pharmacodynamic effect in elderly; adverse effects include constipation (Rx at start), nausea, sedation, respiratory depression. Tolerance and addiction may occur.

usually associated with insulin use and is particularly troubling for older adults. Basal insulin therapy alone without rapid acting insulin usually provided may be preferred during disaster or pandemic conditions as it requires less glycemic testing and dosing. Although newer therapies are available, the familiarity of insulin therapy is often preferred. Managing glucoses using a sliding scale of insulin therapy is outmoded as a reactive treatment regimen.

▌MANAGEMENT OF TRANSITIONS IN CARE

The transfer of patients from one setting to another often requires a change in providers, equipment, pharmacy, and protocols. This provides opportunities for fragmentation of care, inefficiencies, miscommunication, and medication errors, potentially resulting in prolonged recovery, rehospitalization, or, worse, morbidity and mortality. Older adults are particularly vulnerable to mishaps in transitional care.[31]

In a disaster or pandemic, post-acute care organizations and institutions may vary in their preparedness to manage patients, thus introducing further complexity into transfer decisions. During the 2020 COVID-19 pandemic, U.S. nursing facilities, home to both long-term care residents and short-term post-acute patients, struggled to safely manage their own residents, and often could not accommodate post-acute transfers from acute care hospitals.[32] Home health agencies faced shortages of personal protective equipment, disinfectants, travel restrictions, and other challenges to providing needed care for homebound patients.[33]

Studies show that appropriately targeted interventions and communication improve the outcomes of transitional care. Prior to hospital discharge, patient and caregiver education, medication reconciliation, discharge planning, timely post-discharge follow-up, communication with the patient's primary care provider, and timely availability of a discharge summary and clear discharge instructions will reduce the likelihood of post-discharge gaps in care.[34] The Care Transitions Intervention,[35] a randomized clinical trial of transitional care, demonstrated that with the assistance of a "transitions coach," assistance with medication self-management, a patient-centered record to facilitate cross-site information transfer, timely follow-up with primary and specialty care and a list of "red flags," with instructions for responding to worsening conditions could reduce subsequent rehospitalization and significantly reduce gaps in the quality of transitional care.

▌ REFERENCES

1. Jenkins JL, Levy M, Rutkow L, Spira A. Variables associated with effects on morbidity in older adults following disasters. *PLoS Curr*. 2014;6:ecurrents.dis.0fe 970aa16d51cde6a962b7a732e494a.

2. Adams V, Kaufman SR, van Hattum T, Moody S. Aging disaster: mortality, vulnerability, and long-term recovery among Katrina survivors. *Med Anthropol*. 2011;30(3):247-270.

3. Ichiseki H. Features of disaster-related deaths after the Great East Japan earthquake. *Lancet*. 2013;381(9862):204.

4. United Nations, Department of Economic and Social Affairs. World Population Aging 2019. Highlights. https://www.un.org/development/desa/pd/sites/www.un.org.development.desa.pd/files/files/documents/2020/Jan/worldpopulationageing2019-highlights.pdf. Accessed July 11, 2020.

5. Farrell TW, Ferrante LE, Brown T, et al. AGS position statement: Resource allocation strategies and age-related considerations in the COVID-19 era and beyond. *J Am Geriatr Soc*. 2020;68:1136-1142.

6. McGuire AL, Aulisio MP, Davis FD, et al. Ethical challenges arising in the COVID-19 pandemic: An overview from the Association of Bioethics Program Directors (ABPD) Task Force. *Am J Bioeth*. 2020;1-13.

7. Secunda K, Wirpsa MJ, Neely KJ, et al. Use and meaning of "Goals of Care" in the healthcare literature: A systematic review and qualitative discourse analysis. *J Gen Intern Med*. 2020;35(5):1559-1566.

8. Ma C, Riehm LE, Bernacki R, Paladino J, You JJ. Quality of clinicians' conversations with patients and families before and after implementation of the Serious Illness Care Program in a hospital setting: A retrospective chart review study. *CMAJ Open*. 2020;8(2):E448-E454.

9. Back AL, Fromme EK, Meier DE. Training clinicians with communication skills needed to match medical treatments to patient values. *J Am Geriatr Soc*. 2019;67(S2):S435-S441.

10. Inouye SK, Westendorp RG, Saczynski JS. Delirium in elderly people. *Lancet.* 2014;383:911-922.

11. Maldonado JR. Acute brain failure: Pathophysiology, diagnosis, management, and sequelae of delirium. *Crit Care Clin.* 2017;33(3):461-519.

12. Cipriani G, Danti S, Nuti A, Carlesi C, Lucetti C, Di Fiorino M. A complication of coronavirus disease 2019: Delirium. *Acta Neurol Belg.* 2020;120(4):927-932.

13. Wei LA, Fearing MA, Sternberg EJ, Inouye SK. The Confusion Assessment Method (CAM): A systematic review of current usage. *J Am Geriatr Soc.* 2008;56:823-830.

14. Trzepacz PT, Mittal D, Torres R, Kanary K, Norton J, Jimerson N. Validation of the Delirium Rating Scale-Revised-98: Comparison with the delirium rating scale and the cognitive test for delirium. *J Neuropsychiatry Clin Neurosci.* 2001;13(2):229-242.

15. Breitbart W, Rosenfeld B, Roth A, Smith MJ, Cohen K, Passik S. The Memorial Delirium Assessment Scale. *J Pain Symptom Manage.* 1997;13(3):128-137.

16. Jones RN, Cizginer S, Pavlech L, et al. Assessment of instruments for measurement of delirium severity: A systematic review. *JAMA Intern Med.* 2019;179(2):231-239.

17. Inouye SK, Bogardus STJr, Charpentier PA, et al. A multicomponent intervention to prevent delirium in hospitalized older patients. *N Engl J Med.* 1999;340(9):669-676.

18. AGS CoCare: HELP. https://www.americangeriatrics.org/programs/ags-cocare-helptm. Accessed July18, 2020.

19. Marcantonio ER. Delirium in hospitalized older adults. *N Engl J Med.* 2017;377:1456-1466.

20. Bergstrom N, Braden BJ, Laguzza A, Holman V. The Braden Scale for predicting pressure sore risk. *Nurs Res.* 1987;36(4):205-210.

21. Moore Z, Patton D, Avsar P, et al. Prevention of pressure ulcers among individuals cared for in the prone position: Lessons for the COVID-19 emergency. *J Wound Care.* 2020;29(6):312-320.

22. Kohanski MA, Lo LJ, Waring MS. Review of indoor aerosol generation, transport, and control in the context of COVID-19. *Int Forum Allergy Rhinol.* 2020;10(10):1173-1179.

23. Tipping CJ, Harrold M, Holland A, Romero L, Nisbet T, Hodgson CL. The effects of active mobilisation and rehabilitation in ICU on mortality and function: A systematic review. *Intensive Care Med.* 2017;43:171-183.

24. Medication Management in PALTC during COVID-19. Version 1 (with supplement). AGS/ADGAP COVID-19 Educational Toolkit. 10 April 2020. https://www.pharmacy.umaryland.edu/centers/lamy/optimizing-medication-management-during-covid19-pandemic/. Accessed July 18, 2020.

25. Scott IA, Hilmer SN, Reeve E, et al. Reducing inappropriate polypharmacy: The process of deprescribing. *JAMA Intern Med.* 2015;175(5):827-834.

26. Fleming TR, Labriola D, Wittes J. Conducting clinical research during the COVID-19 pandemic. Protecting scientific integrity. *JAMA.* 2020;324:33-34.

27. Fassbender M. FDA outlines renewed efforts to include older adults in clinical trials. August 19, 2019. https://www.outsourcing-pharma.com/Article/2018/07/17/FDA-outlines-renewed-efforts-to-include-older-adults-in-clinical-trials#. Accessed July 12, 2020.

28. World Health Organization. Managing ethical issues in infectious disease outbreaks. 2016. https://apps.who.int/iris/bitstream/handle/10665/250580/9789241549837-eng.pdf;jsessionid=5DFDA746D9183D858BF9050FBD916B5A?sequence=1. Accessed July 12, 2020.

29. American Diabetes Association. Diabetes care in the hospital: Standards of medical care in diabetes-2019. *Diabetes*. 2019; 42(suppl 1):S173-S181.

30. Coleman EA. Falling through the cracks: Challenges and opportunities for improving transitional care for persons with continuous complex care needs. *J Am Geriatr Soc*. 2003;51:549-555.

31. Grabowski DC, Mor V. Nursing home care in crisis in the wake of COVID-19. *JAMA*. 2020;324(1):23-24.

32. Shang J, Chastain AM, Perera UGE, et al. COVID-19 Preparedness in US home health care agencies. *J Am Med Dir Assoc*. 2020;21(7):924-927.

33. Hansen LO, Young RS, Hinami K, Leung A, Williams MV. Interventions to reduce 30-day rehospitalization: A systematic review. *Ann Intern Med*. 2011;155(8):520-528.

34. Coleman EA, Parry C, Chalmers S, Min SJ. The care transitions intervention: Results of a randomized controlled trial. *Arch Intern Med*. 2006;166(17):1822-1828.

35. Oh ES, Fong TG, Hshieh TT, Inouye SK. Delirium in older persons. Advances in diagnosis and treatment. *JAMA*. 2017;318(12):1161-1174.

36. Hshieh TT, Inouye SK, Oh ES. Delirium in the elderly. *Clin Geriatr Med*. 2020;36(2):183-199.

PSYCHIATRIC ISSUES 15

Francis Aguilar, MD

▌ INTRODUCTION

The impact of disaster and crisis events encompass all aspects of a patient's being. The physical injuries are clear and obvious. However, the new or underlying mental health issues that arise from a crisis or trauma may not become as apparent in an acute situation. This is applicable not only for the patient but to the care team and the family of those affected. Pandemics and violent traumas are obvious precipitating factors for mental health illnesses, and acute changes in mental health and behaviors are expected. The factors involved in the aforementioned crisis situations that perpetuate the mental health and behavioral comorbidities become the challenge clinically moving forward in a patient's care. Over time, many of the memorable and devastating world events have highlighted the need to address and manage psychiatric comorbidities. World War II, mass shootings, natural disasters, and global pandemics all have left an indelible impression on the mental health of patients, their families, the medical care team, and the hospital system. In this day and age where information comes fast and often, the recent COVID-19 pandemic has further emphasized the many mental health issues that affect the community during times of an ongoing disaster. The media coverage from the disastrous COVID-19 pandemic has highlighted how hospital systems around the world have been overwhelmed. Hospital systems are struggling with not only addressing how to contain the pandemic but also the difficulty addressing issues such as Personal Protective Equipment resources, allowing family members to see their sick loved ones, medical staffing, physical space to handle patient volume, and the degree of complexity the patient themselves present with during this pandemic. All of these issues bring about stress and strain to all those involved, which in turn has the ability to precipitate or exacerbate mental health comorbidities. This chapter hopes to serve as a conceptual guide for the evaluation, management, and treatment of various psychiatric issues that arise for patients, their families, and the medical team in an acute critical care setting.

EVALUATION OF PSYCHIATRIC DISORDERS IN CRITICAL CARE SETTINGS

Typical psychiatric disorders that are recognized in the critical care setting typically consist of the following: delirium, anxiety disorders (from a reactionary or anticipatory anxiety to panic disorder with agitation and restlessness), adjustment disorders with depressive mood, brief psychotic disorders with or without persecutory delusions, and acute stress or post-traumatic stress disorders. The manifestations of psychiatric disorders occur not only during the stay in the intensive care unit (ICU) but also after transfer from ICU and possibly even several months after discharge from hospital.

In a critical care setting, a significant precipitating factors for the acute appearance of psychiatric symptoms are largely thought to be due to organic or toxic causes (metabolic disturbances, electrolyte imbalance, withdrawal syndromes, infection, vascular disorders, and head trauma) despite even having a preexisting psychiatric comorbidity. The critical care environment or setting itself can precipitate much of what is perceived as an exacerbation of a patient's psychiatric symptoms. Once a patient becomes more lucid and the patient's senses begin to return, the visual and auditory senses alone can trigger an acute stress response. It is imperative to first stabilize a patient's physical medical condition before determining whether or not the preexisting psychiatric disorder is the driving force in the patient's perceived psychiatric presentation. Delirium is typically the cause for the acute change in a critical care patient's change in mental status.

Being mindful of the overall clinical context of how the patient's delirium is presenting before determining that the suspected psychiatric symptom is primarily due to any underlying psychiatric comorbidity is vital in management moving forward. Lack of improvement or decline in health status may not be due to an existing primary psychiatric illness. If the patient's presentation is in fact due to self-injurious behavior or impulsive behavior that caused harm to the patient while in the hospital, stabilizing the patient's physical and medical injuries still must remain the priority. The patient's physiological response to injury will impact the brain's response to stress and injury, which in turn, can impact any preexisting mental health diagnoses.[1]

The psychophysiological mechanisms related to acute changes in mental status, especially in the delirium and disruptive behavior, can be explained in the physiologic concepts that trigger fear and threat responses. These concepts have been studied in psychopathologies such as post-traumatic stress disorder (PTSD). It has been long studied in neuroscience that the amygdala and the hippocampus play a function in regulating and processing how the brain interprets a situational context and how to trigger and process a fear response. The amygdala is known to regulate cortical arousal and neuroendocrine responses to surprising and ambiguous stimuli. The hippocampus has a role not only in memory but is rich in corticosteroid receptors that can play a role in regulatory feedback to the hypothalamus-pituitary-adrenal axis. These connections between the aforementioned neuroanatomy feed into the prefrontal cortex, which subsequently mediates intellectual or executive functions. The prefrontal cortex's complex connectivity patterns, electrophysiological activity, neuroimaging findings, and associated clinical manifestations all reinforce the elaborate role of the prefrontal cortex in mediating higher order behaviors.

In a baseline cognitive state, the alert, non-stressed brain benefits from a hierarchical management system. The medial prefrontal cortex (mPFC) down-regulates amygdala-driven fear conditioning through stimulation of inhibitory γ-aminobutyric (GABA) interneurons in regions of the amygdala. In contrast, the stressed brain is marked by a diminished capacity of the mPFC and the hippocampus to act as checkpoints on the excitatory flow that emerges from the amygdala. Consequently, the primitive brain circuits in the limbic system can take over and override the circuitry, which precipitates a more reflexive and habitual response that manifests as agitation or restlessness[2] (Figure 15-1).

Understanding fully the physiologic changes related to the patient's illness or injuries can assist in determining the possible medication management required in quelling the acute change in a patient's mental status causing a disruption in care while in a critical care setting.[21]

The highly monitored critical care units are surrounded by a multitude of possible environmental and situational triggers to precipitate delirious, anxious, and agitated states. Possible environmental and situational triggers can include high sound levels, sleep deprivation, sensory deprivation, the inability for intubated patients to talk, pain associated with acute medical procedure, and the possibility to witness other patients' death. To face the anxiety, many patients may have psychological defense mechanisms such as regression and denial that may impede on executing optimal patient care in the ICU. When attempts to restart a patient's previous psychotropic medications fail or standard behavioral interventions to decrease the intensity of anxiety, irritability, and behavioral outbursts have not been successful; a consultation with the Psychiatry Consult Liaison (Psychosomatic Medicine) service would be beneficial. The collaboration with the psychiatrist will help to optimize care but also help determine causal factors.

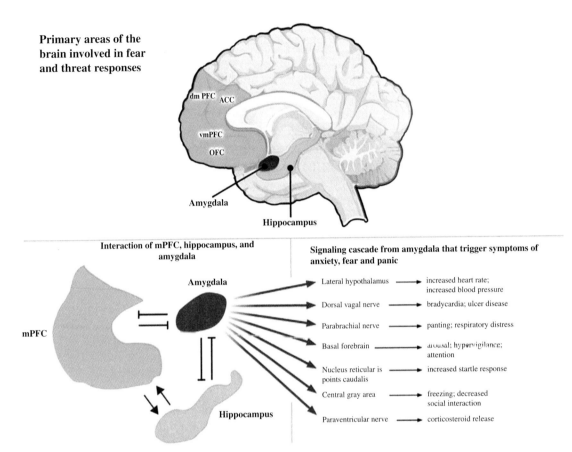

Figure 15-1 • Schematic diagram of neural circuitry involved in fear conditioning and post-traumatic stress disorder. Primary brain regions involved in regulating fear and threat responses are the amygdala, the hippocampus, and the medial prefrontal cortex, which includes the dorsal (dmPFC) and ventral (vmPFC) subdivisions, the orbitofrontal cortex (OFC), and the anterior cingulate cortex (ACC). The amygdala is central in the neural circuit involved in regulating fear conditioning. Interactions between the mPFC and the hippocampus regulate the amygdala's output to subcortical brain regions involved in activating a "fear" reflex. The vmPFC is thought to inhibit amygdala activity and reduce subjective distress, while the hippocampus plays a role both in the coding of fear memories and in the regulation of the amygdala. The hippocampus and mPFC also interact in regulating context and fear modulation. (Used, with permission, from Kim MC, Fricchione GL, Akeju O. Accidental awareness under general anaesthesia: Incidence, risk factors, and psychological management. *BJA Education*. 2021; 21(4):154-161.)

▌ PSYCHOTROPIC MEDICATION MANAGEMENT FOR PATIENTS IN A CRITICAL CARE SETTING

Whether the patient is ill due to a global pandemic or penetrating trauma, critically ill patients undergo a multitude of processes and procedures during their hospitalization. At times, these critically ill patients are on medications to address their chronic mental health comorbidities prior to the presenting disastrous life event. The management of their psychiatric medications while acutely stabilizing the patient may be a source of confusion or trepidation during their hospitalization for the medical team.

High quality supportive care in critical illness aims to achieve many parameters in the patient care, such as sedation, volume status, High Flow Nasal Cannula/Bilevel Positive Airway Pressure electrolyte imbalances, pain management, gastrointestinal prophylaxis, and nutrition. Much of these supportive care processes can influence the absorption, distribution, metabolism, and excretion of psychotropic medications, thereby affecting steady state levels and efficacy.[3] Common psychiatric medications such as lithium, valproic acid, tricyclic antidepressants, and many of the second generation antipsychotics such as Seroquel rely heavily on the status of the renal system, GI physiology, and liver metabolism. If any of these systems are not functioning optimally, the medication's pharmacodynamics and pharmacokinetics can be affected. Subsequently, this can affect the patient's recovery and delay in a return to an expected cognitive baseline.

It has long been routine in the practice of psychiatry to obtain serum levels of several psychotropic medications. The practice standard was either obtaining a 12- or 24-hour post-dose level, or in some cases, a trough level before the morning dose. It may be optimal to obtain blood serum levels of psychotropic medications early in the hospitalization to assist in setting goals and expectations of medication management. Many hospital systems can obtain these blood levels in a timely manner, which will allow for more information in regards to potential toxicity or suboptimal medication management. Therapeutic drug monitoring through the course of a patient's critical care stay can be useful in avoiding toxicity (as many psychotropic medications have narrow therapeutic indices), particularly that due to interactions with other compounds (Table 15-1).[4]

Pharmacokinetic and pharmacodynamic variables affect the ultimate steady-state serum level of psychiatric drugs. The reasons in a critical care stay for obtaining a serum drug level include but are not limited to the following:[4]

- Patient with severe adverse effects in context of what is considered a low dose
- Monitor adherence
- Acute mental status change: rule out drug toxicity or withdrawal
- Predischarge once psychiatrically stable to compare with post-discharge if clinical picture changes
- Pre-GI surgery or procedures to obtain an effective baseline while stable, to assist in drug dosage changes post-surgery

Table 15-1 FACTORS THAT CAN AFFECT THE RELIABILITY AND INTERPRETATION OF PSYCHOTROPIC SERUM DRUG LEVELS

Nonadherence
Variability in drug absorption
Genetic polymorphism of CYP or UGT metabolic enzymes
Drug to drug interactions
Requirement for specific caloric intake to maximize drug absorption
Time serum level is obtained post-dose
Formulation of drug (immediate release, slow release, extended release)
Half-life and time to maximum concentration of the drug
Medical comorbidities affecting drug metabolism
Steady state status of the drug
CYP, cytochrome p450; UGT, (UDP-glucuronosyltransferase)

Serum levels of psychotropic medications can serve as a useful tool to monitor a patients' response to medications and adjust dosing appropriately (Table 15-2).

Discussing the patient's medication regime with the clinical pharmacologist can also be helpful, especially if the patient is unable to tolerate oral medications. There can be dosage equivalencies or formulations that are appropriate for a particular patient undergoing critical care management.

Many of the patients in this setting are unable to participate in a full verbal interview and much of the history of that patient's psychiatric comorbidities are obtained from chart review or collateral information from a family member, friend, or documentation from a transferring facility. Most common topics to discuss about medication management can include the following:

- When did the patient take the last known dose?
- How was the patient doing prior to the current hospitalization?
- Did the patient experience any adverse effects when starting the medication?
- What psychopathology or diagnosis did the medication address for the patient?

Table 15-2 GENERALLY ACCEPTED SERUM LEVELS* OF PSYCHOTROPIC MEDICATIONS	
Drug	Reference range
Lithium	0.6–1.2 mEq/L
Carbamazepine	4–12 µg/mL
Valproic acid	50–125 µg/mL
Lamotrigine	2.5–15 ng/mL
Clozapine	200–700 ng/mL
Amitriptyline and nortriptyline	80–200 ng/mL

*Serum level does not necessarily correlate with clinical efficacy
Source: Adapted from Jacobson SA. *Laboratory Medicine in Psychiatry and Behavioral Science.* 2012.

Confirming the aforementioned information may provide reassurance to the critical care team if the benefit outweighs the risk to continue the patient's at home medication regime. In addition, when brought into the case, the psychiatry consultation team can find this information invaluable as well to assess risks versus benefits.

In restarting or initiating psychotropic medications in the critical care setting, one must be mindful of serotonin syndrome and neuroleptic malignant syndrome (NMS). These are well known emergencies that are expertly managed by the critical care team (Table 15-3).[5] Clinical presentations can be similar and results from the clinical work up may also be similar. Review of a patient's current medication list or reviewing a medication administration record over a short period can at times be overlooked.

Management of "Agitation"

Delirium and associated agitation in critically ill patients has long been known to be associated with adverse clinical outcomes. Episodes of delirium may contribute to prolonged time on mechanical ventilation, impaired cognition, and increased hospital and ICU length of stay.[6] The management of the delirium in the critical care setting can at times be challenging depending on what exactly physiologically or behaviorally precipitated the associated restlessness or agitation during a patient's hospital course. It can be due to the medical condition itself, intoxication/withdrawal, environmental changes (staffing changes, medical monitoring sounds, etc.) and possibly any underlying psychiatric comorbidities.[7] Critical care teams are very skilled to handle delirium and agitation for

Table 15-3 DRUG INDUCED SYNDROMES[1-10]			
Disease	Offending Medication	Shared Clinical Features	Distinguishing Clinical Features
Serotonin syndrome	Serotonergic medications (e.g., SSRI, MAOI, linezolid, tramadol)	Hypertension	Clonus, hyperreflexia, hyperactive bowel sounds
Neuroleptic malignant syndrome	Dopamine antagonists (e.g., typical and atypical antipsychotics, metoclopramide)	Tachycardia	No clonus or hyperreflexia, bradykinesia
Anticholinergic toxicity	Acetylcholine antagonist	Hyperthermia	No clonus or hyperreflexia Dry skin, absent bowel sounds
Malignant hyperthermia	Halogenated anesthetics Succinylcholine	Altered mental status	Extreme muscular rigidity

high risk medically compromised patients. The recent COVID-19 pandemic has shown the immediate cognitive decompensation from acute respiratory distress syndrome (ARDS). The risk of hyperactive delirium increases as ICU hospitalization is prolonged. Hyperactive delirium is commonly defined as the following: increased motor activity, loss of control of activity, restlessness.

Critical care teams have clinical pathways and algorithms that can assess for levels of delirium. Hyperactive delirium with a mixed motor type can be a difficult clinical scenario that can result in a prolonged critical care length of stay or possibly precipitate re-intubation. As the patient continues to recover and improve, a hyperactive delirium can move to a lesser intensity but still prove to be difficult to manage, such is the case in the other end of the spectrum with hypoactive delirium. This subtype of delirium can be very subtle but prove to be challenging in attempting to get a patient stepped down to a lower level of care from ICU/CCU setting. A patient's hypoactive delirium can be characterized by drowsiness, decreased physical activity, sleep–wake pattern disruption, and decreased cognitive function. A patient's limitations include but are not limited to disorganized thinking and speech, which leads to inability to communicate, psychomotor agitation with sensation of extreme fatigue, and a patient with a restricted affect. In addition, there can be residual neurological abnormalities such as slurred speech to frank dysarthria and decreased muscular tone. Overt psychiatric symptoms such as delusions, misperceptions, and hallucinations may be absent with hypoactive delirium. A patient's hypoactive delirium can be active even in the absence or improvement of metabolic abnormalities, infections, hematologic abnormalities, cardiopulmonary abnormalities, or other disorders that would be explaining the delirium.[8] Deciding which pharmacologic treatment to address hyper, mixed, or hypoactive delirium can be a challenge (Table 15-4).

The 2018 Society of Critical Care Medicine practice guidelines recommended a benzodiazepine-sparing approach to manage sedation in ICU patients. Dexmedetomidine in the critical care setting has long been used as a non-benzodiazepine pharmacological treatment to facilitate sedation, especially in the context of agitation secondary to delirium. Dexmedetomidine's ability to inhibit the release of norepinephrine at the presynaptic α_2 receptors aims to help mitigate agitation and restlessness by reducing the hyperadrenergic activity a patient may experience while the patient's awareness and cognitive ability begin to improve. This pharmacologic choice is determined by the critical care team's decision on the individual patients' sedation goals. Sedation strategies vary among each ICU; propofol has been known to be the preferred continuous infusion sedative. Institutional dexmedetomidine stewardship programs can assist in confidently using dexmedetomidine as an alternative to propofol. There are varying protocols or nurse driven screening tools that assist with determining medication management.[9] The Richmond Agitation Sedation Scale (RASS), the Confusion Assessment Method for the ICU (CAM-ICU), or the MINDS Alcohol Withdrawal Scale or Glasgow Modified Alcohol Withdrawal Scale (GMAWS) are common ones used. The implementation of a stewardship program can help evaluate a patient's sedation goals and reassess the need for dexmedetomidine, particularly for use beyond the FDA-approved 24 h.[12] Dexmedetomidine as a centrally acting α_2 agonist that is approved by the Food and Drug Administration (FDA) in adults for procedural sedation and for sedation of intubated and mechanically ventilated patients for up to 24 h.[10] Although approved for up to 24 h, it is often used for longer durations. Discontinuation of dexmedetomidine has been associated with withdrawal symptoms due to sympathetic hyperactivity.[11] At times, the psychiatry consultation team is

Table 15-4 CLINICAL CHARACTERISTICS OF HYPOACTIVE DELIRIUM WITHOUT A CLINICALLY IDENTIFIABLE CAUSE

- Syndrome meets DSM-V criteria for delirium
- Clinical syndrome presents as an acute change over a few days to a few weeks
- Prodrome characterized by insomnia and daytime drowsiness
- Cognitive deficits:
  - Preservation of orientation regarding time, space, and person, except in severe impairment
  - Attention deficits: decreased ability to read, watch television, make telephone calls, and so on
  - Short-term memory is affected early on
  - Disorganized thinking and speech, leading to an inability to communicate with family members or friends
  - Documented cognitive failure on formal testing
- Psychomotor retardation with sensation of extreme fatigue
- Neurological abnormalities
  - From slurred speech to frank dysarthria
  - From decreased muscular tone to completely bed bound
- Absence of delusions, misconceptions, and hallucinations
- Absence of agitation
- Absence of metabolic, infection, hematologic, cardiopulmonary, or other disorders explaining the delirium
- Medication unlikely to be the cause of the delirium

asked to assist when attempts to wean off of dexmedetomidine proves to be challenging, especially in the context of a patient having a psychiatric comorbidity that may contribute to a patient's presentation.

Patients with a previous psychiatric history on their medical chart tend to cloud the clinical picture when agitation and restlessness continue despite the primary medical team determining the source of the delirium has resolved or is improving. A quick assessment may lead a clinician to assume that an underlying psychiatric condition is worsening the current presenting symptoms or is starting to present itself now the physical ailment is "improving." Although this can occur, the fact remains that the patient is still recovering from a serious physical illness or trauma, and the body's attempt to achieve homeostasis can be complicated by physiological responses to stress.[12,13] A patient's source of agitation can be associated with an imbalance in the autonomic nervous system, which may lead to an increase in sympathetic activity, termed paroxysmal sympathetic hyperactivity. PSH has been defined as "a syndrome, recognized in a subgroup of survivors of severe acquired brain injury, of simultaneous, paroxysmal transient increases in sympathetic (elevated heart rate, blood pressure, respiratory rate, temperature, sweating) and motor (posturing) activity.[14] Anoxic brain injury or a low volume state may precipitate this sequela as well. PSH has been suspected in various literature to be involved in the mechanism of post-traumatic agitation. As the patient's condition continues to improve, the need to extubate becomes a priority in the patient's recovery. However, the transition from propofol or dexmedetomidine may be challenging depending on the patient's clinical circumstances. Medications such as Seroquel, Haldol, benzodiazepines, and clonidine have been supported in much of the evidence-based literature to help with agitation. Each pharmacologic option carries a risk and the possibility of being ineffective in decreasing the incidence of agitation and/or need of physical restraints.

Second generation antipsychotics have been used to assist in agitation. Quetiapine (Seroquel), typically used for psychotic and mood disorders like schizophrenia and bipolar, at low doses, has a strong affinity for anti-histamine receptors, which contribute to initiating sedation. In addition, quetiapine has alpha 1 blocking properties that can cause dizziness, sedation, and hypotension. It also has anticholinergic properties that can cause or worsen dry mouth, constipation, and sedation. These effects may not be desired with critical care patients, and the risk may not outweigh the benefit. Seroquel has been used off label for behavioral disturbances in dementias (Lewy body) and Parkinson's disease when the behavioral disturbances are primarily due to psychosis not due to delirium.

Haldol, which is a first generation antipsychotic medication, has long been used to address agitation. Haldol carries significant cardiovascular risk, which can require close cardiac monitoring for QTc prolongation with risk of an arrhythmia. Therefore, the traditional use of antipsychotics for agitation comes with fairly significant risk for patients in critical care settings. When deciding on medication management for agitation, identifying a precipitating cause will be helpful especially if there is an underlying psychiatric condition. Determining the risks and benefits of the aggressive use of antipsychotic medications can be challenging due to the difficult balance of treating severe emotional lability and aggressive behavior with the possibility of precipitating adverse effects such as hemodynamic instability.

Second generation antipsychotics' primary mechanism of action is dopamine blockage, which can help quickly alleviate a patient's agitation if due to a primary psychotic disorder such as schizophrenia, where the particular areas of the brain (mesolimbic area) are overwhelmed with dopamine, which can precipitate sensory disturbances such as auditory and visual hallucinations. These symptoms in turn can precipitate agitation and restlessness. In this case, the use of antipsychotics will prove to be beneficial and efficacious because of its dopamine blocking mechanism of action that is needed to address the very specific pathophysiology. If there is no underlying primary psychotic disorder, the use of a dopamine blocker is theorized to help the neurochemical imbalances in the prefrontal cortex and associated areas to assist with the ability to process information to hopefully achieve calmness and allow a patient to hopefully be verbally redirected. The sedation properties of varying antipsychotics are derived from antihistamine, anticholinergic, α_1 blocking properties and some specific 5HT receptor activation in the hypothalamus. This is a feature of psychopharmacology that can precipitate adverse effects and prescribing patterns in psychiatry aim to avoid oversedation.

The traditional use of antipsychotics may not meet the expectations of quelling an episode of agitation. Agitation may continue because the precipitating factor has not been identified. Alcohol withdrawal, primary psychosis, abrupt discontinuation of sedation medications, and even a patient's baseline personality issues all have different physiologic causes. If primary physiologic factor is not identified, the selected treatment may not provide the expected results.

In the situation where dexmedetomidine is used, agitation can mask the possibility of dexmedetomidine withdrawal. Dexmedetomidine withdrawal symptoms can be unresponsive to benzodiazepines or any of the antipsychotic medications administered.[14] Transitioning from dexmedetomidine to oral/enteral clonidine may be a safe and cost-effective way to continue sedation with a centrally acting α_2 agonist in patients who are hemodynamically stable and have a functional gastrointestinal tract (GI).[15] In a study by Gagnon and colleagues, clonidine doses of 0.3 mg every 6 h were found to be optimal to transition patients from higher dexmedetomidine rates of 1.0 µg/kg/h.[16] Starting doses of clonidine within their studied cohort were primarily 0.1 mg three times a day (TID) and titrated on a dose-by-dose basis dependent on hemodynamic response and sedation parameters. This may explain the increased time needed to transition patients on higher dexmedetomidine infusion rates to clonidine than those starting at lower dexmedetomidine infusion rates. Dexmedetomidine was weaned as soon as patients were responding to clonidine with appropriate RASS, CAM-ICU score, and hemodynamic changes. Once there is an acceptable level of agitation and the patient is appropriate to be stepped down to an appropriate level of care, low dose clonidine can be continued while assessing the need for any additional psychotropic medications that need to be restarted or started for the patient. It is well known that clonidine discontinuation reactions are common and sometimes severe. Sudden discontinuation can result in nervousness, agitation, headache, and tremor, with rapid rise in blood pressure. Therefore, a taper schedule is recommended. Generally, clonidine can be tapered over 2–4 days or longer to avoid rebound effects (nervousness, increased blood pressure). If administered with a beta blocker, stop the beta blocker first for several days before the gradual discontinuation of clonidine.[16] If clinically significant hypotension or bradycardia occurs, one can adjust hemodynamically active drugs (e.g., b-blockers, calcium channel blockers, or digoxin) or decrease the clonidine dose depending on the clinical situation. Clonidine tapering can generally be achieved within several days, following the use of clonidine as a primary sedative agent.[16]

Critical care patients have multiple sources where agitation and restlessness can derive from. Adverse outcomes that the critical care team addresses include self-extubation and unintentional removal of medical devices, post-traumatic stress, nosocomial infections, and increased economic and psychological burden for caregivers. For these reasons, it is vital to identify and manage effectively.

Post-ICU Neuropsychiatric Sequelae

In immediate post ICU care, patients can experience an exacerbation or new onset of psychiatric sequelae. Reactionary anxiety and depressed mood are frequent after ICU stays, and may be mixed with symptoms of PTSD, which can include fear, feelings of horror, helplessness, avoidance, neuro-vegetative symptoms, and intrusive thoughts. This may be a normal variant due to the circumstances and reasonable in the context of a patient's worry post ICU care. As the patient recovers in the same hospitalization, any new onset of psychiatric symptoms disrupting care should be appropriately evaluated before quickly determining that the patient is suffering from a new diagnosis of a mental health disorder. At times, a patient's reactionary and anticipatory anxiety and associated sad mood and affect are appropriate and supportive interviewing, empathy, and validation are needed more so than aggressive initiation of psychotropic medication.

Patients who were admitted to the ICU when followed after critical stay can be found to be experiencing a number of neuropsychiatric long-term effects. The COVID-19 pandemic showed that patients in the ICU with ARDS and severe illness experienced mild cognitive impairment that can present as psychiatric symptoms of depressed mood, low every, sleep disturbance, poor concentration, and an associated low tolerance of frustration. The COVID-19 pandemic may likely follow or worsen this trend in regards to cognitive functioning for patients admitted to the ICU with COVID-19 and patients may feel the virus' effects for years to come.

Patients who have recovered from pandemic illness or crisis events have reported experiences with a wide range of psychiatric issues, including PTSD, depression, insomnia, anxiety, and even suicide. A significant risk factor for these patients was the presence of premorbid psychiatric illnesses. Mental health symptoms causing disruption in activities of daily living become concerning and no longer can be considered a reactionary mood or anxiety response to the traumatic event and hospitalization. Psychotropic medications should be continued (where possible) or restarted in patients with preexisting psychiatric conditions. Medication selection should be based upon the existing guidelines associated with the various psychiatric illnesses.

CARE FOR HEALTH CARE WORKERS DURING CRISIS

The COVID-19 pandemic has affected our health care workers in how they view taking care of patients. Traditionally, patient centered care has been the priority. The extent of the COVID-19 pandemic has added more complexity to that single priority. Medical providers have now highlighted the need to address the common good; assessing the risks and benefits to society as a whole, rather than on a single patient. An intensive care unit team member who is accustomed to caring for a certain number of patients may need to take on more because it is a public health crisis. As a crisis continues, health care providers are being asked to work extra shifts as colleagues fall ill, or become exhausted or overwhelmed. The need to treat the increasing number of actively ill patients in an appropriate time adds more stress and anxiety to all members of the care team. The topic of burnout in the health care setting has long been discussed and studied. Health care workers have the expectation to work hard and maintain ideals about providing the best care possible. Burnout in health care is often used to describe the effects of the ongoing stress among health care workers battling the crisis. Mental health experts have recently begun to transition to calling it moral trauma as a more descriptive term. This moral trauma can be so long-lasting and pervasive that it becomes moral injury.[18,19]

In traumatic or unusually stressful circumstances, people may perpetrate, fail to prevent, or witness events that contradict deeply held moral beliefs and expectations. What the COVID-19 pandemic has shown us is that when health care providers have to launch a "crisis standard" of care, they are forced to make difficult decisions in the allocation of resources

(PPE, staffing, and available care space), which magnified and challenged members of a critical care team in how to care for critically ill patients. Health care providers, altruistically, tend to be more concerned with not being able to meet patient care needs at the expense of their own well-being and self-care.[17] Being constantly inundated with difficult decisions on how to distribute health care resources that ultimately affect the quality of a patient's life or the extent of the patient's illness can be traumatic for a health care provider. This can lead to burnout or moral injury. Individuals of the care team may also experience betrayal from leadership, others in positions of power, or peers that can also result in adverse outcomes. Moral injury is the distressing psychological, behavioral, social, and sometimes spiritual aftermath of exposure to such events. A moral injury can occur in response to acting or witnessing behaviors that go against an individual's values and moral beliefs. Many of the past health care crises, and now especially the COVID-19 pandemic, have brought this to the forefront. A preventive psychological approach to support staff at risk of moral injury is suggested.[20] The World Health Organization (WHO) has provided mental health and psychosocial considerations during the COVID-19 pandemic, but it can be applied to all types of crises. Each hospital system has tailored a "psychological first aid" for their providers and especially those in the critical care settings. Interventions can include reinforcing social bonds between colleagues and supervisors, meeting basic staff needs, being alert to early signs of distress, and avoiding "medicalization" of uncomfortable responses to trauma. The following has been suggested for critical care team leaders by the WHO:

- Adjusting staffing by partnering inexperienced workers with more experienced colleagues, who can provide support, monitor stress, and reinforce safety practices.
- Offer access to psychosocial support. Providing specific staff in the critical care setting with access to sources of psychosocial support.
- Regular monitoring and review of staff member well-being to identify risks and emerging issues and adaptively respond to their needs.
- Create an environment of open communication by encouraging staff to speak openly about their concerns. Provide brief, regular forums to update staff on the status of the practice and how management is addressing challenges.

The COVID-19 pandemic has put great stress on the health care system in a way that has not been experienced in decades. From public health preparedness to the structure and efficiency of our medical facilities, it all has precipitated immense stress not only for the patients but the medical providers working to hold up the health care system. A mindful approach to mental health comorbidities during a pandemic with lessons learned from the past can provide guidance. Mental health services play a vital role in treating patients, family members, first responders, and health care professionals.[21]

The impact of any disaster or crisis can have lasting effects for many years. PTSD, depression, anxiety, and other disorders remain among post-9/11 first responders and many others nearly 20 years after the devastating event. The community that dealt with post-Katrina effects experienced lack of medications, medical care, safety, and bereavement that acted as the main stress predictors for PTSD, psychological distress, and physical symptoms. The belief that an individual's life was in danger continued to predict PTSD at 12 years after the disaster. Both 9/11 and Hurricane Katrina were comparatively shorter in duration to the COVID-19 pandemic, but all these disastrous events have had long-term health consequences. Learning from past disasters, health care systems need to minimize any lapses in services for both physical and mental health care. Psychiatrists and other mental health professionals prepare for the short-term and long-term management of patients and others affected by crisis. Psychiatry has faced unusual tasks during the COVID-19 pandemic, with increasing distress among our society that has led to increasing rates of depression, anxiety, and other mental health conditions not only in their patients but in their colleagues who have been on the front lines. This trend will likely continue, and in the critical setting close collaboration between critical care providers and mental health professionals will be needed to provide optimal care for all those involved.

▌ REFERENCES

1. Guidelines for the Prevention and Management of Pain, Agitation/Sedation, Delirium, Immobility, and Sleep Disruption in Adult Patients in the ICU. *Crit Care Med*. 2018;46(9):e825-e873.

2. Kim MC, Fricchione GL, Akeju O. Accidental awareness under general anaesthesia: Incidence, risk factors, and psychological management. *BJA Education*. 202121:154-161.

3. Woods JC, Mion LC, Connor JT, et al. Severe agitation among ventilated medical intensive care unit patients: Frequency, characteristics and outcomes. *Intensive Care Med*. 2004;30(6):1066-1072.

4. Mitchell PB. Therapeutic drug monitoring of psychotropic medications. *Br J Clin Pharmacol*. 2000;49(4):303-312.

5. Francescangeli J, Karamchandani K, Powell M, Bonavia A. The serotonin syndrome: From molecular mechanisms to clinical practice. *Int J Mol Sci.* 2019;20(9):2288.

6. Jaber S, Chanques G, Altairac C, et al. A prospective study of agitation in a medical-surgical ICU: Incidence, risk factors, and outcomes. *Chest.* 2005;128(4):2749-2757.

7. Skrobik Y, Ahern S, Leblanc M, et al. Protocolized intensive care unit management of analgesia, sedation, and delirium improves analgesia and subsyndromal delirium rates. *Anesth Analg.* 2010;111(2):451-463.

8. Hosker C, Ward D. Hypoactive delirium. *BMJ.* 2017;357:j2047.

9. Strom T, Stylsvig M, Toft P. Long-term psychological effects of a no-sedation protocol in critically ill patients. *Crit Care.* 2011;15(6):R293.

10. Barr J, Fraser GL, Puntillo K, et al. Clinical practice guidelines for the management of pain, agitation, and delirium in adult patients in the intensive care unit. *Crit Care Med.* 2013;41(1):263-306.

11. Lonardo NW, Mone MC, Nirula R, et al. Propofol is associated with favorable outcomes compared with benzodiazepines in ventilated intensive care unit patients. *Am J Respir Crit Care Med.* 2014;189(11):1383-1394.

12. Hall RI, Sandham D, Cardinal P, et al. Clinical investigations in critical care. Propofol vs midazolam for ICU sedation: A Canadian multicenter randomized trial. *Chest.* 2001;119:1151-1159.

13. Glaess SS, Attridge RL, Christina Gutierrez G. Clonidine as a strategy for discontinuing dexmedetomidine sedation in critically ill patients: A narrative review. *Am J Health Syst Pharm.* 2020;77(7):515-522.

14. Hughes JD, Rabinstein AA. Early diagnosis of paroxysmal sympathetic hyperactivity in the ICU. *Neurocrit Care.* 2014;20(3):454-459.

15. Terry K, Blum R, Szumita P. Evaluating the transition from dexmedetomidine to clonidine for agitation management in the intensive care unit. *SAGE Open Med.* 2015;3. doi: 10.1177/2050312115621767.

16. Gagnon DJ, Riker RR, Glisic EK, et al. Transition from dexmedetomidine to enteral clonidine for ICU sedation: An observational pilot study. *Pharmacotherapy.* 2015;35(3):251-259.

17. Czerwonka AI, Herridge MS, Chan L, et al. Changing support needs of survivors of complex critical illness and their family caregivers across the care continuum: A qualitative pilot study of towards RECOVER. *J Crit Care.* 2015;30(2):242-249.

18. Karnatovskaia LV, Johnson MM, Benzo RP, et al. The spectrum of psychocognitive morbidity in the critically ill: A review of the literature and call for improvement. *J Crit Care.* 2015;30(1):130-137.

19. Litz BT, Stein N, Delaney E, et al. Moral injury and moral repair in war Veterans: A preliminary model and intervention strategy. *Clin Psychol Rev.* 2009;29(8):695-706.

20. Shay J. Moral injury. *Psychoanalytic Psychology.* 2014;31(2):182-191.

21. Griffin BJ, Purcell N, Burkman K, et al. Moral injury: An integrative review. *J Trauma Stress.* 2019;32(3):350-362.

16 CHILDREN'S MENTAL HEALTH ISSUES IN CRITICAL CARE

Aurora Tompar Tiu, MD

▌ INTRODUCTION

Early detection and intervention of emerging psychiatric comorbidity in serious medical illness is as important as saving the life of a child in critical care. Anxiety disorders, PTSD, and depressive disorders are among the common psychiatric comorbidity that can develop in hospitalized patients or children of hospitalized patients.[1,2] Delay or failure in identifying the psychiatric disorders and giving prompt intervention may result in poor treatment outcome and delay in recovery because of possible poor compliance, refusal of treatment, and exaggeration of symptoms. Prevention of deterioration of psychiatric disorder and/or exacerbation of pre-existing mental disorders is a challenge but can be achieved by careful assessment and a comprehensive treatment plan. Any serious or life-threatening medical illness is a crisis in a child's life and family. It can disrupt the child's total growth and development—physical, emotional, intellectual, social, and spiritual. The severity and the nature of impact of serious medical illness in children may depend on multiple vulnerability factors that include separation from parents or primary caregiver, developmental age or problems/delay, pre-existing mental disorders, having special needs (e.g., autism, Down syndrome), educational problems (e.g., poor grades, drop-outs), financial difficulties in the family, divorce or separation of parents, parental health, and psychopathology. Several studies indicated that the most common mental disorders in children critical illness survivors were post-traumatic stress disorder (PTSD) (10–28%) and major depression (7–13%).[3] The current COVID-19 pandemic with the emerging multisystem inflammatory syndrome in children (MIS-C)[4] is expected to increase the prevalence of anxiety and depressive disorders in children in critical care. Stressors like separation from the family and friends, fear and worry about COVID-19 infection, feelings of helplessness, loneliness and boredom, history of violence and child abuse, neglect, and deprivation increase financial problems in the family. Loss of learning time and space for play in school lockdown will predispose children to more psychiatric disorders including risk of suicide, psychotic disorders, and drug and alcohol abuse in adolescents. Using the biopsychosocial model with cultural and spiritual considerations in the intervention of psychiatric comorbidity in children in critical care is essential to ensure effective treatment outcome and prompt recovery. Early collaboration with family or primary caregiver, child psychiatrist, psychologist, therapist, social worker, school counselor, as well as spiritual advisers in the initial, subsequent, and discharge treatment planning or as the need arises will have better prognosis of psychiatric comorbidity and help prevent life-time impairments and disabilities. The presence and active participation of the mother or her surrogate or significant caregiver in a child's critical care is a positive and protective factor against the development of psychiatric comorbidity in a child with serious medical illness. Children who are resilient can have positive adaptation despite significant traumatic experiences or adversity. Having a nurturing family relationship with responsive and warm supportive parenting promotes resilience in children and is essential in the prompt and complete recovery of children with life-threatening illnesses and in the prevention of psychiatric comorbidity.

CLINICAL PRESENTATION

Anxiety Disorder

Anxiety disorder is the most common of all psychiatric disorders of children and adolescents with lifetime prevalence (estimated) of 15% to 20% (Table 16-1). In children with medical illnesses, the prevalence of anxiety disorder is 20% to 35%.[2] Anxiety is anticipation of future threat, but fear is the emotional response to real or perceived imminent threat.[5] Anxiety is the emotional, physiological, behavioral, and cognitive responses to a real or imagined threat that occurs in the future.[6] Fear and anxiety can be adaptive emotions that will help prepare for future challenges and are often transitory in nature. Anxiety disorders develop when anxiety is

Table 16-1 CLINICAL DIAGNOSTIC FEATURES OF ANXIETY DISORDER[5]

1. Anxiety is excessive or persistent with disturbance in behavior
2. Accompanied by physical symptoms usually referring to specific organs (e.g., shortness of breath, palpitations) and autonomic nervous system
3. Symptoms impair functioning
4. Not due to medical disorders, other psychiatric disorders, and drug abuse

excessive and causes psychic distress, impairment of function, and persistence "beyond developmentally appropriate periods." Physical signs and symptoms of anxiety include stomachache, "butterflies" in stomach, headache, dizziness, paresthesia, hyperventilation, diarrhea, faintness, nausea, vomiting, anorexia, muscle tension, palpitation, urinary frequency, flushing, dyspnea, and chest pain or tightness of chest. Children in critical care experience more anxiety because of exposure to a new, unfamiliar environment with strangers, perceived and real danger to self, uncomfortable and painful procedures, separation from family and friends, the uncertainty about their illness and future, and fear of death. Genetic, environmental, and sociocultural factors play a significant role in the development of anxiety disorders.

Separation Anxiety Disorder

Separation anxiety is a part of normal development of a child starting around eight months of age and usually diminishes toward the second year. Separation anxiety disorder is the most common anxiety disorder in children below age 12. It is a persistent, developmentally inappropriate, and excessive anxiety or distress concerning separation from a significant attachment figure or caretaker or from home.[5] Children with separation anxiety disorder have excessive worry about losing their significant figures or possible injury to them. They worry about being injured or becoming ill themselves or being kidnapped or having an accident that will separate them from the attachment figure. In a critical care setting, they have clinging behavior, are more distressed when the mother or the primary caregiver is not available, and repeatedly seek reassurance and frequent attention. They may refuse to go to school or sleep alone and may have somatic symptoms and nightmares regarding separation. Separation anxiety disorder decreases in prevalence from childhood through adolescence. It usually presents after serious illness of the child or a parent or injury or death of parent or significant caregiver and other traumatic events in the child's life. Separation anxiety disorder causes significant impairment in educational, social, and other areas of functioning. If hospitalization is prolonged, allow the child to have their favorite toy and put pictures of family and friends in the room.

Panic Disorder

Panic disorder is defined by having experienced unexpected and recurrent panic attacks with no clear, identifiable precipitant (diagnostic and statistical manual of mental disorders fifth edition [DSM-5]). Panic attack is a sudden feeling of extreme fear or discomfort reaching peak about 10 to

15 minutes, usually accompanied by somatic symptoms such as sweating, palpitations, shortness of breath, chest pain, nausea, abnormal distress, feelings of choking, dizziness, fear of dying, losing control or going crazy, and paresthesia (e.g., tingling and numbing sensation) and dissociative symptoms. Panic disorder causes impairment of social, emotional, and academic functions and other significant functions and is not diagnosed if the symptoms of panic attacks are due to physiological presentation of medical conditions like hyperthyroidism, seizure disorders, and cardiopulmonary condition.

Generalized Anxiety Disorder (GAD)

GAD is excessive and persistent anxiety or impairing worry about several ordinary activities or events lasting for 6 months.[5] Anxiety about anticipated dangerous situations like possible COVID-19 infection of family members, storms, and school or sports performance is common. Admission in critical care with possible threat to self together with isolation and loneliness aggravate GAD. Associated symptoms of GAD are insomnia, apprehension, poor concentration, irritability, restlessness, and physical symptoms like headache and muscle tension. There is psychosocial and academic impairment of functions in GAD, and disturbance is not due to physiologic effects of medical conditions and drug abuse. Panic disorder and depressive disorders are common comorbidities of GAD.

Phobia

Simple phobias are marked fears circumscribed to the presence of specific objects (e.g., animals, insects, spiders, needles, and blood) or situations (heights, flying, water, storms, blood drawing and infusion).[5] The phobic stimulus that would provoke extreme anxiety often is actively avoided. Phobia is usually out of proportion to the actual danger to the specific object or situation. It causes significant impairment in psychosocial and other areas of functioning. It is not due to other mental disorders or traumatic events. In children, the marked fear may be manifested by tantrums, clinging behaviors, crying, and freezing.[5] In critical care, the most common phobia is fear of injections, blood, and needles, which is often manifested by vasovagal fainting or almost fainting response. In the current COVID-19 pandemic, a new phobia called "corona phobia" was reported. It is an excessive fear of being infected by COVID-19 that results to refusal to go out of the home or go to school or work. Simple phobia usually has comorbidity that include other anxiety disorders and depressive disorders.

Social Anxiety Disorder

Social anxiety disorder usually starts at age 8–15 years (DSM-5). It may be precipitated by stressful events or humiliating situations like being a victim of bullying. It is manifested as intense anxiety or fear of social situations in which there is possible observation by others with negative evaluation especially during performance. Children with Social anxiety disorder may have tantrums, crying episodes, clinging behavior, or difficulty in speaking when placed in the feared social situation, which is usually avoided. Some other children with Social anxiety disorder refuse urinating in public bathrooms when others are around. This refusal is called paruresis or "shy bladder syndrome."[5] In critical care, the nurses may have problems handling this type of patient and may need extra support from the primary caregiver or parent.

Selective Mutism

Selective mutism frequently starts before age 5 years old. Children with selective mutism refuse to speak in some situations (e.g., hospital settings or in front of strangers) but will speak at home or with close family members and friends.[5] The refusal to speak is not due to communication disorder, autism, or psychotic disorder. In critical care, selective mutism becomes a barrier in identification of locations and severity of pain especially in younger children who may refuse to speak to a stranger (e.g., nurse). Close collaboration with the parents or significant caregiver will encourage the child to cooperate and to communicate through gestures or writing or drawing. Separation anxiety disorder and panic disorder are common comorbidities of selective mutism.

Agoraphobia

Agoraphobia is an intense anxiety or fear precipitated by exposure to anticipated or real situations like enclosed places (e.g., movie houses, buses, trains), open spaces (e.g., bridges), crowds, or being away from home alone.[5] These situations are avoided due to marked fear that escape might not be possible, or help may not be available when panic-like symptoms or humiliating symptoms occur.[5] The intense anxiety or avoidance is usually out of proportion to the real danger posed by the feared situation. Panic disorder is the most common comorbidity. Children with agoraphobia will have marked anxiety when undergoing diagnostic work up like MRI or CT and may refuse to cooperate with the procedures. "Dry-run" with the procedure showing the MRI machine and explaining the purpose in cooperation with the parent or caregiver helps minimize the fear.

Intervention of Pediatric Anxiety Disorders

The first important challenge in critical care is to minimize or prevent occurrence or exacerbation of anxiety disorders in children. Patients and their families are reassured of their safety and that appropriate safety precautions are implemented to prevent hospital acquired infection like COVID-19 considering the current COVID-19 pandemic. Early detection of signs and symptoms of anxiety disorder help facilitate early intervention with appropriate treatment. Prompt consultation with a consult-liaison child psychiatrist is necessary so that further evaluation is done and treatment recommendation is implemented. Cognitive behavioral therapy (CBT) is considered the first-line treatment for anxiety disorder in children.[7] CBT is based on the principle that "how we think and act both affect how we feel." Patients and their families receive psychoeducation about anxiety as part of CBT. The most effective pharmacologic treatments for pediatric anxiety disorder are selective serotonin reuptake inhibitors (SSRIs)[7] (Table 16-2). A combination of SSRI and CBT is considered the best treatment option in children with severe and impairing anxiety disorder with less exacerbation of symptoms and relapse.[6] Close collaboration with parents or significant caregiver, therapist, social worker, school counselor, or spiritual advisor as the need arrives will help promote the best treatment outcome of anxiety disorders in children in critical care.

Post-traumatic Stress Disorder (PTSD)

PTSD is a syndrome that occurs after exposure to life-threatening or traumatic events like severe injury, serious medical illness (e.g., cancer), and sexual violence. The exposure could be directly experiencing the life-threatening event, witnessing the traumatic event in another person as it happened, or learning that the life-threatening event happened to a parent, significant caregiver, close sibling, or friend.[5] The symptoms of PTSD include re-experiencing the traumatic event and in children, reenactment of trauma, specifically in play. Symptoms seen in children include avoidance of specific situations relating the traumatic event, presence of negative changes of mood and cognitions manifested by social withdrawal, decreased participation in important activities or decrease in play activities, and intrusion symptoms such as dreams and nightmares. Hyperarousal symptoms such as hypervigilance, irritability, self-destructive behavior, poor concentration, startle response exaggeration, and disturbance in sleep are also the common symptoms of PTSD. PTSD may occur within three months after the traumatic event or could be delayed. Dissociative symptoms and reactions (e.g., flashbacks) may

Table 16-2 MEDICATIONS USED TO TREAT PEDIATRIC ANXIETY DISORDER		
Class	Medication (Brand name)	Common dose range (mg/day)
SSRI	Citalopram/escitalopram (Celexa/Lexapro)	10/5–40/20
	Fluvoxamine (Luvox, Luvox CR)	100–300
	Sertraline (Zoloft)	25–200
	Fluoxetine (Prozac, Sarafem)	10–60
	Paroxetine (Paxil, Pexeva)	10–50
SNRI	Venlafaxine ER (Effexor)	37.5–225
	Duloxetine (Cymbalta)	30–120
	Atomoxetine (Strattera)	10–100
Tricyclic antidepressant	Clomipramine (Anafranil)	75–250
	Imipramine (Tofranil, Tofranil-PM)	
Benzodiazepine	Alprazolam (Xanax, Alprazolam Intensol)	0.5–1.5
	Clonazepam (Klonopin)	0.5–3
	Lorazepam (Ativan, Lorazepam Intensol)	1–2

also occur in PTSD. Duration of PTSD disturbance is more than one month. Acute stress disorder has the same symptoms and manifestations as PTSD after exposure to life-threatening or traumatic events, but disturbance duration is shorter, lasting three days to one month after exposure to traumatic events.[5]

Intervention of PTSD

Occurrence of PTSD during and after critical care in children with serious medical illness is common. Early detection of the signs and symptoms of PTSD requires prompt referral to a child psychiatrist and therapist for further evaluation and treatment recommendation. Trauma-focused cognitive behavior therapy (TF-CBT) is considered the first line of intervention for pediatric PTSD. So far, no strong evidence of the efficacy of SSRIs in PTSD in children has been reported, but they can be used with comorbidity of anxiety and depressive disorders that usually occur with PTSD.[6] In the current COVID-19 pandemic, children in critical care may have pre-existing PTSD before admission to critical care due to death of a family member or significant caregiver with COVID-19 infection. Exacerbations of pre-existing PTSD symptoms may occur in critical care. Psychoeducation and supportive therapy for the patient and their family will help facilitate optimum treatment outcome.

Major Depressive Disorder

One of the most common psychiatric comorbidities in serious medical illness is major depressive disorder.[1] It can occur during critical care or after critical care of the serious medical illness. Pre-existing major depressive disorder may be exacerbated in critical care. Clinical diagnostic criteria include the following:[5]

1. Irritable mood in children and adolescents, or depressive mood present for two weeks with loss of interest in pleasurable activities
2. Vegetative symptoms—low or increased appetite, low or increased weight, insomnia or hypersomnia, and fatigue
3. Poor concentration and decreased attention, cognitive dysfunctions, feeling of worthlessness and guilt, and poor behavioral performance
4. Suicidal ideations or attempts
5. Psychotic symptoms in severe major depressive disorder with delusion and paranoia with suspiciousness and ideas of reference
6. Symptoms are not due to medical disorder, other psychiatric disorders (e.g., schizophrenia), and drug abuse
7. Symptoms impair functioning including academic and social functions

Intervention of Major Depressive Disorder

Prevention of suicide is the first important task to be implemented in patients with major depressive disorder. Suicidal ideations and attempts as well as psychotic symptoms should be monitored. Urgent referral to consult liaison child psychiatrist for further evaluation and treatment

Table 16-3 MEDICATIONS USED FOR PEDIATRIC DEPRESSION AND ANXIETY		
	Starting dose (mg/d)	Typical dose range (mg/d)
Selective serotonin reuptake inhibitors		
Citalopram	10 to 20	20 to 40
Escitalopram	5 to 10	10 to 40
Fluoxetine	10 to 20	20 to 80
Fluvoxamine	25 to 50	50 to 300
Paroxetine	10 to 20	20 to 60
Sertaline	25 to 50	100 to 200
Serotonin-norepinephrine reuptake inhibitors		
Venlafaxine	37.5	150 to 225
Duloxetine	30	40 to 60
Desvenlafaxine	25	25 to 45
Atypical antidepressants		
Bupropion	75 to 100	100 to 300
Mirtazapine	7.5 to 15	15 to 45
Vortioxetine	5	5 to 20

recommendation is essential to prevent suicide and exacerbation of symptoms. For mild depressive disorder, psychotherapy is the first line of intervention. Antidepressant medications (see Table 16-3) are given to moderate and severe patients with or without psychotic features together with psychotherapy and supportive therapy to patients and their families. Antipsychotic medication like olanzapine is added to SSRIs along with psychotherapy in the treatment of severe major depression with psychotic features.

Bipolar Disorder

Pediatric bipolar disorder, like other psychiatric comorbidities in serious medical illness in critical care, disrupts the child's total growth and development. It increases the risk of suicide attempts, psychosis, dangerous risk-taking behavior, drug abuse, as well as impairment of academic and psychosocial functioning. Bipolar disorder has distinct depressive and manic (type I) or hypomanic episodes (type II). Clinical diagnostic criteria of manic episodes include the following:[5]

1. Distinct behavior with elevated or expansive mood and increases goal-directed energy lasting for at least one week
2. Mood disturbances include irritability, mood lability, and grandiosity
3. Cognitive disturbances include destructibility, flight of ideas, racing thoughts, poor judgement, and distractibility
4. Increased sexual and destructive activities with possible painful and harmful consequences
5. Symptoms impair functioning (e.g., academic and psychosocial)
6. Symptoms are not due to medical conditions, other psychiatric disorders, and drug abuse

Hypomanic symptoms are like manic episodes but less severe with shorter duration (four days) with less severe impairment of psychosocial and academic functions. Symptoms of pre-existing bipolar disorder may exacerbate in critical care. Manic and hypomanic episodes may be precipitated with the use of SSRIs for depressive and anxiety disorder.

Intervention of Bipolar Disorder

Mood stabilizers (e.g., lithium, Depakote, carbamazepine) and atypical antipsychotics (e.g., Abilify and Zyprexa) are used in the acute treatment of manic and hypomanic episodes. Bupropion together with mood stabilizers or atypical antipsychotics are used in depressive episodes. SSRI medication without current concomitant use of mood stabilizers may trigger manic and hypomanic episodes. Supportive psychotherapy and psychoeducation for patients and their families are important for bipolar disorder intervention. Consultations with a consult liaison child psychiatrist and therapist will be necessary for further evaluation and treatment recommendation for bipolar disorder in children.

Adjustment Disorder

Adjustment disorder is a response to an identifiable stressor manifested with depressed or anxious mood as well as behavior and somatic disturbances. It is "wholly situational" and will eventually resolve when the stressors are resolved and positive adaptation to the stressful situation has been demonstrated.[5] The onset of serious medical illness may trigger to the development of adjustment disorder, which will eventually resolve once the medical illness is completely treated. Reassurance of safety, competence of doctors and nurses, and appropriate treatment of medical illness will help promote prompt resolution of adjustment disorder in critical care. Brief supportive therapy and psychoeducation are essential for complete resolution of the symptoms of adjustment disorder.

Psychotic Disorders in Children

Psychotic disorders in children are not common but may occur or be precipitated in critical care. Symptoms of psychotic disorder include disorganized and gross disturbance of behavior and thinking with disorganized speech and display of inappropriate affect.[5] Hallucinations (audible, visual, and tactile) and delusions are common symptoms with impaired reality testing reported in psychotic disorder. Psychotic disorders in children are reported to be more severe and devastating to the patient and family. Hostility and aggression may accompany psychotic disorders. Pediatric psychotic disorders can be functional or organic.[8] Schizophrenia and related disorders, and psychotic symptoms in affective disorders (major depression and bipolar disorder) are functional psychotic syndromes. Organic psychosis could be due to central nervous system lesions in different medical conditions, trauma, and substance abuse disorders. Recently, synthetic (laboratory made analog of tetrahydrocannabinol) cannabinoids, known as "spice," "K2," and "Black Mamba" are used by adolescents who develop psychotic symptoms with delusions, hallucinations, and other neuropsychiatric symptoms including seizure.[9] Common antipsychotic medications used in children include Risperidone (starting dose 0.5–2 mg/day, range 1–6 mg/day), Quetiapine (starting dose 2.5–5 mg/day, range 5–20 mg/day), and Aripiprazole (starting dose 2–5 mg/day, range 5–30 mg/day).[10] Regular monitoring of adverse side effects of antipsychotic medications, such as metabolic syndrome (high triglycerides, elevated fasting blood sugar, increased blood pressure, large weight) and weight gain, is necessary. Evaluation of psychotic symptoms and immediate intervention of psychotic disorders will prevent or decrease aggression with possible harm to self and others. Appropriate treatment with antipsychotic medication, considered first-line treatment for psychosis,[10] in consultation with a consult liaison child psychiatrist, will decrease the negative impact of psychiatric disorders in the child and improve treatment outcome.

REFERENCES

1. Glazer JP, Pao M, Sclionfield DJ. Life-threatening illnesses, palliative care, and bereavement. In: Martin A, Block MH, Volkman F, eds. *Lewis's Child and Adolescent Psychiatry*. 5th ed. Philadelphia, PA: Wolters Kluwer; 2018:946-956.

2. Pao M, Boslc A. Anxiety in medically ill children/adolescent. *Depress Anxiety*. 2011;28:40-49.

3. Daugdow D. Richardson L, Zatzick D, et al. Psychiatric morbidity in critical illness survivors: A comprehensive review of the literature. *Arch Pediatric Adolescent Med*. 2010;164(4):377-385.

4. Clark E, Shandera W. Viral and richettsial infections. In: Papadakils M, McPhee S, eds. *Current Medical Diagnoses and Treatment*. 60th ed. New York, NY: McGraw Hill; 2021:1455.

5. American Psychiatric Association. *Diagnostic and Statistical Manual of Mental Disorders*. 5th ed. Arlington, VA: American Psychiatric Association; 2013.

6. Taylor J, Lebrowitz E, Silverman W. Anxiety disorders. In: Martin A, Block MH, Volkmar F, eds. *Lewis's Child and Adolescent Psychiatry*. 5th ed. Philadelphia, PA: Wolters Kluwer; 2018:509-518.

7. Walkup JT, Albano AM, Piacentini J, et al. Cognitive behavioral therapy, sertraline or a combination in childhood anxiety. *N Engl J Med*. 2008;359(26):2753-2766.

8. Prince J, Wilens T, Biederman J, et al. Psychopharmacology in children and adolescents. In: Stern T, FricChione G, Cassen N, et al., eds. *Handbook of General Hospital Psychiatry*. 5th ed. Mosby, Inc.; 2014:441-445.

9. Pintori N, Loi B, Mereu M. Synthetic cannabinoids: The hidden side of spice drugs. *Behavioral Pharmacology*. 2017;28(6):4-19.

10. Block MH, Beyer C, Scahill L, et al. Antipsychotics. In: Martin A, Block MH, Volkman F, eds. *Lewis's Child and Adolescent Psychiatry*. 5th ed. Philadelphia, PA: Wolters Kluwer; 2018:733-744.

17 TREATING CRITICALLY ILL PEDIATRIC PATIENTS

Reut Kassif Lerner, MD, Oshri Zaulan, MD and
Itai M. Pessach, MD, PHD, MPH, MHA

▌ KIDS ARE NOT SMALL ADULTS, EVEN DURING CRISIS

Some of the most basic instincts of any biological group is the need to protect the progeny in time of peril. Most human cultures see the care for children as one of the highest values. As children have distinctive biological, physiological, psychological, and developmental attributes, it is crucial that pediatric needs are incorporated into every facet of disaster, mass casualties, and preparedness planning. Furthermore, emergency responders, medical professionals, and health care entities may not always have adequate pediatric-adjusted resources, training, equipment, or facilities available, and therefore preparedness must include the ability to provide the special expertise and training that ensure optimal care of children.[1]

Children exhibit significantly higher rates of mortality during disasters as compared to the adult population. This trend probability increases further for children under five years of age.[2]

Part of the reason for this observation rests in the different physiological makeup of children. Children are smaller in size and therefore, absorb higher impact from external forces that are generated during a disaster. Their organs are proportionately larger, closer together, and not as well-protected as are adult organs, further rendering them at greater risk for traumatic injuries. Fluid and electrolyte balance may be difficult to maintain in young children, and they have less circulatory reserve due to smaller circulating volumes. Therefore, young children are at greater risk for severe dehydration and circulatory collapse when exposed to diarrhea, vomiting, hypovolemia, or blood loss. Children also metabolize drugs differently, thereby requiring varying dosages of drugs, antidotes, and specialized equipment for medication administration. Their increased body surface area-to-mass ratio and decreased subcutaneous tissue make them more vulnerable to hypothermia. Furthermore, children are more susceptible to the effects of radiation exposure and require a more vigorous medical response in these occasions.[3]

The biological response to various infectious pathogens may be significantly different in children than that of adults, resulting in a significantly different immunologic response, clinical presentation, or treatment requirement. Their decreased herd immunity also makes them more susceptible to many infectious agents.

Children have a higher metabolic rate, faster heart rate, higher respiratory rate, and less subcutaneous tissue compared to adults. This increases their susceptibility to airborne chemicals and biological agents that may more readily and promptly be absorbed through children's skin or mucosal barriers and more rapidly spread throughout their circulatory system. Chemical agents with high vapor density that are heavier than air, including certain gases such as sarin and chlorine, settle close to the ground, in the "airspace" used by children.[1–3]

These unique pediatric traits are not always fully considered in planning and preparedness efforts and may not be sufficiently addressed during disaster response. This is especially true for the specific challenges such as biological, chemical, or nuclear threats.

▌PEDIATRIC SPECIFIC VULNERABILITIES IN DISASTERS AND MASS CASUALTY EVENTS

Children have unique psychosocial needs that increase their vulnerability in disasters. These vulnerabilities need to be accounted for in pediatric disaster planning. Depending on the age or developmental stage of a child, children may lack the ability to communicate or follow directions. Developmentally, young children are particularly vulnerable because of physical and mental limitations based on developmental milestones. Even if toddlers are able to walk, they may not have the cognitive ability to understand the presence of risk and therefore may not escape or be able to decide in which direction to flee. In the worst-case scenario, a young child may actually be attracted toward the event out of curiosity. Because young children depend on adults for sustenance, security, and socialization, they are among the most susceptible community members when catastrophes occur.[4]

Some of the basic daily needs of young children differ significantly from those of adults. The need for specific food, such as baby formula, specific medication and preparation (liquid emulsions), diapers, and various other needs may not be easily met during crisis situations.

Infants, toddlers, and young children lack the self-preservation and cognitive skills that enable them to appropriately react and may be unable to describe their symptoms or communicate their needs. They may be limited in their ability to recognize danger, escape, and seek assistance. The coping skills are less developed than are those of adults. Their psychological response is also related to their development and attenuated by their caregivers' responses. Children with special health care needs are exceptionally vulnerable.[5]

A child's mental health is affected not only by direct exposure to traumatic events but from indirect exposure as well. Psychological stress impedes growth and development patterns. The chaos associated with disaster events may invoke a crippling sense of fear or anxiety in children. Stress and anxiety are augmented in children when their parents suffer from similar psychological afflictions. Children may have a greater risk of developing post-traumatic stress disorders and other enduring behavioral disturbances. This is further amplified when children are separated from caregivers, either temporarily or permanently. Based on the psychological variations that children present in a disaster response, clinicians must plan on using age-appropriate treatment tactics.[2–5]

▌PEDIATRIC TRIAGE AND PEDIATRIC ILLNESS SEVERITY SCORING SYSTEMS

As in adults, pediatric triage and treatment during mass casualty is different from the routine triage and management of patients. While usual standards of care should be maintained as long as feasible, it is possible that the demand for treatment will significantly exceed the supply during crises. In such situations, the failure to plan and alter standards of care could result in excess deaths.[6]

"Crisis standards of care" (CSC) is a term established to describe the most extreme condition of a medical crisis when efforts fail to care for every patient. Scarce resources are allocated during CSC to those most likely to survive. In comparison to random allocation or first-come first-served selection, allocation of critical care resources to those patients who are likely to survive with brief and focused critical care support may improve overall outcomes. Resources may be triaged when they are initially allocated or they may be reallocated at future points in time. While patients are continually re-evaluated to determine whether they have sufficiently improved such that they no longer require critical care, they could also be re-evaluated at fixed periods of time or if their clinical status significantly deteriorates. Pediatric-specific resources are usually more limited and in lower availability and hence their allocation must be done carefully and most efficiently.[7]

Triage protocols can assist in distributing available resources impartially by prioritizing patients who are more likely to benefit from the limited critical care resources available. Although some patients may not receive all that they could possibly "benefit from," the use of a balanced, unbiased, and agreed upon triage tool assists in maintaining the ethical backbone of decision making. In some cases, children may be prioritized by these tools, depending on ethical and cultural considerations; however, most triage systems and tools have been developed for adult patients based on adult physiology and vital signs. Pediatric mass triage systems exist but are still in development and have been less rigorously tested than those designed for the general population. Furthermore, current literature does not provide validity for the use of triage tools on non-traumatic mass casualty events such as biologic or chemical exposures. Advanced training is required for triage officers to effectively implement the triage protocol. Pediatricians in the community can assist in both triage and treatment of patients.[7–10]

Multiple systems have been suggested as the guiding directive for critical care triage decisions in adult patients during CSC. Several algorithms recommend a two-step process. The first includes diversion of resources to patients without chronic underlying conditions that limit their potential for long-term survival. The second step includes assessment for risk of mortality based on Sequential Organ Failure Assessment (SOFA) scores. Patients with predicted mortality in excess of 90% are denied critical care.[11]

Such protocols cannot be adopted to the pediatric population for multiple reasons including the invalidity of the SOFA and similar scores as mortality predictors in pediatric patients as well as ethical considerations regarding children with pre-existing conditions. As a result of the above, a task force of pediatric expert advisory to the CDC that evaluated several pediatric protocols that use exclusion criteria based on pre-existing conditions concluded that it could not endorse these protocols. The primary difficulty with the proposed exclusion criteria was that they would exclude a very small portion of patients so that no significant impact on resource availability was likely to be gained. Although the task force declined to recommend a specific PICU triage protocol, they did emphasize the need for empirical research and evidence-based pediatric outcome prediction tools to be used in such events.[9,12]

"Jump START" is a common and long standing prehospital pediatric adjusted disaster triage system, predominantly used throughout the United States. This protocol is derived from the "START" protocol used for adults and was found to outperform other triage systems. It provides guidance for triage personnel making potential life-and-death decisions that otherwise may be influenced by emotional issues when triaging children. The triage sorts patients into acuity levels by colors: green, yellow, red, and black/expectant. Green patients are walking wounded who can wait to be treated. Yellow patients are patients who sustained serious injuries that require urgent but not immediate intervention for survival. Red refers to patients who sustained life-threatening injuries that are potentially salvageable with immediate medical attention, in contrast to patients labeled as black/expectant, patients who died or who are likely to die despite immediate intervention.

However, triaging pediatric patients to critical care requires a more complex system for evaluation of benefit and resource utilization. These systems may be objective or subjective, based on statistical analysis, expert opinion, or clinical judgment. Since objective systems sometimes incorporate subjective data elements and vice versa, this distinction is only relative. It has been shown that subjective tools tend to estimate mortality in excess; however, several studies have shown that both objective and subjective estimates preform similarly in discriminating critical from non-critical patients. But in light of the restricted precision of existing systems, especially for pediatric patients, some individuals will be inappropriately triaged not to receive critical care although they may benefit from such treatment. Nevertheless, the ability to exclude those that will not benefit from critical care usually outweighs these limitations. Although bias may be decreased by training and practical safeguards, objective tools are predominantly preferred. Existing pediatric scoring systems, such as the Pediatric Risk of Mortality and the Pediatric Index of Mortality, have many limitations, including the use of intricate formulas, reliance on laboratory test results, and inapplicability at the time of admission to the intensive care unit. Therefore, in most cases in times of crisis, there is a need for expert opinion to minimize biases in light of the lack of a simple, practical, and validated pediatric scoring system.[8–10]

Toltzis and colleagues have proposed a mass casualty population-outcome predictive tool that includes a pediatric-specific scheme that is informed by prediction equations based on data from actual critically ill children. Unlike adult schemes, the pediatric scheme considers the utilization of resources (length of stay and days of mechanical ventilation) as well as risk of mortality when considering PICU admission during CSC and did not exclude children based on pre-existing comorbidities. The study used machine learning methodology and a large scale database to develop the proposed protocol.[7] Further work by the same group extended this by simulating a pandemic crisis offering triage thresholds that maximize population survival and PICU bed occupancy over a range of patient volumes and resource availability. The model effectiveness was established by comparison with a first come, first served triage strategy. Despite the promise of this approach that is based on large scale databases and sophisticated algorithms, the suggested protocols are still not widely accepted. One major limitation that is common to all predictive tools that are based on from population analyses is the limited accuracy of the prediction for any individual patient. This may result in mis-triage in real-time CSC conditions and may have significant ethical and cultural implications. Furthermore, when faced with a previously unknown pandemic or a less common trigger for the crisis event, it is possible that the performance of any illness severity prediction tool may be affected.[10]

A universally excepted and validated pediatric critical care triage tool for CSC conditions is yet to be accepted. There is further need to develop and use pediatric-specific triage systems that address primary, secondary, and tertiary triage. These should address all aspects of disaster triage, including psychological triage, triage for weapons of mass destruction, and triage for children with special health care needs.

SPECIAL CONSIDERATION AND SURGE CAPACITY PLANNING FOR PEDIATRIC DISASTERS

Disaster and crisis planning must consider the needs of children in various settings, including children who for various reasons cannot be reunited with their families. Children with special health care needs are particularly vulnerable, especially if their survival depends on medications or technologies (e.g., respirators) that may not be readily available during an emergency. The literature addressing the needs of children in disasters and disaster planning is sparse and even more so when dealing with pediatric critical care preparedness. The body of literature concerning disaster events, or response and planning for disasters, almost exclusively addresses the needs of adults. Only recently have professional organizations begun to develop policy guidelines considering the needs of children during and after disasters. Such policies tend to focus on the roles of specific providers in disaster planning, preparation, and response as well as training and equipment allocation.[11,12]

Crisis situations that affect a large number of children could quickly overwhelm any health care system given the limited number of pediatric specialty hospitals. This is especially true for pediatric critical care capacity that is even scarcer. Achieving preparedness requires health care facilities to implement measures focusing exclusively the pediatric population. Conducting pediatric intensive care drills, improving pediatric surge capacity, and ensuring that the needs of children are incorporated into all levels of disaster plans is fundamental. During a disaster or terrorist event, children will undoubtedly arrive at general hospitals, so all hospitals must be prepared for a greater number of pediatric victims than usual. Specialty centers must also be prepared for increased pediatric needs. Staff and physician volunteer programs that are key to ensuring adequate numbers of providers must also recognize the need for more pediatric-trained providers. Furthermore, emergency preparations should include plans for storage of sensitive medications and supplies. In this aspect it is important for hospitals to consider the needs of children including, but not limited to, equipment, medications, decontamination equipment, and the ability to handle non-ambulatory children as well as special food, diapers, and other supplies. In addition, hospitals must be prepared to handle situations in which patients will be cared for as a family unit and children will not be able to be separated from adults, such as in a quarantine situation. This will require all hospitals to have the capability to handle children, and all children's hospitals must possess the ability to care for adult patients who will be staying with their children.[11–15]

Surge capacity planning involves the development of additional resources to meet all needs in a disaster. Some surge capacity may be created through modified processes of care. Disaster planning for pediatric critical care has trailed behind that for prehospital and emergency pediatric care. Despite the increasing attention to mass casualty care, scarce evidence is available to support planning of the capacity that will be required in different surge scenarios. The unique needs of children might have been anticipated; however, an evidence-based projection of critical pediatric critical care needs and its implication on existing pediatric hospital resources is still lacking.[14–16]

Children and Disasters 2010 recommended that additional resources provide a "formal regionalized pediatric system of care to support pediatric surge capacity" and emphasizes that children's hospitals are central to such regionalization.[17] However, as children's hospitals usually operate close to capacity, little available reserve exists for even a modest surge. Many hospitals have developed surge capacity response plans that will allow freeing up as many pediatric critical care beds as possible as well as have the potential of setting up more PICU beds in locations other than the PICU. This is achieved by diverting patients, using alternative infrastructure such as recovery and intermediate care units, and using rapidly deployed tents. Further increase in pediatric critical care surge capacity may be achieved by diverting equipment and personnel from adult units. However, sensitive life supporting equipment such as ventilators, syringe pumps, and monitors must be adjusted for use on pediatric patients. Alarms and limits should be appropriately attuned based on age and weight, automated medication protocols should be adjusted, and appropriate measures should be instated to prevent possible harm when using "adult" equipment. Protocols for repurposing of equipment to pediatric use should be instated in advance and implemented upon activation of the crisis response.

Modeling studies predict that even a moderate pandemic would briefly exceed the intensive care ordinary surge capacity in a typical region, in any hospital pediatric bed, or specifically in PICU beds. This may result in the need to alter the standard of care in all levels of care. If altering standards of care is implemented to accommodate patient surges in disasters, cautious consideration should be given to explicit guidelines and measures ratifying such alteration.[13,14]

Crisis preparedness plans must also focus on treatment of pediatric patients outside of the hospital, through establishing pediatric triage centers and strategies for mobilizing pediatric health care providers. Most hospitals and networks can increase critical care capacity by using ordinary surge methods and still provide normal care. It is assumed that shortening of the critical care length of stay for both crisis patients and ordinary patients could be achieved.[14,15]

Crisis situations that produce overwhelming numbers of critically ill children are sporadic and rare, yet in many cases unexpected. The rapid presentation of a surge of critically ill children on the doorstep of any medical system will necessitate extreme measures with significant medical, financial, and ethical consequences. Planning for an unknown event that may never happen is an extraordinary logistical and fiscal challenge, but in light of the special considerations and measures that these events necessitate, advanced planning and preparations are essential.

EDUCATION AND TRAINING FOR A PEDIATRIC CRISIS INCIDENT

By definition, a crisis incident is an event that overwhelms the response capacity of the local health care system for a period of time. A pediatric crisis incident presents even bigger challenges as it confronts the local health care systems with specific and unique vulnerabilities to this population. It is well accepted that during disasters all hospitals and all providers should be prepared to deliver care to pediatric patients.

Therefore, in order to optimize the response to a pediatric crisis, hospitals need to engage in routine training and education in all aspects of pediatric-specific response ranging from logistical to refining medical expertise.

A meta-analysis by Skryabina and colleagues looked at the evidence regarding the effectiveness of public health emergency preparedness exercises and found that exercises were effective at improving participants' knowledge of emergency activities, policies, and procedures and improving overall competence and confidence.[18] Skill specific training, such as accurately triaging trauma patients, is also effective as demonstrated by Vargas and colleagues.[19]

Several strategies were developed to effectively train for those relatively low frequency yet high impact events. Those include short introductory lessons, tabletop drills, full scale large drills, demonstrations, and practical training, video, and computer simulations and analysis of real events.

An important aspect of training and preparedness for pediatric mass events includes the need to divert non-pediatric trained staff to treating pediatric patients. Hence, basic training in pediatric care should be considered as part of preparedness training programs of providers from all disciplines.

Data regarding the overall effectiveness of training programs are scarce; hence, developing a program that includes a mixture of training models seems to be a well-balanced approach.

A full-scale exercise (FSE) is usually a multi-agency, multi-jurisdictional, multi-organizational exercise that validates all aspects of preparedness. They include EMS, hospitals, police and fire departments, as well as city, state, and at times national command centers and agencies. The objective of an FSE is to examine and analyze the implementation of plans, policies, and protocols that were previously developed and drilled in smaller exercises.

Such mega exercises present complex and realistic problems that require critical thinking, rapid problem solving, and effective responses by trained personnel. They also enable stakeholders to test local responses and identify weaknesses, vulnerabilities, and bottlenecks.

FSEs in pediatric mass casual incident (MCI) needs to be scripted in a fashion that confronts the systems with all the unique challenges in pediatrics while mirroring real life events. Patients in a myriad of age groups and injury patterns as well as troubleshooting issues in pediatric transport, psychological stress, and locating and updating the child's parents/legal guardian add an extra layer of complexity in an already stressful event.

FSEs, however, are resource-intensive and time-consuming and should therefore be utilized wisely and infrequently only once individual players drill and implement localized response, thus allowing the full scale exercise to drill higher-level aspects such inter-agency communication, coordination, transport, city wide surge capacity management, etc.

Furthermore, including pediatric scenarios in such exercises may add significant complexity and cost.

Tabletop drills are useful in testing health system response to crisis events while preserving resources. It is highly effective in testing specific aspects of the response such as patients' triage, resource allocation, and prioritizations as well as illustrating system vulnerabilities and response to bottlenecks. They can be enacted in varying levels of an MCI response, ranging from a national command center to a hospital emergency department. There are, however, innate weaknesses using this methodology given the gap between the theoretical response and real-life implementation.

Functional lower scale exercises should be used to practice such "real-life" challenges. Scenario-based drills in a department to a hospital level enable evaluating a range of components in the emergency response. Those include notification of the event, activation of protocols for additional staffing, patients' triage and flow, charting in electronic medical records, communication, utilization of hospital specific protocols such as mass transfusion, usage of equipment reserved for disasters, and simulating the actual patient care.

Given that such drills interrupt hospitals' daytime activity, they should be planned during times when such interruptions are minimized. Scheduling such drills in seasons and times when hospital capacity is lower has proven to be helpful in mitigating those challenges.

Any drill, regardless of its size, needs to be appropriately debriefed and analyzed in order to extract conclusions efficiently. Several methods are routinely used to optimize such debriefing, including video recording of the exercise, inspections by observers with pre-made checklists, interviews of medical staff, self-evaluations, and audits by subject matter experts.[20]

Performing high frequency drills is limited by resources and their impact on hospitals' workflow. Other methods such as online modules and computer-based simulations can be used to train health care providers in different aspects of the response. Such computer simulations are an economical method to educate key hospital decision makers and improve hospital disaster preparedness before implementation of a full-scale drill.[21]

To appropriately address pediatric-specific aspects in preparedness training and education, experts in pediatric care from various disciplines should be integrated in the authorities responsible for planning and executing the training programs. Specialists in pediatric emergency medicine, pediatric critical care, social workers, emergency managers, and others with specific training, interest, and experience in pediatric specialty care should be included.

In order to familiarize hospital staff with resources and protocols, different strategies can be implemented, including seminars and lectures as well as online modules with integrated evaluations of the learners. Using such modules prior to wider scale drills would optimize the efficacy of such drills given that participants will approach such exercises better prepared.

THE MANAGEMENT OF PEDIATRIC TRAUMA IN MASS CASUALTY INCIDENTS

Children have greater susceptibility to injuries during a mass casualty incident for various physiological, psychological, and behavioral reasons. In the Oklahoma City bombing in 1995, of the 19 children who died, 90% had sustained a head injury, which illustrates, as an example, how a higher head-body ratio increases the likelihood for head injury.[22]

Children's mental and psychological features, especially in a mass casualty situation, also play a significant role in their susceptibility to injuries. A diminished sense of self-preservation and a lack of certain cognitive and physical skills contribute to the diminished capacity to react appropriately to signs of danger or to follow instructions. Compared to most adults, children possess fewer coping skills and can sometimes lack the situational awareness that might prove crucial in avoiding injury during a mass shooting, for example.

Analysis of mass trauma incidents and disasters, such as Hurricane Katrina in 2005, demonstrates that many injured children would be evacuated via transport services that lack the equipment and expertise to deal with pediatric trauma victims to medical centers that are challenged, due to limited resources and expertise, to treat a bulk of injured children.

Mass casualty incidents challenge health care infrastructure by creating an imbalance between the number and severity of victims and the available resources. An MCI that involves a large number of pediatric patients might overwhelm the response even further given that the management of pediatric trauma is highly specialized. The first step of an effective pediatric mass casualty plan begins in the prudent triaging of those patients and evacuating them to the appropriate center in a manner that takes into account multiple parameters. As an example, broken limbs can be effectively treated in an adult hospital; however, some injuries to the chest and head would potentially be better managed in a center with specialized pediatric surgeons.

As in adults, the goals of initial trauma management in children are to rapidly assess the injuries, determine management priorities, and provide critical interventions. Achieving these goals requires a systematic and logical approach according to the guidelines of advanced trauma life support (ATLS).

It is important to remember, however, certain unique features in pediatric trauma that will assist the care provider in proper assessment and management of those injured children.

First, indices of blood pressure, pulse rate, and respiratory rate are age dependent and drug dosages are calculated by weight in the child, whereas in the adult more standard therapy may be given. There is also a physiological difference in children's response to blood loss, thus rendering the diagnosis of hemorrhagic shock in children more challenging. Children with significant bleeding will maintain a relatively normal BP by a steep rise in their vascular tone and moderating the drop in cardiac output by elevating the heart rate (Figure 17-1).[23] Hypotension, therefore, will be a late finding and will suggest a decompensated hypovolemic shock. Diagnosing hypovolemic shock might be more challenging in infants compared to toddlers and older children or adults. In infants such shock may manifest as hyperventilation or hypoventilation, skin mottling, erratic cardiovascular measures, glucose intolerance, or metabolic instability.[24] As such, clinical suspicion of significant hemorrhage should prompt IV access and crystalloid infusion or blood transfusion.

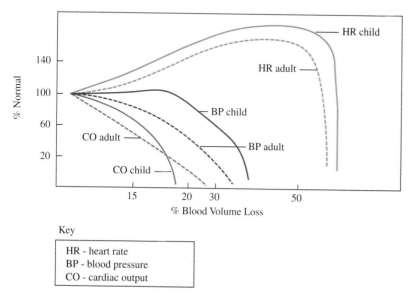

FIGURE 17-1 • Hemodynamic response to hypovolemia. (Adapted from Carcillo JA, Han K, Lin J, Orr R. Goal-directed management of pediatric shock in the emergency department. *Pediatric Emergency Medicine*. 2007;8(3):165-175.

The injury pattern is different as well; children have increased chest wall elasticity and less developed abdominal musculature and therefore can sustain more significant trauma to abdominal solid organs and sustain blunt thoracic injuries with limited rib or sternal fractures. As such, severe parenchymal thoracic injuries may be present with minimal or no signs of external trauma.

Health care providers should therefore have high index of suspicion and should investigate alternations in vital signs, abnormal breathing patterns, or signs of inadequate perfusion. Healthy children also have high cardiac and respiratory reserve, which may obscure signs of injury; however, due to high metabolic demand once a threshold had been crossed and signs of hypoxia or hypotension present, rapid deterioration may follow. The approach to resuscitation of these patients is similar to that in adults. However, because of the above factors, children are more likely to need airway control and assisted ventilation.[25]

Another important and unique feature of pediatric trauma is the higher tendency of children with traumatic brain injury, in comparison to adults, to develop intracranial hypertension and lower tendency to develop lesions with mass effect.[26,27] Severe traumatic brain injury in children should be therefore suspected to cause elevated intracranial pressure (ICP) and should be managed promptly (with elevation of the head, head in the midline position, airway support, oxygenation, hyperventilation, and hyperosmolar therapy) to reduce the secondary brain injury from cerebral edema. In the setting of a mass casualty incident, this realization is of the utmost importance as those immediate actions are far more important in the initial stabilization of the patient than neurosurgical care that would be limited as are other resources in an MCI.

The unique characteristics of head, abdominal, and chest injuries in children are important because these injuries account for most of the disability and death among injured children. During the response to a mass casualty incidence, we need to acknowledge that some of the medical care would be done with limited resources and personnel who are less familiar with injuries in these age groups.

With appropriate initial resuscitation and follow-up care, most injured children can be expected to have a good outcome. Recognition of the fact that children are different from adults and preparation for the therapeutic implications of these differences are the important first steps in management. Hospitals and EMS services planning for disasters and mass casualty effects need to make the appropriate preparation and education to account for the unique characteristics outlined above.

EMOTIONAL AND SOCIAL CONSIDERATION IN PEDIATRIC CRISIS INCIDENTS

Classically, in face of a disaster, pandemic, or mass casualty incident, relief efforts focus on the physical consequences of the event by providing immediate medical attention and addressing health and environmental services (water supply, sewage disposal, and shelter). The short and long-term consequences on mental health and psychosocial well-being of children and their families must also be taken into consideration.

The psychological well-being of an individual child is influenced by the type and intensity of exposure to the event, the availability of family and community support during the event and during recovery, the degree of day-to-day life disruption, the amount of social disorganization and chaos, and the extent to which community social cohesion is maintained (Table 17-1). In addition, vulnerability depends on individual characteristics of the child, the social and economic circumstances of the family and community, and the available resources in the surrounding environment and community.

In the event of disaster or a mass casualty incident, health care providers should acknowledge the importance of reuniting children with their parents or caregivers. Following Hurricane Katrina in 2005, many children who were evacuated got separated from their families only to reunite with them months later. One of those children, a 7-year-old girl, was rescued from the floodwaters by boat and placed in a shelter apart

Table 17-1 FACTORS THAT INFLUENCE THE EMOTIONAL IMPACT ON CHILDREN IN DISASTER SITUATIONS

- Characteristics, extent, and duration of the disaster
- Direct exposure to disaster
- Earlier exposure to disaster and chronic adversity
- Perception of life-threat to self or significant other
- Separation from caregivers
- Physical injury
- Effects on parents or caregivers
- Inner resources of the family, and relation and communication patterns among the family members
- Exposure of children to mass media
- Cultural and context differences
- Degree of disorganization and loss of social control in the community
- Community response

from her family. She had multiple cigarette burns when reunited with her family. In the first two years after the storm, she attended five different schools. Her symptoms included chronic bedwetting, hyperventilation, and self-injurious behavior. She was diagnosed with post-traumatic stress disorder.[28]

In a mass casualty event, affected children would be frightened, possibly in pain or ill, confused, overwhelmed, and potentially desperate. Those children might be going through this experience without their primary support system, which will be an additional destabilizing stressor. When a child is exposed to a disaster, the emotional responses can range from minimal distress to inattention, fear, anhedonia, anxiety, and depressed mood, to symptoms of re-experiencing, avoidance, hypervigilance, and disruptive behavior. In many instances these symptomatic reactions are considered normal responses to a traumatic experience and are time-limited. Children, however, may also have significant impairment and chronic symptomatology.

Health care providers need to learn how to recognize those emotional reactions, reduce the emotional impact of the stressor, and facilitate emotional recovery. The first necessary step of any health care providers taking care of children in a face of disaster is to take charge; this will have a stabilizing effect on a child in the midst of chaos. Provide support, comfort, and emotional care; acknowledge and accept the behavior as normal adaptations to stress; and engage in explaining to the child the situation and what's expected to happen in an age appropriate fashion. Constant reassuring is key in the management of children during such stressful events.

Acute stress reactions should be addressed as soon as possible by focused psychological support provided by skill personnel, as early intervention has the potential to attenuate the psychological long-term sequela. Such response will require enhancing pediatric disaster mental and behavioral health training for professionals and paraprofessionals, including psychological first aid, cognitive-behavioral interventions, social support interventions, and bereavement counseling and support.

In October 2010, after acknowledging that children's mental and behavioral health needs are virtually ignored across federal and state disaster planning efforts, the National Commission on Children and Disasters recommended in their report to the U.S. president and Congress that "Federal agencies and non-Federal partners should enhance pre-disaster preparedness and just-in-time training in pediatric disaster mental and behavioral health, including psychological first aid, bereavement support, and brief supportive interventions, for mental health professionals and individuals, such as teachers, who work with children."

Some logistical consideration in the midst of the MCI response can further mitigate the emotional burden. Health care providers need to obtain pertinent information, such as names of family and how to make contact, and give information in a language the child can understand regarding what happened, the length of time it takes for tests and treatment, and when updates are expected. It is crucial to protect children from undue excitement and stimulation such as onlookers and the media.

Until there is an adequate support system available to the child, efforts should be made to avoid exposing the child to any news of trauma or loss of any friend or relative, and if possible, try to keep the child from hearing other children's rendition of what happened.

During the medical management of the injured child, certain steps will alleviate additional stress and will improve cooperation. Children should receive warning prior to painful procedures. Make additional effort in explaining to the child why certain actions are taking place and provide constant reassurance that the child is doing a good job. When necessary, give the child firm direction to get their cooperation. Asking implies that the person has a choice in the matter. The child could feel fooled or deceived when asked to make a choice where there is none. In such instances, rather provide support, encouragement, and reassurance.

Once reunited with their families or caregivers, health care providers need to acknowledge that they might benefit themselves from emotional first aid. Initial steps should always be providing updated information about their child's condition and what should they expect in the near future.

ETHICAL ISSUES IN PEDIATRIC MASS CRITICAL CARE

Emergency preparedness, in general, entails significant ethical consideration from planning to medical care. In light of recent events such as natural disasters and pandemics, emergency preparedness with all of its aspects has become an increasing priority but in spite of this increased focus, children have received limited attention.

Historically, allocation of scarce resources was always a significant part of the debate in emergency preparedness. Several frameworks (based on philosophical principles) have been suggested to tackle this ethically loaded issue.

The COVID-19 pandemic highlighted some of those issues especially since the pediatric population was less affected. Despite the pandemic, children still required specialized care for complex chronic conditions, congenital anomalies, and prematurity to name a few. Nonetheless, governments and authorities needed to prioritize procedures and medical care based on their urgency, prioritize distribution of disposable and durable equipment, allocate hospital beds, and deploy health professionals to care for affected adults.

There is a general agreement that the guiding principle is resource allocation, providing the greatest benefit to the greatest number of individuals while the fewest resources are used. Other principles such as creating a fair, transparent, and consistent systems are key. It is also imperative to keep in mind that especially during a disaster, vulnerable populations are likely to suffer the greatest impact and hence measures should be taken to even those inequities during public health emergencies as well.

The Task Force for Pediatric Emergency Mass Critical Care recommended in 2009 that surge planning should provide resources for children in proportion to their percentage of the population. Alternatively if data are available, resources should preferably be allocated based on the percentage of those affected by the disaster.

In order to rapidly allocate resources during a mass casualty incident, disaster, or pandemic, health care providers rely on triage protocols to grade the severity of patients. Most protocols, however, are designed for adult patients for whom standardized clinical scoring methods are commonly used. This imbalance creates the potential for inquorate triaging of children that might result in unfair resource allocation.[29]

An ethical dilemma that couldn't not be overstated relates to whether age should be a determinate in favoring patients in resource allocation. Historically, it has been argued that some priority should be given to younger people given the argument that with all other things being equal, those who have not experienced as many life stages and utilized less societal resources so far should have the opportunity to do so.[30] Others, however, suggest the "complete lives system," which prioritizes adolescents and young adults, providing the argument that the death of an adolescent is a greater loss than the death of a toddler or an infant.

During the COVID-19 pandemic that disproportionally affected older populations, some countries instituted age limits for intensive care measures such as intubation or ECMO. This, however, prompted accusations of ageism arguing that a simple age cut-off is an unfair discriminator.[31]

Any system that will be implemented eventually should be a product of a comprehensive deliberation and public discussion, and the framework should be transparent.

Health professionals might also experience higher moral distress in withholding or withdrawing treatment during critical care mass incidents. This might be amplified in the eyes of some clinicians while dealing with pediatric patients in the face of scarce resources.[32] Planning should include providing support mechanisms to clinicians on the front line who are facing such dilemmas.

The COVID-19 pandemic highlighted another ethical dilemma that is unique in pediatrics.[33] In recent years, family centered care had been the focus in pediatrics. This concept originated from the idea that many unique changes that children encounter are mitigated by the presence of their family members at the bedside. In normal circumstances, family centered care fosters increased access to the patient and providers. Parents and caregivers are encouraged to stay with the hospitalized child, including, sometimes during, medical procedures. Families are routinely present during rounds and are encouraged to communicate with medical team members. The medical providers are expected to support families' choices and respect the family wishes in decision making.

During a pandemic, however, this framework is challenged by concerns of disease spreading and other concerns such as the potential that the needs of one family would conflict with those of another family or patient. Those deviations from routine measures should be anticipated. As in many other ethical dilemmas, transparency and equity should mitigate, to some degree, these concerns as well.

REFERENCES

1. Burke RV, Iverson E, Goodhue CJ, et al. Disaster and mass casualty events in the pediatric population. *Semin Pediatr Surg.* 2010;19(4):265-270.
2. Brandenburg MA, Watkins SM, Brandenburg KL, Schieche C. Operation Child-ID: Reunifying children with their legal guardians after Hurricane Katrina. *Disasters.* 2007;31:277-287.
3. Allen GM, Parrillo SJ, Will J, Mohr JA. Principles of disaster planning for the pediatric population. *Prehosp Disaster Med.* 2007;22:537-540.
4. Columbia University, Mailman School of Public Health. Pediatric preparedness for disasters and terrorism: A National Consensus Conference, 2003.
5. Kanter RK, Moran JR. Pediatric hospital and intensive care unit capacity in regional disasters: Expanding capacity by altering standards of care. *Pediatrics.* 2007;119:94-100.
6. Sills MR, Hall M, Fieldstone ES, et al. Inpatient capacity at children's hospitals during pandemic (H1N1) 2009 outbreak, United States. *Emerg Infect Dis.* 2011;17(9):1685-1691.
7. American Academy of Pediatrics Committee on Pediatric Emergency Medicine, American Academy of Pediatrics Committee on Medical Liability, Task Force on Terrorism. The pediatrician and disaster preparedness. *Pediatrics.* 2006;117:560-565.

8. Gilchrist N, Simpson JN. Pediatric disaster preparedness: Identifying challenges and opportunities for emergency department planning. *Curr Opin Pediatr*. 2019;31(3):306-311.

9. Blake N, Stevenson K. Reunification: Keeping families together in crisis. *J Trauma*. 2009;67:S147-S151.

10. Markovitz BP. Pediatric critical care surge capacity. *J Trauma*. 2009;67(2): S140-S142.11.

11. Antommaria AH, Powell T, Miller JE, Christian MD; Task Force for Pediatric Emergency Mass Critical Care. Ethical issues in pediatric emergency mass critical care. *Pediatr Crit Care Med*. 2011;12(6 Suppl):S163-S168.

12. King M, Dorfman M, Einav S, Niven A, Kissoon N. Grissom C. Evacuation of Intensive care units during disaster: Learning from the Hurricane Sandy experience. *Disaster Med Public Health Prep*. 2016;10(1):20-27.

13. Kanter RK. Pediatric mass critical care in a pandemic. *Pediatr Crit Care Med*. 2012;13(1):e1-e4d.

14. Christian MD, Hawryluck L, Wax RS, et al. Development of a triage protocol for critical care during an influenza pandemic. *CMAJ*. 2006;175(11):1377-1381.

15. Toltzis P, Soto-Campos G, Kuhn E, Hahn R, Kanter RT, Wetzel R. Evidence-based pediatric outcome predictors to guide the allocation of critical care resources in a mass casualty event. *Pediatr Crit Care Med*. 2015;16(7):e207-e216.

16. Christian M, Toltzis P, Burkle FM, et al. Treatment and triage recommendations for pediatric emergency mass critical care. *Pediatr Crit Care Med*. 2011;12(6):S109-S119.

17. Gall C, Wetzel R, Kolker A, Kanter R, Toltzis P. Pediatric triage in a severe pandemic: Maximizing survival by establishing triage thresholds. *Crit Care Med*. 2016;44(9):1762-1768.

18. Skryabina E, Reedy G, Amlôt R, Jaye P, Riley P. What is the value of health emergency preparedness exercises? A scoping review study. *Int J Disaster Risk Reduct*. 2017;21:74-283.

19. Vargas JP, Hubloue I, Pinzón JJ, Duque AC. The effect of training and experience on mass casualty incident triage performance: Evidence from emergency personnel in a high complexity university hospital. *Am J Disaster Med*. 2019;14(2):113-119.

20. Kaji AH, Langford V, Lewis RJ. Assessing hospital disaster preparedness: A comparison of an on-site survey, directly observed drill performance, and video analysis of teamwork. *Ann Emerg Med*. 2008;52(3):195-201, 201.e1-12.

21. Hsu EB, Jenckes MW, Catlett CL, et al. Training of hospital staff to respond to a mass casualty incident: Summary. 2004 Apr. In: *AHRQ Evidence Report Summaries*. Rockville, MD: Agency for Healthcare Research and Quality (US);1998-2005:95. Available at https://www.ncbi.nlm.nih.gov/books/NBK11911/.

22. Mallonee S, Shariat S, Stennies G, et al. Physical injuries and fatalities resulting from the Oklahoma City bombing. *JAMA*. 1996;276(5):382-387.

23. Carcillo JA, Han K, Lin J, Orr R. Goal-directed management of pediatric shock in the emergency department. *Pediatr Emerg Med*. 2007;8(3):165-175.

24. Crone RC. Acute circulatory failure in children. *Pediatr Clin North Am*. 1980;27:525-538.

25. Kissoon N, Dreyer J, Walia M. Pediatric trauma: Differences in pathophysiology, injury patterns and treatment compared with adult trauma. *CMAJ*. 1990;142(1):27.
26. Walker ML, Storr BB, Mayer TA. Head injuries. In: Mayer, ed. *Emergency Management of Pediatric Trauma*. Philadelphia: Saunders; 1985:272-286 38.
27. Bruce DA, Schut L, Bruno LA et al. Outcome following severe head injuries in children. *J Neurosurg*. 1978;48:679-688.
28. Olteanu A, Arnberger R, Grant R, Davis C, Abramson D, Asola J. Persistence of mental health needs among children affected by Hurricane Katrina in New Orleans. *Prehosp Disaster Med*. 2010;26(1):3-6.
29. National Commission on Children and Disasters. 2010 Report to the President and Congress; https://archive.ahrq.gov/prep/nccdreport/nccdreport.pdf.
30. Daugherty Biddison EL, Faden R, Gwon HS, et al. Too many patients... a framework to guide statewide allocation of scarce mechanical ventilation during disasters. *Chest*. 2019;155(4):848-854.
31. Williams A. Intergenerational equity: An exploration of the "fair innings" argument. *Health Econ*. 1997;6(2):117-132.
32. Laventhal N, Basak R, Dell ML, et al. The ethics of creating a resource allocation strategy during the COVID-19 pandemic. *Pediatrics*. 2020;146(1):e20201243.
33. Antommaria AH, Powell T, Miller JE, Christian MD; Task Force for Pediatric Emergency Mass Critical Care. Ethical issues in pediatric emergency mass critical care. *Pediatr Crit Care Med*. 2011;12(6 Suppl):S163-S168.
34. Dwyer OM. The ethical allocation of resources during a pediatric emergency mass critical care event. *Curr Treat Options Peds*. 2017;3:293-303.

18 COPING STRATEGIES

Aurora Tompar Tiu, MD and Anna C. Go, MD

▌ GENERAL CONSIDERATIONS

Understanding the coping strategies of critical care patients and their families or primary care providers is vital in helping facilitate the use of effective and healthy ways to cope with their illnesses and their consequences. The suddenness of onset of acute life threatening illness, unavailability of family and social support, feelings of aloneness, and uncertainty about the illness and its implications for the patient's ability to cope with demands of personal life and maintaining family and social relationship are the stressors that critical care patients and their families/primary care givers experience. The current COVID-19 pandemic and its consequences (e.g., lock down, isolation, feelings of uncertainty, fear of getting infected, and loss or decrease of financial and social resources) magnify and increase the stressors of hospitalization. How are the patients and their families coping? Coping is best defined as problem-solving behaviors and thoughts intended to manage both external and internal stressors and to help bring about resolution and relief.[1,2] It is a process of appraisal, self-instruction and correction, performance, and self-rehearsal as well as guidance and help from outside sources.[1] Cultural and religious practices need to be considered and understood for individuals' coping strategies. There are four major categories of coping,[2] which include:

1. Emotion-focused: aims to decrease negative emotions associated with the stressors like fear, anger, anxiety, and depression. Ask patients what aspects of their illnesses and their treatment that they are most worried or afraid about and understanding where their emotions are coming from.
2. Problem-focused: addresses the main problem causing the distress (e.g., COVID-19 pandemic and its consequences).
3. Meaning-focused: uses cognitive strategies "to derive and manage the meaning of the situation." Religious and cultural practices play a role in their type of coping.

4. Social coping support: seeking from family and medical community emotional and instrumental support. Open communication is important in their type of coping.

Preliminary data on coping strategies gathered from interviews of patients and their families, physicians, primary care providers, and other health care providers as well as from data of existing literature on coping strategies are included and arranged here from A to Z. Each person has developed their own coping strategies and what works for them may not work for other people. Effective copers are usually optimistic, practical, flexible, resourceful, and composed when facing difficult situations to avoid impairment of judgment. Bad copers or ineffective copers are usually rigid and inflexible with very high self-expectation and with excess denial and extreme rationalization and failed to focus on important problems. Negative or maladaptive coping strategies include abuse of alcohol and drugs, overspending or too much "retail therapy," overeating, oversleeping, self and family neglect with failure to follow up with medical appointments with poor compliance, intimate partner abuse/violence, and indiscriminate, unprotected sex and other reckless and self-destructive behaviors. Effective coping strategies mitigate acute and chronic stress, which is the body's respond to stressors from different situations and events. The stress reaction can be physical, emotional, mental, and social. Acute stress is self-limiting like an inability to contact a primary care physician. Chronic stress can be due to prolonged duration of stressors like chronic pain due to arthritis or ongoing problems with a spouse or intimate partner. It can cause chronic headaches, hypertension, muscle tension, irritability, anxiety, lack of motivation, depression, aggression, and withdrawal from friends and family. The following coping strategies are considered positive or effective according to the individual's choices and experience that they may find useful to cope with the stressors.

COPING STRATEGIES

Acceptance
The ability to accept the reality of the stressors like illness and its severity and possible complications or situations like the COVID-19 pandemic without denial or minimizing the stressor or situation. Studies have indicated that acceptance was associated with lower levels of anxiety and stress.[3]

Acknowledgement
To acknowledge one's capability, limitations, and the resources available and the capability and limitation of others as well. This will minimize

frustration due to a high level of expectations and the failure to cope with the stressors. Lower expectations when necessary.

Appreciation

The ability to appreciate, identify, and value the positive aspects of the events or situation the person experiences in spite of the many difficulties encountered. Expressing appreciation of the patients' efforts to cooperate and cope with their illness is valuable. Extend appreciation to physicians, nurses, and other health care providers as well as family members who are supportive especially during critical events when one is in need the most.

Assessment

Evaluate the critical aspects of the problem or stressors involved to plan appropriately the necessary solutions. Assess the recourses available that may be helpful in the solution of the problem or stressor.

Attention

Giving attention to the important details of the stressor like the life-threatening illness and possible complications will provide information that will help mitigate anxiety and help prepare oneself to accept the situation. It is also important to pay attention to one's needs and emotional response to stressors. When an emotional response like anxiety and depression is overwhelming, consulting a professional will prevent further deterioration of function and prevent disability.

Beliefs

Sharing positive cultural and religious beliefs will help buffer the negative impact of stressful life events. Knowing and understanding these beliefs assist health care providers in their care of patients.

Be Positive

Seeing difficulties and obstacles in coping with stressors as opportunities to learn from and to gain confidence in one's coping strategies.

Communication

Open communication between patients and their families with their health providers will facilitate improved compliance with treatment plans and enhance the morale of patients and their families/primary care providers. Family members and their patients are encouraged to communicate with each other about their concerns and plans in the future.

"Circle of Friends"

Nurturing and expanding the "circle of friends" and supporters who provide emotional support during crisis and other stressful life events mitigate emotional distress.

Creative Activities

Arts and craft relax the mind and divert attention from stressful situations. Painting, coloring, drawing, and creating useful items are some activities that are helpful in promoting mental health.

Development of Plan

Planning for immediate and future action to address the current or ongoing stressors and to find appropriate and feasible solutions to decrease the negative impact of the stressors. Making a daily schedule of activities gives a sense of stability and security especially with children who need predictability as a stabilizing force, particularly in the current COVID-19 pandemic that has disrupted routine activities.

Drawing

Many children use drawing as a means to express their feelings and experiences and to decrease boredom.

Exercise

Physical activity and other forms of exercise is associated with decreased anxiety and depression.[11] The release of endorphins during exercise improves mood.

Encourage Each Other

Caring for others and encouraging each other benefit both the recipient and the giver. Mutual love and kindness lift the spirit of each and decrease anxiety and depression.

Family

Close, familiar ties become a buffer of the negative impact of stressful situations. Nurturing the family relationship and providing mutual support of each other is vital in the behavioral of family members and maintaining good mental health.

Finding Your Sanctuary

Having a special place like a church or a garden to give you respite from the stressful situation enhances your capabilities and insight on what is the best strategy to cope with your current stressors.

Friendship

True friends provide valuable emotional support no matter what the circumstances without judgment or criticism.

Good Deeds

Doing good deeds to others without expecting any returns strengthen the spirit and enhances the morale especially during stressful events.

Gratitude

Feelings of thankful appreciation for services and favors received during stressful situations increases strength and confidence to manage stressors.

"Strive to be Happy"

Finding happiness in whatever stressful situation is enjoying every little achievement or being happy in whatever you have and with people who care about you.

Hope

A feeling that what is wanted will happen—"To leap up in expectation." To hope for healing, recovery, and resolution of the problem gives courage and determination to find the best solution.

Humor

The ability to perceive, appreciate, and express what is funny, amusing, or ludicrous. In difficult moments, having a good sense of humor helps alleviate suffering. To be able to laugh at oneself requires confidence and belief that one is good enough despite limitations and failure.

Inspire Others

By good example in work and deeds, inspire anybody who may be facing stressful situations. Inspiring others to help them rise above their difficulties is a rewarding experience.

Involvement

Being involved in the diagnostic and treatment process by providing accurate information help the health care providers in providing the best treatment options.

Joy

"A very glad feeling"—rejoicing in every part of recovery and healing. Joyful feelings improve immune system and give hope and confidence.

Kindness

Being kind in words and deeds brings out the goodness of others. Kindness begets kindness, which is much needed in stressful situations.

Laughter

Laughter is considered the best medicine. It improves the immune system[12] and has a positive effect on the emotional, mental, and physical aspects in the body. It releases endorphins, the natural feel good chemicals that promote a good sense of well-being, and decreases depression. It relieves stress and eases tension and anxiety. It also strengthens friendship and relationship. It lowers stress hormones.

Love

Love surpasses many trials and difficulties in life. It gives strength and hope. It helps the healing of anger, depression, anxiety, and resentment. It forgives.

Mindfulness

"Mindfulness is attending to and accepting the present experiences, thoughts, behavior and feelings without engaging in judgmental thoughts about them."[13] It reduces depressive symptoms and improves self-esteem and interpersonal sensitivity.

Music

Preferred music improves mood and increases motivation. It decreases pain and suffering especially in stressful situations.

Nutrition

A well-balanced diet is positively correlated with improved mental health and decreased risk of cognitive decline.[4] Proper nutritional intake can also improve the immune system and mitigate the effects of infection.[5] With the current COVID-19 pandemic, good nutrition is a preventive measure against infection stressors. Maintenance of adequate nutrition status is essential to support a healthy immune system and mitigate the effects of infection. This involves the intake of foods rich in nutrients that fight against free radicals and inflammation, proper hydration, and avoiding sugary, salty, or fatty foods. Certain dietary patterns with an emphasis on nutrient dense foods and low or minimal intake of processed meats and food products, such as a Mediterranean diet, have anti-inflammatory properties. Other diets such as the Western diet, associated with high intake of processed foods, red meat, fried foods, sugar, and salt increase risk of inflammation and disease.[6] Consultation with a physician for appropriate amounts and vitamin dosage is recommended depending on the person's age, lifestyle, nutrition status, inborn enzyme deficiencies, food allergies, and underlying comorbidities. Nutrient dense foods with positive effects on the immune system include fruits, vegetables, meat, poultry, fish, eggs, milk and dairy products, whole grains, seeds and nuts, and oils. Many nutrients help promote immunity and prevent or decrease the effects of infection, either alone or in combination with other nutrients, and many nutrients encompass several food groups. The following summarizes more common nutrients that have been shown to improve immunity as well as their common sources. Vitamin A (found in orange vegetables and fruits rich beta carotene, such as carrots or squash, and several varieties of green vegetables) promotes the proliferation and differentiation of T lymphocytes that stimulate the antibody response and increase the production of surfactant. Alpha and beta carotene in fruits and vegetables, converted to vitamin A, have antioxidant prosperities and decrease the production of reactive oxygen species. Vitamin B9 (found in dark green leafy vegetables, such as spinach, and other green vegetables) plays a role in DNA synthesis. Vitamin B9, along with vitamin B6 (found in meat, fish, or vegetables) and B12 (found in meat, fish, poultry, or dairy products), can alleviate the severity of viral infections through modulation and support of T lymphocyte activity, increased natural killer cell activity, and decrease inflammation. Vitamin C (found in citrus fruits, red and green peppers, or berries) has a protective effect on cells, functions in the clearance of macrophages, decreasing inflammation and reducing activity of reactive oxygen species. Vitamin D (found in eggs, oily fish, fortified foods and milk, synthesized in the skin via sunlight) interacts with angiotensin converting enzyme 2 (ACE2) to reduce viral entry and activity and reduce cytokine storm activity, reducing inflammation. Vitamin E (found in nuts, seeds, and vegetable oils) reduces damage to cell membranes by decreasing the activity of reactive oxygen species and promotes clearance of free radicals and macrophages.[7-9] Trace elements such as selenium (found in fish, eggs, meat, and nuts), zinc (found in meat, and grains), copper (found in nuts, grains, and vegetables), and iron (found in meat, nuts, and grains) function as cofactors for enzymes in the oxidative burst pathway, thus supporting immune efficiency and decreasing the risk or susceptibility of microbial infections.[7,8,10]

Optimism

The tendency to take the most hopeful view of matters and to expect the best outcome. Optimism encourages courage and determination not to give up even if a person experiences failure. It also promotes resiliency.

Pets

Pets reduce stress and anxiety. They give a sense of security and companionship. They decrease depressive symptoms and have a calming effect on their owners. They buffer stressful events and promote socialization with other pet owners.

Prayer and Meditation

One of the most common coping strategies is prayer and meditation. Faith in God and his healing mercy is powerful to overcome the feeling of uncertainty in life threatening illnesses and gives hope. God answers all heartfelt and sincere prayers according to his will in his own ways and according to his own time. There is increased cerebral blood flow during meditative prayer.[14] Prayer also promotes insight and gives peace.

Quality Time

Spending quality time with family and friends enriches our experiences and enhances the feeling of security.

Quiet

Finding quiet time to rest your mind and to prevent distractions. Peace and quiet invigorate the spirit.

Recreation

Recreation refreshes the mind and body. It promotes a feeling of well-being and encourages socialization, which buffers stress and anxiety. Movies and reading are positive coping strategies.

Safety

Safety is priority during the current COVID-19 pandemic. The use of personal protective equipment (e.g., masks), social distancing, and hand washing are mandatory to protect individuals and communities from the viral infection.

Therapy

Talk with a professional or someone when emotions like anxiety and depression are overwhelming and impairing.

Universality

"We are together, and this too shall pass." There is a universal feeling of uncertainty with the COVID-19 pandemic, but one is not alone in coping with this universal viral infection.

Volunteer

Volunteering in religious and civic organizations increases self-esteem and promotes a sense of well-being and satisfaction.

Win New Friends

Increasing socialization gains emotional support during crises or stressful situations.

X-hale/letting go

Letting go of grudges and resentments promotes mental health. Forgiveness gives peace and feelings of well-being.

Yearning

Longing for resolution of stressful situations and recovery from life threatening illness.

Zero In What Is Important

Prioritize energy and resources to deal with stressors that may have life-long negative impact.

Zoom

Using Zoom technology to reach out to friends and family for emotional support and to have fun.

REFERENCES

1. Schlozman S, Droves J, Weisman A. Coping with illness and psychotherapy of true medically ill. In: Stern T, Fricchione G, Cassem N, et al., eds. *Handbook of General Hospital Psychiatry*. 5th ed. Philadelphia, PA: Mosby; 2004:61-68.
2. Folkman S, Moskowitz JT. Coping: Pitfalls and promise. *Annul Rev Psychol*. 2004;55:745-749.
3. Gurvich C, Thomas N, Thomas EH, et al. Coping styles and mental health in response to societal changes during the Covid-19 pandemic (published online ahead of print,2020 Oct 4). *Int Social Psychiatry*. 2020.20764020961790.
4. Adam RAH, Van der Beck EM, Buitelaan JK, et al. Nutritional psychiatry: Towards improving mental health by what you eat. *Eur Neuropsychopharmacology*. 2019;29 (12):134-1332.
5. Calder PC, Cair AC, Dombaut AF, Eggersdofer M. Optimal nutritional status for a well-functioning immune system is an important factor to protect against vital infections. *Nutrients*. 2020;12(4):1181.

6. Zabetaskis I, Lordan R, Norton C, Tsoupras A. Covid-19: The inflammation link and the role of nutrition in protentional mitigation. *Nutrients*. 2020;12(5):1466.

7. Iddir M, Brito G, Dingeo G, et al. Strengthening the immune system and reducing the inflammation and oxidative stress through diet and nutrition: Considerations during the Covid-19 crisis. *Nutrients*. 2020;12(6):1562.

8. Calder PC. Nutrition, immunity and Covid-19. *BMJ Nutr Prev Health*. 2020;3(1):74-92.

9. Jovic TH, Ali SR, Ibrahim N, et al. Could vitamins help in the fight against Covid-19? *Nutrients*. 2020;12(9):2550.

10. Calder PC. Feeding the immune system. *Proc Nutr Soc*. 2013;72(3):299-309.

11. Ashdown-Frank G, Firth J, Carvey R, et al. Exercise on medicine for mental and substance use disorders A meta-review of the benefits for neuropsychology and cognitive outcomes. *Sports Med*. 2020;50:151-170.

12. Bennett MP, Lengachen CA. Humor and laughter may influence health. History and background. *Evid Based Complement Alternat Med*. 2006;3:61-63.

13. Minjanez MB, Montague RA, Fox EA, Piacentinic J. Cognitive and behavior therapies. In: Martin A, Block M, Volkman F, eds. *Lewis's Child and Adolescent Psychiatry*. 5th ed. Philadelphia, PA: Wolters Kluwer; 2018:757-785.

SECTION II
Crises in Pandemics

SARS AND MERS 19

Jerry Jomi, MD and Taaran Ballachanda, MD

▌INTRODUCTION

Coronaviruses are associated with the common cold as well as severe acute respiratory syndrome coronavirus (SARS-CoV-1) and Middle Eastern Respiratory Syndrome (MERS). These viruses belong to the family *Coronaviridae* which falls under the *Nidovirales* order. The coronaviruses are positive strand RNA viruses that range from 80–120 nm in diameter. The RNA genome forms a helical capsid with an N protein and has at least 3–4 surface proteins, which give it its crown or "corona"-like appearance under electron microscopy, from which it derives its name.[1]

There remains a large deficit in our understanding of the novel coronavirus infections that have infected humans because of the lag between the emergence of a new strain that infects human beings from animal reservoirs, isolating the animal host from which the new strains are thought to have emerged, and understanding how these novel viruses cause disease in human beings. It is hypothesized that the emergence of novel infectious viruses through zoonotic transmission from animals to humans is a consequence of climate change.[2]

The SARS-CoV-1 virus is thought to have emerged from bats, more specifically horseshoe bats (*Rhinolophus sinicus*) whose close interaction with unsanitary "wet markets" in the Guangdong province in China is thought to have been the origin of the SARS CoV-1 viral epidemic in 2003.[3] Antibodies for SARS-CoV-1 have also been found in masked palm civet (*Paguma larvata*) populations and isolated cases have been described from exposure to these mammals.[4] The zoonotic reservoir for MERS-CoV is the dromedary camels (*Camelus dromedarius*) that have been found to carry neutralizing antibodies to MERS-CoV and have interactions with humans and densely populated marketplaces.[5]

EPIDEMIOLOGY

The first cases of SARS-CoV-1 were noted in Guangdong Province in south eastern China in November, 2002. It soon spread from the southern and eastern provinces of China as well as Hong Kong to more countries in Asia and then to Europe, Canada, and the United States.[6] The initial cases were traced to exotic meat markets and resulted in local community spread in China. Index cases in new hotspots thereafter were traced to people who had traveled from the provinces of China as well as to healthcare institutions which is displayed in the fact that healthcare workers and their contacts were disproportionately affected during the epidemic.

The novel virus was successfully isolated and identified between February and March 2003.[7] During the major SARS epidemic from 2002–2003 a total of 8,096 cases were reported in 29 countries with 774 deaths. Of these 1,706 cases were reported among healthcare workers.[8] Since the end of the major epidemic, small outbreaks have been traced to laboratories working with the SARS virus[9,10] as well as unrelated cases from presumed exposure to infected animals.[11]

The MERS CoV epidemic is thought to have started in April 2012 and the index case of MERS-CoV was a male patient from Jeddah, Saudi Arabia in June 2012.[12] Since that time there have been several outbreaks and clusters of cases. A majority of the cases are seen in the Arabian Peninsula.[13] In May 2015 another large outbreak occurred in South Korea and the index case was identified to be a male patient who had traveled extensively to countries in the Middle East.[14] Dromedary camels are thought to be the reservoir of the disease. Close contact between humans and these camels appears to be the primary mode of animal to human transmission and the reason for high sustained prevalence in Saudi Arabia and its neighboring countries. This is of course followed by person to person spread. Cases have also been described that are imported to other countries and then lead to clusters of cases described usually in household and community contacts or in healthcare settings. This has led to ongoing cases and clusters described around the world. As of November 2020, 2,562 laboratory confirmed cases of MERS- CoV have been reported in 27 countries.

RISK FACTORS

In both SARS CoV-1 and MERS, mortality is linked with advanced age, especially in cases where the patient is more than 60 years old, with an increase in risk for every 10 years added. Diabetes mellitus, lung disease, kidney disease, obesity, and an immunocompromised state were also noted to be associated with increased mortality and increased incidence of adverse outcomes.[15,16]

For SARS CoV-1, additional factors associated with adverse outcomes include severe lymphopenia, high neutrophil count at presentation, prolonged thromboplastin time, elevated urea, lactate dehydrogenase level > 450 IU/l, and multilobar infiltrates on radiograph.[17-19] Other factors include high inflammatory markers on admission, elevated viral titers during the first week of disease, and low antibody titers during the second week of disease.[20]

PATHOPHYSIOLOGY

SARS CoV-1 interacts with cells through the metallopeptidase, ACE2[21,22] and the distribution of ACE2 by immunohistochemical staining does, in general, reflect the pattern of infected organs[23] (Figure 19-1). However, the lack of ACE2 receptors on immune cells, some epithelial cells and neuronal cells, where SARS CoV-1 infection is described suggest other receptors, co-receptors or mechanisms are involved.[24] ACE2 itself is dependent on cathepsin L which is a pH sensitive proteolytic enzyme and activity differs in each organ.[25-27]

The first 10 days of the infection involves direct cytopathic effects of the virus. This has been best described in the lower respiratory tract as well

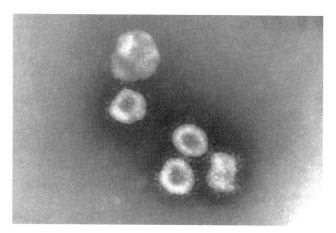

Figure 19-1 • Transmission electron microscopic image of coronavirus virions, each surrounded by its characteristic corona due to the presence of viral spike peplomers emanating from the proteinaceous capsid. (*Courtesy of the CDC.* https://phil.cdc.gov/Details.aspx?pid=16331.)

as the immune cells and lymphoid tissue. Infection of the T-lymphocytes and monocytes/macrophages in the blood, lymph nodes, lungs, and spleen and resulting apoptosis, autophagy, aberrant cell honing and destruction of bone marrow precursors help explain the lymphopenia noted early on in the disease.[28] The involvement of T-lymphocytes and monocytes which are integral components of both the innate and cell mediated immune responses can also help explain the compromised immune status of infected patients.[29]

Both cytokines and chemokines are believed to play important roles in the progression of SARS CoV-1 infection. A dysregulation of these proteins is believed to lead to immune related injury which is supported by clinical deterioration of cases in the second week despite down-trending viral titers. An increase in levels of several cytokines and immunosuppressive chemokines such as prostaglandin E2 and transforming growth factor B have been described.[30,31] In addition, there is impairment of macrophage phagocytosis, which makes the patient prone to secondary bacterial infections.[32]

Autoantibodies against pulmonary epithelial cells and systemic vascular endothelium, causing pneumonitis and vasculitis, have been described. This mechanism is thought to be caused by either direct SARS CoV-1 viral cytopathic effect as well as cytokine directed organ damage.[33] Studies have also described a difference in disease severity in certain populations that has been linked to different HLA haplotypes.[34]

Although the description of clinical manifestations of MERS CoV and SARS CoV-1 infections may seem very similar, in vitro and ex vivo studies have shown significant differences in their growth characteristics, their receptor usage, and expected host responses suggesting differing pathogenesis (Figure 19-2).[35] Using spectral microscopy, Hocke et al. studied human lung tissue that had been infected ex vivo by the MERS CoV and described the expression of viral antigen on the surfaces of type I and type II alveolar cells, ciliated and non-ciliated bronchial epithelium, pulmonary vascular endothelial cells, and rarely even in alveolar macrophages.[36] The receptor Dipeptidyl peptidase 4 (DPP4) or also named CD26 has been recognized as the receptor used by the MERS-CoV virus.[37] These are exopeptidases but their proteolytic activity is not thought to be required for the virus to bind to the cell or to enter it.[38] DPP4 is widely distributed over type I and type II alveolar cells, bronchial epithelium, submucosal glands, pulmonary vascular endothelium as well as alveolar macrophages and leukocytes. This correlates well with the findings of tropism noted in the ex vivo and cell line in vitro studies.[39] Studies of other species show that the MERS-CoV binding site on the DPP4 receptor differs. Hence, different species are

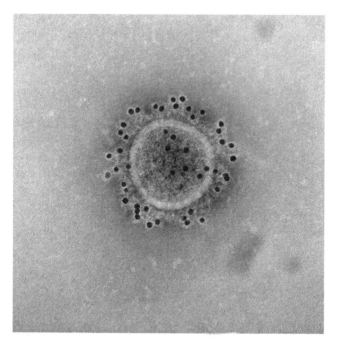

Figure 19-2 • Transmission electron microscopic image of MERS-CoV showing a single, spherical shaped virion. (*Courtesy of the CDC.* https://phil.cdc.gov/Details. aspx?pid=18108.)

affected differently and findings for other species cannot directly be applied to explain findings in humans.[40]

MERS-CoV appears to have a much more significant cytopathic effect compared with SARS-CoV-1 early in the infection and this may explain its increased susceptibility to prophylactic and therapeutic agents in vitro.[41] In addition MERS-CoV causes significant dysregulation of immune pathways, specifically by down-regulating genes involved in the antigen presentation pathway that further impairs adaptive immune mechanisms.[42] Unfortunately, the lack of autopsy studies means that we do not know which cytokine and chemokine responses are the most responsible for the MERS-CoV infection and clinical picture.

CLINICAL MANIFESTATION

SARS-CoV-1

The mean incubation period is 5.29 days with a variance of 12.33 days with approximately 90% of the patients having onset of symptoms before 11.58 days.[43] Time from onset of patients' clinical symptoms to admission to hospital is between 3 and 5 days.[44] During the epidemic, WHO estimated the maximum incubation period to be 10 days.[45]

The major clinical characteristics of SARS on presentation include fever (> 38°C), non-productive cough, myalgia, chills/rigors, and dyspnea.[46-48] Symptoms such as diarrhea, nausea and vomiting, sputum production, dizziness are less commonly seen on initial presentation. In addition, upper respiratory symptoms (sore throat, rhinorrhea) are less often seen. Watery diarrhea is found later in the disease process; up to 73% of patients in one prospective study in Hong Kong had watery diarrhea at one point.[49] Diarrhea was also noted as one of the only complaints for initial presentation later during the epidemic. Case reports revealed neurological manifestations of SARS including SARS as a possible etiology for resulting status epilepticus.[50] The elderly population may present atypically. They may present afebrile, with poor appetite, falls, and encephalopathy.[51] The pediatric population typically had milder symptoms with no recorded mortality.[52]

A meta-analysis revealed that the overall seroprevalence for the general population (other than wild animal handlers) was 0.10% (95% CI, 0.02–0.18). The analysis revealed healthcare workers and close contacts had a higher seroprevalence of 0.23% (95% CI, 0.02–0.45) when compared with healthy blood donors or non-SARS patients recruited from a healthcare setting.[53]

On initial presentation, the physical exam revealed fevers above 38°C.[54] Auscultation of the lungs may have produced crepitus, however this is seldom heard. Surprisingly, the exam typically did not correlate with the radiographic findings.[55]

Blood analysis commonly reveals lymphocytopenia, and less often thrombocytopenia and isolated prolonged activated partial thromboplastin time. Lymphocytopenia in particular was seen among 98% of patients in a retrospective study from Hong Kong.[56] Elevated lactate dehydrogenase, creatinine kinase, and alanine aminotransferase are also possible.

Chest X-ray had abnormal findings in approximately 71–87% of the SARS patients.[57-60] Two different patterns may emerge: unifocal, peripheral airspace opacification (typically peripherally); or lobar consolidation or bilateral consolidation resembling acute respiratory distress syndrome (ARDS). In one retrospective study evaluating chest X-rays of SARS patients, 64.8% of the images had lower lung zone involvement.[61] Although the findings were nonspecific, especially in the early part of the epidemic, having an abnormal chest X-ray in the accompaniment of relevant clinical labs and history aided in the diagnosis.

The most common findings on CT are ground glass opacities or consolidation, or both. Findings such as pleural effusion, cavitation, reticular/nodular opacification, calcification, and lymphadenopathy are not found on a review of over 100 CT scans in any of the SARS patients.[62] Twelve percent of patients developed pneumomediastinum spontaneously unrelated to intubation or positive-pressure ventilation.[63] Patients may have normal CXR but 67% may have abnormal CT.[63]

It is believed that SARS has a disease progression in a couple of phases. The first phase is believed to be directly from the viral replication and its direct effect. This is the typical presentation of fevers, coughs, myalgias as mentioned above. A majority of these patients have clinical improvement of their symptoms and are discharged. By the second week, approximately 30% of the patients will require admission to the intensive care unit with 20% of them even advancing to ARDS requiring invasive mechanical ventilation. The patients that deteriorate are believed to have a second phase that is theorized to be a result of host immunopathological damage or what we refer to now as "cytokine storm"; by the second week, the viral load has significantly decreased.

MERS-CoV

The mean incubation period is 5.2 days with a range of 1.9 to 14.7 days.[64-68] Interestingly, a study from Korea analyzed the incubation period for 170 patients and found a correlation of having a shorter incubation period associated with increased mortality.[69]

The major clinical characteristics of MERS on presentation include fever (> 38°C), chills/rigors, non-productive cough, and dyspnea. In additions, patients may present less commonly with upper respiratory symptoms (sore throat, rhinorrhea), headache, myalgias, or gastrointestinal disturbances such as diarrhea, nausea, and vomiting.[52-56] Other non-pulmonary manifestations include neurological features. Three cases from Saudi Arabia were noted to have presentations of confusion, ataxia, and focal deficits.[70] MERS affecting the pediatric population was less commonly seen. Of the pediatric population affected, 42% were asymptomatic.[71,72] In total, 298 cases of laboratory confirmed MERS have been reported to WHO as asymptomatic.[73]

On initial presentation, the physical exam for the symptomatic patients revealed documented fevers above 38°C. In one retrospective chart review of 51 patients from Saudi Arabia, 15.7% of the patients had hypotension, 76.9% of the patients had tachypnea, and 33% patients had hypoxia noted during the physical exam.[74]

A review of laboratory findings revealed lymphocytopenia as a common finding. In addition, blood analysis may reveal thrombocytopenia, leukocytosis, transaminitis, elevated LDH, and elevated markers indicative of disseminated intravascular coagulation.[75–78]

Chest X-ray abnormalities, such as ground glass, consolidations and cavitary lesions, were found in between 83 and 100% of the cases.[79] The most common location was the right lower lobe.[79] CT also revealed ground glass and consolidations. Nearly half the patients in one retrospective study showed pleural effusions. The presence of pleural effusion was associated with increased mortality. Tree in bud, cavitation, and lymph node enlargement are not as commonly seen although they do exist.[80,81]

MERS for most patients involved a rapid and severe deterioration to respiratory and multi-organ failure. The study determined that median time to mechanical ventilation was 7 days (range 3–11).[82–84] Mortality was determined to be a staggering 60%.[82–84] Attempts were made to place patients on non-invasive ventilation as a trial. An analysis from 14 different centers showed that around 92.4% of patients placed on non-invasive ventilation ended up requiring invasive ventilation and no change in outcome compared to early invasive ventilation strategy.[85] Strategies for managing the acute hypoxic respiratory failure on the ventilator consisted mainly of ARDS. Ventilator settings were altered to ensure lung protection was the highest priority including low tidal volumes and low plateau pressures.[86] A retrospective analysis concluded that the use of ECMO as a rescue therapy indicated lower mortality for MERS patients with refractory hypoxemia.[87]

DIAGNOSIS

SARS-COV-1

Clinical presentation is non-specific and often epidemiologic correlation can aide with diagnosis. Reverse transcriptase PCR (RT-PCR) could be completed on samples obtained from respiratory tract secretions (upper and lower), serum, stools, and urine specimens. RT-PCR used early in the epidemic had poor sensitivity in the first 5 days of illness so a negative result did not exclude the diagnosis.[88] In addition, upper respiratory samples had a poorer yield than lower respiratory samples which can be explained by the low upper respiratory compromise of the infection. Completing repeated RT-PCR on different specimens did lead to a higher diagnostic rate.

Viral culture was not ideal as it required processing in Biosafety Level 3 facilities and the results would take too long to alter management.

Antibody assays such as ELIZA, IFA have better specificities when conducted 2–4 weeks after onset of infection and thus relayed as a use for confirmation that a patient had SARS in the past.[89,90]

MERS-CoV

Lack of distinguishing symptoms, laboratory findings, or radiological differences forced clinicians to use epidemiology and clinical suspicion stemming from case definition to aid in diagnosis.

An early definition released by WHO which clinicians adopted included a person with acute respiratory syndrome having fevers ($> 38°C$) and cough. In addition, these suspected patients required hospitalization and indicated clinical/radiological suspicion of lower respiratory airway involvement not explained by any other etiology. Epidemiology played a huge role as the suspected patient should have close contact with MERS within 10 days.[91]

Laboratory modes of diagnosis included real time reverse transcriptase PCR (rRT-PCR) assay for detection of the viral RNA, viral cultures, and serological testing for the antibodies. Samples obtained for nucleic acid amplification and viral cultures required upper or lower respiratory tract specimens. DPP4 was determined to be a key cellular receptor for MERS. This cellular receptor is located primarily in the non-ciliated bronchial epithelial cells, alveolar epithelial cells, and macrophages of the lower respiratory tract. Therefore, lower respiratory tract specimens such as those obtained from bronchoalveolar lavage, sputum aspirates, and tracheal aspirates resulted in a higher diagnostic yield, which should always be sought.[92] A combination of both upper and lower respiratory specimens obtained was recommended by WHO.

rRT-PCR was quickly developed after the initial sighting of MERS.[93] The rapid process time with high sensitivity made it a great tool for screening and confirmation of MERS infection. Three rRT-PCR assays were produced: one assay targeting upstream of the E protein gene (upE), one assay targeting open reading frame 1b (ORF1b), and one assay targeting open reading frame 1a (ORF1a). In addition, assays can target the MERS nucleocapsid (N) protein gene. The assay targeting upE was considered the ideal screening tool with its very high sensitivity profile. Positive results from assays targeting two different genomic locations were considered confirmation of the presence of MERS infection.

Removal of isolation precautions was vital to conserve resource consumption. During the endemic, if two repeated rRT-PCR were negative, that was indicative of clearance of the virus. Viral cultures was not considered a preferred tool as this required processing in Biosafety Level 3 facilities which were not readily available.[94] Serological detection of antibodies can be helpful for diagnosing prior MERS infection. If used for patients on presentation, this required two separate samples; the first sample obtained within the first week of illness and the second sample 3–4 weeks after onset.

TREATMENT

SARS-COV-1

There was and still no definitive treatment/cure for SARS. Most clinicians provided empiric antibacterial antibiotics covering for typical and atypical sources of community acquired pneumonias as it was difficult to differentiate from SARS.

Numerous institutions enacted protocols that included providing a mix and match of several medication combinations mentioned below that made retrospective analysis very difficult. This was mostly due to quick development of the epidemic that forced clinicians to provide treatment options based on theoretical models or in-vitro results. Due to that, there were no randomized, placebo-controlled clinical trials completed. An extensive systematic review was published in 2006 outlining 54 trials during the epidemic regarding management. A vast majority of the studies were considered inconclusive with several signaling harm to the patient.[95] Here we will briefly discuss some of the medications that were used in the acute management of SARS throughout the epidemic.

Ribavirin

As it was unclear which specific organism was causing SARS in the earlier part of the pandemic, Ribavirin was initially provided as it had broad anti-viral properties. Many of the studies were considered inconclusive. Several studies revealed the treatment arms with Ribavirin resulted in increased occurrence of hemolytic anemias.[96] In one study from Toronto, in addition to 49% of the patients on a higher Ribavirin dose experiencing drops in hemoglobin (66% of these were found to be secondary to hemolysis), transaminitis was noted in 40% of the patients, and bradycardia in 14%.[97] The significant adverse effects made the use of Ribavirin fall off.

Corticosteroids

In attempts made to control the immunopathological damage triggered by SARS, the use of corticosteroid was evaluated. The typical choice was IV methylprednisolone, sometimes given in pulse. A total of 15 studies were analyzed during the systemic analysis, and 13 were deemed to be considered inconclusive. The other two studies signaled harm to the patient; one study showed inability to decrease viral load,[98] and another study had a correlation with psychosis.[99] The timing and dosing of corticosteroids varied widely and was considered a controversial topic.[100]

Protease Inhibitors

The combination of choice during the epidemic was lopinavir-ritonavir. Promising results from in-vitro labs to SARS prompted use of this medication duo. Two larger retrospective matched cohort studies, although deemed inconclusive due to selection bias and treatment allocation, did show promising results. One study with early administration of lopinavir-ritonavir in addition to Ribavirin and corticosteroid was associated with reduced mortality (2.3%) compared to the control arm of only Ribavirin and corticosteroid use with mortality of 15.6%.[101] The other study compared 41 patients that received lopinavir-ritonavir and Ribavirin to 111 patients that did not receive lopinavir-ritonavir. This study showed association of decreased ARDS or death for the lopinavir-ritonavir arm.[102]

Interferon

Interferon was another option that had good yields from in-vitro studies that clinicians were hoping to translate clinically to patients. In an open label study in Toronto, nine patients given interferon alpha plus corticosteroids were compared with 13 patients given only corticosteroids. The interferon alpha treatment group showed quicker resolution of lung imaging abnormalities, improved oxygen saturation, resolved dependency on supplemental oxygen quicker, and smaller increase in creatine kinase levels.[103]

Convalescent Plasma/Immunoglobulins

One of the novel treatment options offered was the administration of convalescent plasma donated by fully recovered SARS patients. There were seven studies evaluated by the systemic analysis and all of them were considered inconclusive. Among them, one was a retrospective study that compared a total of 40 patients after receiving a course of Ribavirin plus pulsed methylprednisolone treatment. Nineteen of these patients were allocated to receive convalescent plasma, and the other group was continued on pulsed corticosteroid. The convalescent plasma arm showed an increased discharge rate (77% vs 23%, p = 0.004), and more importantly reduced mortality (0% vs 23.8%, p = 0.049).[104]

Lack of an adequate treatment protocol forced major emphasis on methods to control an outbreak. WHO provided guidance on containing outbreaks:

- prompt detection of cases through good surveillance networks and including an early warning system;
- isolation of suspected or probable cases;
- tracing to identify both the source of the infection and contacts of those who are sick and may be at risk of contracting the virus;
- quarantine of suspected contacts for 10 days;
- exit screening for outgoing passengers from areas with recent local transmission by asking questions and temperature measurement; and
- disinfection of aircraft and cruise vessels having SARS cases on board using WHO guidelines.

Personal preventive measures to prevent the spread of the virus include frequent hand washing using soap or alcohol-based disinfectants. For those with a high risk of contracting the disease, such as health care workers, use of personal protective equipment, including a mask, goggles and an apron is mandatory. Whenever possible, household contacts should also wear a mask.[105]

MERS-CoV

A definitive treatment/cure for MERS was never found. Management consisted mostly of supportive care. Most guidelines recommended the use of empiric antibacterial antibiotics covering for typical and atypical sources of community acquired pneumonias. MERS had up to 23.6% co-infection from bacterial sources such as streptococcus pneumonia and legionella pneumophila. Macrolides was considered as an antibiotic option, but was considered controversial with its side effect profile—especially cardiac arrhythmias. One retrospective study saw no changes in mortality with the use of macrolides.

During the endemic, institutions created protocols and made investigational choices on their use of drugs to combat MERS. This made the formation of a formal randomized, placebo-controlled clinical trial nonexistent. No conclusive trial exists to support the use of any drug against MERS. Here we will briefly discuss some of the medications that were used during the endemic.

Corticosteroids

Studies on corticosteroid use during the SARS pandemic reduced the frequency of corticosteroid use during the MERS endemic. The benefits seen from the MERS era also appear to be insufficient. In a retrospective analysis of 151 patients from 14 different Saudi Arabia health centers, a study published in the American Journal of Respiratory and Critical Care Medicine determined that corticosteroid use effected no change in mortality and in fact was associated with delayed MERS coronavirus RNA clearance.[106] Corticosteroids were used however for their benefit in distributive shock through the formulation of hydrocortisone.

Interferon and Ribavirin

Administration of interferon analogues was thought to help combat the suppressed interferon response induced by the MERS infection. In-vitro studies had positive findings that led to clinical application. Ribavirin also had inhibitory effects seen in-vitro, but in very high doses. Patients typically received a combination of interferon with Ribavirin. Data collected consisted mostly of case series and several small population retrospective trials with inconsistent efficacy. One retrospective study on the use of interferon + ribavirin early in the endemic conferred a positive 14-day mortality; however, no change in mortality at 28 days.[107–109]

Convalescent Plasma/Immunoglobulins

Positive trends seen during the SARS pandemic led to development of the use of plasma/immunoglobulins for the MERS endemic. The high mortality and lack of any treatment forced WHO to take the position early in the endemic that this should be a highly sought-after treatment option with trials required immediately.[110] Early animal studies showed a significant improvement of lung histological changes and viral clearance after administration of high-titer MERS immune serum. Evidence on the use of plasma/immunoglobulins for MERS is very minimal. The lack of a large pool of donors became an obstacle for any large interventional trial that could be planned.[111]

Vaccines

A vaccine for SARS-CoV-1 was considered due to the discovery of a less severe variant from Guangzhou, China, that resembled the palm civet SARS-CoV virus. It was hypothesized that neutralizing antibodies from the less severe form is effective against the original strain. Targets included blockade of ACE receptors and S protein. Other vaccine candidates included recombinant vaccines like the recombinant Baculovirus with the full length S protein or its extracellular domain,[112] the modified vaccinia Ankara virus expressing the S protein,[113] and attenuated parainfluenza virus expressing SARS coronavirus spike proteins.[114] Some studies also tested the immunogenicity of portions of the spike protein to elucidate which would be the most immunogenic.[115,116] None have been successful.

MERS-CoV

Most of the vaccine candidates for MERS-CoV have focused on the spike protein, specifically the receptor-binding domain which interacts with the human cell receptors for viral entry into cells. Nanoparticles, recombinant protein subunits, DNA, and recombinant viral vectors are among the modalities that have been developed and tested on mice and non-human primates.[117–121] Most of these studies remain in the pre-clinical phases and only a few have reached phase I/II human trials.[122] Greater success has been noted in vaccine candidates that have used whole DNA material or a combination of DNA material and subunit protein for booster purposes as opposed to simply using protein subunits.[123] Unfortunately, despite work on vaccines against MERS-CoV starting in 2012 after the discovery of the virus, thus far a viable vaccine candidate has not yet been brought to market.

▌ REFERENCES

1. Weiss SR, Navas-Martin S. Coronavirus pathogenesis and the emerging pathogen severe acute respiratory syndrome coronavirus. *Microbiol Mol Biol Rev*. 2005;69(4):635-664.
2. Coleman CM, Frieman MB. Coronaviruses: important emerging human pathogens. *J Virol*. 2014;88(10):5209-5212.
3. Kan B, Wang M, Jing H, et al. Molecular evolution analysis and geographic investigation of severe acute respiratory syndrome coronavirus-like virus in palm civets at an animal market and on farms. *J Virol*. 2005;79(18):11892-11900.
4. Shi Z, Hu Z. A review of studies on animal reservoirs of the SARS coronavirus. *Virus Res*. 2008;133(1):74-87.
5. Azhar EI, El-Kafrawy SA, Farraj SA, et al. Evidence for camel-to-human transmission of MERS coronavirus. *N Engl J Med*. 2014;370(26):2499-2505.
6. Christian MD, Poutanen SM, Loutfy MR, Muller MP, Low DE. Severe acute respiratory syndrome. *Clin Infect Dis*. 2004;38(10):1420-1427.
7. Ksiazek TG, Erdman D, Goldsmith CS, et al. A novel coronavirus associated with severe acute respiratory syndrome. *N Engl J Med*. 2003;348(20):1953-1966.
8. https://www.who.int/publications/m/item/summary-of-probable-sars-cases-with-onset-of-illness-from-1-november-2002-to-31-july-2003. Accessed December 18, 2020.

9. Lim PL, Kurup A, Gopalakrishna G, et al. Laboratory-acquired severe acute respiratory syndrome. *N Engl J Med*. 2004;350(17):1740-1745.

10. https://www.who.int/csr/don/2004_04_30/en/.

11. https://www.who.int/csr/don/archive/disease/severe_acute_respiratory_syndrome/en/.

12. Zaki AM, Van Boheemen S, Bestebroer TM, Osterhaus AD, Fouchier RA. Isolation of a novel coronavirus from a man with pneumonia in Saudi Arabia. *N Engl J Med*. 2012;367(19):1814-1820.

13. Bermingham A, Chand MA, Brown CS, et al. Severe respiratory illness caused by a novel coronavirus, in a patient transferred to the United Kingdom from the Middle East, September 2012. *Euro Surveill*. 2012;17(40): 20290.

14. Kim SW, Yang TU, Jeong Y, Park JW, Lee KJ, Kim KM. Middle East respiratory syndrome coronavirus outbreak in the Republic of Korea, 2015. *Osong Public Health Res Perspect*. 2016;6(4):269-278.

15. Garbati MA, Fagbo SF, Fang VJ, et al. A comparative study of clinical presentation and risk factors for adverse outcome in patients hospitalised with acute respiratory disease due to MERS coronavirus or other causes. *PloS One*. 2016;11(11):e0165978.

16. Garbati MA, Fagbo SF, Fang VJ, et al. A comparative study of clinical presentation and risk factors for adverse outcome in patients hospitalised with acute respiratory disease due to MERS coronavirus or other causes. *PloS One*. 2016;11(11):e0165978.

17. Chan JWM, Ng CK, Chan YH, et al. Short term outcome and risk factors for adverse clinical outcomes in adults with severe acute respiratory syndrome (SARS). *Thorax*. 2003;58(8):686-689.

18. Hui DS, Azhar EI, Kim YJ, Memish ZA, Oh MD, Zumla A. Middle East respiratory syndrome coronavirus: risk factors and determinants of primary, household, and nosocomial transmission. *Lancet Infect Dis*. 2018;18(8):e217-e227.

19. Garbati MA, Fagbo SF, Fang VJ, et al. A comparative study of clinical presentation and risk factors for adverse outcome in patients hospitalised with acute respiratory disease due to MERS coronavirus or other causes. *PloS One*. 2016;11(11):e0165978.

20. Hong KH, Choi JP, Hong SH, et al. Predictors of mortality in Middle East respiratory syndrome (MERS). *Thorax*. 2018;73(3):286-289.

21. Gu J, Korteweg C. Pathology and pathogenesis of severe acute respiratory syndrome. *Am J Pathol*. 2007;170(4):1136-1147.

22. Li W, Moore MJ, Vasilieva N, et al. Angiotensin-converting enzyme 2 is a functional receptor for the SARS coronavirus. *Nature*. 2003;426(6965):450-454.

23. Sims AC, Baric RS, Yount B, Burkett SE, Collins PL, Pickles RJ. Severe acute respiratory syndrome coronavirus infection of human ciliated airway epithelia: role of ciliated cells in viral spread in the conducting airways of the lungs. *J Virol*. 2005;79(24):15511-15524.

24. Hamming I, Timens W, Bulthuis MLC, Lely AT, Navis GV, van Goor H. 2004. Tissue distribution of ACE2 protein, the functional receptor for SARS coronavirus. A first step in understanding SARS pathogenesis. *J Pathol*. 2004;203(2):631-637.

25. Huang IC, Bosch BJ, Li F, et al. SARS coronavirus, but not human coronavirus NL63, utilizes cathepsin L to infect ACE2-expressing cells. *J Biol Chem*. 2006;281(6):3198-3203.

26. Jeffers SA, Tusell SM, Gillim-Ross L, et al. CD209L (L-SIGN) is a receptor for severe acute respiratory syndrome coronavirus. *Proc Natl Acad Sci.* 2004;101(44):15748-15753.

27. Marzi A, Gramberg T, Simmons G, et al. DC-SIGN and DC-SIGNR interact with the glycoprotein of Marburg virus and the S protein of severe acute respiratory syndrome coronavirus. *J Virol.* 2004;78(21):12090-12095.

28. Gu J, Gong E, Zhang B, et al. Multiple organ infection and the pathogenesis of SARS. *J Exp Med.* 2005;202(3):415-424.

29. Yen YT, Liao F, Hsiao CH, Kao CL, Chen YC, Wu-Hsieh BA. 2006. Modeling the early events of severe acute respiratory syndrome coronavirus infection in vitro. *J Virol.* 2006;80(6):2684-2693.

30. Nicholls JM, Poon LL, Lee KC, et al. Lung pathology of fatal severe acute respiratory syndrome. *Lancet.* 2003;361(9371):1773-1778.

31. Hamming I, Timens W, Bulthuis MLC, Lely AT, Navis GV, van Goor H. Tissue distribution of ACE2 protein, the functional receptor for SARS coronavirus. A first step in understanding SARS pathogenesis. *J Pathol.* 2004;203(2):631-637.

32. Tseng CTK, Perrone LA, Zhu H, Makino S, Peters CJ. Severe acute respiratory syndrome and the innate immune responses: modulation of effector cell function without productive infection. *J Immunol.* 2005;174(12):7977-7985.

33. Yang YH, Huang YH, Chuang YH, et al. Autoantibodies against human epithelial cells and endothelial cells after severe acute respiratory syndrome (SARS) associated coronavirus infection. *J Med Virol.* 2005;77(1):1-7.

34. Ng MH, Lau KM, Li L, et al. Association of human-leukocyte-antigen class I (B*0703) and class II (DRB1*0301) genotypes with susceptibility and resistance to the development of severe acute respiratory syndrome. *J Infect Dis.* 2004;190(3):515-518.

35. Van Den Brand JM, Smits SL, Haagmans BL. Pathogenesis of Middle East respiratory syndrome coronavirus. *J Pathol.* 2015;235(2):175-184.

36. Hocke AC, Becher A, Knepper J, et al. Emerging human middle East respiratory syndrome coronavirus causes widespread infection and alveolar damage in human lungs. *Am J Respir Crit Care Med.* 2013;188(7):882-886.

37. Raj VS, Mou H, Smits SL, et al. Dipeptidyl peptidase 4 is a functional receptor for the emerging human coronavirus-EMC. *Nature.* 2013;495(7440):251-254.

38. Delmas B, Gelfi J, L'Haridon R, Sjöström H, Laude H. Aminopeptidase N is a major receptor for the enteropathogenic coronavirus TGEV. *Nature.* 1992;357(6377):417-420.

39. Chan RW, Chan MC, Agnihothram S, et al. Tropism of and innate immune responses to the novel human betacoronavirus lineage C virus in human ex vivo respiratory organ cultures. *J Virol.* 2013;87(12):6604-6614.

40. Raj VS, Smits SL, Provacia LB, et al. Adenosine deaminase acts as a natural antagonist for dipeptidyl peptidase 4-mediated entry of the Middle East respiratory syndrome coronavirus. *J Virol.* 2014;88(3):1834-1838.

41. de Wilde AH, Raj VS, Oudshoorn D, et al 2013. MERS-coronavirus replication induces severe in vitro cytopathology and is strongly inhibited by cyclosporin A or interferon-α treatment. *J Gen Virol.* 2013;94(Pt 8):1749.

42. Josset L, Menachery VD, Gralinski LE, et al. Cell host response to infection with novel human coronavirus EMC predicts potential antivirals and important differences with SARS coronavirus. *MBio.* 2013;4(3):e00165-13.

43. Cai Q-C, Xu Q-F, Xu J-M, Guo Q, Cheng X, Zhao G-M. Refined estimate of the incubation period of the severe acute respiratory syndrome and related influencing factors. *Am J Epidemiol.* 2006;163(3):211-216.

44. Donnelly CA, et al. Epidemiological determinants of spread of causal agent of severe acute respiratory syndrome in Hong Kong. *Lancet.* 2003;361(9371):1761-1766.

45. World Health Organization. Update 49 - SARS case fatality ratio, incubation period. 2003, May 07. Available at https://www.who.int/csr/sars/archive/2003_05_07a/en/.

46. Hui DSC, Zumla A. Severe Acute Respiratory Syndrome: Historical, Epidemiologic, and Clinical Features. *Infect Dis Clin North Am.* 2019;33(4):869-889.

47. Peiris JS, Lai ST, Poon LL, et al. Coronavirus as a possible cause of severe acute respiratory syndrome. *Lancet.* 2003;361(9366):1319-1325.

48. Lee N, Hui D, Wu A, et al. A major outbreak of severe acute respiratory syndrome in Hong Kong. *N Engl J Med.* 2003;348(20):1986-1994.

49. Leung WK, To KF, Chan PK, et al. Enteric involvement of severe acute respiratory syndrome-associated coronavirus infection. *Gastroenterology.* 2003;125(4):1011-1017.

50. Lau KK, Yu WC, Chu CM, Lau ST, Sheng B, Yuen KY. Possible central nervous system infection by SARS coronavirus. *Emerg Infect Dis.* 2004;10(2):342-344.

51. Wong KC, Leung KS, Hui M. Severe Acute Respiratory Syndrome (SARS) in a Geriatric Patient with a Hip Fracture. *J Bone Joint Surg Am.* 2003;85(7):1339-1342.

52. Hon KLE, Leung CW, Cheng WT, et al. Clinical presentations and outcome of severe acute respiratory syndrome in children. *Lancet.* 2003;361(9370):1701-1703.

53. Leung GM, Lim WW, Ho LM, et al. Seroprevalence of IgG Antibodies to SARS-Coronavirus in Asymptomatic or Subclinical Population Groups. *Epidemiol Infect.* 2006;134(2): 211-221.

54. Booth CM, Matukas LM, Tomlinson GA, et al. Clinical Features and Short-term Outcomes of 144 Patients with SARS in the Greater Toronto Area. *JAMA.* 2003;289(21):2801-2809.

55. Peiris JS, Lai ST, Poon LL, et al. Coronavirus as a possible cause of severe acute respiratory syndrome. *Lancet.* 2003;361(9366):1319-1325.

56. Wong RSM, Wu A, To KF, et al. Haematological manifestations in patients with severe acute respiratory syndrome: retrospective analysis. *BMJ.* 2003;326:1358.

57. Wong KT, Antonio GE, Hui DS, et al. Severe acute respiratory syndrome: radiographic appearances and pattern of progression in 138 patients. *Radiology.* 2003;228(2):401-406.

58. Chan JWM, Ng CK, Chan YH, et al. Short term outcome and risk factors for adverse clinical outcomes in adults with severe acute respiratory syndrome (SARS). *Thorax.* 2003;58:686-689.

59. Tsang KW, Ho PL, Ooi GC, et al. A cluster of cases of severe acute respiratory syndrome in Hong Kong. *N Engl J Med.* 2003;348(20):1977-1985.

60. Peiris JS, Chu CM, Cheng VC, et al. Clinical progression and viral load in a community outbreak of coronavirus-associated SARS pneumonia: a prospective study. *Lancet (London, England).* 2003;361(9371):1767-1772.

61. Antonio GE, Wong KT, Chu WC, et al. Imaging in severe acute respiratory syndrome (SARS). *Clin Radiol.* 2003;58(11):825-832.

62. Antonio GE, Wong KT, Hui DS, et al. Imaging of severe acute respiratory syndrome in Hong Kong. *AJR Am J Roentgenol.* 2003;181(1):11-17.

63. Grinblat L, Shulman H, Glickman A, Matukas L, Paul N. Severe acute respiratory syndrome: radiographic review of 40 probable cases in Toronto, Canada. *Radiology*. 2003;228(3):802-809.

64. Zumla A, Hui DS, Perlman S. Middle East respiratory syndrome. *Lancet*. 2015;386(9997):995-1007.

65. Al-Abdallat MM, Payne DC, Alqasrawi S, et al. Hospital-associated outbreak of Middle East respiratory syndrome coronavirus: a serologic, epidemiologic, and clinical description. *Clin Infect Dis*. 2014;59(9):1225-1233.

66. Assiri A, McGeer A, Perl TM, et al. Hospital outbreak of Middle East respiratory syndrome coronavirus. *N Engl J Med*. 2013;369(5):407-416.

67. Arabi YM, Arifi AA, Balkhy HH, et al. Clinical Course and Outcomes of Critically Ill Patients with Middle East Respiratory Syndrome Coronavirus Infection. *Ann Intern Med*. 2014;160:389-397.

68. World Health Organization. Investigation of cases of human infection with Middle East respiratory syndrome coronavirus (MERS-CoV). 2018, June. Available at https://apps.who.int/iris/bitstream/handle/10665/178252/WHO_MERS_SUR_15.2_eng.pdf;sequence=1.

69. Virlogeux V, Park M, Wu JT, Cowling BJ. Association between Severity of MERS-CoV Infection and Incubation Period. *Emerg Infect Dis*. 2016;22(3):526-528.

70. Arabi YM, Harthi A, Hussein J, et al. Severe neurologic syndrome associated with Middle East respiratory syndrome corona virus (MERS-CoV). *Infection*. 2015;43(4):495-501.

71. Al-Tawfiq JA, Kattan RF, Memish ZA. Middle East respiratory syndrome coronavirus disease is rare in children: An update from Saudi Arabia. *World J Clin Pediatr*. 2016;5(4):391-396.

72. Memish ZA, Al-Tawfiq JA, Assiri A, et al. Middle East respiratory syndrome coronavirus disease in children. *Pediatr Infect Dis J*. 2014;33(9):904-906.

73. Grant R, Malik MR, Elkholy A, Van Kerkhove MD. A Review of Asymptomatic and Subclinical Middle East Respiratory Syndrome Coronavirus Infections. *Epidemiol Rev*. 2019;41(1):69-81.

74. Al Ghamdi M, Alghamdi KM, Ghandoora Y, et al. Treatment outcomes for patients with Middle Eastern Respiratory Syndrome Coronavirus (MERS CoV) infection at a coronavirus referral center in the Kingdom of Saudi Arabia. *BMC Infect Dis*. 2016;16:174.

75. Azhar EI, Hui DSC, Memish ZA, Drosten C, Zumla A. The Middle East Respiratory Syndrome (MERS). *Infect Dis Clin North Am*. 2019;33(4):891-890.

76. Chan JF, Lau SK, To KK, Cheng VC, Woo PC, Yuen KY. Middle East respiratory syndrome coronavirus: another zoonotic betacoronavirus causing SARS-like disease. *Clin Microbiol Rev*. 2015;28(2):465-522.

77. Saad M, Omrani AS, Baig K, et al. Clinical aspects and outcomes of 70 patients with Middle East respiratory syndrome coronavirus infection: a single-center experience in Saudi Arabia. *Int J Infect Dis*. 2014;29:301-306.

78. Assiri A, Al-Tawfiq JA, Al-Rabeeah AA, et al. Epidemiological, demographic, and clinical characteristics of 47 cases of Middle East respiratory syndrome coronavirus disease from Saudi Arabia: a descriptive study. *Lancet Infect Dis*. 2013;13(9):752-761.

79. Das KM, Lee EY, Al Jawder SE, et al. Acute Middle East Respiratory Syndrome Coronavirus: Temporal Lung Changes Observed on the Chest Radiographs of 55 Patients. *AJR Am J Roentgenol.* 2015;205(3):W267-W274.

80. Ajlan AM, Ahyad RA, Jamjoom LG, Alharthy A, Madani TA. Middle East respiratory syndrome coronavirus (MERS-CoV) infection: chest CT findings. *AJR Am J Roentgenol.* 2014;203(4):782-787.

81. Das KM, Lee EY, Enani MA, et al. CT correlation with outcomes in 15 patients with acute Middle East respiratory syndrome coronavirus. *AJR Am J Roentgenol.* 2015;204(4):736-742.

82. Yin Y, Wunderink RG. MERS, SARS and other coronaviruses as causes of pneumonia. *Respirology (Carlton, Vic.).* 2018;23(2):130-137.

83. Senga M, Arabi YM, Fowler RA. Clinical spectrum of the Middle East respiratory syndrome coronavirus (MERS-CoV). *J Infect Public Health.* 2017;10(2):191-194.

84. Arabi YM, Al-Omari A, Mandourah Y, et al. Critically Ill Patients With the Middle East Respiratory Syndrome: A Multicenter Retrospective Cohort Study. *Crit Care Med.* 2017;45(10):1683-1695.

85. Alraddadi BM, Qushmaq I, Al-Hameed FM, et al. Noninvasive ventilation in critically ill patients with the Middle East respiratory syndrome. *Influenza Other Respir Viruses.* 2019;13(4):382-390.

86. Khalid I, Alraddadi BM, Dairi Y, et al. Acute Management and Long-Term Survival Among Subjects With Severe Middle East Respiratory Syndrome Coronavirus Pneumonia and ARDS. *Respir Care.* 2016;61(3):340-348.

87. Alshahrani MS, Sindi A, Alshamsi F, et al. Extracorporeal membrane oxygenation for severe Middle East respiratory syndrome coronavirus. *Ann Intensive Care.* 2018;8(1):3.

88. Chan KH, Poon LL, Cheng VC, et al. Detection of SARS coronavirus in patients with suspected SARS. *Emerg Infect Dis.* 2004;10(2):294-299.

89. Wu HS, Chiu SC, Tseng TC, et al. Serologic and molecular biologic methods for SARS-associated coronavirus infection, Taiwan. *Emerg Infect Dis.* 2004;10(2):304-310.

90. Centers for Disease Control and Prevention. Public Health Guidance for Community-Level Preparedness and Response to Severe Acute Respiratory Syndrome (SARS) Version 2/3. Centers for Disease Control and Prevention. Available at https://www.cdc.gov/sars/guidance/f-lab/assays.html. Accessed November 10, 2020.

91. World Health Organization. Case definition for case finding severe respiratory disease associated with novel coronavirus. 2012, Sept. Available at https://www.who.int/csr/disease/coronavirus_infections/case_definition_25_09_2012/en/. Accessed November 10, 2020.

92. World Health Organization. Laboratory Testing for Middle East Respiratory Syndrome Coronavirus. Interim guidance(revised). 2018, January. Available at https://apps.who.int/iris/bitstream/handle/10665/259952/WHO-MERS-LAB-15.1-Rev1-2018-eng.pdf?sequence=1&isAllowed=y. Accessed November 20, 2020.

93. Corman VM, et al. Detection of a novel human coronavirus by real-time reverse-transcription polymerase chain reaction. *Eurosurveillance.* 2012;17(39,27), doi:10.2807/ese.17.39.20285-en.

94. Arabi YM, Arifi AA, Balkhy HH, et al. Clinical Course and Outcomes of Critically Ill Patients With Middle East Respiratory Syndrome Coronavirus Infection. *Ann Intern Med.* 2014;160(6):389-397.

95. Stockman LJ, Bellamy R, Garner P. SARS: systematic review of treatment effects. *PLoS Med.* 2006;3(9):e343.

96. So LK, Lau AC, Yam LY, et al. Development of a standard treatment protocol for severe acute respiratory syndrome. *Lancet (London, England).* 2003;361(9369):1615-1617.

97. Booth CM, Matukas LM, Tomlinson GA, et al. Clinical Features and Short-term Outcomes of 144 Patients With SARS in the Greater Toronto Area. *JAMA.* 2003;289(21):2801-2809.

98. Lee N, Allen Chan KC, Hui DS, et al. Effects of early corticosteroid treatment on plasma SARS-associated Coronavirus RNA concentrations in adult patients. *J Clin Virol.* 2004;31(4):304-309.

99. Lee DT, Wing YK, Leung HC, et al. Factors associated with psychosis among patients with severe acute respiratory syndrome: a case-control study. *Clin Infect Dis.* 2004;39(8):1247-1249.

100. Tai DYH. Pharmacologic treatment of SARS: current knowledge and recommendations. *Ann Acad Med Singap.* 2007;36(6):438-443.

101. Chan KS, Lai ST, Chu CM, et al. Treatment of severe acute respiratory syndrome with lopinavir/ritonavir: a multicentre retrospective matched cohort study. *Hong Kong Med J.* 2003;9(6): 399-406.

102. Chu CM, Cheng VC, Hung IF, et al. Role of lopinavir/ritonavir in the treatment of SARS: initial virological and clinical findings. *Thorax.* 2004;59(3):252-256.

103. Loutfy MR, Blatt LM, Siminovitch KA, et al. Interferon alfacon-1 plus corticosteroids in severe acute respiratory syndrome: a preliminary study. *JAMA.* 2003;290(24):3222-3228.

104. Soo YO, Cheng Y, Wong R, et al. Retrospective comparison of convalescent plasma with continuing high-dose methylprednisolone treatment in SARS patients. *Clin Microbiol Infect.* 2004;10(7):676-678.

105. World Health Organization. Severe Acute Respiratory Syndrome (SARS): Treatment. Updated August 13, 2003. Available at https://www.who.int/health-topics/severe-acute-respiratory-syndrome#tab=tab_3. Accessed October 13, 2020.

106. Arabi YM, Mandourah Y, Al-Hameed F, et al. Corticosteroid Therapy for Critically Ill Patients with Middle East Respiratory Syndrome. *Am J Respir Crit Care Med.* 2018;197(6):757-767.

107. Omrani AS, Saad MM, Baig K, Bahloul A, et al. Ribavirin and interferon alfa-2a for severe Middle East respiratory syndrome coronavirus infection: a retrospective cohort study. *Lancet Infect Dis.* 2014;14(11):1090-1095.

108. Al-Tawfiq JA, Memish ZA. Update on therapeutic options for Middle East Respiratory Syndrome Coronavirus (MERS-CoV). *Expert Rev Anti Infect Ther.* 2017;15(3):269-275.

109. Mo Y, Fisher D. A review of treatment modalities for Middle East Respiratory Syndrome. *J Antimicrob Chemother.* 2016;71(12):3340-3350.

110. World Health Organization. WHO-ISARIC joint MERS-CoV Outbreak Readiness Workshop: Clinical management and potential use of convalescent plasma. 2013 December. Available at https://www.who.int/csr/disease/coronavirus_infections/MERS_outbreak_readiness_workshop.pdf.

111. Arabi Y, Balkhy H, Hajeer AH, et al. Feasibility, safety, clinical, and laboratory effects of convalescent plasma therapy for patients with Middle East respiratory syndrome coronavirus infection: a study protocol. *Springerplus*. 2015;4:709.

112. He Y, Li J, Heck S, Lustigman S, Jiang S. Antigenic and immunogenic characterization of recombinant baculovirus-expressed severe acute respiratory syndrome coronavirus spike protein: implication for vaccine design. *J Virol*. 2006;80(12):5757-5767.

113. Chen Z, Zhang L, Qin C, et al. Recombinant modified vaccinia virus Ankara expressing the spike glycoprotein of severe acute respiratory syndrome coronavirus induces protective neutralizing antibodies primarily targeting the receptor binding region. *J Virol*. 2005;79(5):2678-2688.

114. Bukreyev A, Lamirande EW, Buchholz UJ, et al. Mucosal immunisation of African green monkeys (*Cercopithecus aethiops*) with an attenuated parainfluenza virus expressing the SARS coronavirus spike protein for the prevention of SARS. *Lancet*. 2004;363(9427):2122-2127.

115. Bosch BJ, Martina BE, Van Der Zee R, et al. Severe acute respiratory syndrome coronavirus (SARS-CoV) infection inhibition using spike protein heptad repeat-derived peptides. *Proc Natl Acad Sci*. 2004;101(22):8455-8460.

116. Jaume M, Yip MS, Kam YW, et al. SARS CoV subunit vaccine: Antibody mediated neutralisation and enhancement. *Hong Kong Med J*. 2012;18(Suppl 2):31-36.

117. Jung SY, Kang KW, Lee EY, et al. Heterologous prime–boost vaccination with adenoviral vector and protein nanoparticles induces both Th1 and Th2 responses against Middle East respiratory syndrome coronavirus. *Vaccine*. 2018;36(24):3468-3476.

118. Pallesen J, Wang N, Corbett KS, et al. Immunogenicity and structures of a rationally designed prefusion MERS-CoV spike antigen. *Proc Natl Acad Sci*. 2017;114(35):E7348-E7357.

119. Chi H, Zheng X, Wang X, et al. DNA vaccine encoding Middle East respiratory syndrome coronavirus S1 protein induces protective immune responses in mice. *Vaccine*. 2017;35(16):2069-2075.

120. Bodmer BS, Fiedler AH, Hanauer JR, Prüfer S, Mühlebach MD. Live-attenuated bivalent measles virus-derived vaccines targeting Middle East respiratory syndrome coronavirus induce robust and multifunctional T cell responses against both viruses in an appropriate mouse model. *Virology*. 2018;521:99-107.

121. Alharbi NK, Padron-Regalado E, Thompson CP, et al. ChAdOx1 and MVA based vaccine candidates against MERS-CoV elicit neutralising antibodies and cellular immune responses in mice. *Vaccine*. 2017;35(30):3780-3788.

122. Xu J, Jia W, Wang P, et al. Antibodies and vaccines against Middle East respiratory syndrome coronavirus. *Emerg Microbes Infect*. 2019;8(1):841-856.

123. Wang L, Shi W, Joyce MG, et al. Evaluation of candidate vaccine approaches for MERS-CoV. *Nat Commun*. 2015;6(1):1-11.

20 COVID-19

Danit Arad, MD, FACP, Anuja Pradhan, MD, and Zhiyong Peng, MD

▌ INTRODUCTION

This chapter addresses the novel Coronavirus disease (COVID-19) during the pandemic. The authors share their clinical experiences diagnosing and treating hundreds of patients and their interpretations of the frequently updated literature. The chapter summarizes currently available data on epidemiology, pathophysiology, clinical features, emerging variants, diagnosis, infection control, treatment, anticoagulation, prognosis, and the recent vaccinations.

▌ EPIDEMIOLOGY

As of this writing, more than 111 million confirmed cases of COVID-19 and 2.4 million related deaths have been reported globally. Since the first reports at the end of 2019 from Wuhan in the Hubei Province of China, cases have been reported in all continents, including Antarctica which reported its first case in December 2020.[1]

Epidemiologic investigation in Wuhan at the beginning of the outbreak identified an initial association with a seafood market that sold live animals, where most patients had worked or visited; the market was subsequently closed for disinfection.[2] However, as the outbreak progressed, person-to-person spread became the main mode of transmission for the SARS-CoV-2 virus[3] (Figure 20-1). Transmission from asymptomatic individuals (or individuals within the incubation period) also is well documented.[4,5] However, detectable viral RNA does not always correlate with isolation of infectious virus; there may be a viral RNA threshold below which infectivity is unlikely.

The risk of transmission after contact with an individual with COVID-19 increases with the closeness and duration of contact and appears highest with prolonged contact in indoor settings.[6] Nevertheless, clusters of

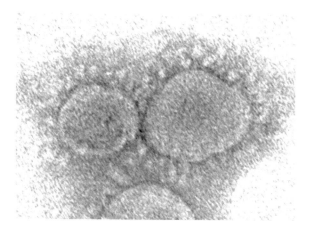

Figure 20-1 • Electronic microscopic image of SARS-CoV-2. (*Courtesy of the CDC.* https://phil.cdc.gov/Details.aspx?pid=23641.)

cases are frequently reported following family, work, or social gatherings where close personal contact can occur.

The virus can affect people of all ages. However, children and younger adults often remain asymptomatic or contract a mild form of the disease. Adults of advanced age are more susceptible to moderate, severe, or even critical illness.

Primary conditions that are considered risk factors for developing severe COVID-19 disease include:

- hypertension
- cardiac conditions (congestive heart failure/coronary artery disease or cardiomyopathies)
- obesity (BMI = 30–40) and severe obesity (BMI > 40)
- diabetes mellitus Type 2
- immunocompromised state from a solid organ or bone marrow transplant or immunosuppressants for other chronic conditions
- chronic lung disease
- cancer
- chronic kidney disease
- sickle cell disease
- smoking status; the relationship between smoking per se and the severity of COVID-19 is unclear; however, patients with underlying smoking-related COPD are at high risk of superimposed respiratory failure from COVID-19.
- Uncontrolled HIV also may be a risk factor.

▌PATHOPHYSIOLOGY

The host receptor for SARS-CoV-2 cell entry is the angiotensin-converting enzyme 2 (ACE2).[7] SARS-CoV-2 binds to ACE2 through the receptor-binding gene domain (RBD) of its spike protein. The S1 subunit of a coronavirus is further divided into two functional domains: an N-terminal domain and a C-terminal domain. Structural and biochemical analyses have identified 211 amino acid regions (amino acids 319–529) at the S1 C-terminal domain of SARS-CoV-2 as the RBD, which plays a key role in virus entry. Heparan sulfate interacts with the RBD of the SARS-CoV-2 spike glycoprotein adjacent to ACE2 and shifts the spike structure to an open conformation to facilitate ACE2 binding. Thus, heparan sulfate is a necessary co-factor for SARS-CoV-2 infection.[8]

The transmembrane serine protease 2 (TMPRSS2) also appears to be important for SARS-CoV-2 cell entry.[9] Following host cell binding, viral and cell membranes fuse, enabling the virus to enter the cell. S-protein priming by TMPRSS2, which may be substituted by cathepsin B/L, is required to facilitate SARS-CoV-2 entry into host cells.[10] SARS-CoV-2 is mostly transmissible through large respiratory droplets, directly infecting cells of the upper- and lower-respiratory tracts, especially nasal ciliated and alveolar epithelial cells. The infection induces cellular death and injury in airway epithelial cells through diverse processes such as pyroptosis.[11] In addition to the lungs, ACE2 is also expressed in tissues such as the small intestine, kidneys, heart, thyroid, testes, and adipose tissue, indicating the virus may directly infect cells of other organ systems when viremia is present.[12]

Viral-mediated cell death causes the release of various damage- and pathogen-associated molecular patterns believed to be recognized by pattern recognition receptors on alveolar macrophages and endothelial cells.[13] These processes foster increased secretion of proinflammatory cytokines and chemokines, such as interleukin 6 (IL-6), type II interferon, monocyte chemoattractant protein 1, and interferon gamma-induced protein 10, and subsequent pulmonary recruitment of immune cells, including macrophages and dendritic cells.[14]

Direct viral infection of macrophages and/or dendritic cells propagate further cytokine and chemokine release, subsequently activating late-phase immune-cell recruitment of antigen-specific T-cells to destroy virally infected alveolar cells.[15] In most COVID-19 patients, the combined immune response of initial cytokine release and activation of the antiviral interferon response, followed by immune-cell recruitment, result in successful SARS-CoV-2 clearance from the lungs.[16] However, as extensively reported, viral infection can progress to severe disease due to a dysregulated immune response. Markedly elevated levels of circulating proinflammatory cytokines and chemokines significantly correlate to disease severity and mortality. Thus, IL-6 has emerged as a candidate treatment target due to its robust association with disease progression.[17]

The reason for lymphopenia in severe COVID-19 is unclear, although T-cell redistribution via pulmonary recruitment and exhaustion and depletion through apoptosis or cytopathic injury have been proposed.[18] Other prevalent and important pathological changes in COVID-19 patients are coagulation abnormalities and high incidence of thrombotic events.[19] Hypercoagulability in severe COVID-19 is notable. Prolonged activated partial thromboplastin time and prothrombin time, elevated D-dimer, thrombocytopenia, and lupus anticoagulant in the circulation have been reported.[20] Fibrin thrombi in pulmonary small arterial vessels suggests the contribution of coagulation in diffuse alveolar and endothelial damage.[21] SARS-CoV-2-induced endothelial damage fosters monocyte recruitment and activation, along with tissue factor exposure, which then activates blood coagulation. SARS-CoV-2 genomes have been found in endomyocardial biopsies, mostly involving immune cell infiltrates.[22] Cardiac injury and failure in patients with greater disease severity have been reported. Increasing cardiac troponin levels are correlated with other inflammatory markers, such as c-reactive protein (CRP), ferritin, and IL-6.[23,24] Cytokine release is known to directly affect cardiomyocytes and cause COVID-19 cardiovascular manifestations. Additionally, some studies describe myocarditis and stress-related cardiomyopathy due to respiratory failure and hypoxemia.[25,26]

Renal involvement manifests as mild proteinuria, minor serum creatinine elevations, acute kidney injury, and renal failure.[27] ACE2 is expressed in the kidney, and direct virulence in tubular epithelium and podocytes has been found.[28] Direct SARS-CoV-2 infection of the renal epithelium is estimated to result in mitochondrial dysfunction, acute tubular necrosis, and protein leakage.[29] Additionally, uncontrolled cytokine release, thrombosis, and ischemia can indirectly result in further kidney dysfunction characterized by intrarenal inflammation, increased vascular permeability, and volume depletion.

There is evidence of direct SARS-CoV-2 gastrointestinal (GI) infection through isolation of viral RNA from GI epithelial cells.[30] The GI manifestations possibly result from SARS-CoV-2 infection of intestinal enterocytes and subsequent dysfunction in the ileum and colon. Studies describe higher rates of liver injury in patients with severe COVID-19.[31]

Abundant SARS-CoV-2 viral particles in hepatocytes have been reported in post-mortem specimens, and systemic inflammatory response may lead to cytotoxic T-cell-mediated necrosis and liver injury.[32] ACE2 is expressed in both the exocrine and islet cells of the pancreas.[33] In one cohort of COVID-19 patients, 17% had serologic evidence of exocrine pancreatic injury, defined as elevated amylase or lipase.[34] Importantly, COVID-19 appears to enhance complications for inpatients with diabetes, likely due to viral-induced pancreatic dysfunction, as well as associated immune dysregulation, vasculopathy, and coagulopathy.[35]

Reported neurological manifestations of COVID-19 include headache, dizziness, confusion, epilepsy, ataxia, and Guillain-Barré syndrome.[36-38] The underlying pathophysiology of neurological injury is direct invasion and indirect effects due to hyperinflammation. The SARS-CoV-2 virus has been detected in the cerebrospinal fluid.[39] Loss of olfactory and gustatory perceptions are due to direct damage to the supporting cells of the olfactory epithelium or olfactory bulb and altered function of the olfactory neurons, altered ACE2-signal transmission, and accelerated gustatory particle degradation by sialic acid.[40] In rare cases, children can be severely affected, and multisystem inflammatory syndrome (MIS) in children (MIS-C) can be induced.[41] The MIS-C is thought to result from immune dysregulation occurring after acute infection has passed.

CLINICAL MANIFESTATIONS

SARS-CoV-2 has an average incubation period of 5 days (range 2–14 days) followed by varied clinical presentations from asymptomatic infection to pneumonia, respiratory failure, and critical illness.

Severe and critical COVID-19 are noted to be a biphasic illness. The first phase is viral, lasting about a week; the second week is the inflammatory phase, with host-mediated organ damage or cytokine storm. Excessive production of pro-inflammatory cytokines, rather than the virus itself, is thought to cause most of the mortality in COVID-19.

Most patients with mild illness present with cough, fever, sore throat, malaise, myalgia, anosmia, and/or dysgeusia. Gastrointestinal manifestations such as anorexia, nausea, and diarrhea are also frequently seen. Mild illness is typically self-limiting and managed on an outpatient basis.

Some patients progress to moderate or severe illness with worsening symptoms of dyspnea, usually in the second week. This is clinically evident with signs of lower-respiratory involvement with hypoxemia, infiltrates on chest X-ray, and increased inflammatory markers.

According to data from China, approximately 81% of patients had mild-to-moderate disease (including people without or with only mild pneumonia), 14% had severe disease, and 5% had critical illness.

Respiratory System

Respiratory features of moderate and severe COVID-19 include tachypnea, hypoxemia, and infiltrates on chest X-rays. Diffuse bilateral opacities in lungs are seen in severe infections from COVID-19 causing an atypical acute respiratory distress syndrome (ARDS).

"Silent hypoxemia" is a baffling presentation in many patients with COVID-19 disease. Patients typically have low oxygen levels with no notable increase in the work of breathing. Several mechanisms have been proposed for this phenomenon, but the exact pathophysiology remains unclear.

Although uncommon, pneumothorax and pneumomediastinum were reported in several cases. Some reports suggest that these can occur in the context of COVID-19 pneumonia, even in the absence of mechanical ventilation-related barotrauma.[42]

Severe and critical COVID-19 infections usually require intensive care unit (ICU) admission. Supplemental oxygen using noninvasive or invasive positive pressure ventilation is warranted for patients who progress to COVID-19-associated ARDS. One striking difference between typical ARDS and COVID-19-associated ARDS is that most COVID-19 patients have relatively normal lung compliance. Further, onset of severe disease is usually 8 to 12 days into the illness, rather than the less than one week onset per the Berlin criteria for typical ARDS.

Although COVID-19 is predominantly a respiratory disease, it can affect other organs.

Central Nervous System (CNS)

Encephalopathy, encephalitis, meningitis, acute disseminated encephalomyelitis, and CNS vasculitis were reported. Although uncommon, peripheral neuropathies such as Guillain-Barré syndrome or rhabdomyolysis, acute ischemic thrombotic stroke, and cavernous sinus thrombosis hemorrhagic stroke, also were noted. We observed patients presenting with syncope, unexplained otherwise but possibly due to a transient acquired autonomic dysfunction.

Cardiovascular System

Acute myocardial injury and myocarditis with elevated troponin were seen in a significant proportion of critically ill patients. Myocarditis has been associated with high viral loads, and mononuclear infiltrates identified on autopsy. Severe systemic inflammation increases the risk of athero-sclerotic plaque rupture and acute myocardial infarction. Also reported were acute heart failure, dysrhythmias, cardiogenic shock, and increased thromboembolic events.

Renal System

Evidence of renal excretion of the virus suggests that the kidneys may be a viral reservoir. It is common to see kidney involvement in COVID-19 patients, manifesting with hematuria and proteinuria to acute kidney injury that warrants replacement therapy. COVID-19-associated acute kidney injury is a risk factor for high mortality in all hospitalized COVID-19 patients.[43]

Cutaneous Manifestations

COVID-19 patients of all ages, including children, have shown diverse cutaneous manifestations, including livedoid, maculopapular, vesicular, petechial, urticarial, and pernio-like lesions. Rashes are also common in Multisystem Inflammatory Syndrome in Children (MIS-C).[44]

Multisystem Inflammatory Syndrome in Children (MIS-C)

Young children were thought to be relatively spared from severe infection, due to either a generally mild course or asymptomatic infection. However, around April 2020, a novel syndrome was described in children and adolescents. Clinical features include fever, rash, conjunctivitis, stomatitis, nausea, vomiting, abdominal pain, and headache. Shock, myocarditis, hyponatremia, renal failure, and hypoxemia, along with the elevated inflammatory markers CRP, ferritin, IL-6, procalcitonin, and D-dimer, were noted with laboratory evidence of current or past infection with SARS-CoV-2. Early infection appears to trigger macrophage activation, followed by stimulation of T-helper cells. This in turn leads to cytokine release, stimulating macrophages, neutrophils, and monocytes along with B-cell and plasma-cell activation with the production of antibodies, leading to a hyperimmune response. This immune dysregulation is thought to be associated with MIS-C rather than directly with SARS-CoV-2 infection. Treatment is directed toward decreasing systemic inflammation and restoring organ function. Intravenous immunoglobulin, aspirin, corticosteroids, anakinra, and tocilizumab have been used.[44]

Multisystem Inflammatory Syndrome in Adult (MIS-A)

Since June 2020, several cases of a similar MIS in adults have been reported. Adult patients of all ages with current or previous SARS-CoV-2 infection can develop a hyperinflammatory syndrome resembling MIS-C, although most patients do not have respiratory symptoms typical of severe COVID-19. The interval between infection and development of MIS-A is unclear because some patients did not have any preceding respiratory symptoms. Those who reported typical COVID-19 symptoms reported MIS-A approximately 2 to 5 weeks later. Treatment is similar to MIS-C with supportive care, corticosteroids, intravenous immunoglobulin, and IL-6 inhibitors.[45]

EMERGING VARIANTS

Several SARS-CoV-2 variants have been identified. Three of them B.1.1.7, B.1.351, and P.1 share the D614G mutation, which seems to allow the virus a faster rate of spread compared with the wild type SARS-CoV-2. Table 20-1 summarizes the main known variants.

DIAGNOSIS

Currently, no available test for the COVID-19 disease has 100% accuracy. Because the field has not yet established a "gold standard" for diagnostics, the validity of current tests is unknown. Therefore, as always in medicine, the first step in diagnosis is identifying the clinical setting and estimating the pretest probability.

Clinical Setting and Pretest Probability

The novel coronavirus disease should be suspected in the presence of new-onset fever, cough and/or dyspnea, loss of taste or smell, pernio-like skin lesions, or other symptoms listed in the clinical features section of this chapter. During surge time, strokes, cardiac injury, syncope, and venous thromboembolism also may be attributed to COVID-19 and should prompt testing. Obviously, the high prevalence of the disease raises the pretest probability even with unusual presentation. We have seen patients who present with hip fractures after a fall, having no respiratory symptoms or fever. However, routine pre-op chest X-rays revealed multilobar ground glass opacities, and reverse transcription polymerase chain reaction (RT-PCR) tests showed positive for COVID-19. It is possible that the fall resulted from a brewing viral illness.

Available Tests

Common available tests include nucleic acid amplification testing (NAAT) with RT-PCR assay or its alternative, antigen testing, as well as serological

Table 20-1 PRIMARY VARIANTS

Variant name	Place first identified	Special characteristics	Number of U.S. cases[a] identified
B.1.1.7[47]	United Kingdom (UK)	• Many mutations detected globally • First US detection at end of December 2020 • Evidence from UK suggests this variant carries a higher risk of death than do the other variants[b]	2,102
B.1.351[47]	South Africa	• First US detection at end of January 2021 • Preliminary reports suggest the Moderna (mRNA-1273) vaccination may be less effective against this variant[b] • Per early in vitro studies, E484K mutation may play help prevent some monoclonal antibodies and convalescent and vaccine sera's neutralizing activity[b]	49
P.1[47]	Brazil	• First identified in Brazilian travelers to Japan, January 2021 • First US detection at end of January 2021. • 28 unique mutations, including three (K417T, E484K, and N501Y) in RBD of the spike protein • Some mutations may affect antibodies' (natural or vaccination) ability to recognize and neutralize the virus[b]	6
B.1.526[48]	New York City	• Novel variant in patients throughout the New York metro area • Patients tended to be older and hospitalized more often	

[a]As of 26 February 2021 (these numbers may be underreported, given that genetic sequencing was not routinely conducted at all sites);
[b]Additional research is required to confirm the preliminary (often, non-peer-reviewed) evidence.

and radiological tests. However, in a setting of high clinical suspicion, no currently available test can adequately rule out a COVID-19 diagnosis.

NAAT with RT-PCR Assay

The currently preferred initial diagnostic test for COVID-19 is the NAAT with RT-PCR assay, which detects SARS-CoV-2 RNA from the upper respiratory tract. Compared to other available tests, the RT-PCR seems to have the highest accuracy. However, its sensitivity is still suboptimal—estimated at 60% to 80%.[49]

We observed patients who first tested negative and later tested positive in the right clinical scenarios. Based on our experience, patients with classic presentations and negative tests should be kept in isolation and have one—and sometimes two—repeat tests, ideally 48 to 72 hr later.

Upper-respiratory samples are the primary specimens for SARS-CoV-2 NAAT. In the United States, the Centers for Disease Control and Prevention (CDC) recommends that healthcare professionals (HCP) collect one of the following specimens.[50]

- nasopharyngeal swab
- nasal swab from both anterior nares (collected by HCP or by the patient on-site or at home)
- nasal or nasopharyngeal wash/aspirate
- oropharyngeal swab

As noted in the Prognosis section, patients may test positive for COVID-19 up to several weeks after recovery. This is thought to be a false positive due to the presence of nonviable virus rather than true virus shedding.

Antigen Testing

Although tests that detect the SARS-CoV-2 antigen seem less sensitive than NAATs,[50] they are relatively inexpensive and can be performed rapidly (within about 15 min) and at the point of care. Manufacturers have begun supplying point-of-care antigen tests with rapid results, and the U.S. FDA has issued emergency use authorizations on some tests that use nasal swabs.[51] Nonetheless, when the pretest probability is high, negative initial antigen tests should be confirmed using NAATs because NAAT sensitivity appears to be greater than that of antigen testing.[52]

Serology Testing (Prior/Late Infection)

Serologic tests detect SARS-CoV-2 antibodies in the blood. Thus, adequately validated serologic tests are especially useful in two scenarios. First, they can aid in diagnosing COVID-19 patients who have been symptomatic for at least a week[53,54] but tested negative on early PCR tests.[52] Second, they are useful for finding evidence of prior infection in currently asymptomatic patients.

Table 20-2, which we developed based on our clinical experiences, presents our interpretations of test results and recommended actions according to the level of clinical suspicion.

Laboratory Workup

Upon admitting a patient, we normally collect a baseline EKG and a lab workup to include:

- basic metabolic panel, magnesium, liver panel
- complete blood count with differential
- CRP, D-dimer, lactic acid, lactate dehydrogenase (LDH), ferritin
- partial thromboplastin time (PTT), prothrombin time/international normalized ratio (PT/INR)
- troponin, creatine phosphokinase (CPK)
- N-terminal pro-B type natriuretic peptide (pro-BNP)

Radiology

Chest X-ray

In many cases, even portable chest X-rays can be adequate. Note that in the early stages of the disease, initial chest X-rays may show normal in

Table 20-2 TEST INTERPRETATION

| Clinical suspicion level | RT-PCR | | | SARS-CoV-2 antigen | |
	Test type/ result Negative	Inconclusive/ indeterminate	Positive	Negative	Positive
Low	Consider as no disease	Maintain infection control precaution; repeat test	Presume positive for COVID-19 disease	Consider as no disease	Presume positive for COVID-19 disease
Intermediate to high	Maintain infection control precautions; repeat test after 24–48 hr	Maintain infection control precautions; repeat test	Positive disease	Maintain infection control precautions; check RT-PCR test	Positive disease

Source: Author developed.

up to 30% of hospitalized COVID-19 patients[55] (Figure 20-2). Table 20-3 compares typical, intermediate, and atypical appearances on chest X-rays.

Chest CT

Although chest X-rays are less sensitive than CT scans (59% vs. 86%),[56] routine CT scans are not recommended because they are unlikely to change the course of the disease management.[57] Chest CTs are used only to exclude alternate or co-occurring conditions including empyema, pulmonary embolism, or abscess (Figure 20-3).

Ultrasonography

A lung ultrasound can show diffuse or focal B-lines with sparing of the uninvolved areas; irregular and thickened pleural lines; and subpleural, alveolar consolidations with air bronchograms. It may help distinguish cardiogenic pulmonary edema from ARDS.[58]

Vetrugno et al.[59] described a broad lung-ultrasound score (LUS) that can be used as a tool to follow patient trajectories. Increases in LUS indicate decreased lung aeration, and vice versa. These may limit the need for chest CT scans or X-rays.[60]

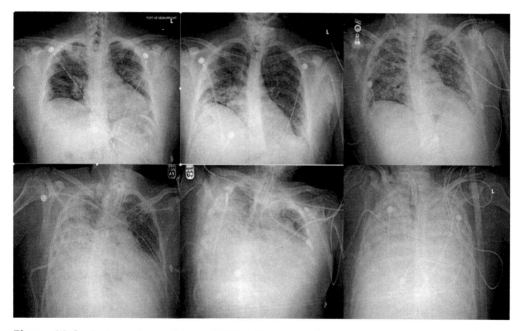

Figure 20-2 • Radiographic evolution of COVID-19 pneumonia from room air, to invasive mechanical ventilation, and to tracheostomy with ECMO.

Table 20-3 APPEARANCES OF CHEST X-RAYS FOR COVID-19 PATIENTS		
Typical	Intermediate (nonspecific)	Atypical
Bilateral, peripheral, basal predominant	Multifocal, perihilar, or unilateral GGO with or without consolidation	Isolated lobar or segmental consolidation without GGO[a]
GGO[a] with or without consolidation	Lacking distribution	Discrete small nodules (centrilobular, "tree in bud")
Bilateral findings in about 85% of patients[23,24]	Nonrounded or nonperipheral	Cavitation
33%–86% predominantly peripheral[23,24]	Few very small GGO, nonrounded and nonperipheral	Smooth interlobular septal thickening with pleural effusions
70%–80% predominantly posterior[23,24]		

GGO = ground glass opacities

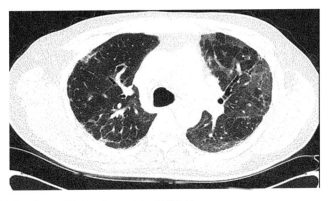

Figure 20-3 • Chest CT of patient with COVID-19.

In the hands of an experienced user, portable ultrasound devices offer the benefit of point-of-care operation rather than needing to transport patients. These devices can be easily disinfected. Operators can evaluate for lung parenchyma, assess for inferior vena cava filling pressure or deep vein thrombosis, and offer a limited bedside echocardiogram.

Transthoracic Echocardiogram (TTE)

A TTE may be useful if a patient is suspected of having a COVID-19-associated cardiovascular disorder. These disorders may include acute cor pulmonale of pulmonary embolism, acute myocarditis, acute coronary syndrome, hypoxic vasoconstriction, and stress-induced cardiomyopathy. Indications of new heart failure or arrhythmia, significant troponinemia, or changes in ECGs can prompt a TTE. Limited TTEs often are sufficient, and bedside TTEs can reduce the risk of transport-related patient decompensation, as well as of contamination during transport.

▌ INFECTION CONTROL

Transmission

Direct person-to-person transmission occurs through close-range contact, mainly via respiratory droplets. The virus released in respiratory secretions—when a person with the infection coughs, sneezes, or talks—can infect another person if the virus makes direct contact with the mucous membranes.[61,62] Infection also might occur if a person whose hands are contaminated by droplets or by touching contaminated surfaces then touches their eyes, nose, or mouth.[63] Aerosolized secretions also may transmit the virus. It has been suggested that aerosolized secretions travel further, remain suspended in the air longer, and are smaller than typical respiratory droplets.[62]

It seems that SARS-CoV-2 can be transmitted before the development of symptoms, as well as throughout the course of illness, particularly early in the course.[64] That is, viral RNA levels from upper-respiratory specimens appear to be higher soon after symptom onset than they are later in the illness.

Personal Protective Equipment (PPE)

Healthcare personnel must adhere to standard safety precautions[65] and should wear the following PPE while treating confirmed or suspected COVID-19 patients:[66]

- fitted respirator (such as N95 or PAPR); if a respirator is not available, use the best alternative, such as a face mask
- face shield
- isolation gown
- gloves

Aerosol-Generating Procedures (AGP)

Procedures such as intubations, cardiopulmonary resuscitation, and nasogastric tube insertions can generate infectious aerosols and should be performed with extreme caution: The number of people within the room should be limited, and healthcare professionals should wear PPE. The procedure should take place in an airborne-infection isolation room whenever one is available, and the procedure room should be sanitized promptly following the AGP.[67]

Environmental Infection Control

Any equipment being used on a confirmed or suspected COVID-19 patient should be dedicated to that specific patient. However, if the equipment is nondedicated or nondisposable, then it must be sanitized in accordance with the facility's policy and manufacturer's instructions. Environmental cleaning must be routine and consistent in all healthcare settings, including patient-care areas in which AGPs are performed.[68]

Healthcare Personnel

Healthcare providers are particularly vulnerable to COVID-19 due to their consistent exposure. As early as July 2020 in the United States alone, over 100,500 cases and 641 deaths among HCP were reported.[69] In a Chinese study[70] of 44,672 subjects, 1,716 (3.8%) were healthcare workers, of whom 1,080 (63%) were working in Wuhan at the time of the outbreak. Of the healthcare workers in the study who were infected with COVID-19, 14.8% were classified with severe or critical symptoms, and five deaths among them were reported.[71]

Protection for HCP should involve providing relevant training and ensuring adequate access to and standards for wearing PPE, including wearing face masks at work and in the community. Whenever feasible, donning and doffing should be observed by an infection control specialist to ensure proper technique. Social-distancing practices should enable HCP to take rest breaks and perform administrative procedures, such as charting, at a safe distance from other team members.

Removal of Isolation

For most patients with COVID-19, non-test-based strategies are sufficient to decide when to discontinue infection-control precautions.[72,73] Non-test-based strategies allow discontinuing precautions when the patient's symptoms improve or at prespecified time intervals. The rationale is that after 10 days from symptom onset, it is rare to isolate a viable virus from recovering patients who had nonsevere infection.[73] Severely immunocompromised patients could remain infectious—that is, produce replication-competent virus—20 days or more after symptom onset or (if asymptomatic) from the date of their first positive viral test. The CDC recommends consulting with an infectious disease specialist for whether to use a test-based or non-test-based strategy and to discontinue precautions.[66]

Obviously, these criteria are symptom-based and cannot apply to asymptomatic patients. The CDC suggests that precautions and home isolation for patients with test-confirmed SARS-CoV-2 infection but no symptoms can be discontinued 10 days after the date of their first positive COVID-19 test—but only if there is no evidence of subsequent illness. If symptoms develop, then the CDC recommends using a symptom-based strategy.[72,73] Similarly, the WHO endorses a non-test-based strategy to end precautions and isolation. However, they suggest that formerly symptomatic patients be without any respiratory symptoms for at least 3 days.[74] Table 20-4 highlights the CDC's discontinuation criteria according to disease severity/immunocompromise.

TREATMENT

Supportive care and clinical monitoring are mostly recommended for mild illness, with therapeutic options for COVID-19 targeted toward the viral or inflammatory phase. Treatments are still under investigation. Table 20-5 summarizes the current therapy benefits suggested by preliminary research.

Anti-Viral Therapy

Viral replication of SARS-CoV-2 is responsible for many clinical manifestations of COVID-19 early in the disease. Many antivirals have been studied in clinical trials. However, it is important to remember that antiviral therapy may provide the greatest benefit *before* the illness progresses to the hyperinflammatory state that is thought to cause severe or critical illness.

Remdesivir is currently the only FDA-approved antiviral medication for COVID-19 for treatment of hospitalized adults and pediatric populations older than 12 years and who weigh more than 40 kg. Remdesivir binds to the viral RNA-dependent RNA polymerase, inhibiting viral replication through premature termination of RNA transcription. Currently, a 5-day course or a course over the duration of admission, whichever is

Table 20-4 CRITERIA TO DISCONTINUE (HEALTHCARE-SETTING) INFECTION-CONTROL PRECAUTIONS BY DISEASE SEVERITY/ IMMUNOCOMPROMISE[66]

Strategy	Mild to moderate illness Non-test-based strategy recommended	Severe to critical illness May consider test-based strategy in consultation with infection control specialist	Severely immunocompromised patients May consider test-based strategy in consultation with infection control specialist
Symptoms[a]			
Days since first symptoms appeared	10	10 (up to 20)	Often 20
Hours since last fever (with fever-reducing medication)	24	24	24
Cough/shortness of breath	Symptoms improved	Symptoms improved	Symptoms improved

Note.[a]Include *all* criteria: days since first symptoms, and hours since last fever, and symptom improvement.

shorter, is recommended. Two key studies led to approval of this antiviral treatment and duration:

(1) The Adaptive COVID-19 Treatment Trial was a double-blind, randomized, controlled trial with intravenous Remdesivir versus a placebo. The study group was hospitalized patients with COVID-19 and evidence of lower-respiratory-tract infection for up to 10 days. The results showed that Remdesivir was superior to the placebo in shortening time to recovery.

(2) An (open label) randomized controlled trial involving hospitalized patients with COVID-19 infection showed no significant difference between a 5-day and 10-day course of Remdesivir in patients with severe illness.

Table 20-5 CHARACTERISTICS OF DIFFERENT SEVERITY OF COVID-19			
Characteristic	**Mild**	**Moderate**	**Severe or Critical**
Clinical feature	Fewer common features	Common features	Multiple organ dysfunction/failure
Dyspnea	Absent	At daily activity	At rest
Chest image	Involvement < 25%	Involvement 25%–50%	Involvement > 50%
Hospitalization	No need	Typically require admission to non-ICU ward	Intensive care admission
Specific medication	Supportive care **Monoclonal antibodies** for those at risk for progression to severe disease **Convalescent plasma with high titer neutralizing antibody** for those at risk for progression to severe disease	**Remdesivir** for hospitalized patients within 10 days of symptoms onset with SpO2 ≤ 94% on room air on low-flow oxygen and with eGFR ≥ 30 mL/min Use for 5 days or for the duration of admission, whichever is shorter. No benefits in clinical trials in patients with severe hypoxemia requiring oxygen delivery through a high-flow device, noninvasive ventilation, mechanical ventilation **Dexamethasone** 6 mg IV/PO daily for up to 10 days in patients with COVID-19 who require supplemental oxygen **VTE prophylaxis with low molecular dose heparin or unfractionated heparin** for all hospitalized patient without contraindication to anticoagulation.	**Dexamethasone** 6 mg IV/PO daily for up to 10 days in patients with COVID-19 who require supplemental oxygen or intubation **IL-6 Inhibitor-Tocilizumab** Patients within 24 (up to 48) hr of progressing to require continuous advanced oxygen support, defined as 100% non-rebreather, high-flow nasal cannula, BIPAP, CPAP, or mechanical ventilation to maintain oxygenation and/or cardiovascular support with vasopressors. Exclude patients with AST/ALT above 5 times upper limit of normal and with Platelet counts < 50,000 mcg/L **VTE prophylaxis with low molecular dose heparin or unfractionated heparin** for all hospitalized patient without contraindication to anticoagulation
Oxygen supplementation	No need	Low-flow oxygen supplement	Oxygen delivery through a high-flow device (preferred when available and sufficient), noninvasive ventilation, mechanical ventilation

Several other antimicrobials, including chloroquine or hydroxychloroquine with or without azithromycin, lopinavir/ritonavir, and Ivermectin, were studied but not proven to show beneficial effect. Thus, current guidelines suggest against using these medications.

Neutralizing Monoclonal Antibodies

Recent studies reported specific monoclonal antibodies neutralizing SARS-CoV-2 infection in vitro and in vivo.[75] However, the high cost and limited capacity of manufacturing and the problem of bioavailability may restrict the wide application of monoclonal antibody therapy.

In the United States, the FDA issued an emergency use authorization (EUA) for bamlanivimab (LY-CoV555) and etesevimab (LY-CoV-016) administered together and for casirivimab/imdevimab (REGN-COV2) to treat mild to moderate COVID-19 in adults and pediatric patients (12 years of age or older weighing at least 40 kg) who are at high risk for progressing to severe COVID-19. However, based on preliminary results, using these neutralizing monoclonal antibodies on patients admitted due to COVID-19 or on COVID-19 patients who require oxygen therapy is not authorized except for in clinical-trial settings.

As of 2 March 2021, the National Institutes of Health treatment guideline panel suggested a preference for bamlanivimab and etesevimab over bamlanivimab alone, as well as over casirivimab/imdevimab. They based this recommendation on better quality data available from the blocking viral attachment and cell entry with SARS-CoV-2 neutralizing antibodies (BLAZE-1) Phase 3 trial, which included a larger sample and more events, in which a benefit of treatment with bamlanivimab plus etesevimab was not observed in patients hospitalized due to COVID-19. Monoclonal antibodies may be associated with worse clinical outcomes when administered to hospitalized patients with COVID-19 who require high-flow oxygen or mechanical ventilation.[76]

Convalescent Plasma with High Titer Neutralizing Antibodies

Convalescent plasma treatment is another potential adjunctive therapy for COVID-19.[77] Preliminary findings suggested improved clinical status after the treatment.[78] Donato et al. showed that convalescent plasma containing high neutralizing antibody titers conferred transfer of antibodies and an earlier viral neutralization while preserving endogenous antibody production.[79] Although preliminary data suggest the intervention is fairly safe, larger trials are ongoing to further explore the risks and benefits.

Anti-Inflammatory Therapy

Corticosteroids

The recent Randomized Evaluation of COVID-19 Therapy (RECOVERY) trial found that dexamethasone reduced mortality by about one-third in hospitalized patients with COVID-19 who received invasive mechanical ventilation, and by one-fifth in patients who received oxygen. By contrast, no benefit was found in patients without respiratory support.[80] In addition, Cai et al. analyzed 12,862 cases and found an index of neutrophils to lymphocytes above 6.12 to be an accurate, robust indicator for initiating corticosteroid treatment for severe COVID-19.[81]

IL-6 inhibitors: Tocilizumab and Sarilumab

Initial studies evaluating the use of IL-6 inhibitors to treat COVID-19 produced conflicting results. EMPACTA was a randomized double-blind placebo-controlled trial to evaluate tocilizumab's safety and efficacy in hospitalized patients with COVID-19 pneumonia not receiving mechanical ventilation.[82,83] The results showed that the likelihood of progression to mechanical ventilation or death at 28 days was significantly lower in the tocilizumab arm, but no improvement in overall survival rates.[83]

In January 2021, the international Randomized, Embedded, Multi-Factorial, Adaptive Platform Trial for Community-Acquired Pneumonia (REMAP-CAP) released early results for patients with severe COVID-19. The results showed an 8.5% reduction in absolute risk of death when IL-6 inhibitors (tocilizumab and sarilumab) were administered within 24 hours of ICU admission.[84] The RECOVERY trial showed 596 (29%) out of 2022 patients who received tocilizumab and 694 (33%) out of 2094 patients the usual care died within 28 days (rate ratio 0.86; 95% CI 0.77–0.96 PP=0.007).[85] The patients receiving tocilizumab were also more likely to be discharged, (57% vs 50% RR 1.22; CI 1.12–1.33 P<0.0001).[85] However, several questions regarding the use of IL-6 inhibitors, such as timing of administration in the course of the disease and whether there is any long-term mortality benefit, remain unanswered. It appears that the greatest benefits are seen when tocilizumab is combined with corticosteroids.[82]

Anticoagulation

Preliminary results from the ATTACC study suggest mortality benefit for full anticoagulation with unfractionated heparin or low molecular weight heparin in hospitalized COVID-19 patients not requiring invasive mechanical ventilation.[86]

Proning

The prone position improves oxygenation, although it is still unclear whether the benefit is temporary or truly affects the disease course. When using proning in sedated patients, it is important to pay extra attention to facial pressure ulcer prevention and to risk of aspiration.

PROGNOSIS

Recovery and Post-Infection Syndrome

Prognoses for patients with COVID-19 vary depending on factors such as age, underlying conditions, and severity of disease. Those with mild illness typically recover within 2 to 10 days. Most show no residual symptoms, but some report continued symptoms 3 weeks after diagnosis,[87] such as general fatigue, persistent cough, dyspnea on exertion, hair loss, and rarely palpitations and intermittent tachycardia.

For patients with moderate to severe disease, the illness duration is longer and commonly followed by post-acute COVID-19 syndrome lasting a month or longer. A U.S. study of 350 patients who had been hospitalized found that only 39% reported being free of symptoms 3 weeks after diagnosis.[88] A similar Italian study of 143 patients showed only 13% returned to baseline health within 2 months.[89] These patients most commonly reported persistent fatigue, dyspnea, joint pain, and chest pain.[87,88]

Mortality

In the study from China of 44,672 confirmed COVID-19 cases, the overall case fatality rate (CFR) was 2.3% (1,023 deaths). Age is significant in prognosis: Patients aged less than 9 years old had 0% CFR, 70 to 79 years had 8%, and older than 80 years had 14.8%. Pre-existing conditions also contribute to high CFRs: Cardiovascular disease had 10 5%, diabetes 7.3%, chronic respiratory disease 6.3%, hypertension 6.0%, and cancer 5.6% CFR.[70] Further associations with a bad prognosis include obesity, chronic kidney disease, and liver disease.[90]

Reports of mortality rates for critical illness vary. The previously mentioned study from China showed a 49% CFR for patients admitted to the ICU with critical symptoms,[70] whereas a New York area study reported an increase to 88.1% if patients with critical symptoms had been intubated.[90] A study from the Lombardy region of Italy identified a 26% CFR for young adults (21 years and younger),[91] and one from Seattle, Washington showed a 50% CFR for older adults.[92]

Immunity

Antibodies to the virus are induced in some patients who become infected. It is reported that seroconversion in COVID-19 patients occurs about 7 to 14 days post-symptom-onset.[93,94] Preliminary evidence suggests that some of these antibodies are protective, but this remains to be definitively established.[95] It is unknown whether all infected patients mount a protective immune response or how long any protective effect will last. Evolving evidence also suggests a significant role of T-cell response in early control of several viral infections, although that role with COVID-19 is still unclear.[96] Some research indicated that specific T-cells may contribute to prolonged COVID-19 symptoms,[97–99] but more studies are needed to define the benefits and drawbacks of these T-cells in various settings.

Reinfection

Symptomatic reinfection of SARS-CoV-2 has been reported. In one case, a different viral strain was identified by genomic analysis. The scope of reinfection is still unclear. However, several studies reported positive RT-PCR tests for SARS-CoV-2 in patients with laboratory-confirmed COVID-19 who clinically recovered and tested negative on two consecutive tests.[7,100] These positive tests occurred shortly after the negative tests and were not associated with worsening symptoms.[101] Most likely, they did not represent a reinfection or an infectious virus,[101] but a false positive from viral shedding that occurred earlier in the illness.[102]

▌VACCINATIONS

The rapid global transmission of SARS-CoV-2 infection has ignited extensive efforts toward developing COVID-19 vaccines that can be used to end the pandemic. Vaccine design includes selection of antigens and vaccination platforms, routes, and regimens.[103] The full-length spike glycoprotein or RBD of virion can prevent host and virus interaction by inducing neutralizing antibodies; hence, it is considered the most important vaccine target antigen.

Most ongoing COVID-19 vaccine development projects are using S-protein as the target antigen. In general, vaccine platforms are divided into six categories: live-attenuated virus, recombinant-viral vectored, inactivated virus, protein subunit, virus-like particles, and nucleic-acid based, which are currently under clinical and preclinical development. Typically, these nonviral platforms require multiple vaccinations to induce protective immunity, whereas live virus-based vaccines can provide "one-shot" immunity. Similar to nonviral platforms, killed-virus vaccines sometimes require the inclusion of an adjuvant and repeated administration for full efficacy.

The vaccination route is an integral consideration of vaccine strategies, particularly for mucosal pathogens such as SARS-CoV-2 and pathogens against which optimal protection requires not only neutralizing antibodies, but also innate and adaptive cellular immunity. The respiratory–mucosal vaccination route is adept at inducing antibodies and resident memory T-cells (T_{RM}-cells) in the respiratory mucosa, as well as macrophage-mediated trained immunity. Most vaccines, however, are administered intramuscularly (or intradermally). These elicit primarily a systemic immune response with less robust protection in the upper-respiratory mucosa than after natural infection.

The safety of a vaccine is generally determined by the adjuvant, administration mode and route, age, and status of pre-existing vaccine immunity.[104–106] For example, replicating live-attenuated virus or viral-vectored vaccines may not be safe for a respiratory–mucosal route. When a prime-boost immunization strategy is required, adverse events are generally more frequent and intense following the booster vaccination. Vaccine strategies for COVID-19, as for some other respiratory viral infections, require additional safety considerations related to the possibility of antibody-dependent disease enhancement and the role of overproduction of proinflammatory cytokines in lung immunopathology.

The aim of the vaccination is to ensure all immune-protective elements are present within the respiratory mucosa before viral entry. This means the vaccination can effectively induce mucosal IgA antibodies or T_{RM} cells in the lungs. Common immunological properties used to evaluate the vaccine's efficacy include neutralizing antibody response, T-cell response (CD4$^+$ T_H-cells, CD8$^+$ T-cells, and lung T_{RM}-cells). Several vaccine candidates have demonstrated immunogenicity without major safety concerns in early-phase human trials. Table 20-6 highlights the effectiveness rates of some common vaccines.

Since the end of 2020 and early 2021, two COVID-19 mRNA vaccines have been used in tens of millions of the global population. Each recipient is given two intramuscular doses separated by a few weeks.

Table 20-6 VACCINES[102,103]			
Vaccine	Manufacturer	Effectiveness in preventing symptomatic COVID-19	Comment
BNT162b2	Pfizer	52.4% after first dose; 95.0% after second dose	mRNA
mRNA-1273	Moderna	94.1% after second dose	mRNA
AstraZeneca	Oxford-AstraZeneca	66.7% after second dose	viral vector
Janssen	Johnson & Johnson	66.3% single dose	viral vector

In large placebo-controlled trials, these vaccines had 95% efficacy in preventing laboratory-confirmed symptomatic COVID-19 after the second dose.[107] Local and systemic adverse effects (pain, fever, fatigue, headache) are common but usually nonsevere. It is not yet known which COVID-19 vaccine strategy will be used or how long the vaccine-induced protection may last in humans. Longer observations are needed to answer these questions.

Data from a mass vaccination setting in Israel compared 592,656 vaccinated individuals to a matched unvaccinated cohort. In the follow-up period (7–21 days after the second dose) after administering the novel BNT162b2 mRNA (Pfizer) vaccine, there was a significant reduction in the number of new COVID-19 cases, related hospitalizations, and related mortality. The vaccine's estimated effectiveness at 7-day follow-up was reported as 92%, 94%, 87%, and 92%, respectively, for documented infections, symptomatic infections, hospitalizations, and severe cases. At 14 to 20 days after the first dose, these respective effectiveness estimates were 46%, 57%, 74%, and 62%; at 21 to 27 days (shifting between first and second doses), the estimates reached 60%, 66%, 78%, and 80%, respectively. Further, effectiveness against COVID-19-related deaths were estimated at 72% during the 14-to-20-day follow-up period, and 84% during the 21-to-27-day follow-up period.[108]

CONCLUSION

COVID-19, characterized with rapid person-to-person transmission, has imposed a huge financial and social burden on the world. Up to 40% of infections are asymptomatic, and severe disease (e.g., with hypoxia and pneumonia) is reported in 15% to 20% of symptomatic infections. Although ARDS is the major complication in patients with severe disease, many other complications—including thromboembolic events, acute cardiac injury, kidney injury, and inflammatory complications—have been reported. A positive NAAT for SARS-CoV-2 confirms the COVID-19 diagnosis, but NAAT sensitivity is still around 60% to 80%. Antigen tests are useful for serial screening for infection in high-risk settings, and serology is a useful adjunctive diagnostic test. The optimal approach to treating COVID-19, focused mainly on symptom relief and organ support, is uncertain. Outcomes relate to age and comorbidities. There is no better way to protect from SARS-CoV-2 than personal preventive behaviors, such as social distancing, wearing masks, and public health measures. Vaccines are considered the most promising approach to control the pandemic.

REFERENCES

1. Stringhini S, Wisniak A, Piumatti G, et al. Seroprevalence of anti-SARS-CoV-2 IgG antibodies in Geneva, Switzerland (SEROCoV-POP): a population-based study. *Lancet*. 2020;396(10247):313-319.
2. World Health Organization. *Novel Coronavirus Situation Report*. 22 January 2020. Available at https://www.who.int/docs/default-source/coronaviruse/situation-reports/20200122-sitrep-2-2019-ncov.pdf. Accessed 16 December 2020
3. Meyerowitz EA, Richterman A, Gandhi RT, Sax PE. Transmission of SARS-CoV-2: a review of viral, host, and environmental factors. *Ann Intern Med*. 2021;174(1):69-79.
4. Rothe C, Schunk M, Sothmann P, et al. Transmission of 2019-nCoV infection from an asymptomatic contact in Germany. *N Engl J Med*. 2020;382(10):970-971.
5. Bai Y, Yao L, Wei Tan, et al. Presumed asymptomatic carrier transmission of COVID-19. *JAMA*. 2020;323(14):1406-1407.
6. Fung HF, Martinez L, Alarid-Escudero F, et al. The household secondary attack rate of SARS-CoV-2: a rapid review. *Clin Infect Dis*. 2020;ciaa1558.
7. Van Elslande Jan, Vermeersch P, Vandervoort K, et al. Symptomatic SARS-CoV-2 reinfection by a phylogenetically distinct strain. *Clin Infect Dis*. 2020;ciaa1330. https://doi:10.1093/cid/ciaa1330.
8. Clausen TM, Sandoval DR, Spliid CB, et al. SARS-CoV-2 infection depends on cellular heparan sulfate and ACE2. *Cell*. 2020;183(4):1043-1057.

9. Bourgonje AR, Abdulle AE, Timens W, et al. Angiotensin-converting enzyme 2 (ACE2), SARS-CoV-2 and the pathophysiology of coronavirus disease 2019 (COVID-19). *J Pathol.* 2020;251(3):228-248.

10. Hoffmann M, Kliene-Weber H, Schroeder S, et al. SARS-CoV-2 cell entry depends on ACE2 and TMPRSS2 and is blocked by a clinically proven protease inhibitor. *Cell.* 2020;181(2):271-280.e8.

11. Nagashima S, Castilho Mendes M, Camargo Martins AP, et al. Endothelial dysfunction and thrombosis in patients with COVID-19: Brief report. *Arterioscler Thromb Vasc Bio.* 2020;40(10):2404-2407.

12. Zhou P, Yang X-L, Wang X-G, et al. A pneumonia outbreak associated with a new coronavirus of probable bat origin. *Nature.* 2020;579(7798):270-273.

13. Bohn MK, Hall A, Sepiashvili L, Jung B, Steele S, Adeli K. Pathophysiology of COVID-19: mechanisms underlying disease severity and progression. *Physiology.* 2020;35(5):288-301.

14. Ragab D, Eldin HS, Taeimah M, Khattab R, Salem R. The COVID-19 cytokine storm: what we know so far. *Front Immunol.* 2020;11(1446). https://doi:10.3389/fimmu.2020.01446.

15. Rydyznski Moderbacher C, Ramirez SI, Dan JM, et al. Antigen-specific adaptive immunity to SARS-CoV-2 in acute COVID-19 and associations with age and disease severity *Cell.* 2020;183(4):996-1012.e19.

16. Sa Ribero M, Jouvenet N, Dreux M, Nisole S. Interplay between SARS-CoV-2 and the type I interferon response. *PLoS Pathog.* 2020;16(7):e1008737.

17. Górgolas Hernández-Mora M, Cabello Úbeda A, Prieto-Pérez L, et al. Compassionate use of tocilizumab in severe SARS-CoV2 pneumonia. *Int J Infect Dis.* 2021;102:303-309.

18. Sánchez-Cerrillo I, Landete P, Aldave B, et al. COVID-19 severity associates with pulmonary redistribution of CD1c+ DCs and inflammatory transitional and nonclassical monocytes. *J Clin Invest.* 2020;130(12):6290-6300.

19. Hill JB, Garcia D, Crowther M, et al. Frequency of venous thromboembolism in 6513 patients with COVID-19: a retrospective study. *Blood Adv.* 2020;4(21):5373-5377.

20. Bowles L, Platton S, Yartey N, et al. Lupus anticoagulant and abnormal coagulation tests in patients with Covid-19. *N Engl J Med.* 2020;383(3):288-290.

21. Ackermann M, Verleden SE, Kuehnel M, et al. Pulmonary vascular endothelialitis, thrombosis, and angiogenesis in Covid-19. *N Engl J Med.* 2020;383(2):120-128.

22. Tavazzi G, Pellegrini C, Maurelli M, et al. Myocardial localization of coronavirus in COVID-19 cardiogenic shock. *Eur J Heart Fail.* 2020;22(5):911-915.

23. Guo T, Fan Y, Chen M, et al. Cardiovascular implications of fatal outcomes of patients with Coronavirus disease 2019 (COVID-19). *JAMA Cardiol.* 2020;5(7):811-818.

24. Zhou F, Yu T, Du R, et al. Clinical course and risk factors for mortality of adult inpatients with COVID-19 in Wuhan, China: a retrospective cohort study. *Lancet.* 2020;395(10229):1054-1062.

25. Kim I-C, Kim JY, Kim HA, Han S. COVID-19-related myocarditis in a 21-year-old female patient. *Eur Heart J*. 2020;41(19):1859.

26. Inciardi RM, Lupi L, Zaccone G, et al. Cardiac involvement in a patient with Coronavirus disease 2019 (COVID-19). *JAMA Cardiol*. 2020;5(7):819-824.

27. Cheng Y, Luo R, Zhang M, et al. Kidney disease is associated with in-hospital death of patients with COVID-19. *Kidney Int*. 2020;97(5):829-838.

28. Ye M, Wysocki J, William J, Soler MJ, Cokic I, Batlle D. Glomerular localization and expression of angiotensin-converting enzyme 2 and angiotensin-converting enzyme: Implications for albuminuria in diabetes. *J Am Soc Nephrol*. 2006;17(11):3067-3075.

29. Ronco C, Reis T, Husain-Syed F. Management of acute kidney injury in patients with COVID-19. *Lancet Respir Med*. 2020;8(7):738-742.

30. Xiao F, Tang M, Zheng X, Liu Y, Li X, Shan H. Evidence for gastrointestinal infection of SARS-CoV-2. *Gastroenterology*. 2020;158(6):1831-1833.e3.

31. Zhang C, Shi L, Wang F-S. Liver injury in COVID-19: management and challenges. *Lancet Gastroenterol Hepatol*. 2020;5(5):428-430.

32. Wang Y, Liu S, Liu H, et al. SARS-CoV-2 infection of the liver directly contributes to hepatic impairment in patients with COVID-19. *J Hepatol*. 2020;73(4):807-816.

33. Liu F, Long X, Zhang B, Zhang W, Chen X, Zhang Z. ACE2 expression in pancreas may cause pancreatic damage after SARS-CoV-2 infection. *Clin Gastroenterol Hepatol*. 2020;18(9):2128-2130.e2.

34. Wang F, Wang H, Fan J, Zhang Y, Wang H, Zhao Q. Pancreatic injury patterns in patients with Coronavirus disease 19 pneumonia. *Gastroenterology*. 2020;159(1):367-370.

35. Drucker DJ. Coronavirus infections and type 2 diabetes-shared pathways with therapeutic implications. *Endocr Rev*. 2020;41(3):bnaa011.

36. Mao L, Jin H, Wang M, et al. Neurologic manifestations of hospitalized patients with Coronavirus disease 2019 in Wuhan, China. *JAMA Neurol*. 2020;77(6):683-690.

37. Helms J. Neurologic features in severe SARS-CoV-2 infection. *N Engl J Med*. 2020;382(23):2268-2270.

38. Toscano G, Palmerini F, Ravaglia S, et al. Guillain-Barré syndrome associated with SARS-CoV-2. *N Engl J Med*. 2020;382(26):2574-2576.

39. Zhou Z, Kang H, Li S, Zhao X. Understanding the neurotropic characteristics of SARS-CoV-2: from neurological manifestations of COVID-19 to potential neurotropic mechanisms. *J Neurol*. 2020;267(8):2179-2184.

40. Vaira LA, Fois AG, Piombino P, De Riu G. Potential pathogenesis of ageusia and anosmia in COVID-19 patients. *Int Forum Allergy Rhinol*. 2020;10(9):1103-1104.

41. Consiglio CR, Cotugno N, Sardh F, et al. The immunology of multisystem inflammatory syndrome in children with COVID-19. *Cell*. 2020;183(4):968-981.e7.

42. Reyes S, Roche B, Kazzaz F, et al. Pneumothorax and pneumomediastinum in COVID-19: a case series. *Am J Med Sci*. [Online ahead of print]. https://doi:10.1016/j.amjms.2020.11.024.

43. Nadim MK, Forni LG, Mehta RL, et al. COVID-19-associated acute kidney injury: consensus report of the 25th Acute Disease Quality Initiative (ADQI) Workgroup. *Nat Rev Nephrol.* 2020;16:747-764.

44. Singh H, Kaur H, Singh K, Sen CK. Cutaneous manifestations of COVID-19: a systematic review. *Adv Wound Care.* 2021;10(2):51-80.

45. Nakra NA, Blumberg DA, Herrera-Guerra A, Lakshminrusimha S. Multisystem inflammatory syndrome in children (MIS-C) following SARS-CoV-2 infection: review of clinical presentation, hypothetical pathogenesis, and proposed management. *Children.* 2020;7(7):69.

46. Bamrah Morris S, Schwartz NG, Patel P, et al. Case series of multisystem inflammatory syndrome in adults associated with SARS-CoV-2 infection: United Kingdom and United States, March–August 2020. *Morb Mortal Wkly Rep.* 2020;69:1450-1456.

47. U.S. Centers for Disease Control and Prevention. *SARS-CoV-2 Variants.* 2021. Available at https://www.cdc.gov/coronavirus/2019-ncov/cases-updates/variant-surveillance/variant-info.html. Accessed 28 February 2021.

48. Annavajhala MK, Mohri H, Zucker JE, et al. A novel SARS-CoV-s variant of concern, B.1.526, identified in New York. medRxiv. 2021:2021.02.23.21252259.

49. Woloshin S, Patel N, Kesselheim AS. False negative tests for SARS-CoV-2 infection: challenges and implications. *N Engl J Med.* 2020;383:e38.

50. U.S. Centers for Disease Control and Prevention. *Interim Guidelines for Collecting, Handling, and Testing Clinical Specimens for COVID-19.* 2020. https://www.cdc.gov/coronavirus/2019-ncov/lab/guidelines-clinical-specimens.html. Accessed 16 December 2020.

51. Perera RAPM, Tso E, Tsang OTY, et al. SARS-CoV-2 virus culture and subgenomic RNA for respiratory specimens from patients with mild coronavirus disease. *Emerg Infect Dis.* 2020;26(11):2701-2704.

52. Patel A, Jernigan DB, 2019-nCoV CDC Response Team. Initial public health response and interim clinical guidance for the 2019 novel coronavirus outbreak: United States, December 31, 2019–February 4, 2020. *Morb Mortal Wkly Rep.* 2020;69(5):140.

53. Cheng MP, Papenburg J, Desjardins M, et al. Diagnostic testing for severe acute respiratory syndrome-related Coronavirus 2: a narrative review. *Ann Intern Med.* 2020;172(11):726-734.

54. Weissleder R, Lee H, Ko J, Pittet MJ. COVID-19 diagnostics in context. *Sci Transl Med.* 2020;12:eabc1931.

55. Wong HYF, Lam HYS, Fong AH, et al. Frequency and distribution of chest radiographic findings in patients positive for COVID-19. *Radiology.* 2020;296(2):e72-e78.

56. Guan W-j, Ni Z, Hu Y, et al. Clinical characteristics of Coronavirus disease 2019 in China. *N Eng J Med.* 2020;382:1708-1720.

57. Simpson S, Kay FU, Abbara S, et al. Radiological Society of North America expert consensus document on reporting chest CT findings related to COVID

19: endorsed by the Society of Thoracic Radiology, the American College of Radiology, and RSNA. *Radiol Cardiothorac Imaging.* 2020;2(2):e200152.

58. Mayo PH, Copetti R, Feller-Kopman D, et al. Thoracic ultrasonography: a narrative review. *Intensive Care Med.* 2019;45:1200-1211.

59. Vetrugno L, Bove T, Orso D, et al. Our Italian experience using lung ultrasound for identification, grading and serial follow-up of severity of lung involvement for management of patients with COVID-19. *Echocardiography.* 2020;37(4):625-627.

60. Bouhemad B, Mongodi S, Gabriele V, Rouquette I. Ultrasound for "lung monitoring" of ventilation patients. *Anesthesiology.* 2015;122:437-447.

61. U.S. Centers for Disease Control and Prevention. *Interim Infection Prevention and Control Recommendations for Healthcare Personnel during the Coronavirus Disease 2019 (COVID-19) Pandemic.* 2020. Available at https://www.cdc.gov/coronavirus/2019-nCoV/hcp/infection-control.html. Accessed 16 December 2020.

62. World Health Organization. *Transmission of SARS-CoV-2: Implications for Infection Prevention Precautions.* 2020. https://www.who.int/publications/i/item/modes-of-transmission-of-virus-causing-covid-19-implications-for-ipc-precaution-recommendations. Accessed 16 December 2020.

63. Ong SWX, Tan YK, Chia PY, et al. Air, surface environmental, and personal protective equipment contamination by severe acute respiratory syndrome Coronavirus 2 (SARS-CoV-2) from a symptomatic patient. *JAMA.* 2020;323(16):1610-1612.

64. Wei WE, Li Z, Chiew CJ, Yong SE, Toh MP, Lee VJ. Presymptomatic transmission of SARS-CoV-2: Singapore, January 23–March 16, 2020. *Morb Mortal Wkly Rep.* 2020;69(14):411-415.

65. U.S. Centers for Disease Control and Prevention. *Core Infection Prevention and Control Practices for Safe Healthcare Delivery in All Settings: Recommendations of the HICPAC.* 2020. Available at https://www.cdc.gov/hicpac/pdf/core-practices.pdf. Accessed 16 December 2020.

66. U.S. Centers for Disease Control and Prevention. *Discontinuation of Transmission-Based Precautions and Disposition of Patients with COVID-19 in Healthcare Settings: Interim Guidance.* 2021. Available at https://www.cdc.gov/coronavirus/2019-ncov/hcp/disposition-hospitalized-patients.html. Accessed 8 March 2021.

67. U.S. Centers for Disease Control and Prevention. *Clinical Questions about COVID-19: Questions and Answers.* 2020. Available at https://www.cdc.gov/coronavirus/2019-ncov/hcp/faq.html. Accessed 16 December 2020.

68. U.S. Environmental Protection Agency. List-N Disinfectants for Coronavirus (COVID-19). 2020. Available at https://www.epa.gov/pesticide-registration/list-n-disinfectants-coronavirus-covid-19. Accessed 16 December 2020.

69. Hughes MM, Groenewold MR, Lessem SE, et al. Update: characteristics of Health Care Providers with COVID-19; United States, February 12–July 16, 2020. *Morb Mortal Wkly Rep.* 2020;69(38):1364-1368.

70. Wu Z, McGoogan JM. Characteristics of and important lessons from the Coronavirus disease 2019 (COVID-19) outbreak in China: summary of a report of 72 314 cases from the Chinese Center for Disease Control and Prevention. *JAMA*. 2020;323(13):1239-1242.

71. The Novel Coronavirus Pneumonia Emergency Response Epidemiology Team. Vital surveillances: the epidemiological characteristics of an outbreak of 2019 novel Coronavirus diseases (COVID-19); China, 2020. *China CDC Wkly*. 2020;2(8):113-122.

72. U.S. Centers for Disease Control and Prevention *Clean and Disinfect*. 2020. Available at https://www.cdc.gov/coronavirus/2019-ncov/prepare/cleaning-disinfection.html. Updated March 1, 2020. Accessed December 15, 2020.

73. U.S. Centers for Disease Control and Prevention. *Interim Guidance for Implementing Home Care of People Not Requiring Hospitalization for 2019 Novel Coronavirus (2019-nCoV)*. 2020. Available at https://www.cdc.gov/coronavirus/2019-ncov/hcp/guidance-home-care.html. Accessed 1 March 2021.

74. U.S. Centers for Disease Control and Prevention. *Duration of Isolation and Precautions for Adults with COVID-19*. 2020. Available at https://www.cdc.gov/coronavirus/2019-ncov/hcp/duration-isolation.html. Accessed 8 March 2021.

75. Shi R, Shan C, Duan X, et al. A human neutralizing antibody targets the receptor-binding site of SARS-CoV-2. *Nature*. 2020;584(7819):120-124.

76. National Institutes of Health *The COVID-19 Treatment Guidelines Panel's Statement on the Emergency Use Authorization of the Bamlanivimab Plus Etesevimab Combination for the Treatment of COVID-19*. 2 March 2021. Available at https://www.covid19treatmentguidelines.nih.gov/statement-on-bamlanivimab-plus-etesevimab-eua/. Accessed 3 March 2021.

77. Piechotta V, Chai KL, Valk SJ, et al. Convalescent plasma or hyperimmune immunoglobulin for people with COVID-19: a living systematic review. (Update). *Cochrane Database Syst Rev*. 2020;10:CD013600.

78. Shen C, Wang Z, Zhao F, et al. Treatment of 5 critically ill patients with COVID-19 with convalescent plasma. *JAMA*. 2020;323:1582-1589.

79. Donato ML, Park S, Baker M, et al. Clinical and laboratory evaluation of patients with SARS-CoV-2 pneumonia treated with high-titer convalescent plasma. *JCI Insight*. [Online ahead of print]. https://doi.org/10.1101/2020.07.20.20156398.

80. RECOVERY Collaborative Group, Horby P, Lim WS, et al. Dexamethasone in hospitalized patients with Covid-19. *N Engl J Med*. 2021;384:693-704.

81. Cai Q, Zeng M, Wu X, Zhan Y, Tian R, Zhang M. CaMKIIα-driven, phosphatase-checked postsynaptic plasticity via phase separation. *Cell Res*. 2021;1:37-51.

82. National Institutes of Health. *Coronavirus Disease 2019 (COVID-19): Treatment Guidelines*. 2021. Available at https://www.covid19treatmentguidelines.nih.gov/. Accessed 22 February 2021.

83. Salama C, Han J, Yau L, et al. Tocilizumab in Patients Hospitalized with Covid-19 Pneumonia. *N Engl J Med*. 2021;384:20-30.

84. REMAP-CAP Investigators. Interleukin-6 Receptor Antagonists in Critically Ill Patients with COVID-19. *N Engl J Med*. 2021;384:1491-1502.

85. RECOVERY Collaborative Group. Tocilizumab in patients admitted to hospital with COVID-19 (RECOVERY): preliminary results of a randomized controlled open label platform trial. *Lancet*. 2021;397:1637-1645.

86. National Institutes of Health. *News release: full-dose blood thinners decreased need for life support and improved outcome in hospitalized COVID-19 patients*. 22 January 2021. Available at https://www.nih.gov/news-events/news-releases/full-dose-blood-thinners-decreased-need-life-support-improved-outcome-hospitalized-covid-19-patients. Accessed 8 March 2021.

87. Tenforde MW, Kim SS, Lindsell CJ, et al. Symptom duration and risk factors for delayed return to usual health among outpatients with COVID-19 in a multistate health care systems network: United States, March–June 2020. *Morb Mortal Wkly Rep*. 2020;69(30):993.

88. Tenforde MW, Billig Rose E, Lindsell CJ, et al. Characteristics of adult outpatients and inpatients with COVID-19: 11 academic medical centers, United States, March–May 2020. *Morb Mortal Wkly Rep*. 2020;69(26):841.

89. Carfi A, Bernabei R, Landi F, for the Gemelli Against COVID-19 Post-Acute Care Study Group. Persistent symptoms in patients after acute COVID-19. *JAMA*. 2020;324(6):603.

90. Richardson S, Hirsch JS, Narasimhan M, et al. Presenting characteristics, comorbidities, and outcomes among 5700 patients hospitalized with COVID-19 in the New York City area. *JAMA*. 2020;323(20):2052-2059.

91. Grasselli G, Zangrillo A, Zanella A, et al. Baseline characteristics and outcomes of 1591 patients infected with SARS-CoV-2 admitted to ICUs of the Lombardy region, Italy. *JAMA*. 2020;323(16):1574-15781.

92. Bhatraju PK, Ghassemieh BJ, Nichols M, et al. Covid-19 in critically ill patients in the Seattle region: case series. *N Engl J Med*. 2020;382(21):2012-2022.

93. Guo L, Ren L, Yang S, et al. Profiling early humoral response to diagnose novel coronavirus disease (COVID-19). *Clin Infect Dis*. 2020;71(15):778-785.

94. Zhao J, Yuan Q, Wang H, et al. Antibody responses to SARS-CoV-2 in patients with novel Coronavirus disease 2019. *Clin Infect Dis*. 2020;71(16):2027-2034.

95. Cao X. COVID-19: immunopathology and its implications for therapy. *Nat Rev Immunol*. 2020;20(5):269-270.

96. Karlsson AC, Humbert M, Buggert M. The known unknowns of T cell immunity to COVID-19. *Sci Immunol*. 2020;5(53):eabe8063.

97. Mathew D, Giles JR, Baxter AE, et al. Deep immune profiling of COVID-19 patients reveals distinct immunotypes with therapeutic implications. *Science*. 2020;369(6508):eabc8511.

98. Juno A, Tan H-X, Lee WS, et al. Humoral and circulating follicular helper T cell responses in recovered patients with COVID-19. *Nat Med*. 2020;26:1428-1434.

99. Kaneko N, Kuo HH, Boucau J, et al. Loss of Bcl-6-expressing T follicular helper cells and germinal centers in COVID-19. *Cell*. 2020;183:143-157.e13.

100. To KK-W, Hung IF-N, Ip JD, et al. COVID-19 re-infection by a phylogenetically distinct SARS-coronavirus-2 strain confirmed by whole genome sequencing. *Clin Infect Dis*. 2020;ciaa1275.

101. Suri T, Mitta S, Tiwari P, et al. COVID-19 real-time RT-PCR: does positivity on follow-up RT-PCR always imply infectivity? *Am J Respir Crit Care Med*. 2020;202(1):147.

102. Wölfel R, Corman VM, Guggemos W, et al. Virological assessment of hospitalized patients with COVID-2019. *Nature*. 2020;581(7809):465-469.

103. Jeyanathan M, Afkhami S, Smaill F, Miller MS, Lichty BD, Xing Z. Immunological considerations for COVID-19 vaccine strategies. *Nat Rev Immunol*. 2020;20:615-632.

104. Rawat K, Kumari P, Saha L. COVID-19 vaccine: a recent update in pipeline vaccines, their design and development strategies. *Eur J Pharmacol*. 2021;892:173751.

105. U.S. Centers for Disease Control and Prevention. *Different COVID-19 Vaccines*. 31 March 2021. Available at https://www.cdc.gov/coronavirus/2019-ncov/vaccines/different-vaccines.html. Updated March 2021. Accessed March 2021.

106. Voysey M, Costa Clemens SA, Madhi SB, et al. Single dose administration, and the influence of the timing of the booster dose on immunogenicity and efficacy of ChAdOx1 nCoV-19 (AZD1222) vaccine: a pooled analysis of four randomised trials. *Lancet*. 2021;397(10277):881-891.

107. Hahn SM, Marks P. *FDA Statement on Following the Authorized Dosing Schedules for COVID-19 Vaccines*. 2021. Available at https://www.fda.gov/news-events/press-announcements/fda-statement-following-authorized-dosing-schedules-covid-19-vaccines. Accessed 6 January 2021.

108. Dagan N, Barda N, Keplen E, et al. BNT162b2 mRNA Covid-19 vaccine in a nationwide mass vaccination setting. *N Engl J Med*. 2021;384(15):1412-1423.

21 INFLUENZA

Steven J. Sperber, MD, FACP, FIDSA

▌INTRODUCTION

The influenza virus wreaks havoc on our healthcare system and infrastructure and regularly requires significant public health resources for the fairly predictable seasonal influenza, and in addition in an unpredictable manner for pandemic influenza. The influenza virus and its epidemiology create optimal conditions for the development of an unanticipated pandemic of unforeseeable severity.

Influenza viruses, 0.08–0.12 microns, belong to the Orthomyxoviridae family and can be classified as types A, B, C, and D. Influenza A and B viruses cause seasonal influenza whereas only influenza A viruses have resulted in pandemics. Influenza C is infrequently recognized as causing relatively mild respiratory disease in humans and is not included in routine influenza virus testing. Influenza D is newly recognized and shares about 50% homology with influenza C.

Influenza A viruses are subclassified based on two surface glycoproteins—hemagglutinin (HA) and neuraminidase (NA). There are currently recognized 18 subtypes of HA (designated H1-18) and 11 subtypes of NA (N1-11). These subtypes circulate in birds. Influenza A(H1N1), A(H2N2), and A(H3N2) have caused seasonal influenza outbreaks. Influenza B has no recognized animal reservoir. The unique features of the influenza A viruses—their ability to undergo antigenic change and ability to infect other species—contribute to their threat as a novel pandemic virus.

Newer scientific methods have permitted the study of past pandemics that was not possible at the time of occurrence or even decades ago. With the recent attention to the 100th anniversary of the 1918–1919 influenza pandemic, it is instructive to look at influenza as a model of a pandemic pathogen that might prove useful in preparing for future pandemics.

EPIDEMIOLOGY

Human influenza viruses are transmitted from person to person via the respiratory tract by coughing and sneezing. Small particle aerosol, large droplet, and fomite are all potential routes of infection. Species of influenza viruses from animals could reach humans via the same routes.

Birds, such as migratory waterfowl, can become infected by influenza viruses. The avian illness may be very mild or asymptomatic; virus shed in the feces has the potential to infect domestic poultry, swine, horses, and marine mammals, which may transmit infection to humans as a zoonosis.

Swine are also recognized as having an important role in the potential development of a pandemic influenza strain. The swine respiratory tract has receptors for both human and avian influenza viruses, which allow for infection with human and avian strains. The pig has been considered a mixing bowl where reassortment of human and avian influenza viruses may occur.

A unique feature of the influenza viruses is their spontaneous antigenic variation. Mutations resulting in minor changes in the protein structure of influenza viruses allow the virus to evade the host immune response. These changes, called antigenic drift, lead to outbreaks with new virus strains, and occur with influenza A and B viruses. Antigenic shift is much rarer and occurs when two different subtypes of influenza A virus infect the same host (such as swine) and undergo reassortment to create a new influenza A virus. The ability of influenza A viruses to infect other species with the potential for reassortment permits the development of novel strains. If the novel strain to which the human population has no immunity is readily transmittable, it can cause an epidemic or pandemic.

Prior Influenza Pandemics

Four pandemics have occurred since the beginning of the last century (Table 21-1).[1] The pandemics of the prior century are occasionally referred to by a common name to indicate the presumed site of origin. The geographic origin of the 1918 "Spanish flu" pandemic is not known but was most likely not Spain.

The 1918 influenza pandemic (Figure 21-1) resulted in approximately 50 million deaths worldwide with 675,000 of them in the United States.[2] This pandemic is frequently referred to as "the mother of all pandemics".[3] Many areas experienced three closely spaced waves. A unique feature of this pandemic is that it did not target the usual victims of seasonal influenza—the elderly and those with traditional risk factors for

Table 21-1   CHARACTERISTICS OF THE MOST RECENT INFLUENZA PANDEMICS

Pandemic year of emergence and common name	Area of origin	Influenza A virus subtype (type of animal genetic introduction/ recombination event)	Estimated case fatality	Estimated attributable excess mortality worldwide	Age groups most affected
1918 "Spanish flu"	Uncertain	H1N1 (unknown)	2–3%	20–50 million	Young adults
1957–1958 "Asian flu"	Southern China	H2N2 (avian)	< 0.2%	1–4 million	All age groups
1968–1969 "Hong Kong flu"	Southern China	H3N2 (avian)	< 0.2%	1–4 million	All age groups
2009–2010 "influenza A(H1N1) 2009"	North America	H1N1 (swine)	0.02%	100,000– 400,000	Children and young adults

Adapted from Global Influenza Programme. *Pandemic influenza risk management: A WHO guide to inform and harmonize national and international pandemic preparedness and response.* Geneva: World Health Organization; 2017. License: CC BY-NC-SA 3.0 IGO.[1]

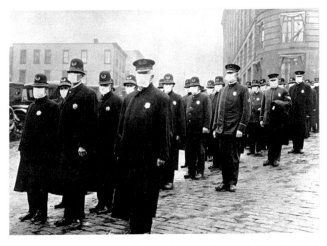

Figure 21-1 • Policemen in Seattle wearing masks made by the Red Cross during the influenza pandemic, December 1918. (*Courtesy National Archives, photo no. 165-WW-269B-25.*)

influenza infection—but took a large toll on the young and previously healthy. Wartime conditions during World War 1 likely provided a unique opportunity for spread of the virus and increased morbidity and mortality. Crowding in military camps and in cities, poor sanitation, and limited medical personnel were contributing factors.[2]

At the time, influenza was widely considered to be a bacterial disease, and *Haemophilus influenzae* was described as the cause; the influenza virus had not yet been identified.[4] *H. influenzae* was found by Richard Pfeiffer in 1892 in the nostrils of patients with flu-like illnesses. It was initially thought to be the etiology of influenza and called *Bacillus influenzae* or Pfeiffer's bacillus.[5] The 1918 pandemic indeed was characterized by a high frequency of bacterial pneumonia from autopsy results.[4] Secondary bacterial infections including pneumonia are sequelae of seasonal influenza and were associated with severe disease during the 1918 pandemic.[4,6] In fact, an early "influenza vaccine" in 1919 included bacteria such as pneumococcus, streptococcus and *H. influenzae*; in a study involving 21,759 men, the risk of death in severe or complicated cases of influenza was 8% in those who received full vaccination compared with 27% of those who did not. As the vaccine could not prevent viral infections the findings highlight the importance of secondary bacterial complications.[7] The H1N1 virus that caused this pandemic was characterized by emergence of antigenic shifts in both HA and NA. The origin of the virus is not known with certainty but may have been a direct introduction from an avian reservoir.[3,7]

The 1957 "Asian flu" pandemic was caused by an A(H2N2) virus, which was a result of reassortment between an avian H2N2 virus and seasonal H1N1 influenza virus and caused at least one million excess deaths worldwide.[8] In contrast to observations during the prior pandemic, underlying chronic cardiac or pulmonary disease was found in most patients, and women in their third trimester pregnancy were recognized to be at increased risk.[9]

The 1968 "Hong Kong flu" pandemic was due to an A(H3N2) virus, which developed from reassortment between an avian H3N2 virus and the H2N2 virus that had been circulating as seasonal influenza since the 1957 pandemic, and contributed to approximately one million or more deaths.[8] This virus has continued to circulate and remains a major cause of seasonal influenza.

The 2009 pandemic was characterized by an outbreak of a novel A(H1N1) virus (named H1N1 pdm09) in Mexico that quickly spread to the United States and the rest of the world (Figure 21-2). This virus represented a quadruple reassortment of two swine strains, one avian strain, and a human strain.[10] The Centers for Disease Control and Prevention (CDC) estimates that during the pandemic there were 60.8 million cases,

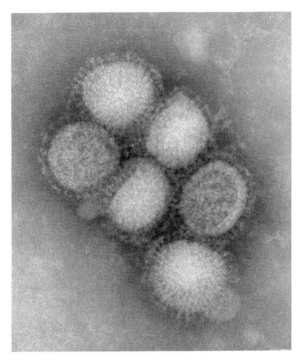

Figure 21-2 • Transmission electron microscopic image of Influenza A(H1N1) surrounded by spikes. (*Courtesy of the CDC.* https://phil.cdc.gov/Details.aspx?pid=11214.)

274,304 hospitalizations, and 12,469 deaths in the United States due to the new virus.[11] Since the pandemic was declared over in 2010, the pandemic A(H1N1) strain has continued to circulate seasonally in the United States.

Surveillance

There is continuous monitoring for the development of human influenza infections caused by animal viruses. This surveillance involves international cooperation and sharing of information at the level of human and animal experts (a One Health approach).[12] When a novel influenza A virus is identified in the human population but not yet circulating widely, the CDC utilizes a tool called the Influenza Risk Assessment Tool[13] to evaluate the potential risk of the new virus. Ten criteria are grouped within three categories (properties of the virus, attributes of the population, and ecology and epidemiology) to stratify the risk and impact on public health.[13] The CDC[14] and World Health Organization (WHO)[1] have stepwise phases to characterize the emergence and spread of new influenza subtypes in the development of a pandemic (Figure 21-3), and these are described later.

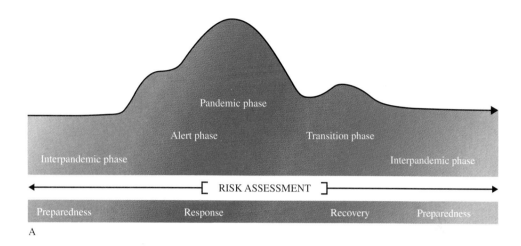

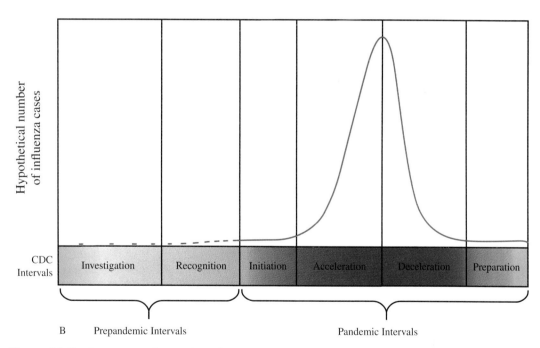

Figure 21-3 • Continuum of a pandemic based on the World Health Organization pandemic phases and interpandemic phases **(panel A)** and the Centers for Disease Control and Prevention pandemic intervals and prepandemic intervals **(panel B)**. (From Global Influenza Programme. *Pandemic influenza risk management: A WHO guide to inform and harmonize national and international pandemic preparedness and response*. Geneva: World Health Organization; 2017 and US Department of Health and Human Services. *Pandemic influenza plan, 2017 update*. https://www.cdc.gov/flu/pandemic-resources/pdf/pan-flu-report-2017v2.pdf.)

Recognized Novel Influenza Viruses of Pandemic Potential

The number of cases of influenza in humans caused by novel influenza viruses has increased significantly over the past decade.[12] This is due not only to increased surveillance, but also the expanding pig and poultry markets with their proximity to populated communities, and air travel which permits rapid worldwide dissemination of novel strains. A number of novel influenza A viruses have emerged with sporadic human cases. Some of the more notable viruses are described below.

Influenza A(H5N1) viruses were recognized in humans in 1997 in Hong Kong and represented the first known fatal cases. There were six deaths among the first 18 confirmed cases. Visiting a live poultry market or exposure to sick or dead poultry were identified as risk factors.[15] Serologic studies suggest unrecognized poultry-to-human transmission had occurred among poultry workers. This led to closure of the live poultry markets, slaughter of 1.5 million chickens and, restrictions on importation of poultry from China. The WHO actively monitors influenza A(H5N1) infections and has identified 861 human infections with 455 deaths between November 2003 and July 2020 (53% mortality).[16] Fortunately, these viruses have not shown that they are readily transmitted from person to person.

In early 2013, human cases of novel avian influenza A(H7N9) were identified in China. Annual epidemics have occurred through 2017, with over 760 cases reported from October 2016 through September 2017. Since then, there have been only a few human infections reported.[17] Most of the human infections were associated with exposure to infected poultry, although this virus is not as pathogenic in birds as in other avian species. Infection in humans is known to result in pneumonia and acute respiratory distress syndrome (ARDS) with mortality of around 39%.[17] A limited number of transmission was reported in China, which thankfully was not associated with sustained human-to-human transmission. Influenza A(H7N9) is considered a potential pandemic strain and is monitored by the WHO. Because of its virulence, the CDC also considers it to have a high potential to cause a pandemic if it changes to acquire the ability for sustained human-to-human transmission.[17]

Human infections caused by avian influenza A(H9N2) viruses are recognized infrequently and tend to cause mild illness. These viruses are considered of potential pandemic concern[18,19] and are included among the avian influenza viruses monitored by the WHO and CDC. Most of the infections have been in children and were associated with poultry exposure.[19]

Sporadic human infections also occur with influenza A viruses that circulate among pigs. These swine strains that infect humans are called "variant" viruses and are designated with a "v" after the subtype. Human infections with A(H1N1v), A(H3N2v), and A(H1N2v) have been reported in the United States. Illnesses with the variant viruses tend to resemble seasonal influenza. The illnesses are milder than those caused by some of the avian influenza viruses, but severe illness and death can occur. Most infections have been associated with exposure to infected pigs, such as on a farm or at a fair; limited non-sustained human-to-human spread have been detected.[19]

RISK FACTORS

Risk factors for serious complications of seasonal influenza are recognized to include age 65 and older or younger than 2 years, pregnancy, American Indians and Alaska natives, nursing home and long-term care residents, asthma or chronic lung disease, neurologic/neuro development conditions, hematologic disorders, heart disease, kidney disease, liver disease, metabolic disorders, obesity, immune disease or immunosuppression, and children receiving aspirin or salicylate-containing medications.[20] Immunization or prior infection with a similar strain may prevent infection or result in a milder illness if infection does occur.

Seasonal influenza is usually associated with a U-shaped epidemic curve with attack rates highest in the young and mortality greatest among older adults.[10] Whereas seasonal influenza viruses are generally predictable in their appearance from fall to spring, pandemic strains may arise at any time. In addition, the pandemic strains may have greater impact on young children or young adults with relative sparing of the elderly, resulting in a W-shaped epidemiological curve. During the 1918 influenza pandemic, an increase in mortality was observed among young adults between the ages of 20 and 40 with a peak in those aged 28 years in many populations.[21] The 2009 influenza pandemic was characterized by higher rates of infections among those aged 24 and younger.[22] Increased mortality among women in the latter part of pregnancy was seen during the 2009 pandemic, similar to observations during other pandemics and with seasonal influenza. Morbid obesity was also recognized as a risk factor for increased mortality.[23]

Transmission

The transmissibility of viruses can be quantified based on the average number of secondary cases that result from one infectious case. The reproduction number (R) represents how many persons a typical case will infect. A value greater than 1 indicates the infection will persist or grow in a population.[24] The median R for seasonal influenza over many years has been calculated to be 1.27. For the 1918 pandemic virus, the median R value was 1.80, with a higher median R value reported in confined settings such as schools, shops, and military camps. During the 2009 pandemic, the median estimate of R was 1.46; a higher value was also reported in confined settings such as military or summer camps, schools, and night clubs. A number of studies have looked at the reproduction number during influenza A(H5N1) outbreaks and reported R values from 0 to 1.14.[24] Prior investigations have found higher cumulative attack rates in populations with increasing R values (from 15%–21% when R=1.13 to 34%–42% when R=2.0).[24]

▌PATHOPHYSIOLOGY

When the influenza virus reaches the respiratory tract and infects the epithelial cells, viral replication and release of virus can occur along with cell death. Viral shedding is detectable prior to the onset of illness and typically for up to 5–10 days, although children tend to shed virus for longer.[10] In experimental influenza models, the severity of illness is proportional to the quantity of virus shedding. Systemic symptoms correlate with the release of cytokines such as interferons, tumor necrosis factor, and interleukins.[10] On autopsy, severe cases show necrotizing tracheobronchitis with ulceration and sloughing of the bronchial mucosa, hemorrhage, and hyaline membrane formation.[10]

The response to infection includes the development of resistance to the homologous strain, and a variable degree of cross-resistance to related strains.[10] This host response includes systemic antibody production, local mucosal antibody stimulation, and cellular responses. Systemic antibodies include those directed against the envelope glycoproteins HA and NA and against the structural proteins. Antibodies to HA prevent virus attachment to the cell and neutralize infectivity. Certain antibodies that are produced appear to have broader cross-reactivity among several HA subtypes that have been categorized together as group 1 (H1, H2, and H5) and group 2 (H3 and H7).[10] The anti-NA antibody reduces the release of viruses from infected cells. HA-specific IgA can be measured in nasal secretions resulting from local production and appears to play a role in resistance to infection. Optimal protection depends on the presence of both serum and local antibodies.[10]

Explanations for the high mortality during the 1918 influenza pandemic have focused on both host and virus specific factors. Tissue specimens dating back to 1918 and 1919 have been analyzed with techniques only available almost a century later to identify the genes of the virus and to reconstruct the pandemic strain.[7] The reconstructed 1918 H1N1 virus has been shown to be highly pathogenic in animals resulting in histopathologic changes in lung tissue that resemble autopsy findings from victims of the 1918 pandemic. Similar changes have been found with avian influenza A(H5N1) and A(H7N9) infections.[25] While these viruses are virulent, this alone may not have been sufficient to account for their high mortality.[7] Cytokines, such as tumor necrosis factor and interleukins, have been detected in non-respiratory tissues following infection of ferrets with the reconstructed 1918 H1N1 virus suggesting a greater role for cytokines and the host response in the pathophysiology.[7] It has been proposed that the increased severity of illness among the young during the 1918 pandemic may in part have resulted from cytokine storm, a dysregulated immune response.[6,7]

The increased mortality of the young and relative protection of the elderly during the 1918 pandemic is also believed to be a result of protective immunity from prior influenza virus infection. The concept of original antigenic sin suggests that infection in early childhood results in T cell and B cell memory that can confer life-long protection.[7] It has been speculated that the elderly might have been born when an H1N1 virus was circulating, whereas those in their 20s–40s during the pandemic were likely exposed when very young to a virus with different HA and NA components, such as H3N8, which would not provide protection later against an H1N1 virus.[7,25] Exposure to a double-heterogenic virus in childhood, such as H3N8, may have induced antibody-dependent cellular cytotoxicity leading to enhanced pulmonary disease contributing to severe illness in the young.[25] These factors likely contributed to the W-shaped mortality curve during the 1918 pandemic. Further evidence of long-term protection was observed during the 2009 influenza A(H1N1) pandemic where older adults who were exposed to the 1918 influenza A(H1N1) virus or immediate descendant virus were protected from infection and severe disease by antibodies that cross-reacted with the 2009 pandemic strain.[6] Malnutrition, immune suppression related to measles, and concurrent infection with malaria have been suggested as additional host factors leading to disease severity during the 1918 pandemic.[6]

The pathogenicity of the virulent influenza A(H5N1) viruses has been under investigation and is not completely understood. Viral and host factors are likely to play a role, with differences compared with seasonal influenza viruses. The target cells for influenza A(H5N1) virus replication include bronchiolar and alveolar cells, not epithelium, which may explain the high frequency of lung involvement. In addition, higher levels of cytokines (such as interleukin-6, interleukin-10, and interferon gamma) are produced by host cells in response to influenza A(H5N1) infection (especially those with a fatal outcome) than with seasonal influenza infection.[26] Comparably high levels of some cytokines are also found in the sera of patients with influenza A(H7N9) infection.[27]

CLINICAL MANIFESTATIONS

Influenza typically begins following an incubation period of 1–2 days with sudden onset of systemic symptoms including feverishness, chills, headache, myalgia, malaise, and anorexia. Higher fever may be associated with more severe headache or myalgia.[10] Non-productive cough, throat pain, rhinorrhea, and nasal stuffiness often accompany the systemic symptoms. Systemic symptoms usually resolve after about 3 days, with persistence of cough. Complete recovery may take 2 or more weeks. There is a wide spectrum of clinical presentations and some patients may have mild illness or asymptomatic infection. Infection in children may be characterized by higher temperature, cervical adenopathy, and croup, whereas infection in the elderly is more frequently complicated by pulmonary manifestations.[10]

Pulmonary complications of influenza virus infection include primary viral pneumonia and secondary bacterial pneumonia. Primary viral pneumonia follows a typical influenza illness with rapid progression of fever, cough, and shortness of breath, rather than recovery. Hypoxia, cyanosis, and diffuse bilateral non-focal radiographic findings are typical. Sputum studies do not reveal a bacterial etiology and the patients do not respond to antibiotics. The mortality from viral pneumonia is high. Patients with rheumatic heart disease, and in particular mitral stenosis, are at highest risk, with increased risk also for patients with other cardiac and pulmonary diseases.[10]

Secondary bacterial pneumonia differs from primary viral pneumonia in that it typically follows a period of recovery from influenza with clinical improvement that lasts several days to 2 weeks. The most common bacterial pathogens are *Streptococcus pneumoniae* and *Staphylococcus aureus*. Infection may be due to community-acquired methicillin-sensitive *Staphylococcus aureus* or methicillin-resistant *Staphylococcus aureus*.[10] Thus, during influenza season, the clinician should be attuned to the risk of community-acquired *Staphylococcus aureus* pneumonia. Empiric antibiotics should be initiated to provide treatment against these organisms and adjusted based on culture results. Some patients have manifestations suggestive of both viral and bacterial pneumonia. Other complications include exacerbation of asthma and chronic bronchitis, sinusitis, and otitis media in children.

Toxic shock syndrome associated with *Staphylococcus aureus* infection or colonization has been reported following influenza infection.[28,29] It has been postulated that the plague of Athens from 430–427 BCE, described by Thucydides, was the result of an epidemic of influenza associated with toxigenic staphylococcus.[30] The term Thucydides syndrome has been proposed for clinical manifestations of toxigenic staphylococcus in association with influenza infection.[30]

Whereas infection with a pandemic influenza virus indicates that the virus has spread globally, the clinical manifestations of pandemic influenza virus infection for the individual patient may be similar to seasonal influenza infection, or they may be more severe as in 1918, or milder as in 2009.

The 1918 influenza pandemic was characterized by infection with a virulent virus.[2,6] Unusual clinical findings that were observed during this pandemic included epistaxis and dark blue cyanosis, probably due to destruction of the respiratory epithelium.[7,21] Both viral pneumonia and secondary bacterial pneumonia were frequent causes of death.[2]

The 2009 influenza pandemic was notable for its lower mortality than prior pandemics. Worldwide, 80% of influenza-related deaths occurred in people younger than 65, compared with approximately 80% of deaths occurring in those 65 and older during typical seasonal influenza epidemics.[11] Prior virus exposure among the older population probably impacted the frequency and severity of illness[6,11] as nearly one third of people over age 60 had antibodies against the virus.[11]

Infection with novel influenza A(H5N1) often presents with severe pneumonia that progresses rapidly to ARDS. In fatal cases the median time from onset to death was 9–10 days. Leukopenia with lymphopenia, thrombocytopenia, and elevated transaminases have been reported in most series. In many cases, the correct diagnosis was not suspected early in the presentation.[26] Patients with novel influenza A(H7N9) are also at risk for development of pneumonia and ARDS. In one series, 76.6% of patients required admission to an ICU. Laboratory findings of lymphopenia, thrombocytopenia, and elevated transaminases have been common. The median time from onset of symptoms to ARDS was 7 days and to death was 14 days.[31]

DIAGNOSIS

The diagnosis of influenza can usually be made based on clinical symptoms and epidemiology. When influenza is confirmed in a community, an adult with typical symptoms of influenza, such as fever and cough, without other obvious cause is likely to have influenza. The symptom complex may be less helpful at the beginning of an outbreak and cannot confirm the particular influenza strain. Various laboratory tests are available to confirm the diagnosis of influenza and may indicate the particular subtype.

Polymerase chain reaction (PCR) tests are presently widely used to detect influenza virus infection (Table 21-2). These have the advantage of sensitivity, can detect a number of predetermined respiratory viruses with the same test, and can often determine the influenza subtype. These tests require specimens to be transported to a lab which may limit their usefulness, especially in the outpatient setting. Rapid antigen tests can be run at the point of care and are less expensive, but they have lower sensitivity which is dependent on specimen collection and timing in the course of illness. Viral isolation by culture has been the gold standard against which other tests are measured, but this requires access to a laboratory and results are not available for 3–10 days, limiting its value in the immediate care of the patient. PCR can also detect the novel avian subtypes if the specific primers are included. Patients with influenza-like illnesses who have traveled to a region with one of the avian subtypes and have had close contact with sick birds or poultry markets or a known case of avian influenza should be tested with the appropriate PCR tests in addition to looking for the more common causes. Serologic testing of acute and convalescent serum for change in virus specific antibody may help with a retrospective diagnosis.

▌TREATMENT

There are currently six antiviral prescription medications approved to treat influenza in the United States. Two of the medications, amantadine and

Table 21-2 INFLUENZA TESTS AND TIME TO RESULTS		
Influenza Test Modality	Method	Time
Molecular Assay	Nucleic Acid Amplification	10–30 minutes
Rapid Influenza Diagnostic Test	Antigen Detection	10–15 minutes
IFA	Antigen Setection	1–4 hours
Rapid Cell Culture	Viral Isolation	1–3 days
Viral Culture	Viral Isolation	3–10 days

rimantadine, are no longer recommended because they target only influenza A viruses and in recent years many circulating influenza A viruses have
shown resistance to these medications. Three of the recommended influenza
medications are neuraminidase inhibitors which are active against both influenza A and B viruses and are administered by different routes—oseltamivir
(oral), zanamivir (inhaled), and peramivir (intravenous). The fourth recommended antiviral drug, baloxavir, is a cap-dependent endonuclease inhibitor
that blocks viral replication and is active against both influenza A and B
viruses.[32] These agents have been approved for treatment, and in some cases
prevention, of influenza in different age groups (Table 21-3). The choice of
agent usually depends on the age of the patient, setting (outpatient, hospital,
critical care) and contraindications (such as to avoid zanamivir in patients
with asthma or chronic obstructive pulmonary disease [COPD]). In general,
oseltamivir is the drug of choice for patients with influenza who are hospitalized, or seriously ill and not hospitalized, or are pregnant. Data from
controlled trials and observational series show that early antiviral treatment
can shorten the duration of fever and symptoms and may reduce the risk of
some complications. Shorter duration of hospitalization and reduced mortality have also been reported.[32]

The antiviral agents are most effective when started early, such as
within 48 hours of symptom onset, and some studies show increased
benefit the earlier they are initiated. Because of the potential for delay
in initiating therapy, the decision to initiate therapy should not await the
results of a diagnostic test if the results are not immediately available and
the clinical presentation and epidemiology suggest influenza infection.
Antiviral therapy should not be withheld from ill hospitalized patients
with longer symptom durations; some studies suggest benefit in this population up to 4–5 days after onset of symptoms.[32] Treatment should be
considered in hospitalized patients as well as outpatients at highest risk
for complications of influenza (see prior discussion of risk factors).

Patients infected with one of the novel avian influenza viruses associated with severe disease should receive antiviral therapy as soon as possible. Outpatient cases under investigation that had close contact with
a confirmed or probable case should also receive antiviral therapy.[33]
Treatment should not be withheld if the duration of symptoms is greater
than 48 hours or while awaiting laboratory confirmation. Most of the
influenza A(H5N1) and A(H7N9) viruses tested have been susceptible to
the neuraminidase inhibitors (oseltamivir, peramivir, and zanamivir), but
not to amantadine or rimantadine. For most patients with these novel
strains oseltamivir is the recommended antiviral drug. The treatment
course for seasonal influenza is 5 days, but longer treatment courses (10
days) should be considered for severely ill hospitalized patients infected

Table 21-3 CURRENT ANTIVIRAL MEDICATIONS RECOMMENDED FOR TREATMENT AND CHEMOPROPHYLAXIS OF INFLUENZA

Antiviral Agent	Activity Against	Use	Recommended For	Dose	Not Recommended For Use With
Oral Oseltamivir	Influenza A and B	Treatment Chemoprophylaxis	Any age 3 months and older	Adults: 75 mg twice a day Children (≥1 year old): ≤15 kg 30 BID 15–23 kg 45 BID 23–40 kg 60 BID >40 kg 75 BID Term 0–11 3mg/kg BID Months	N/A N/A
Inhaled Zanamivir	Influenza A and B	Treatment Chemoprophylaxis	7 years and older 5 years and older	Age ≥7: 10 mg (two inhalations of 5 mg) twice a day	underlying respiratory disease (e.g., asthma, COPD) underlying respiratory disease (e.g., asthma, COPD)
Intravenous Peramivir	Influenza A and B	Treatment Chemoprophylaxis	2 years and older Not currently recommended	Age >13: 600 mg IV over 15–30 minutes Age 2–12: 12 mg/ kg dose (600 mg max) over 15–30 minutes	N/A N/A
Oral Baloxavir	Influenza A and B	Treatment Chemoprophylaxis	12 years and older Not currently Recommended	≥40–80 kg 40 mg ≥80 kg 80 mg	N/A N/A

COPD = chronic obstructive pulmonary disease; N/A = not applicable.

Adapted from Centers for Disease Control and Prevention. *Influenza antiviral medications. Summary for clinicians.* Updated August 31, 2020. https://www.cdc.gov/flu/professionals/antivirals/summary-clinicians.htm.

with one of these viruses.[33] For patients with progressive lower respiratory disease despite treatment with oseltamivir or peramivir, consideration should be given to the potential development of a drug resistant virus. These oseltamivir/peramivir resistant viruses may retain their susceptibility to zanamivir, and intravenous zanamivir may be an option if it is available. Questions related to the diagnosis or management of suspected antiviral resistance in this setting should be directed to the CDC Influenza Division.[33]

A concern during a pandemic or concurrent severe epidemics would be to ensure an adequate supply of antiviral medication, especially if longer treatment courses are indicated or if the same medication is recommended for prophylaxis. Early recognition of the emergence of a potential pandemic strain may afford some time for increased production and distribution of antiviral medications. A strategy utilizing probenecid to reduce the renal clearance of oseltamivir, allowing reduced antiviral dosing[34] might be an option but has not been fully evaluated.

Treatment during the 1918 pandemic was limited to a significant degree to supportive care. The armamentarium of antiviral drugs, and even antibiotics, was not available. Bacterial pneumonia played a significant role as a cause of death. Since the introduction of antibiotics there has been a reduction in excess influenza mortality.[35] Management of respiratory failure by mechanical ventilation and extracorporeal membrane oxygenation in the intensive care unit have also contributed to a decrease in influenza mortality.[35]

Convalescent plasma containing passively delivered anti-influenza antibodies was utilized as a treatment modality during the 1918 influenza pandemic. A meta-analysis of eight studies suggested, despite significant methodologic limitations, that convalescent plasma may have been associated with a reduction in mortality in patients with influenza pneumonia.[36] Convalescent plasma which has been employed in other epidemics and pandemics (such as Ebola and COVID-19), could be an effective, timely, and widely available treatment for patients during influenza outbreaks or pandemics with influenza H5N1[36] or other novel influenza strains.

▍PREVENTION

The CDC's Influenza Risk Assessment Tool[13] can be utilized to plan and prioritize pre-pandemic preparedness activities. Since it is specific for a particular virus it allows for development, stockpiling, and distribution of diagnostic tests and supplies, vaccines, and antiviral agents.[12]

Vaccines

Vaccination is the most effective strategy for preventing seasonal influenza illness and infection. Yet the protection from annual influenza immunization is far from ideal. A number of factors contribute to the deficiencies of current influenza vaccines. Among the most important are the continuous antigenic change that the virus undergoes, and the relatively slow process of vaccine development and production that requires about 6 months for most influenza vaccines. This means that the vaccine composition is based on circulating virus in the other hemisphere and is a best guess as to what will be coming next. Immunity is narrow, not broad, and is not long lasting so the vaccine must be administered each year.

Traditional influenza vaccines have been grown in eggs and some influenza viruses undergo mutations during this process which may affect the level of protection achieved. Recently, cell culture-derived, and recombinant vaccines have been introduced. In certain populations, especially those who would benefit most from immunization, such as the elderly and immunocompromised, the vaccines are not sufficiently antigenic. Higher dose, and adjuvant vaccines have been introduced which elicit increased immunogenicity in older adults.

The production of vaccines for use during a pandemic creates even greater challenges than during seasonal influenza. During the 2009 H1N1 pandemic, vaccines became available late in the pandemic.[12,37] Some of the avian viruses are pathogenic for chicken eggs so they do not replicate well when grown in chicken eggs. Because a pandemic strain is a newly introduced virus in the population, there is no (or very limited) pre-existing immunity and two doses of vaccine may be needed. One proposed approach involving "split strategy" consists of administering a single dose of an H5 or H7 vaccine pre-pandemic to prime the immune response. A subsequent dose that is matched to the pandemic strain could be administered when available.[37] This would allow only one dose, rather than two doses, at the time of the pandemic which would spare doses in addition to generating a quicker protective immune response. The use of adjuvants which permit use of smaller amounts of antigen may also result in the availability of more doses of vaccine.[37]

There continues to be interest in the development of an effective ideal "universal" influenza vaccine that would provide long-term protection against a broader range of influenza viruses within and across subtypes[12]; such vaccines would not have to be reformulated seasonally and may offer protection against an emerging novel virus. The development of a potentially effective vaccine in relation to a new pandemic would most likely be associated with lack of adequate supply for the targeted population. The

CDC has provided guidance for stepwise vaccination based on high-risk population and occupation dependent on severity of the pandemic and vaccine supply[38] (Figure 21-4).

The ability of a vaccine program to succeed in establishing herd immunity depends on a number of factors including the reproduction number (R) for the virus, vaccine effectiveness, availability of the vaccine, as well as willingness of the population to be vaccinated. For a highly susceptible population, as during a pandemic, a greater proportion of the population would need to be vaccinated to achieve herd immunity than with a comparably transmissible seasonal influenza virus against which some of the population is protected. A greater number would need to be vaccinated for a vaccine with lower effectiveness, or for a virus with a higher R value (more transmissible).[39]

Post-Exposure Antiviral Prophylaxis

The use of antiviral therapy for prophylaxis is another approach to prevent influenza virus infection in certain circumstances during seasonal influenza outbreaks.[32] Post-exposure prophylaxis has been suggested by the CDC for asymptomatic workers who had unprotected exposure to a patient with a novel influenza A virus associated with severe human disease and are needed to return to work.[40] Oral oseltamivir and inhaled zanamivir are the two agents approved for use as chemoprophylaxis for seasonal influenza (Table 21-3).

Non-Pharmaceutical Interventions

Coordination of human and animal influenza surveillance globally with sharing of information is essential for enacting time sensitive control measures. Action to control the spread of novel avian influenza viruses has included closure of the live poultry markets, mass slaughter of poultry, restructuring the markets, and poultry vaccination programs.[12,15]

The identification of a novel influenza virus from humans and the stages outlined by the Pandemic Intervals Framework (Figure 21-3) provides recommendations for actions to control the further spread of the virus. For example, non-pharmacologic interventions such as social distancing, and school and daycare closures might be recommended as a community enters the Acceleration phase of a pandemic.[14]

Social distancing and restrictions on mass gatherings were imposed in many cities in the United States during the 1918 influenza pandemic. The restrictions were effective in reducing mortality while they were in effect, but the mortality again increased when they were lifted.[6,41] Efforts to decrease the virus in the community or reduce its entry into the population

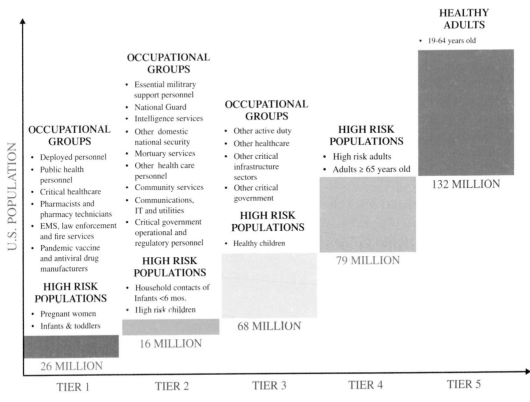

Figure 21-4 • Vaccination tiers and population groups based on occupation and high-risk populations during a high or very high level of pandemic severity. (From Centers for Disease Control and Prevention. *Interim updated planning guidance on allocating and targeting pandemic influenza vaccine during an influenza pandemic.* https://www.cdc.gov/flu/pandemic-resources/pdf/2018-Influenza-Guidance.pdf.)

may need to be continued for a longer period of time. Similarly, closure of schools during the 2009 pandemic was associated with reduced influenza transmission, but an increase in transmission was temporally related to the re-opening of the schools.[6,41] Further investigation is necessary to understand how to optimize each of these strategies as well as contact tracing during an influenza pandemic.[42]

Restrictions on travel to prevent the spread of influenza can take the form of temporarily recommending against travel to a geographic area with an outbreak due to a novel influenza virus, or more global restrictions on travel or screening of incoming travelers during a pandemic. In 1918, many countries imposed restrictions on incoming ships, but these were mostly unsuccessful in controlling the spread of influenza.[6] By comparison, analogous measures today would involve travel by all modes of transportation including land, sea, and air.

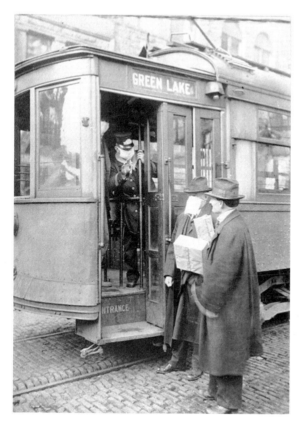

Figure 21-5 • Street car conductor in Seattle in 1918 not allowing passengers aboard without a mask. (*Courtesy National Archives, photo no. 165-WW-269B-11.*)

Personal hygiene, such as handwashing and/or use of hand sanitizer and avoiding touching one's face are recommended to reduce the transmission of influenza virus but additional studies are needed to determine the benefit of these interventions in both pandemic and seasonal influenza.[43] Facemasks were worn during by many during the 1918 pandemic (Figures 21-3 and 21-5), and in some localities were mandatory. Mortality data was not significantly different in cities with mask requirements than those without the requirements.[6] Requirements for wearing a mask may not have been successful because of poor compliance (Figure 21-5), improper fitting, or inappropriate material.[6]

INFECTION CONTROL

The CDC recommends a higher level of infection control precautions for the novel influenza A viruses associated with severe disease than for seasonal influenza.[40] The recommendations attempt to minimize the risk to healthcare workers upon exposure to a confirmed case, possible case, or case under investigation. Planning prior to an encounter with a symptomatic patient includes educating the patient on respiratory hygiene and cough etiquette, placement of a face mask on the patient at entry, and implementation of airborne isolation precautions, in addition to standard and contact precautions.[40] Exposed healthcare workers should be monitored for symptoms. In healthcare facilities, isolation precautions should continue for 7 days after illness or 24 hours after resolution of fever and respiratory symptoms, whichever is longer. Even asymptomatic healthcare workers with an unprotected exposure could be excluded from work or allowed to work while wearing a face mask at all times for 10 days and while taking prophylactic anti-influenza medications.[40]

Stricter infection control practices for these novel influenza viruses include hand hygiene, gloves, gowns, and respiratory protection. Respiratory protection in this context consists of an N95 respirator and eye protection (goggles or face shields). The patient should be placed in an airborne infection isolation room. Caution is recommended when performing potentially aerosol-generating procedures. Screening of visitors and limitations or restrictions may be necessary.[40]

During the 2009 H1N1 influenza pandemic the CDC issued guidance to reduce the risk of transmission in the healthcare environment. These recommendations included limiting and screening of visitors, education regarding respiratory hygiene and cough etiquette, mask wearing by patients with respiratory illnesses consistent with influenza when outside their room and limiting patient transport as feasible. For healthcare workers in close contact with a suspected or confirmed case, N95 respirators and gloves were specified. Prioritization was described for respirator shortages in various exposure settings. Gowns and eye protection were added for activities with the potential to generate splashes or infectious aerosols. If available, an airborne infection isolation room should be used for aerosol-generating procedures.[44]

COMPLICATIONS

The medical complications of influenza virus infection were outlined earlier. The initial viral infection may be followed by viral pneumonia or one of a number of bacterial secondary infections including pneumonia, otitis media or sinus infection. In some instances, pandemic viruses may be associated with an increased frequency of viral pneumonia. Persistent lung dysfunction has been identified in survivors a year or longer after infection with influenza A(H7N9).[45]

Known cardiac sequelae after seasonal influenza include myocarditis and pericarditis.[10,46] A number of studies have shown an increase in hospitalizations and death due to ischemic heart disease during the influenza season, with a significant increase during epidemics.[46] Similarly, influenza vaccination has been associated with a reduction in acute myocardial infarctions.[46]

Neurological complications of influenza infection include progressive encephalopathy that has been reported more often in pediatric than adult patients.[10] Post-influenza encephalopathy occurs after resolution of the respiratory symptoms and may be associated with metabolic encephalopathy, a dysregulated immune response, and/or genetic predisposition.[46] Guillain-Barré syndrome is considered to be caused by an autoimmune response to a variety of infections including influenza. Similarly, cases of acute disseminated encephalomyelitis and transverse myelitis have been reported after influenza infection.[46] An increase in the incidence of narcolepsy was observed in China following the 2009 H1N1 pandemic.[46]

Symptoms of Parkinsonism were reported associated with the 1918 influenza pandemic and some studies have suggested that transient Parkinson symptoms may infrequently follow influenza infection.[46] Encephalitis lethargica, characterized acutely by fever, excessive sleepiness, and motility disorders followed by a chronic phase with Parkinsonism-like symptoms, were first described in 1917 although some of the cases appeared as early as 1915. Peaks in recognized cases occurred in 1920 and 1924, and during this time an estimated one million people worldwide may have been afflicted.[47] Many suffered permanent neurologic damage. The disease surfaced as an epidemic around the same time as the 1918 influenza pandemic and was thought to be a sequela of influenza. Serologic studies and examination of brain tissue have not consistently supported the hypothesis of influenza as the etiology.[47] Reye's syndrome is associated with acetylsalicylic acid use and influenza infection. With the recognition of the role of aspirin in causing Reye's syndrome, other antipyretics are utilized instead, and influenza vaccination is recommended for children who require long-term aspirin use. As a result, there has been a significant decline in the incidence of Reye's syndrome.

Hepatic involvement as measured by transaminase elevations has been observed most commonly during severe cases of influenza due to avian influenza A(H5N1) and A(H7N9) infections. Liver injury may also be strain specific as elevated alanine aminotransferase and aspartate aminotransferase were reported more often during 2009 influenza A(H1N1) infection than with seasonal influenza.[46]

Conjunctivitis has been observed during some influenza outbreaks and appears to be related to specific strains. Avian influenza H7 viruses other than influenza A(H7N9) have been associated with cases of conjunctivitis.

Conjunctivitis, optic neuritis, acute retinitis, and uveal effusion syndrome have been reported associated with the 2009 influenza A(H1N1) virus.[46]

Rhabdomyolysis and myositis can occur during the course of influenza virus infection and may result in renal failure. Renal insufficiency during influenza virus infection may also be secondary to acute illness and hypoperfusion.[46] Influenza virus infection may serve as an infrequent trigger of hemophagocytic syndrome, thrombotic thrombocytopenic purpura, and complications of diabetes mellitus.[46]

Infection with influenza during gestation has been described as a risk for the development of schizophrenia. This has been investigated serologically and in animal studies. It has been suggested that influenza along with other infections may play a role in the etiology of schizophrenia, perhaps through some common pathways and genetic factors.[48]

The long-term effects of an influenza pandemic in a community in terms of social and psychological well-being cannot be easily quantified. Social isolation, disruption to school or work schedules, unemployment, and financial difficulty are potential sequelae of a pandemic. In addition, psychological effects may linger related to prolonged physical manifestations of influenza and loss of family members and friends. First time hospitalizations with mental illnesses attributed to influenza were observed to increase in Norway by an annual factor of 7.2 in the 6 years following the influenza pandemic of 1918.[49]

PROGNOSIS

Most patients infected with influenza will completely recover. Risk factors for more severe disease are described earlier, with mortality from seasonal influenza highest in infants and the elderly, especially those who are unvaccinated. When a novel pandemic virus arises, age-related mortality will depend on when the last antigenically related virus circulated. The pandemic of 1918 has been regarded as the "mother of all pandemics" with about 500 million infections worldwide and a case fatality rate of greater than 2.5%.[3] In contrast, overall mortality during the 2009 influenza pandemic was approximately 0.02% (Table 21-1). By comparison, for influenza A(H5N1) which is not readily transmitted between humans, mortality is over 50%.[16,19]

CONCLUSION: LESSONS LEARNED FROM PAST INFLUENZA PANDEMICS

What have we learned from past influenza pandemics? How can this information help us prepare for and navigate a future influenza pandemic or pandemic caused by a different as of yet unknown novel pathogen, such as "Disease X"?[50]

Some aspects of a new pandemic may resemble prior pandemics. A novel pathogen may cause significant morbidity and mortality and be readily spread from person to person by the respiratory route. At the beginning as the pandemic takes hold on a community and then on many communities, the full extent of the pandemic to unfold will not be known. At the time, the identity of the pathogen may or may not be known. Scientific advances, none of which were present in 1918, may allow us to identify and sequence a virus, develop diagnostic tests, and begin preparation of a vaccine. At first, specific medical interventions may be limited. For a viral pathogen, targeted antiviral therapy may or may not be readily available. Methods to prevent spread by non-pharmaceutical intervention such as social distancing, closure of schools and workplaces, and requirements for face coverings such as masks, may be employed to buy time for the development of a vaccine. In the case of the 2009 influenza pandemic, the development of a vaccine came late in the course of the pandemic. A system to prioritize the distribution of a vaccine when available, could allocate who would first receive a vaccine in limited supply (Figure 21-4). And what if there was skepticism about the safety of the vaccine?

Working in parallel with vaccine development for prevention would be the study of the pathogenesis of disease with the goal of developing effective treatment. In the case of influenza viruses, the severity of illness may be due directly to viral replication, or to an exaggerated host response, or possibly due to secondary bacterial infections, or to a combination of factors. Each of these would present opportunities to target therapy. In 1918, the viral etiology of influenza was not yet known, nor was there a clear understanding of immune response to infection, and antibiotics for treating bacterial infections were not available.

Our global community of the 21st century allows for rapid worldwide spread of a novel pathogen as well as rapid dissemination of information, and potentially misinformation. We now have much more sophisticated surveillance for the emergence of novel pathogens capable of causing a pandemic that relies on a One Health approach among human and animal experts and global communication, cooperation, and information sharing. The CDC and WHO have pre-pandemic and pandemic phases that provide guidance for associated actions as an evolving pandemic is recognized (Figure 21-3). This process could be impeded by the lack of free exchange of information.

Through scientific advances, we may have more knowledge to build upon the experiences of prior influenza pandemics to more quickly and effectively respond to a future threat. Will we have sufficient stockpiles of protective equipment, medications, other supplies, and potential vaccines? Only in the future will we know if we have the organization, infrastructure, manpower, reagents, etc. for the healthcare system to appropriately and optimally manage large numbers of sick patients. One major constant feature of influenza is its unpredictability at the level of the virus and related to its impact on individuals and society in terms of severity and extent of illness (mild disease/localized, mild disease/pandemic, severe disease/localized or severe disease/pandemic). These unique characteristics add to the challenges in preparing for the next influenza pandemic.

ACKNOWLEDGMENT

The author thanks Paula Cortez for assistance with the preparation of the manuscript.

REFERENCES

1. Global Influenza Programme. *Pandemic influenza risk management: a WHO guide to inform and harmonize national and international pandemic preparedness and response.* Geneva: World Health Organization; 2017.
2. Jester B, Uyeki T, Jernigan D. Readiness for responding to a severe pandemic 100 years after 1918. *Am J Epidemiol.* 2018;187(12):2596-2602.
3. Taubenberger JK, Morens DM. 1918 Influenza: the mother of all pandemics. *Emerg Infect Dis.* 2006;12(1):15-22.
4. Dunning J, Thwaites RS, Openshaw PJM. Seasonal and pandemic influenza: 100 years of progress, still much to learn. *Mucosal Immunol.* 2020;13(4):566-573.
5. Van Epps HL. Influenza: exposing the true killer. *J Exp Med.* 2006;203(4):803.
6. Short KR, Kedzierska K, van de Sandt CE. Back to the future: Lessons learned from the 1918 influenza pandemic. *Front Cell Infect Microbiol.* 2018;8:343.
7. Oxford JS, Gill D. Unanswered questions about the 1918 influenza pandemic: origin, pathology, and the virus itself. *Lancet Infect Dis.* 2018;18(11): e348-e354.
8. Kain T, Fowler R. Preparing intensive care for the next pandemic influenza. *Crit Care.* 2019;23(1):337.
9. Kilbourne ED. Influenza pandemics of the 20th century. *Emerg Infect Dis.* 2006;12(1):9-14.
10. Treanor JJ. Influenza viruses, including avian influenza and swine influenza. In: Bennett JE, Dolin R, Blaser MJ, eds. *Mandell, Douglas, and Bennett's Principles and Practice of Infectious Diseases.* 9th ed. New York, NY: Elsevier; 2020:2143-2168.
11. Centers for Disease Control and Prevention. 2009 H1N1 pandemic (H1N1pdm09 virus). https://www.cdc.gov/flu/pandemic-resources/2009-h1n1-pandemic.html. Accessed August 29, 2020.

12. National Academies of Sciences, Engineering, and Medicine; Health and Medicine Division; Board on Global Health; Forum on Microbial Threats. Global progress to prepare for the next influenza pandemic. In: Nicholson A, Shah CM, Ogawa VA, eds. *Exploring Lessons Learned from a Century of Outbreaks: Readiness for 2030: Proceedings of a Workshop*. Washington (DC): National Academies Press; May 8, 2019:23-41.

13. Centers for Disease Control and Prevention. Influenza risk assessment tool (IRAT). https://www.cdc.gov/flu/pandemic-resources/national-strategy/risk-assessment.html. Accessed August 27, 2020.

14. US Department of Health and Human Services. Pandemic influenza plan, 2017 update. https://www.cdc.gov/flu/pandemic-resources/pdf/pan-flu-report-2017v2.pdf. Accessed August 28, 2020.

15. Levitt A, Messonnier N, Jernigan D, et al. Emerging and reemerging infectious disease threats. In: Bennett JE, Dolin R, Blaser MJ, eds. *Mandell, Douglas, and Bennett's Principles and Practice of Infectious Diseases*. 9th ed. New York, NY: Elsevier; 2020:170-173.

16. World Health Organization. Cumulative number of confirmed human cases for avian influenza A(H5N1) reported to WHO, 2003–2020. https://www.who.int/influenza/human_animal_interface/2020_10_07_tableH5N1.pdf. Accessed August 29, 2020.

17. Centers for Disease Control and Prevention. Asian lineage avian influenza A(H7N9) virus. https://www.cdc.gov/flu/avianflu/h7n9-virus.htm.

18. Carnaccini S, Perez DR. H9 Influenza viruses: an emerging challenge. *Cold Spring Harb Perspect Med*. 2020;10(6):a038588.

19. Centers for Disease Control and Prevention. Viruses of special concern. https://www.cdc.gov/flu/pandemic-resources/monitoring/viruses-concern.html. Accessed August 26, 2020.

20. Centers for Disease Control and Prevention. People at high risk for flu complications. https://www.cdc.gov/flu/highrisk/. Accessed August 26, 2020.

21. Shanks GD. Insights from unusual aspects of the 1918 influenza pandemic. *Travel Med Infect Dis*. 2015;13(3):217-222.

22. Jhung MA, Swerdlow D, Olsen SJ, et al. Epidemiology of 2009 pandemic influenza A(H1N1) in the United States. *Clin Infect Dis*. 2011;52(Suppl 1):S13-S26.

23. Van Kerkhove MD, Vandemaele KA, Shinde V, et al. Risk factors for severe outcomes following 2009 influenza A(H1N1) infection: a global pooled analysis. *PLoS Med*. 2011;8(7):e1001053.

24. Biggerstaff M, Cauchemez S, Reed C, Gambhir M, Finelli L. Estimates of the reproduction number for seasonal, pandemic, and zoonotic influenza: a systematic review of the literature. *BMC Infect Dis*. 2014;14:480.

25. McAuley JL, Kedzierska K, Brown LE, Shanks GD. Host immunological factors enhancing mortality of young adults during the 1918 influenza pandemic. *Front Immunol*. 2015;6:419.

26. Abdel-Ghafar AN, Chotpitayasunondh T, Gao Z, et al. Update on avian influenza A(H5N1) virus infection in humans. *N Engl J Med*. 2008;358(3):261-273.

27. Zhou J, Wang D, Gao R, et al. Biological features of novel avian influenza A(H7N9) virus. *Nature*. 2013;499(7459):500-503.

28. MacDonald KL, Osterholm MT, Hedberg CW, et al. Toxic shock syndrome. A newly recognized complication of influenza and influenzalike illness. *JAMA*. 1987;257(8):1053-1058.

29. Sperber SJ, Francis JB. Toxic shock syndrome during an influenza outbreak. *JAMA*. 1987;257(8):1086-1087.

30. Langmuir AD, Ray CG. The Thucydides syndrome. *JAMA*. 1987;257(22):3071.

31. Gao HN, Lu HZ, Cao B, et al. Clinical findings in 111 cases of influenza A(H7N9) virus infection. *N Engl J Med*. 2013;368(24):2277-2285.

32. Centers for Disease Control and Prevention. Influenza antiviral medications. Summary for clinicians. Accessed September 15, 2020. https://www.cdc.gov/flu/professionals/antivirals/summary-clinicians.htm. Updated August 31, 2020. Accessed September 15, 2020.

33. Centers for Disease Control and Prevention. Interim guidance on the use of antiviral medications for treatment of human infections with novel influenza A viruses associated with severe human disease. https://www.cdc.gov/flu/avianflu/novel-av-treatment-guidance.htm. Accessed September 15, 2020.

34. Holodniy M, Penzak SR, Straight TM, et al. Pharmacokinetics and tolerability of oseltamivir combined with probenecid. *Antimicrob Agents Chemother*. 2008;52(9):3013-3021.

35. Morens DM, Taubenberger JK, Harvey HA, Memoli MJ. The 1918 influenza pandemic: lessons for 2009 and the future. *Crit Care Med*. 2010;38 (4 Suppl):e10-e20.

36. Luke TC, Kilbane EM, Jackson JL, Hoffman SL. Meta-analysis: convalescent blood products for Spanish influenza pneumonia: a future H5N1 treatment. *Ann Intern Med*. 2006;145(8):599-609.

37. Trombetta C, Piccirella S, Perini D, Kistner O, Montomoli E. Emerging influenza strains in the last two decades: A threat of a new pandemic. *Vaccines*. 2015;3(1):172-185.

38. Centers for Disease Control and Prevention. Interim updated planning guidance on allocating and targeting pandemic influenza vaccine during an influenza pandemic. https://www.cdc.gov/flu/pandemic-resources/pdf/2018-Influenza-Guidance.pdf. Updated August, 2018. Accessed January 4, 2021.

39. Plans-Rubió P. The vaccination coverage required to establish herd immunity against influenza viruses. *Prev Med*. 2012;55(1):72-77.

40. Centers for Disease Control and Prevention. Interim guidance for infection control within healthcare settings when caring for confirmed cases, probable cases, and cases under investigation for infection with novel influenza A viruses associated with severe disease. https://www.cdc.gov/flu/avianflu/novel-flu-infection-control.htm. Updated January 23, 2014. Accessed September 15, 2020.

41. Rashid H, Ridda I, King C, et al. Evidence compendium and advice on social distancing and other related measures for response to an influenza pandemic. *Paediatr Respir Rev*. 2015;16(2):119-126.

42. Fong MW, Gao H, Wong JY, et al. Nonpharmaceutical measures for pandemic influenza in nonhealthcare settings-social distancing measures. *Emerg Infect Dis.* 2020;26(5):976-984.

43. Xiao J, Shiu EYC, Gao H, et al. Nonpharmaceutical measures for pandemic influenza in nonhealthcare settings-personal protective and environmental measures. *Emerg Infect Dis.* 2020;26:967-975.

44. Centers for Disease Control and Prevention. Interim guidance on infection control measures for 2009 H1N1 influenza in healthcare settings, including protection of healthcare personnel. https://www.cdc.gov/flu/pandemic-resources/2009-h1n1-pandemic.html. Updated June 11, 2019. Accessed January 5, 2021.

45. Wang Q, Jiang H, Xie Y, et al. Long-term clinical prognosis of human infections with avian influenza A(H7N9) viruses in China after hospitalization. *EClinicalMedicine.* 2020;20:100282.

46. Sellers SA, Hagan RS, Hayden FG, Fischer WA. The hidden burden of influenza: A review of the extra-pulmonary complications of influenza infection. *Influenza Other Respir Viruses.* 2017;11(5):372-393.

47. Hoffman LA, Vilensky JA. Encephalitis lethargica: 100 years after the epidemic. *Brain.* 2017;140(8):2246-2251.

48. Brown AS, Derkits EJ. Prenatal infection and schizophrenia: a review of epidemiologic and translational studies. *Am J Psychiatry.* 2010;167(3):261-280.

49. Mamelund S. The impact of influenza on mental health in Norway 1872-1929. Presented at: Historical Influenza Pandemics: Lessons Learned Meeting and Workshop. Copenhagen: May 3–7, 2010, 30.

50. Simpson S, Kaufmann MC, Glozman V, Chakrabarti A. Disease X: accelerating the development of medical countermeasures for the next pandemic. *Lancet Infect Dis.* 2020;20(5):e108-e115.

22 PLAGUE

Robert Lee, MD

▌INTRODUCTION

Yersinia pestis causes the plague, a devastating infection that has resulted in pandemics both in the past and recently. It continues to be a concern with sporadic natural surges throughout the world and as a form of bioterrorism.

▌EPIDEMIOLOGY

Y. pestis is a facultative, anaerobic, gram-negative bacteria shaped like a coccobacillus and with a safety pin appearance.[11] (Figure 22-1). *Y. pestis* has caused three pandemics, in 6th century AD (541–760) causing 100 million deaths, the Black Death in 1347–1353 with 50 million deaths, and the Oriental plague starting in 1894 causing 12 million deaths.[2-6] It has also been used as a biological weapon.[9,10]

The main reservoir of *Y. pestis* are rodents in different geographical foci around the world. Predators such as birds can also spread the vectors over long distances.[14] Cats, dogs, bandicoots, and shrews can also act as reservoirs. Humans are only incidental hosts and not the primary host in nature.[4] Fleas from rodents, such as *Xenopsylla ceopis* and sylvanic or forest cycle fleas, are vectors and bite humans.

In the USA most cases occur in the southwest; New Mexico, Arizona, Colorado, Utah, Nevada, Idaho, Wyoming, Montana, and California in rural areas and semi-rural areas. It occurs in any season but mostly in late spring to early fall. The last major USA outbreak was in Los Angeles in 1924–1925.[7] Outbreaks occurred in the mid-1960s, 1970s, and 1980s. From 2010 to 2015, 3,248 cases were reported to the World Health Organization (WHO) of which there were 584 deaths. Active foci of plague are currently mainly in Madagascar, Congo, southern China, Myanmar, Vietnam, Indonesia, and Peru. Plague has been found in all continents currently with the exception of Australia and Antarctica.[8]

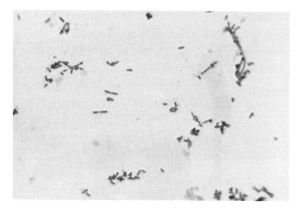

Figure 22-1 • Gram-stained image of gram negative rod shaped *Yersinia pestis* bacteria. (*Courtesy of the CDC*. https://phil.cdc.gov/Details.aspx?pid=21563.)

Climate is known to play an important role in *Y. pestis* infections. Temperature, rainfall, and humidity can factor into the timing of outbreaks. Humidity levels between 60 and 80% were associated with plague outbreaks.[16]

PATHOPHYSIOLOGY

Y. pestis infects a host without causing severe immune response. After the infection has spread in the bubonic or pneumonic form, the bacteria multiply inside the cells and then suddenly the host goes into the septicemic form of plague.

The type III secretion system (T3SS), which is an important virulence factor, is not yet expressed by the bacteria at 26°C, which is the temperature in fleas. There is a lack of a pre-inflammatory phase of infection as a result. Once the *Y. pestis* is taken up to the lymph nodes where the temperature is higher, the bacteria proliferate. Various genes in *Y. pestis* are switched on at 37°C at the target lymph nodes and organs.[13]

There the bacteria's weapons including yersinia outer membrane proteins (YOPS) are acquired via a plasmid pYV/pCD1. pCD1 encodes for the type III secretion system (T3SS) which allows YOPS to translocate into the host cell's cytoplasm. This is an important part of *Y. pestis*' infectivity and helps *Y. pestis* infect macrophages. Other bacterial proteins inhibit Rho GTPases as well as damaging cell cytoskeletons, thereby preventing phagocytosis by neutrophils in target organs. Local inflammatory cytokines important in defense are also inhibited by YOPS.[13] YopE and YopH have been shown to inhibit neutrophil primary granule release, stopping the granules from being released against the *Y. pestis* bacteria.

The primary granules/azurophilic granules contain myeloperoxidases that otherwise would form antibacterial compounds.[17]

The Pla protease is encoded by the pPla/pPCP1 plasmid. It has several characteristics that allow *Y. pestis* to attach to cells and invade cells, helping it to spread into deeper tissues. Additionally the protease has fibrinolytic and coagulase properties, interfering with coagulation. It can break down various plasminogens, antiplasmin, and C3 complement that are supposed to fight the infection too.[13]

There is a third virulence plasmid pFra/pMT1 which inhibits bacterial uptake by inhibiting adhesion.[13] In the lymph node, *Y. pestis* can cause apoptosis and necroptosis which results in the rupture of infected cells causing the bacteria to spread further. *Y. pestis* can also overcome nutritional immunity by cells. The bacterium has the siderophore yersiniabactin (Ybt) which helps defend *Y. pestis* from metals such as iron and zinc which are supposed to protect against bacteria. Eventually when there is sufficient spread of the bacteria, the patient becomes septic and goes into shock.[13]

In the pneumonic form of plague, the infection develops slightly differently. The pneumonic form occurs at a higher initial temperature of 37°C. Macrophages in the lung are targeted first and then neutrophils in later stages. Yersinia can secrete IL-1 and IL-RA receptor blockers preventing an inflammatory response to IL-1B/IL-18. Neutrophil chemo-attractants G-CSF, MIP-2, and KC are inhibited by *Y. pestis*. The macrophages undergo apoptosis. The neutrophils finally come in to attack Yersinia but release inflammatory mediators leading to diffuse lung injury, cytokine storm, sepsis, and death. YopM inhibits neutrophil death and the subsequent release of bactericidal neutrophil contents.[13]

Additional virulence factors are being studied but their roles are not yet fully understood—phage shock system PspAB, protein YPO0862, esterase YPO1501, and nitrite transporter NirC.[13] Other mediators are being studied too, including cyclic AMP receptor protein (Crp) as well as an RNA chaperone (Hfq).

In places where there are other enterobacteria it may be possible for *Y. pestis* to acquire other plasmids. It is thought that in 1995 a strain of *Y. pestis* in Madagascar received a plasmid that gave it resistance to tetracycline and aminoglycosides.[4]

CLINICAL MANIFESTATIONS

The five forms of *Y. pestis* infection in humans are bubonic, pneumonic, septicemic, meningeal, and pharyngeal.[4,8] As few as 10 bacteria can cause infection in a person.[4] The bubonic form is the most common. Patients have red painful infected swollen nodes in the axilla, groin, neck, and other places (Figure 22-2). These nodes are known as buboes. Buboes can become open sores filled with pus and can become fluctuant. Patients also have headache, weakness, fever, and chills. Incubation is 2–6 days. Infection from person to person in the bubonic form of plague is rare.[8] There is also a milder form of bubonic plague called pestis minor when the fever and buboes are relatively minor.[6] Approximately 80% of USA cases are the bubonic form.[7]

Pneumonic plague is caused by inhaling droplets. Incubation is 1–7 days, but usually 3–5 days. Patients may develop pneumonia with hemoptysis, chest pain, and shortness of breath. This can lead to acute respiratory distress syndrome (ARDS) and shock. It is the only form that can usually spread from people to people.[8] CDC unpublished data showed a 40% mortality rate in 2005 with treatment vs the nearly 100% mortality if untreated.[6]

Septicemic plague can be the initial presentation or it can develop after the bubonic or pneumonic forms.[8] Patients may have nausea, vomiting or diarrhea as well. Because the symptoms are nonspecific, the diagnosis is sometimes not even suspected until the blood cultures come back positive. Mortality was an estimated 30% in the USA from 1960 to 2004 with treatment. Patients will often have DIC and ARDS.[6]

Complications include clots from disseminated intravascular coagulation, gangrene (DIC), ARDS, multisystem organ failure (MOF), meningitis, endophthalmitis, and abscesses in the liver or spleen[8] (Figure 22-3).

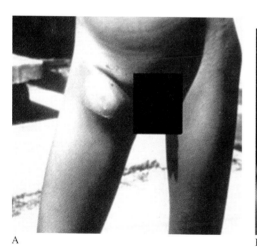
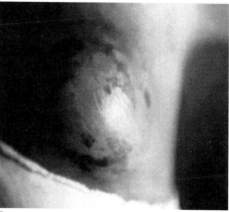

A   B

Figure 22-2 • A: Close view of swollen lymph node in patient with bubonic plague. (*Courtesy of the CDC.* https://phil.cdc.gov/Details.aspx?pid=20546.) **B:** Close view of right inguinal swollen lymph node. (*Courtesy of the CDC.* https://phil.cdc.gov/Details.aspx?pid=20544.)

Hemorrhagic changes and cyanosis from pneumonia cause the skin in the extremities to become cyanotic and darkened. Hence, the name "black death."[18]

Meningeal plague is a rare and late complication. Survival was 78% with treatment. Before antibiotic therapy, there was a chronic relapsing form of meningeal plague that lasted for months. It presented as bacterial meningitis.[6] Pharyngeal plague is an infection that starts in the throat with fever, sore throat, and adenopathy. Buboes may develop later. It may look like any other pharyngitis.[6]

▌DIAGNOSIS

Infection with *Y. pestis* is associated with elevated leukocytes and thrombocytopenia while eosinophilia may be found during recovery.[4] The WHO has a rapid diagnostic test (RDT) using a dipstick. F1 test strips are based on either polyclonal antibodies or the superior paired Mab using lateral flow assay (LFA) technique. These tests detect the capsule-like surface antigen or F1 antigen. Test strips are fast, cheap, and sensitive and can be very useful for epidemiological investigation of outbreaks.[1] Direct fluorescent antibody (DFA) and polymerase chain reaction (PCR) tests are available as well. Multiplex real-time PCR was used in Madagascar in 2017. Uncertain cases had to be confirmed by PCR testing of additional targets. Matrix-Assisted Laser Desorption/Ionization-Time of Flight (MALDI-TOF) mass spectrometry can also be utilized for faster results.[4] Cultures from blood, sputum, and lymph node aspirate can be performed. Serologies maybe helpful if cultures are negative.[7]

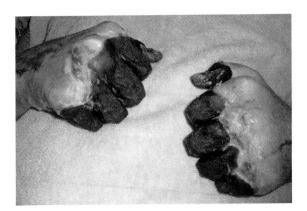

Figure 22-3 • Gangrenous fingers of patient infected with *Yersinia pestis*. (*Courtesy of the CDC.* https://phil.cdc.gov/Details.aspx?pid=16552.)

TREATMENT

Streptomycin is the most effective antibiotic but not commonly available in the USA (Table 22-1). It is especially effective for the pneumonic form.[3] The streptomycin treatment dose for adults is 1 g per day in two divided doses given IM for 10 days or 3 days after temperature is normal. For children the dose is 30 mg/kg/day. The duration of treatment is for 10 days or until the patient is afebrile for 3 days. Gentamicin is a good

Antibiotic	Dose/Interval	Adult 70 kg	Duration	Notes
Aminoglycosides				
Streptomycin	Adults 2 g/day Children 30 mg/kg/day Two divided doses	1 gm IM q12h	10 days	Not commonly available in USA
Gentamicin	Adults 5 mg/kg daily or 2 mg/kg loading dose + 1.7 mg/kg q8h Children 7.5 mg/kg/day In three divided doses Infants 7.5 mg/kg/day	120 mg IM/IV q8h	10 days	Used in pregnancy
Chloramphenicol	Adults 25 mg/kg/ every 6h Children > 2 years of age, 25 mg/kg/day Four divided doses	25 mg/kg IV q6h		Best for meningitis Can use with aminoglycoside Not commonly available in USA
Tetracyclines	Adults 2 gm/day Children 15 mg/kg loading dose then 25–50 mg/kg/day Four divided doses	1 gm PO loading then 500 mg PO q6h	10 Days	Bacteriostatis
Doxycycline	Adults 200 mg/day Children 200 mg/day 1–2 divided doses	200 mg PO daily or 100 mg PO q12h	10 days	Used in pregnancy
Levofloxacin	Adults 500 mg/day Children 8 mg/kg q12h	500 mg PO/IV daily	10 days	Limited data

Table 22-1 ANTIBIOTICS FOR *YERSINIA PESTIS*[3,7]

(Continued)

Table 22-1 ANTIBIOTICS FOR *YERSINIA PESTIS*[3,7] (*CONTINUED*)

Antibiotic	Dose/Interval	Adult 70 kg	Duration	Notes
Ciprofloxacin	Adults 800–1200 mg/day IV 2–3 divided doses 1000–1500 mg/day PO Two divided doses Children 15 mg/kg IV q12h 20 mg/kg PO q12h	400 mg IV q8-12h 500–750 mg PO q 12h	10 days	Used in pregnancy
Moxifloxacin	400 mg PO/IV daily	400 mg PO/IV daily	10 days	
Sulfadiazine	2–4 gm loading dose 1 gm q4-6h	1 g q4-6h	10 days	

Post-exposure prophylaxis

Antibiotic	Dose/Interval	Duration	Notes
Tetracycline	Adult 1–2 gm/day Children 25–50 mg/kg/day Two divided doses	7 days	
Doxycycline	Adults 100–200 mg/day Children 100–200 mg/day 1–2 divided doses	7 days	Used in pregnancy at 100 mg/day
Ciprofloxacin	Adults 500 mg bid Children 20 mg/kg bid	7 days	Used in pregnancy

choice in the USA. Gentamicin can be used in pregnancy and for children. The adult dose is 5 mg/kg/day daily or a loading dose of 2 mg/kg followed by 1.7 mg/kg IM or IV every 8 hours for 10 days or 3 days after temperature is normal. For children the dose is 6.0–7.5 mg/kg/day divided into three doses every 8 hours. For infants and neonates the dose is 7.5 mg/kg/day.

Chloramphenicol is a good alternative choice to streptomycin. It has better penetration into tissues for meningitis, pleuritis, and endophthalmitis. The dose is 50 mg/kg per day given in four divided doses. Chloramphenicol can also be used in combination with aminoglycosides such as streptomycin. Tetracycline/doxycycline are also effective. These drugs are bacteriostatic and best used for uncomplicated cases.

Tetracycline for adults is 2 g/day in four divided doses orally. For children the dose is 25–50 mg/kg/day in four divided doses for 10 days. Doxycycline is 200 mg/day divided into one or two doses orally. For children $\geq$ 45 kg, the dose is the same as adults. If the weight < 45 kg, the dose is 2.2 mg/kg twice a day. Sulfonamides have also been used. However, they are not as effective according to some studies. Patients have a higher mortality and longer duration of fever. Sulfadiazine is given as a loading dose at 2–4 g then 1 g every 4–6 hours for 10 days. Bactrim has also been used. Quinolones have been effective in vitro but have not been extensively studied in vivo for treatment of plague.[8] For levofloxacin the dose is 500 mg once daily IV or PO. For ciprofloxacin the dose is 400 mg every 8–12 hours IV or 500–750 mg bid for PO.[7]

For children, the same antibiotics can be used but the doses have to be adjusted. For pregnancy, gentamicin, doxycycline, and ciprofloxacin have been used. For children and pregnant women, there is increased risk of complications, but the benefits likely outweigh the risk given the high mortality of *Y. pestis*.[7] Close contacts of patients with pneumonic plague may need abortive treatment with tetracycline, chloramphenicol, or Bactrim for 7 days. Prophylaxis to prevent infection can be useful for healthcare workers or researchers involved with plague.[3]

INFECTION CONTROL AND PREVENTIVE MEASURES

Personal Protective Equipment (PPE)

Protection against blood, fluids, and secretions should be used. Surgical masks should be used. Standard precautions include gloves, gowns, and splash protection.[3] Persons under investigation (PUI) should be placed in respiratory droplet isolation or a negative air pressure room. Patients should be monitored for at least 48 hours for fever and symptoms after treatment is started. The effective distance for transmission is 2 meters.[1] DEET can be used as a flea repellant. *Y. pestis* has low resistance to the environment. Sun, high temperatures, desiccation, and disinfectants containing Lysol or chlorine can kill Yersinia within 1 to 10 minutes.[3]

Public Health Measures

Controlling an Outbreak

Controlling the vector and rodent population is best done with expert supervision (Tables 22-2 and 22-3). Controlling the vector is the priority, more so than controlling the rodent population. It is felt that controlling the rodent population would lead to the vectors fleeing to new hosts and

Table 22-2 ROLE OF THE WHO[20]

Confirmed cases should be reported to the WHO
Advise on diagnosis, testing, and treatment
Identify the source
Determine the extent of epizootic activity
Assess for possible additional human cases
Provide information to healthcare workers
Implement control and prevention measures

Table 22-3 PLAGUE OUTBREAK MANAGEMENT PER WHO[3]

Find and stop the source
Protect healthcare workers
Correct treatment for active patients/chemoprophylaxis to exposed patients
Isolate patients
Surveillance
Obtain specimens
Disinfection
Safe burial practices
Maintain surveillance and control

would not establish good control. Use of poison for the fleas is considered the best way to control the spread of the vector.

Insecticide dust can be applied in and around rodent burrows and runways. Also bait traps can be used with insecticide. The rodents get the insecticide dust on their fur and carry it back to their burrows. There are a variety of insecticides available as well as a test kit from the WHO for insecticide resistance.[3]

After vector control has been accomplished, control of the rodent population is the next goal. The type of rodent or species of rat is particularly important. Rodent populations can be controlled with rodenticide, poisons, anticoagulants, or fumigants like cyanide gas.[3] Plague is one of the three infections that are covered by international health regulations. Cases should be reported and investigated by the WHO.

Vaccination

Y. pestis vaccine was of poor effectiveness and no longer available.[7] The vaccine has since been withdrawn from the USA. A live vaccine using *Y. pestis* EV76 is available in Asia and Russia, and is effective against both bubonic and pneumonic plague.[13] Side effects include headache, malaise, and pyrexia, sometimes leading to hospitalization.[12] Newer vaccines are directed at pneumonic plague as it is a possible bioweapon.

Molecular vaccines have been developed—rF1-V (USA), RypVax (UK), and SV1 (China). They use the F1 and V antigens. These vaccines are patented but not under license. rF1-V and SV1 have completed phase II trials only. Other candidates have been suggested but not developed. A live *Y. pseudotuberculosis* vaccine VTnF1 might also be useful. A single dose was effective for mice against *Y. pestis*.[13] Since current vaccination effectiveness is not well studied, all possible patients should be treated with antibiotics anyway. Therefore, the vaccine does not obviate the need for treatment in cases of exposure or actual disease.

REFERENCES

1. Hsu HL, Chuang CC, Liang CC, et al. Rapid and sensitive detection of Yersinia pestis by lateral-flow assay in simulated clinical samples, *BMC Infect Dis*. 2018;18:402.

2. Farndon J. *The Sickening History of Medicine*. Minnesota, MN: Lerner Publishing; 2017.

3. World Health Organization. Plague Handbook B. Available at https://www.who.int/csr/resources/publications/plague/whocdscsredc992b.pdf?ua=1. Accessed October 25, 2020.

4. Raoult D, Mouffok N, Bitam I, Piarroux R, Drancourt M. Plague: History and contemporary analysis. *J Infect*. 2013;66:18-26.

5. Mordechai L, Eisenberg M, Newfield TP, Izdebski A, Kay JE, Poinar H. The Justinianic Plague: An inconsequential pandemic? *PNAS*. 2019;116(51): 25546-25554.

6. Guerrant RL, Walker DH, Weller PF. *Tropical Infectious Diseases*. Elsevier; 2011. Dennis DT, Mead PS. Chapter 42 Plague.

7. Centers for Disease Control and Prevention. Plague. Available at https://www.cdc.gov/plague/index.html. Accessed October 25, 2020.

8. World Health Organization. Plague Handbook A. Available at https://www.who.int/csr/resources/publications/plague/whocdscsredc992a.pdf. Accessed October 25, 2020.

9. Wikipedia. Plague. Available at https://en.wikipedia.org/wiki/Plague_(disease). Accessed October 31, 2020.

10. Byrne JP. *The Black Death*. Westport, Connecticut: Greenwood Press; 2004.

11. Wikipedia. Yersinia pestis. Available at https://en.wikipedia.org/wiki/Yersinia_pestis. Accessed October 31, 2020.

12. Pechous RD, Sivaraman V, Stasulli NM, Goldman WE. Pneumonia Plague: The Darker Side of Yersini a pestis. *Trends Microbiol*. 2016;24(3):190-197.

13. Demeure CE, Dussurget O, Fiol GM, Guern A, Savin C, Pizarro-Cerda J. Yersina pestis and plague: an updated view on evolution, virulence determinants, immune subversion, vaccination, and diagnostics. *Genes Immun.* 2019;20:357-37021.

14. Yang R, Anisimov A, eds. Yersinia pestis: Retrospective and Perspective, Advances in Experimental Medicine and Biology 918, Chapter 5.

15. Hinnebusch BJ, Erickson DL. Yersinia pestis biofilm in the flea vector and its role in the transmission of plague. *Curr Top Microbiol Immunol.* 2008;322:229-248.

16. Tennant W, Tildesley MJ, Spencer S, Keeling MJ. Climate drivers of plague epidemiology in British India, 1898-1949. *Proc Biol Sci.* 2020; 287(1928).

17. Eichelberger KR, Jones GS, Goldman WE. Inhibition of Neutrophil Primary Granule Release during Yersinia pestis Pulmonary Infection. *mBio.* 2019;10(6):e02759-19.15.

18. Mayo Clinic. Plague. Available at https://www.mayoclinic.org/diseases-conditions/plague/symptoms-causes/syc-20351291. Accessed on October 29, 2020.

19. World Health Organization. Plague. Available at https://www.who.int/health-topics/plague#tab=tab_1. Accessed October 25, 2020.

20. World Health Organization. Plague Handbook C. Available at https://www.who.int/csr/resources/publications/plague/whocdscsredc992c.pdf?ua=1. Accessed October 25, 2020.

21. Bruki T. Plague in Madagascar. *Lancet Infect Dis.* 2017;17(12):1241.

22. Inglesby TV, Dennis DT, Henderson DA, et al. Plague as a Biological Weapon Medical and Public Health Management. *JAMA.* 2000;283(17):2281-22902.

23. Stenseth NC, Atshabar BB, Begon M, et al. Plague: past, present, and future. *PLoS Med.* 2008;5(1):e3.

TULAREMIA 23

Han Nguyen, MD

▌INTRODUCTION

Tularemia is a rare zoonotic disease caused by *Francisella tularensis*, a Gram-negative, non-motile, non-spore forming, facultative intracellular bacterium. The genus *Francisella* comprises seven species, and *F. tularensis* can be subdivided into four subspecies, *F. tularensis* (type A strains), *F. holartica* (type B strains), *F. mediasiatica*, and *F. novicida*. *F. tularensis* and *F. holartica* are the only two subspecies to cause tularemia worldwide.

Transmission occurs via ticks, deer flies, and, in some regions (e.g., Sweden and Finland), mosquitoes. Small mammals such as rabbits, hares, and muskrats act as reservoir hosts. Modes of transmission to humans are direct transmission from the animal reservoir, arthropod bites, and through contaminated water and soil. Infection in the US and Canada is mainly due to *F. tularensis* while in Europe and the rest of the northern hemisphere infection is caused by *F. holartica*.[1–3] In the United States, most of the cases are found in the northwest, and parts of Massachusetts including Martha's Vineyard. The first case of Tularemia-like disease was reported in Norway in 1653.[1] In 2008–2018 the incidence of the disease in the United States per 100,000 residents was 0.07.[1–3]

Occupational risk includes veterinarians, butchers, farmers, and landscapers. The first human case was reported 2 years later from a butcher suffering lymphadenopathy and conjunctival ulcer in Ohio.[1,2] One study determined the seroprevalence of Tularemia as 7.57% among farmers in Ilam Province, a region in western Iran.[4] Another study identified 8.6% of landscapers as having antibodies to Tularemia compared to 1.0% of the general population.[5] One study noted infection mainly through contact with rodents or game (21.4%), through tick bites (12.9%), and outdoor leisure activities (20.9%).[6]

Pathogenesis

Francisella is a small gram-negative pleomorphic coccobacillus that is catalase-positive and an intracellular pathogen (Figure 23-1). Tularemia virulence is due to its ability to invade macrophages and replicate intracellularly. The organism escapes the phagosomal compartment of the macrophage and multiplies in the cytosol. The bacterial lipopolysaccharide (LPS) does not trigger an inflammatory response in the macrophages, and thus reduces the host immune response.

Clinical Manifestations

Incubation is 3–6 days. Initial symptoms include fever myalgia, headache, and/or cough and eventually develop maculopapular lesions. Temperature-pulse dissociation is common as is gastrointestinal or pulmonary involvement. There are six known syndromes: ulceroglandular, glandular, oculoglandular, oropharyngeal, pneumonic, and typhoidal. (Figures 23-2 and 23-3) Ulceroglandular syndrome involves formation of skin ulcer at the inoculation site with localized lymphadenopathy. Glandular is an isolated tender lymphadenopathy without skin manifestations. Oropharyngeal occurs when individuals ingest the bacteria causing pharyngitis, fever, and cervical lymphadenopathy.[7] Oculoglandular occurs due to direct contact of contaminated hands, or via bodily fluids of animals or contaminated water.[7] Pneumonic can be primary after inhalation of the bacteria or secondary after hematogenous spread. Typhoidal usually presents with high fever, splenomegaly, and hepatomegaly and is less common. These individuals do not have lymphadenopathy or ulcerations. Typhoidal and pulmonary tularemia have high mortality.

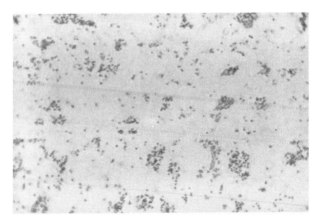

Figure 23-1 • *Francisella tularensis* via methylene-blue stain. (*Courtesy of the CDC.* https://phil.cdc.gov/Details.aspx?pid=10526.)

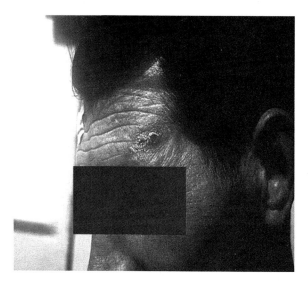

Figure 23-2 • This photograph depicts a left lateral view of a patient's forehead, which reveals an ulcerative lesion. The man happened to be a Vermont muskrat trapper, who had contracted tularemia. The bacterium responsible for causing the disease tularemia, *Francisella tularensis*, can often be found in rodents, including rabbits, hares, and musk-rats. (*Courtesy of the CDC.* https://phil.cdc.gov/Details.aspx?pid=6465.)

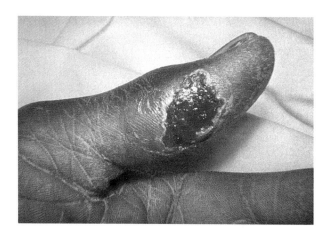

Figure 23-3 • Ulcerative lesion on the lateral aspect of the thumb. (*Courtesy of the CDC.* https://phil.cdc.gov/Details.aspx?pid=1344.)

Diagnosis

Diagnosis initially can be presumptive based on exposure, clinical manifestations, and epidemiological risk factors. Treatment should not be delayed. Although cultures can confirm the diagnosis, they are rarely positive. Serologic changes at least 2 weeks from onset of symptoms can be used to confirm diagnosis and include: (1) four-fold increase between acute and convalescent specimen; (2) $\geq$ 1:160 titer with tube agglutination test; and (3) $\geq$ 1:128 titer with microagglutination.[8] Polymerase chain reaction (PCR) tests can be performed but are not routinely available.

Treatment

Untreated tularemia has fatality rates of between 30 and 70% but with antibiotics, rates drop to 2%.[1–8] The first line of therapy for severe disease is the aminoglycosides, streptomycin (1 g IM/IV every 12 hours for 7–10 days) or gentamicin (5.0 mg/kg IV every 8 hours for adults or 2–5 mg/kg IV every 8 hours for children for 10 days). Duration can be extended depending on clinical course. Treatment for meningitis is aminoglycoside + chloramphenicol 50–100 mg/kg/day IV in four divided doses.[9–16]

For mild to moderate disease, ciprofloxacin (400 mg IV or 740 mg PO twice a day for adults and 10–15 mg/kg PO twice a day in children for 14–21 days), levofloxacin (500 mg PO daily for 14 days in adults) or doxycycline (100 mg PO/IV twice a day for adults and 2.2 mg/kg PO twice a day for children for 14–21 days) may be used.

Prophylaxis recommendations include doxycycline 100 mg PO BID or ciprofloxacin 500 mg PO daily for 14 days or ciprofloxacin 500 mg PO BID for 14 days.

Pregnancy

There is insufficient data to establish treatment recommendation; however, case reports suggest streptomycin or chloramphenicol for at least 14 days.

REFERENCES

1. Nigrovic LE, Wingerter SL. Tularemia. *Infect Disc Clin North Am*. 2008;(3):489-504.
2. Hirschmann JV. From Squirrels to Biological Weapons: The Early History of Tularemia. *Am J Med Sci*. 2018;356(4):319-328.
3. Maurin M, Gyuranecz M. Tularaemia: Clinical Aspects in Europe. *Lancet Infect Disc*. 2016;16(1):113-124.
4. Esmaeili S, Ghasemi A, Naserifar R, et al. Epidemiological Survey of Tularemia in Ilam Province, West Iran. *BMC Infect Disc*. 2019;19(1):502.
5. Feldman KA, Stiles-Enos D, Julian K, et al. Tularemia on Martha's Vineyard: seroprevalence and occupational risk. *Emerg Infect Dis*. 2003;9:350-354.

6. Darmon-Curti A, Darmon F, Edouard S, et al. Tularemia: A Case Series of Patients Diagnosed at the National Reference Center for Rickettsioses From 2008 to 2017. *Open Forum Infect Dis.* 2020;7(11):ofaa440.

7. Dietrich T, Garcia K, Strain J, Ashurst J. Extended-Interval Gentamicin Dosing for Pulmonic Tularemia. *Case Rep Infect Dis.* 2019;2019:9870510.

8. Chairnat V, Djordjevic-Spasic M, Ruettger A et al. Performance of seven serological assays for diagnosing tularemia. *BMC Infect Dis.* 2014;14:234.

9. Hofiner DM, Cardona L, Mertz GJ, Davis LE. Tularemic meningitis in the United States. *Arch Neurol.* 2009;66(4):523-527.

10. Maurin M. Francisella tularensis, Tularemia and Serological Diagnosis. *Front Cell Infect Microbiol.* 2020;10:512090.

11. Dennis DT, Inglesby TV, Henderson DA, et al. Tularemia as a biological weapon: medical and public health management. *JAMA.* 2001;285(21):2763-2773.

12. Yeni DK, Buyuk F, Aashraf A, Shah MSUD. Tularemia: a re-emerging tick-borne infectious disease. *Folia Microbiol (Praha).* 2020;1-14.

13. Pulavendran S, Prasanthi M, Ramachandran A, et al. Production of Neutrophil Extracellular Traps Contributes to the Pathogenesis of Francisella tularemia. *Front Immunol.* 2020;11:679.

14. Larson MA, Sayood K, Bartling AM, et al. Differentiation of Francisella tularensis Subspecies and Subtypes. *J Clin Microbiol.* 2020;58(4).e01495-19.

15. Hennebique A, Boisset S, Maurin M. Tularemia as a waterborne disease: a review. *Emerg Microbes Infect.* 2019;8(1):1027-1042.

16. Yanes H, Hennebique A, Plloux I, et al. Evaluation of In-House and Commercial Serological Tests for Diagnosis of Human Tularemia. *J Clin Microbiol.* 2017;56(1):e01440-17.

24 EBOLA AND MARBURG VIRUS

Armand Gottlieb, MD

▌INTRODUCTION

Ebola virus disease is caused by infection with the filovirus *Ebolavirus*. Five different species have been identified, and the vast majority of cases and outbreaks have been caused by the Zaire species. The Ebola virus was first recognized during outbreaks in Sudan and Zaire in 1976.[1] Since then, intermittent outbreaks caused by the virus have occurred mostly in sub-Saharan Africa. The largest known outbreak occurred between 2013 and 2016, producing an epidemic in West Africa with nearly 29,000 known or suspected cases and over 11,000 deaths.[1] Ebola virus disease has also proven to be highly contagious, and appropriate infection control measures have been essential in managing epidemics in Africa as well as in preventing spread where cases have been identified and managed in the United States and Europe.[1] Early diagnosis and prompt initiation of supportive care are essential to decreasing both mortality and transmission of the virus. This chapter will also discuss the closely related Marburg virus, which was the first identified filovirus, but has been much less commonly encountered in recent years.

▌EBOLA

Epidemiology and Risk Factors

The Ebola virus has caused more than 20 outbreaks in sub-Saharan Africa since it was first identified in 1976 (Figure 24-1). Most Ebola virus disease outbreaks have occurred in small and isolated regions of central Africa or Sudan. While often devastating to the local populations, these outbreaks have generally not caused widespread epidemics, likely due to low population density and limited travel by infected populations. The largest outbreak occurred in West Africa from 2013 to 2016, primarily in Guinea,

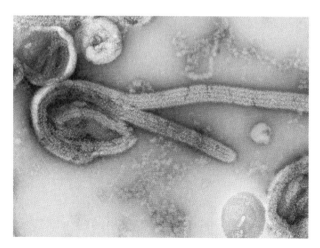

Figure 24-1 • Electron microscopic image of Ebola Virus. (*Courtesy of the CDC.* https://phil.cdc.gov/Details.aspx?pid=23186.)

Sierra Leone, and Liberia, causing more than 11,000 deaths, though due to under-reporting the toll could have been considerably higher.[1-3] This recent epidemic showed that the virus has a potential for wide and rapid spread both in urban areas and across international borders. A few secondary infections were noted in the nurses of Spain and the United States, who had cared domestically for infected patients returning from endemic areas.[3] Since 2018, there have been multiple outbreaks in the Democratic Republic of the Congo as well, with over 2,000 deaths reported.[1-3]

Ebola virus disease is thought to be a zoonotic disease, possibly residing in fruit bats though this has not been rigorously proven. Initial human infection is likely caused by either the handling of infected wild animals such as chimpanzees and gorillas for meat, or by exposure to infected bats. Human-to-human transmission occurs via contact with mucous membranes or broken skin with infected body fluids, primarily blood, feces, and vomit. Sexual transmission has also been reported. The potential for aerosol and airborne transmission is debated.[2]

Treating infected patients and handling dead bodies have been identified as particularly high risk for transmission. Washing the deceased's body, a common ritual in endemic areas was thought to contribute to the West African epidemic. High nosocomial transmission rates have been noted both early in outbreaks before the cause is identified and when appropriate protective equipment is not used or available.[2] The West African epidemic caused an estimated 881 infections and 513 deaths among healthcare workers in Guinea, Liberia, and Sierra Leone.[3]

Pathogenesis

Ebola virus is a filamentous virus, 80 nanometers in diameter and up to 14,000 nanometers in length depending on the particle. The virus causes host cell damage both through direct cytotoxic effects as well as indirect effects on the host immune system. Ebola virus first enters the body through mucous membranes or breaks in the skin. Macrophages and dendritic cells are quickly infected and are the sites of rapid viral replication. Serum viral levels then increase exponentially, often from undetectable to $> 10^5$ viral particles/mL in the first three days after symptom onset.[4]

The virus produces a complex interaction with the host immune system resulting in both immune suppression and over-activation in various parts of the immune system. Early evasion of host immune responses is essential to early rapid viral replication. Ebola virus proteins suppress host Type I interferon responses as well as the maturation of dendritic cells. Type I interferon is one of the primary pathways through which the immune system interferes with viral replication, and dendritic cells are essential antigen presenting cells that link the innate and adaptive immune systems. Under these conditions the virus is able to replicate quickly in macrophage and dendritic cells, which then necrose and release large quantities of the virus into the bloodstream.[4]

Later in the clinical course, the Ebola virus may produce a systemic inflammatory response syndrome mediated by a large release of inflammatory cytokines. This overactive immune response likely contributes significantly to the high mortality seen with severe disease. The release of pro-inflammatory mediators contributes to the development of disseminated intravascular coagulation, vascular endothelial dysfunction, and eventually shock with multisystem organ failure.[5]

Patients suffering from Ebola virus infection commonly experience severe diarrhea and vomiting, which may progress to volume depletion and eventually shock. The profuse watery diarrhea induced by the Ebola virus is highly contagious, and if handled without appropriate protective equipment contributes to a rapid spread of the virus. It is not known whether these gastrointestinal symptoms are due to direct viral infection of gastrointestinal tract cells or mediated by systemically distributed inflammatory cytokines.[4]

Severe Ebola virus infection may lead to disseminated intravascular coagulation and life-threatening coagulopathy. Tissue factor is released by infected macrophages as well as non-infected macrophages reacting to high levels of pro-inflammatory cytokines. This leads to rapid consumption of endogenous coagulation factors and severe coagulopathy.

Hepatocellular necrosis is also often seen in infected patients, and progressive hepatic injury may contribute to coagulopathy as well.[6]

Additionally, adrenocortical infection and necrosis have also been noted with Ebola virus infection. The resulting loss of hormone synthesis may lead to hypocortisolemia and mineralocorticoid deficiency contributing to progressive volume depletion and shock.[6]

Clinical Manifestations

Previously, infection with the Ebola virus was called "Ebola hemorrhagic fever" as the confirmed cases tended to be severe infections that often featured major hemorrhage and fever. During the recent 2014–2016 epidemic, the broader range of identified infections included many milder and even asymptomatic cases, leading to the disease being reclassified as "Ebola virus disease" to acknowledge the larger spectrum of clinical findings.[7]

After exposure, there is typically an incubation period ranging from 2 to 21 days depending upon the mode of transmission, with most patients falling ill between 6 and 12 days after exposure. Initial signs and symptoms include fever, malaise, and headache. These nonspecific symptoms often lead to missed diagnosis and the ongoing transmission, especially early in an outbreak[8] (Table 24-1).

Gastrointestinal symptoms are also common in the first week after illness onset, and include nausea, vomiting, abdominal pain, and diarrhea.

Table 24-1 COMMON SYMPTOMS OF EBOLA VIRUS DISEASE[9]	
Fever	87%
Fatigue	76%
Vomiting	68%
Diarrhea	66%
Loss of Appetite	65%
Headache	53%
Abdominal Pain	44%
Joint Pain	39%
Muscle Pain	39%
Chest Pain	37%

The diarrhea may be profuse and watery, as much as 5 to 10 liters per day. The combination of vomiting, diarrhea, and anorexia may result in significant fluid loss and acute kidney injury. In severe cases this may progress to hypovolemia and shock.[8] A diffuse nonpruritic, erythematous, maculopapular rash may also be noted in the first week of infection. The rash may be difficult to observe in dark-skinned individuals, and the reported prevalence of the rash has varied widely between studies and outbreaks.[9,10] Subsequently, patients may develop a variety of other symptoms, including chest pain, shortness of breath, confusion, and conjunctival injection. Seizures and cerebral edema have been reported as well.[11]

Bleeding may be present later in the illness, most commonly seen as blood in the stool. Patients may also develop petechiae, ecchymosis, oozing from venipuncture sites, and mucosal hemorrhage. Clinically significant hemorrhage may be seen in fulminant disease or during pregnancy.[11]

Laboratory abnormalities are common. Leukopenia may be seen initially with progression to leukocytosis and atypical lymphocytosis. Thrombocytopenia is common while marked anemia is rare on presentation. Elevated liver transaminase levels, with AST > ALT may be seen. Gastrointestinal losses may lead to multiple electrolyte abnormalities including hypokalemia, hyponatremia, hypomagnesemia, hypocalcemia, and acidemia, any of which may become life threatening. Severe cases progressing to renal insufficiency or failure present with typical findings of elevated creatinine and BUN and associated electrolyte derangements. As above, severe cases may progress to disseminated intravascular coagulation and have elevated PT and PTT.[7]

Diagnosis

Making the diagnosis of Ebola virus infection can be difficult due to the usually nonspecific presentation of infected individuals. Clinicians need to be wary of other febrile illnesses common in West and Central Africa, including malaria, typhoid, Lassa fever, Marburg virus, and leptospirosis. Other viral and bacterial causes of gastroenteritis, including hepatitis and influenza need to be considered as well. However, high clinical suspicion for Ebola virus infection in the appropriate setting is critical both to treating patients at high risk for decompensation and preventing transmission of the virus.[7]

Ebola virus RNA is usually detectable by RT-PCR in the blood samples of infected patients within 3 days from the onset of symptoms. Repeat testing should be considered for patients with negative tests performed early in their illness course. Rapid viral antigen testing by ELISA has been deployed in some regions, though confirmatory testing with

RT-PCR is generally recommended. Serum IgM or IgG levels can also be useful for checking for past infection, but are less useful for diagnosis of acute infection.[7]

Patients should be tested if they are symptomatic and have either a history of travel to an area known to have active Ebola disease cases or contact with a person possibly infected within the 21 days prior to symptom onset. Additionally, symptomatic patients who are under investigation require isolation. Infection control measures are discussed in detail in the "Infection Control and Preventative Measures" section. Asymptomatic individuals with an exposure to Ebola virus need to be carefully monitored for 21 days for suspicious symptoms, but do not require immediate testing.[12]

Treatment

Treatment of Ebola virus infection centers on supportive care to prevent severe complications, isolation, and preventative measures to avoid spread of disease. Early diagnosis and early supportive care appear to increase survival, as patients who present with significant volume depletion or other severe features are at increased risk of death. Very recently, the first Ebola virus-specific medication has received FDA approval, and other experimental therapies remain under investigation. Prevention measures and isolation techniques will be discussed in the next section.

Ebola virus outbreaks have almost exclusively occurred in resource-poor settings, where sufficient personal protective equipment (PPE), laboratory and monitoring equipment, and even diagnostic testing supplies are not readily available. Providing critical care in this setting can be extremely challenging, and outbreaks in Africa have yielded case fatality rates ranging from 40 to 90%.[8] However, data from a small series of patients treated for Ebola virus disease outside Africa showed a mortality rate of just 18.5%, suggesting a large survival benefit from modern supportive critical care for this patient population.[13] Mobilizing modern critical care infrastructure on a system level to affected areas as much as possible is ideal, though often providers must improvise due to severely limited resources.

Volume Resuscitation

Vomiting and profuse diarrhea leave many Ebola virus patients with profound hypovolemia. Fluid resuscitation is essential to prevent development of shock and renal failure. Hemodynamic monitoring and intravenous fluid resuscitation are ideal when available. Lactated ringers or other balanced crystalloid solutions are preferred over normal saline given the often large volume of required parenteral resuscitation and the risk of causing hyperchloremic metabolic acidosis with normal saline. Resuscitation with albumin may also be considered for patients with hypoalbuminemia. Oral rehydration and electrolyte replacement may be administered to patients in resource-poor settings, and may be sufficient for patients with only mild symptoms or early in their clinical courses. Parenteral resuscitation is still preferred when available, especially for patients with severe presentations. Some patients additionally may not have sufficient blood pressure response to fluid resuscitation alone and may require intravenous vasopressor therapy.[7]

Gastrointestinal Distress

Anti-emetics and anti-diarrheal medications may be useful in preventing ongoing gastrointestinal volume losses. It should be noted that the safety of anti-diarrheal medications in Ebola virus infection is uncertain, and anti-diarrheal medications have not been shown to be efficacious in cholera, which causes a similar large volume watery diarrhea.[7]

Respiratory Failure

Most respiratory failures seen in Ebola virus infection appear to be secondary to altered mental status, hemodynamic instability, metabolic acidosis from gastrointestinal losses and acute kidney injury, rather than from a primary pulmonary insult. The need for aggressive fluid resuscitation combined with increased vascular permeability may also lead to pulmonary edema or acute lung injury requiring respiratory support. This may pose additional challenges in resource-poor settings where ventilatory support may not be available. Where available, respiratory failure is preferentially managed with intubation over non-invasive ventilation given the potential for aerosol generation and transmission of virus.[7]

Renal Failure and Metabolic Derangements

Patients who develop shock may develop acute renal injury and failure, and may require renal replacement therapy. The massive gastrointestinal losses may also precipitate multiple life-threatening metabolic abnormalities, including hypokalemia, hyponatremia, hypomagnesemia, hypocalcemia, and acidemia, which often need aggressive repletion and frequent monitoring.[7]

Coagulopathy

Thrombocytopenia is common, though platelet levels typically do not fall below 50,000 to 100,000/microliter.[11] Patients who develop hemorrhage require transfusion of appropriate blood products to correct anemia, thrombocytopenia, and coagulopathy.[7]

Coinfection and Superinfection

Antimicrobial therapy should be considered for possible coinfection and superinfection. In endemic areas, antimalarial treatment should be considered upfront, as well as broad-spectrum antibiotics for patients with suspected bacterial superinfection or sepsis. As with other types of critically ill patients, those with severe infection are at risk for catheter associated infections, ventilator associated pneumonia, translocation of bacteria from the gut into the bloodstream, as well as colitis from *Clostridium difficile.*[7]

Ebola Virus-Specific Therapies

Investigational therapies for the treatment of Ebola virus infection have aimed to inhibit viral replication. Experimental therapies have included convalescent plasma, monoclonal antibody cocktails, nucleoside analogs, and interfering RNA molecules. In October 2020, a monoclonal antibody cocktail combining atoltivimab, maftivimab, and odesivimab-ebgn became the first Ebola virus-specific treatment to receive FDA approval.[14] The drug showed an absolute mortality reduction of 17.8% at 28 days in a clinical trial in which 154 patients were randomized to receive the study drug and 168 patients received another investigational control. Another monoclonal antibody, labeled MAb114 also showed a similar efficacy as part of the same clinical trial, but has not received FDA approval.[15]

At the time of this writing the precise indications for use of Ebola virus-specific therapies have not yet been determined, and the expense and availability of novel drugs may make it impractical for widespread use in the resource-limited settings where Ebola virus outbreaks typically occur. Clinicians with access to novel therapeutics should monitor local institutional and organizational guidelines for updated recommendations for their use (Table 24-2).

Infection Control

In addition to the treatment of infected individuals, controlling an Ebola virus outbreak also hinges on a multitude of healthcare system measures

Table 24-2 APPROVED EBOLA VIRUS-SPECIFIC DRUGS AND VACCINES[14,15,20,21]

Drug	Trade Name	Description	Approval
rVSV-ZEBOV vaccine	Ervebo	Live, attenuated vaccine. Delivered in single dose. Available data shows 97.5% effectiveness.	Approved by FDA December 2019
Ad26.ZEBOV/ MVA-BN-Filo vaccine	Zabdeno/Mvabea	Two dose vaccine series, must be delivered 56 days apart.	Recommended for approval by European Medicines Agency May 2020
Cocktail of atoltivimab, maftivimab, and odesivimab-ebgn	Inmazeb	Monoclonal antibody cocktail. Demonstrated 17.8% absolute mortality reduction in randomized trial	Approved by FDA October 2020

and coordinated public health efforts. Healthcare system preparedness, strict isolation practices, public health outreach, and vaccination programs each play a key role in halting Ebola virus outbreaks.

Personal Protective Equipment and Healthcare Setting Practices

Infection control measures to prevent transmission is essential to prevent nosocomial spread. Ebola virus has been detected in blood, urine, feces, vomit, sweat, tears, saliva, mucus, breast milk, and semen. Serum viral loads appear to correlate closely with the timing of symptoms, and the infectious dose is thought to be low, potentially fewer than 10 viral particles. Transmission is thought to primarily be through contact with infected bodily fluids or fomites, and potentially by airborne transmission or aerosolization, though this is debated. Careful measures to protect healthcare workers and other patients in healthcare settings is critical to preventing spread.[7]

The CDC recommends standard, contact, and droplet precautions when caring for patients with known or suspected Ebola virus infection. This includes an impermeable gown or coverall, double gloving, respiratory protection with either an N95 with a surgical hood and disposable face shield or powered air purifying respirator (PAPR), boot covers, and an additional apron on top if the patient is vomiting or has diarrhea. Healthcare workers should have no exposed skin when caring for Ebola virus patients.[16]

Donning and doffing of PPE requires careful institutional training and monitoring. Removal of PPE in particular is a potentially hazardous process and should be supervised by a trained observer and potentially assisted by a fully protected assistant. If aerosol-generating procedures such as intubation or bronchoscopy are required, a negative pressure room and high efficiency particulate absorbing filters may help decrease the risk of transmission, and their use is recommended by the CDC for any patients with prominent cough, vomiting, diarrhea, or hemorrhage.[16,17]

The CDC recommends routine cleaning and meticulous sterilization of surfaces in hospital areas where Ebola virus patients are cared for. Ebola virus can be eliminated from hospital surfaces and materials with a variety of strategies. The virus is sensitive to heat, and can be eradicated by heating to 60°C for 60 minutes, 72–80°C for 30 minutes, or submersion in boiling water for 5 minutes. The virus is also sensitive to UV light, as well as many common chemical agents, including bleach, alcohols, ammonia, and peroxides.[18]

Hospitals should create specialized clinical care teams to care for Ebola virus patients, and staffing plans need to account for the added strain of providing care in this setting. Working shifts in full PPE creates increased difficulty in providing patient care due to reduced dexterity, altered sensory input, and increased fatigue. Additionally, given the high viral load in infected bodily fluids and low dose required for transmission, the margin for error is low. A National Institutes of Health multidisciplinary team concluded that caring for one critically ill Ebola virus patient for one week requires 12 full-time nurses, six full time physicians, and six full time PPE adherence monitors.[7]

Blood sampling is necessary but should be minimized as much as possible. Teams should consider placing central or peripherally inserted central catheters to minimize needle sticks. Point of care laboratory testing within the containment area is a potential strategy to decrease risk of exposures. Transporting patients for studies and procedures must be minimized, and the use of portable diagnostic equipment for testing is preferred whenever possible.[7]

Public Health Measures

Public health measures to halt community transmission is crucial to achieve control of an Ebola virus outbreak. This includes early case identification, rapid isolation, safe burial practices, community engagement, and coordination of services.[2]

Early case identification requires a vast surveillance system and community education programs. The population at risk needs to know what symptoms to look out for and needs to be willing to engage with the healthcare system. Ebola outbreaks often occur in remote areas where the disease is unknown and outsiders are not trusted without buy-in from local community leaders. Additionally, a robust testing infrastructure needs to be able to rapidly identify the infected individuals and communicate the results so that they can be quickly received and reviewed by the coordinating agencies. Contact tracing can help to both identify cases and prevent spread as well. This requires both human and physical resources to be in coordination at a regional or national level.[2]

Identified cases should be isolated as rapidly as possible. Creation of Ebola Treatment Centers (ETC) as close as possible to affected communities can help quickly isolate patients and facilitate communication and trust with the local community. As resources permit, families should be kept informed and be able to visit, as both these help patients cope with the psychological ramifications of Ebola virus infection and relevant isolation, as well as builds trust with families and the community.[2]

Traditional funeral practices, which include ritual washing of the body have been thought to contribute significantly to the spread of Ebola virus infection. A single funeral in Guinea was linked to 85 subsequent confirmed cases.[19] Permitting attendance to funerals and allowing for traditional ceremonies, with the provision of taking necessary safety precautions can increase community acceptance and adherence to recommended safe burial practices.[2]

Vaccination

Vaccination to prevent Ebola virus infection was not available until very recently. Two vaccines have been used in the most recent epidemic. The first to be widely used was Ervebo, a single dose live attenuated vaccine that received FDA approval in December 2019. This vaccine has been delivered to over 300,000 people in the Democratic Republic of the Congo, with a reported 97.5% efficacy. A small case series has also described the use of this vaccine for post-exposure prophylaxis, though it has not received approval for this use.[20]

The other vaccine in use is a two-dose series branded as Zabdeno and Mvabea, which received recommendation for approval by the European Medicines Agency in May 2020, though it has not been approved by the FDA. This newer vaccine requires the two doses to be given 56 days apart, though potentially it may produce a longer lasting response.[21]

Complications

After convalescing from acute Ebola virus infection, recovering patients may have persistent symptoms for more than 2 years after the initial episode. Several large cohort studies have documented ongoing complications in Ebola virus infection survivors. These patients may suffer from ongoing urinary frequency, headache, fatigue, myalgia, memory loss, and arthralgia. Uveitis is also common and may be persistent.[22]

Ebola virus RNA may persist in immunologically privileged sites such as the eyes, central nervous system, and testes for far longer than the initial acute illness. Persistent viral load in these sites, where the body's antiviral immune response is less robust, is associated with ongoing symptoms and even viral transmission.[2] Thirty percent of surviving males have detectable Ebola virus RNA in their semen, and sexual transmission from convalescent patients has been documented. In one case, Ebola virus RNA was documented in a patient's semen 40 months after the initial acute illness.[22] A case of meningoencephalitis has also been documented 9 months after initial recovery from Ebola virus infection.[2]

Long term functional limitations have been documented, with many patients reporting decreased ability to work for more than 1 year after their initial illness.[23] Post-traumatic stress disorder, depression, and anxiety have also been documented among Ebola virus infection survivors. One case series has documented the ongoing neurocognitive effects for more than 2 decades after initial presentation.[24]

Surviving patients should be connected to comprehensive follow-up care, with special focus on monitoring rheumatological, auditory, and ocular function. Mental health screening should be offered with social and psychological support provided as needed. Male survivors should have seminal fluid screening for viral RNA, and be counseled on safe sex practices.[2]

Prognosis

Ebola virus infection carries a high case fatality rate, which has been documented in the 40–90% range in West African epidemics. However, a significant portion of this mortality may be related to the resource-limited settings in which the vast majority of Ebola virus patients receive care.[8] Several variables have been shown to correlate with the prognosis for individual patients. Older age has been associated with worse outcomes. A small study of patients in Sierra Leone found that patients under 21 years old had a 57% chance of mortality, while patients over 45 years old had a striking mortality rate of 94%.[25]

The presence of gastrointestinal distress at presentation has also been shown to be associated with mortality, possibly due to profuse diarrhea being a significant driver of the development of hemodynamic collapse. The same study above noted that the patients with diarrhea at time of presentation had a 94% rate of mortality, compared with 65% for those who did not.[25]

High viral load at time of presentation has also been associated with worse prognosis. Several studies have found that viral loads greater than 10 million copies per milliliter at time of presentation is a significant predictor of mortality.[25,26]

▌ MARBURG VIRUS

Marburg virus is a filovirus closely related to Ebola virus (Figure 24-2). As there have been multiple recent large Ebola virus outbreaks compared to the relative rarity of Marburg virus, significantly more resources have been devoted to researching the pathophysiology and clinical management of Ebola virus. The current understanding of Marburg virus is largely extrapolated from available Ebola virus data, and the epidemiology, pathogenesis, clinical presentation, and treatment of the two viruses are felt to be similar.

The first recognized outbreak of Marburg virus occurred in Germany and Yugoslavia in 1967 following the importation of infected vervet monkeys from Uganda for use in vaccine production. The case fatality rate in this outbreak was 23%.[27] All subsequent outbreaks of Marburg virus have occurred in Africa, and case fatality rates have been as high as 80–90%.[28] As with Ebola virus, the strikingly different case fatality rates between African and European case series may suggest that mortality from the infection is significantly affected by the availability or lack of modern critical care resources.

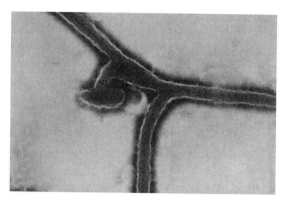

Figure 24-2 • Transmission electron microscopic image (TEM) of the Marburg virus. (*Courtesy of the CDC.* https://phil.cdc.gov/Details.aspx?pid=1245.)

The largest outbreak occurred in Angola in 2004, which appears to have been promulgated through contaminated transfusion equipment on an inpatient pediatric ward. Nearly 400 cases were identified with a mortality rate around 90%.[29] Since 2004, Marburg virus disease cases have only been identified in Uganda.

Like Ebola virus, Marburg virus is thought to asymptomatically infect species of fruit bats that reside across central Africa. Several outbreaks of Marburg virus have been traced to individuals with known bat exposures. Transmission is thought to spread from person to person in a similar fashion to Ebola virus, through direct contact with contaminated body fluids. Traditional funerals and ritual washings have been implicated in viral transmission as well. Available information suggests the pathogenesis is similar to what is described above for Ebola virus infection.[2]

The clinical presentation and clinical course are similar to that of Ebola virus. After a brief incubation period, patients generally initially develop non-specific symptoms that may quickly progress to shock and multi-system organ failure (Figures 24-3 and 24-4). Change to management is based on supportive care and strict isolation. Public health outreach and contract tracing are essential in controlling a developing epidemic. Specific recommendations for isolation of patients with Marburg virus disease are the same as for Ebola virus.[10]

There are no FDA approved specific therapies for Marburg virus disease, and vaccinations are in development but have not yet been deployed to human subjects. Lastly, testing for Marburg virus by RT-PCR and ELISA exists only in the research laboratory setting, and no rapid diagnostic tests have been field tested yet.

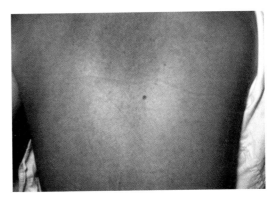

Figure 24-3 • Maculopapular rash on the back from a patient infection with Marburg virus that blanches with pressure and appears around the 5th day of onset of symptoms. This might be difficult to see in dark skinned patients. (*Courtesy of the CDC.* https://phil. cdc.gov/details.aspx?pid=6570.)

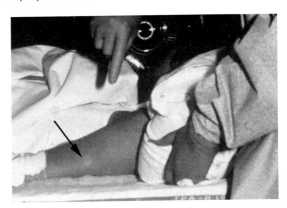

Figure 24-4 • Patient is infected with Marburg virus. Notice how skin blanches after pressure. (*Courtesy of the CDC.* https://phil.cdc.gov/Details.aspx?pid=6562.)

CONCLUSION

Ebola Virus and Marburg virus are some of the most virulent human pathogens known and have shown a capability for rapid transmissibility with high case fatality rates. Managing outbreaks requires coordinated public health measures as well as careful isolation of infected and potentially infected individuals. The recent introduction of effective vaccines in the last several years will hopefully help both in preventing its spread and controlling ongoing outbreaks. Treatment is predominantly supportive care. The first Ebola virus-specific drug has just received FDA approval at the time of this writing, and clinicians with access to this and other novel therapeutics should monitor local guidelines for how to incorporate these into their treatment plans.

REFERENCES

1. World Health Organization. Interim Infection Prevention and Control Guidance for Care of Patients with Suspected or Confirmed Filovirus Haemorrhagic Fever in Health-Care Settings, with Focus on Ebola. https://apps.who.int/iris/bitstream/handle/10665/130596/1/WHO_HIS_SDS_2014.4_eng.pdf?ua=1&ua=1&ua=1. Accessed October 15, 2020.

2. Malvy D, McElroy AK, de Clerck H, et al. Ebola virus disease. *Lancet.* 2019; 393:936-948.

3. World Health Organization. Ebola virus disease: Democratic Republic of the Congo. External situation report 42. https://apps.who.int/iris/bitstream/handle/10665/324843/SITREP_EVD_DRC_20190521-eng.pdf?ua=1. Accessed October 15, 2020.

4. Baseler L, Chertow DS, Johnson KM, et al. The Pathogenesis of Ebola Virus Disease. *Annu Rev Pathol.* 2017;12:387.

5. Mahanty S, Bray M. Pathogenesis of filoviral haemorrhagic fevers. *Lancet Infect Dis.* 2004;4:487.

6. Feldmann H, Geisbert TW. Ebola haemorrhagic fever. *Lancet.* 2011;377:849.

7. West TE, von Saint André-von Arnim A. Clinical presentation and management of severe Ebola virus disease. *Ann Am Thorac Soc.* 2014;11:1341.

8. Leligdowicz A, Fischer WA, Uyeki TM, et al. Ebola virus disease and critical illness. *Crit Care.* 2016;20:217.

9. WHO Ebola Response Team. Ebola virus disease in West Africa: the first 9 months of the epidemic and forward projections. *N Engl J Med.* 2014;371:1481-1495.

10. Kortepeter MG, Bausch DG, Bray M. Basic clinical and laboratory features of filoviral hemorrhagic fever. *J Infect Dis.* 2011;204(Suppl 3):S810.

11. Centers for Disease Control and Prevention. Ebola virus disease information for clinicians in U.S. healthcare settings. http://www.cdc.gov/vhf/ebola/hcp/clinician-information-us-healthcare-settings.html. Accessed October 15, 2020.

12. Centers for Disease Control and Prevention. Review of human-to-human transmission of Ebola virus. http://www.cdc.gov/vhf/ebola/transmission/human-transmission.html. Accessed October 15, 2020.

13. Uyeki TM, Mehta AK, Davey RT Jr, et al. Clinical Management of Ebola Virus Disease in the United States and Europe. *N Engl J Med.* 2016;374:636.

14. Food and Drug Administration. FDA Approves First Treatment for Ebola Virus. https://www.fda.gov/news-events/press-announcements/fda-approves-first-treatment-ebola-virus. Accessed October 15, 2020.

15. Mulangu S, Dodd LE, Davey RT Jr, et al. A Randomized, Controlled Trial of Ebola Virus Disease Therapeutics. *N Engl J Med.* 2019;381:2293.

16. Centers for Disease Control and Prevention. Guidance on personal protective equipment (PPE) to be used by healthcare workers during management of patients with confirmed Ebola or persons under investigation (PUIs) for Ebola who are clinically unstable or have bleeding, vomiting, or diarrhea in U.S. hospitals, including procedures for donning and doffing PPE. https://www.cdc.gov/vhf/ebola/healthcare-us/ppe/guidance.html. Accessed October 15, 2020.

17. Centers for Disease Control and Prevention. Guidelines for Environmental Infection Control in Health-Care Facilities. https://www.cdc.gov/infectioncontrol/pdf/guidelines/environmental-guidelines-P.pdf. Accessed October 15, 2020.

18. Centers for Disease Control and Prevention. Information on the Survivability of the Ebola Virus in Medical Waste. https://www.cdc.gov/vhf/ebola/clinicians/cleaning/ebola-virus-survivability.html. Accessed October 15, 2020.

19. Victory KR, Coronado F, Ifono SO, et al. Ebola transmission linked to a single traditional funeral ceremony—Kissidougou, Guinea, December, 2014–January 2015. *MMWR Morb Mortal Wkly Rep*. 2015;64:386.

20. Food and Drug Administration. First FDA-approved vaccine for the prevention of Ebola virus disease, marking a critical milestone in public health preparedness and response. https://www.fda.gov/news-events/press-announcements/first-fda-approved-vaccine-prevention-ebola-virus-disease-marking-critical-milestone-public-health. Accessed October 15, 2020.

21. Burki T. DRC getting ready to introduce a second Ebola vaccine. *Lancet Infect Dis*. 2019;19:1174.

22. PREVAIL III Study Group, Sneller MC, Reilly C, et al. A Longitudinal Study of Ebola Sequelae in Liberia. *N Engl J Med*. 2019;380:924.

23. Clark DV, Kibuuka H, Millard M, et al. Long-term sequelae after Ebola virus disease in Bundibugyo, Uganda: a retrospective cohort study. *Lancet Infect Dis*. 2015;15:905.

24. Kelly JD, Hoff NA, Spencer D, et al. Neurological, Cognitive, and Psychological Findings Among Survivors of Ebola Virus Disease From the 1995 Ebola Outbreak in Kikwit, Democratic Republic of Congo: A Cross-sectional Study. *Clin Infect Dis*. 2019;68:1388.

25. Schieffelin JS, Shaffer JG, Goba A, et al. Clinical illness and outcomes in patients with Ebola in Sierra Leone. *N Engl J Med*. 2014;371:2092.

26. Fitzpatrick G, Vogt F, Moi Gbabai OB, et al. The Contribution of Ebola Viral Load at Admission and Other Patient Characteristics to Mortality in a Médecins Sans Frontières Ebola Case Management Centre, Kailahun, Sierra Leone, June–October 2014. *J Infect Dis*. 2015;212:1752.

27. Martini GA. Marburg virus disease. *Postgrad Med J*. 1973;49:542.

28. Glaze ER, Roy MJ, Dalrymple LW, Lanning LL. A Comparison of the Pathogenesis of Marburg Virus Disease in Humans and Nonhuman Primates and Evaluation of the Suitability of These Animal Models for Predicting Clinical Efficacy under the 'Animal Rule' *Comp Med*. 2015;65:241.

29. Centers for Disease Control and Prevention. Marburg Virus Disease. https://www.who.int/news-room/fact-sheets/detail/marburg-virus-disease. Accessed October 15, 2020.

DENGUE, YELLOW FEVER, CHIKUNGUNYA, LASSA FEVER, AND CRIMEAN-CONGO HEMORRHAGIC FEVER

25

Lopa Maharaja, MD

INTRODUCTION

Families of RNA viruses such as *Flaviviridae* (Dengue and Yellow Fever), *Togaviridae* (Chikungunya), *Arenaviridae* (Lassa Fever) and *Bunyaviridae* (Crimean-Congo Hemorrhagic Virus) can lead to hemorrhagic fevers with limited treatment options.

DENGUE

Dengue virus is transmitted by the arthropod *Aedes aegypti* (Figure 25-1) to humans at an increasingly rapid rate, with cases found mostly in warm tropical climates. Reports in the past several years have indicated that this viral infection is no longer being contained to tropical areas and have been reported in the southern border of the United States in Texas and in Hawaii also.[1,2] Data from the World Health Organization (WHO) has identified 796 cases of dengue in the United States during the period of 2001–2007.[2] Dengue virus has caused high morbidity throughout the world. Symptomatic disease has been estimated in as high as 96 million cases of annually reported worldwide infections and overall as high as 390 million dengue viral infections have been reported yearly.[1]

Pathogenesis

Dengue virus is a single stranded RNA genome consisting of seven non-structural proteins (NS1, NS2A, NS2 B, NS3, NS4A, NS4B, and NS5),

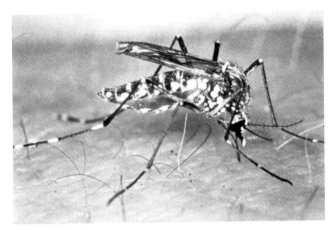

Figure 25-1 • Female Aedes aegypti mosquito. (*Courtesy of the CDC.* https://phil.cdc. gov/Details.aspx?pid=2740.)

structural envelope, membrane, and capsid viral structural proteins[3] (Figure 25-2). The envelope protein plays a key role in the viral pathogenicity with receptor binding, activation of immunological responses, and antibodies as well as agglutination of red cells.[3] NS1 increases vascular permeability through its various interactions with the vascular endothelium, activates of the complement cascade, and the amount of NS1 and Sc5b-9 in serum may be related to severity.[3–5]

Dengue virus has four serotypes (DENV-1, DENV-2, DENV-3, and DENV-4). DENV-2 is associated with Dengue Shock Syndrome.[6–9] Infection from one of the four serotypes does not prevent infection from the other serotypes, but provides immunity from re-infection from the original serotype.[10,11]

Susceptibility to severe infection includes obese persons, females, children and obese persons, females, children, human major-histocompatibility complex class I related sequence B, and phospholipase C epsilon1 genes.[4,11]

Clinical Manifestations

Dengue virus infection becomes symptomatic after 5–7 days of incubation. The clinical state is divided into three phases. The first phase is biphasic febrile illness, which is associated with constitutional symptoms, such as vomiting, malaise, severe headache, pharyngitis, retro-orbital pain, and conjunctivitis with associated flushing, and it lasts for 2–7 days.[4,11] Petechiae, Ecchymosis, and palpable liver can also often be found.[4,11] Most patients improve after fevers resolve.[4,11]

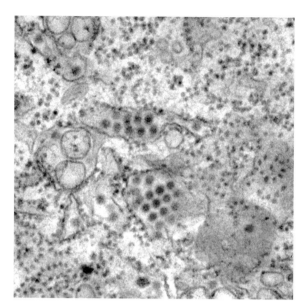

Figure 25-2 • Dengue Virus under transmission electron microscopic image (TEM). (*Courtesy of the CDC*. https://phil.cdc.gov/Details.aspx?pid=12493.)

The second phase begins when the patient defervesces and lasts for 24–48 hours. This is the critical phase, where there is an extensive plasma leakage due to increased capillary permeability and dysfunction.[2] Pleural effusions and ascites can develop subsequent hypotension and DSS with multiorgan dysfunction.[4] Hemorrhagic complications, liver failure, myocarditis, and encephalopathy occur.[4] Significant bleeding from the skin and mucosa can be triggered often with minimal plasma leakage and no inciting factors.[4,7] The last phase is the convalescent phase. This is where the plasma leakage subsides. Improvement with support care will occur within 48–72 hours, but desquamatic and pruritic rash, fatigue, and weakness may persist for several weeks.[4,11]

Dengue is diagnosed if there are ≥ 2 clinical findings in a patient who has traveled to an endemic area. Severe dengue (SD) is suggested if associated with shock or other cardiac dysfunction, pulmonary dysfunction such as respiratory distress, bleeding, elevated liver function test, or altered mental status.

Diagnosis

The febrile illness can be associated with laboratory derangements such as thrombocytopenia and leukopenia.[11] Worsening hematocrit with concurrent worsening thrombocytopenia can be seen as symptoms progress

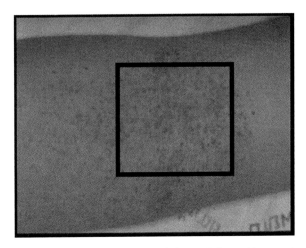

Figure 25-3 • Tourniquet test. (*Courtesy of the CDC.* https://www.cdc.gov/dengue/training/cme/ccm/page73112.html.)

during impending shock.[7] Small rise in the activated partial-thromboplastin time and a decrease in fibrinogen levels are often seen.[7] In shock states, patients may have an increase in white blood cell count with decrease in hematocrit secondary to bleeding.[2] Abnormalities in liver function studies and hypoalbuminemia can be seen.[11]

The Tourniquet test is a marker of capillary fragility, and may suggest dengue. It is performed by taking the patient's blood pressure. Then the cuff is inflated to a point midway between systolic blood pressure (SBP) and diastolic blood pressure (DBP) and maintained for a few minutes. The pressure is slowly reduced and an observation is made after 2 minutes. The number of petechiae below the antecubital fossa is counted and considered positive if ≥ 10 per 1 square inch (Figure 25-3).

If available, serologies can be obtained. In the initial phase of illness up to Day 5, detection of viral antigens by ELISA or viral RNA by nucleic acid amplification tests (NAAT), or virus isolation in cell culture can be performed.[2] Dengue virus and its antigens are likely undetectable after Day 5 of disease onset.[2] IgM levels can persist for up to 6 months and IgG can always remain positive and be used as a marker for previous DENV infection.[2] NS1 antigen detection can persist for a few days after fevers resolve; therefore, it can be used as a diagnostic tool.[2] The sensitivity of NS1 antigen testing detection is lower in patients with prior dengue infections, suggesting immune mediated memory activation.[4]

Management

Supportive care with appropriate resuscitation has to be performed. Full laboratory panels with complete blood counts, and chemistries including liver function studies and lactate should be monitored.[2] Patients not exhibiting the warning signs and tolerating oral intake without signs of significant dehydration, stable hematocrit, white blood cell counts, and platelets can be sent home with vigilant observation by their healthcare providers and home caregivers.[2] These patients should be advised to return to the hospital immediately, if there is any worsening in their clinical status.[2] Individuals with warning signs should be admitted and given intravenous hydration with isotonic solutions and supportive care with close monitoring for severe dengue.[2] Patients with hypotension, organ dysfunction, and lab derangements such as renal failure, changes in hematocrit, platelets or signs of bleeding should be managed in an intensive care unit setting for any organ-specific treatments, transfusion of blood products, and intravenous hydration for treatment of severe dengue/DSS.[2]

The first dengue virus vaccine was licensed by Sanofi Pasteur. The CYD-TDV vaccine or known by its brand name Dengvaxia is a live virus vaccine and was approved by the FDA in May 2019.[12] The vaccine is approved in patients with a prior history of dengue infection.[12] No isolation is needed with dengue infection.

Prognosis

Overall prognosis is good for most patients who recover with adequate oral intake and supportive care.[13] Those patients with risk factors, and presenting with warning signs of progression to SD must be monitored closely.[13] If SD develops, patients have improved outcomes with adequate hydration, and supportive care for associated bleeding and organ dysfunction.[13] Those who do not seek medical attention or delayed in the diagnosis of their febrile illness are more likely to have poor outcomes including death.[13]

▌CHIKUNGUNYA

There have recently been outbreaks of Chikungunya in India, southern United States in the regions of Texas and Florida, Puerto Rico, and the Caribbean Islands.[13–17] *Aedes albopictus* and *Aedes aegypti* are two of the predominant mosquito species associated with transmission.[13–17] Maternal fetal transmission has occurred with transmission rates of up to 50% reported.[18,19]

Pathogenesis

The RNA genome of Chikungunya has the nonstructural protein NSP3 which promotes virulence[13,14,20] (Figure 25-4). Type I Interferon may block viral replication; as suggested by animal models where lack of Interferon Type I signaling was associated with increased viral growth and activity.[14,18] The specific interferon stimulating gene associated with Chikungunya is OAS3, though other ISG likely exist that have not been identified.[14,18]

Clinical Manifestations

Disease manifestations can be divided into acute and chronic. Acute infections occur with intermittent fevers which can be as high as 104°F/40°C starting in the first 2 weeks.[21] They are accompanied by severe joint pains involving the large joints of the upper and lower extremities.[21] Eighty percent of patients will also develop a diffuse, sometimes bullous, full body maculopapular rash between 2nd and 5th of illness.[18,21] Myelitis, neuropathies, encephalitis, hepatitis, myocarditis, conjunctivitis, retinitis, and uveitis have been reported.[18,21] The chronic phase is associated with polyarthralgia lasting for several months to a year or more.[21]

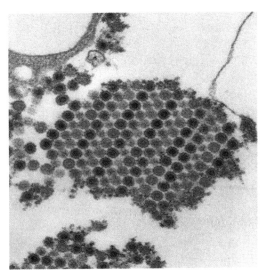

Figure 25-4 • Transmission electron microscopic image of Chikungunya virus shows it is 50 nm in diameter and composed of a central dense core surrounded by viral envelope. (*Courtesy of the CDC.* https://phil.cdc.gov/Details.aspx?pid=17550.)

Diagnosis

Patients with Chikungunya may have hypocalcemia, transaminitis, thrombocytopenia, and lymphopenia.[18] Inflammatory markers and antibody titers can be followed in those with chronic illness.[18]

Diagnosis can be made by serum and cerebrospinal fluid (CSF) PCR, viral culture or paired acute and convalescent antibodies.[18,21] Serum IgM will be positive by Day 5 or sooner.[18,21] IgG titers which rise by 4-fold from acute to convalescent titers is also a positive diagnosis.[18,21] When macrophages and synovial fluid were evaluated in patients showing signs of chronic arthritis the presence of viral proteins and genetic material could be found up to a year and half out from the inciting illness.[22,23]

Treatment

There is no effective vaccine or medication specifically for treating Chikungunya infection. Prevention of mosquito bites is a key method of limiting viral spread and infection.[17] Wearing protective clothing and the use of insecticide and mosquito repellent help to curtail spread of disease.[18] Supportive treatment with nonsteroidal anti-inflammatory drugs (NSAIDS) and acetaminophen are mainstays of therapy.[17] Steroids have been used in those refractory to NSAIDS treatment.[17] For those patients with chronic arthritis and changes similar to rheumatoid arthritis the use of Disease Modifying Anti-Rheumatic Drugs (DMARDS) such as methotrexate has been found to be effective.[24,25] Biologics have also been used and evaluated in severe cases.[26] Antiviral medications have been studied but promising results in human clinical trials have not come to fruition as a successful treatment option.[26] Fingolimod, a drug used in the treatment of multiple sclerosis, has been showing some promise in Chikungunya treatment.[26] Vaccines are currently being researched but none has successfully come to market.[26]

Prognosis

The overall prognosis for survival is good with very few deaths reported.[27] Rare reports of fatalities are associated with those with underlying medical conditions.[18]

▌YELLOW FEVER

Yellow fever is a mosquito-borne (*Aedes aegypti*) illness found in Africa and South America with 200,000 annual cases reported on average.[28–30]

In modern times, outbreaks have been described in Brazil, Angola, and the Democratic Republic of the Congo.[28–30]

Pathogenesis

Yellow fever virus is a single stranded RNA virus and replicates in the cytoplasm of infected cells[31] (Figure 25-5). The virion contains structural proteins (C,M,E) and nonstructural proteins (NS1, NS2A, NS2B, NS3, NS4A, NS4B, and NS5).[32] The E glycoprotein is responsible for membrane binding and activities to promote and prepare for viral invasion of the host cells.[31,32] NS1 has been shown to hamper the host complement cascade.[32,33] NS3 plays a vital part in sustaining the yellow fever life cycle.[32] NS3 and NS5 help create viral replication units on membranes.[32,34]

Clinical Manifestations

Incubation period is 3–6 days.[32] Eighty eight percent of the patients remained asymptomatic or had mild disease and may serve as vectors for

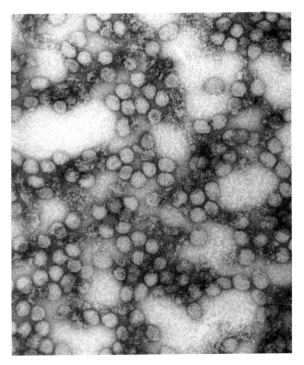

Figure 25-5 • This photogram shows yellow fever virions. (*Courtesy of the CDC.* https://phil.cdc.gov/Details.aspx?pid=8239.)

world-wide transmission.[35] Symptoms include generalized vague symptoms of nausea, vomiting, myalgias, dizziness, and fevers.[31] Individuals can develop Faget's sign with high fevers and bradycardia.[31] This acute phase is a period of infectivity when the virus can be transmitted via a new mosquito bite on the infected person and passed along to a new host.[32]

This is followed by "period of remission" where symptoms will improve and serum antibodies are formed.[32] In approximately 15–25% of infected individuals there will be a secondary phase called "the intoxication phase," in which more severe manifestations of the disease occur.[31] These will have severe vomiting, abdominal pain, liver failure, renal failure, hemorrhagic complications, altered mental status, and shock.[32] Patients can have release of cytokine storms and secondary bacterial infections can occur as well during the "intoxication period."[31] Those who develop the combination of liver and renal dysfunction have higher death rates of up to 50% within 10 days of symptom onset.[31]

For those who survive this phase chronic symptoms can last for several months and are likely to have a slow recovery.[31] These patients will complain of lethargy and feelings of weakness for several weeks as well remaining jaundiced.[31]

Diagnosis

Diagnosis confirmation is by positive IgM titer or evaluation of IgG titers with paired titers, antigen detection by immunohistochemistry or PCR, and positive cultures (Figure 25-6).[32]

Treatment

Treatment is mostly supportive care based on specific organ dysfunction.[31] Animal studies on Ribavirin have not shown benefit.[31] Use of Interferon-γ have only shown some benefit in early post exposure prophylaxis.[31] Prevention is an important component in this disease. A phase 1 clinical trial conducted in Singapore for a monoclonal antibody for yellow fever has demonstrated some promise for potential drug therapy.[36] Participants in this trial were found to have decreased levels of viremia in persons who received the drug, denoting potential for this drug to be used in post or pre exposure prophylaxis.[36] Yellow fever vaccine 17D which is a live vaccine developed from chick embryos has been a highly effective vaccine, possibly providing lifelong immunity after one dose.[31] Vaccine recipients seroconverted; producing neutralizing antibodies within 3 days for 90% of recipients and up to 99% 30 days post vaccination.[31] Vaccination is indicated for travelers who are traveling

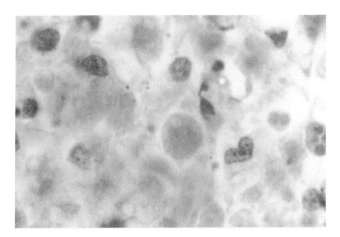

Figure 25-6 • Hematoxylin-eosin stained photograph of liver tissue of yellow fever patient showing cytoarchitectural changes showing councilman bodies from fatty degeneration. Diagnosis confirmation is based on parenchymal disorganization, midzonal necrosis, acidophilic degeneration and the fatty degeneration. (*Courtesy of the CDC.* https://phil.cdc.gov/Details.aspx?pid=13009.)

or living in endemic countries for more than 9 months.[36,37] The World Health Organization has stated that a single dose of vaccine is sufficient for lifelong immunity but ACIP still recommends a booster dose after 10 years in certain situations.[38]

Contraindications for vaccination include: 1) people with egg allergies; 2) infants less than 6 months old; and 3) impaired immune systems secondary to underlying diseases or those requiring administration of medications which can impair immunity.[37] These include individuals with malignancies, organ transplantation, thymus disorders, immunodeficiency syndromes or those taking immuno-modifying or suppressive medications.[37] People older than 60, pregnant or breastfeeding women, and HIV patients who have CD4+ T-lymphocytes greater than 400/mm[3] are advised to discuss the risks and benefits with their healthcare providers.[37]

Vaccine side effects have been widely reported and these include neurological and vaccine associated multiorgan dysfunction.[32] Yellow fever Associated Neurological Disease (YEL-AND) was reported as post vaccination encephalitis found to occur mostly in children less than 7 months of age.[31] Guillain-Barré syndrome, acute disseminated encephalitis, and meningoencephalitis have been described in adults especially those over age 60.[39]

Yellow fever vaccine-associated viscerotropic disease was described in 100 cases of vaccinations in 2001 with noted high levels of viral replication in multiple organs leading to organ dysfunction or failure with some reported deaths.[39] Those older than 70 appear to be more susceptible to this adverse vaccine reaction.[39]

Prognosis

Risk of developing severe disease is low with only 12% of those infected progressing to severe disease.[30] However, those patients who develop multiorgan dysfunction or failure have death rates as high as 50%.[31]

▌ LASSA FEVER

Lassa Fever is a viral illness, which is predominantly found in the West African countries of Nigeria, Sierra Leone, Guinea, and Liberia.[40–42] Reporting estimates suggest up to 300,000 cases annually with 5000 deaths.[40–42] The vector is *Mastomys natalensis*, a multimammate rodent with infection occurring after consumption of these rats or exposure to rat feces or urine.[43] Person-to-person transmission can occur.

Pathogenesis

Lassa virus is a single stranded RNA virus with four different strains.[42,44] It is a fast-replicating virus and the actual mechanism is unknown.[45] It can slow the production of spike proteins, macrophages, and dendritic cells.

Clinical Manifestations

The incubation period is 6–21 days and 80% of patients can be asymptomatic.[44] Symptoms include fever, malaise, headaches, myalgias, pharyngitis, pleurisy, back pain, seizures, altered mental status, sensorineural hearing loss, and hemorrhagic complications.[45–47] The fever can be as high as 40°C, is more prominent toward the day, and can last > 10 days.

Diagnosis

Diagnosis is via ELISA (Enzyme-Linked Immunosorbent Assay) or RT-PCR (Reverse Transcriptase Polymerase Chain Reaction), and tissue cultures can be used to identify the infection.[48] ELISA IgM antibody testing and antigen testing has 88% sensitivity and 90% specificity during the early stages of illness.[48,49] Biopsies maybe necessary.

Treatment

Treatment begins with supportive care and Ribavirin, an antiviral drug which is a guanosine analog that helps to improve disease outcomes by decreasing viral loads when administered during the initial phases of illness.[49] Intravenous administration doubles drug efficacy. Early administration by Day 6 of disease onset can have a dramatic effect on death rates, decreasing them by up to 90%.[44] Oral Ribavirin can be given as post exposure prophylaxis and there is currently no vaccine.[47,48]

CRIMEAN-CONGO HEMORRHAGIC FEVER

Crimean Congo Hemorrhagic Fever (CCHF) a tick-borne illness found in Africa, the Middle East, and Eastern Europe and is caused by the genus *Nairovirus* of the order *Bunyaviridae*.[49] The virus maintains an enzootic tick-vertebrate-tick cycle circulating pattern.[49] The virus is carried by members of the family of hard ticks Ixodidae of which the members of the genus *Hyalomma* are the most common carriers.[49]

Drinking unpasteurized milk and contact with the blood and tissues of infected animals are the methods of transmission.[49] Large outbreaks have occurred in farmers and agricultural workers.[50] Veterinarians and slaughterhouse workers are also two at risk groups.[51] Human to human transmission can occur via contact with mucus membranes, skin sites or bodily fluids of patients with CCHF.[52,53]

Contact with infected bodily fluid and blood of hospitalized individuals with CCHF puts healthcare personnel at risk.[52,54], Injection sites can be a location of viral spread.[53] Outdoor activities such as camping and hiking are also risk factors.[51] Animal trading markets in large city areas can be a high risk location of acquisition as are rural areas.[52,55] Outbreaks have been reported in Eastern Europe (Greece, Turkey, and Georgia) and the Middle East (Iran) in the early 2000s.[52,56,57]

Pathogenesis

CCHF is a negative sense single stranded RNA virus with three genomes: small (S), medium (M), and large (L).[52,58] The medium gene segment of the virus has been found to be important in viral pathogenicity and host immunity.[52,59,60] There are two envelope glycoproteins, Gn and Gc.[52] The Gc glycoprotein is thought to facilitate entry into host cells by binding the host cellular receptors.[52,61] The assembly of new virions occurs at the Golgi membrane of host cells.[52]

CCHF is a fast-replicating virus that attacks Kupffer cells, hepatocytes in the liver, and hepatic endothelial cells.[52] It causes destruction and injury to the host vascular endothelial structure and lymphoid organs.[49] Platelet dysfunction occurs as well as activation of the intrinsic coagulation cascade.[50] DIC is noted as a key component of the disease.[49] Rash can occur secondary to failure of hemostasis due to endothelial injury.[52] Interleukin 6 (IL-6) and tumor necrosis factor-alpha (TNF-α) is key to severity.[49,62]

Clinical Manifestations

There are four phases: incubation, pre hemorrhagic, hemorrhagic, and convalescent period.[49] Incubation periods range from 3 to 7 days.[49] The pre hemorrhagic phase consists of fevers, myalgias, headaches, nausea, diarrhea, abdominal pain, facial and trunk hyperemia, and conjunctivitis.[49,50] The hemorrhagic phase occurs around days 3–6 with petechiae and ecchymosis and overt hemorrhage of multiple organs and mucus membranes in the oropharyngeal cavity and gastrointestinal tract[52] (Figure 25-7). Hepatomegaly and splenomegaly can occur in up to a third of infected individuals.[62,63] The convalescent stage occurs between days 10 and 20 of illness.[49] During this stage infected individuals have described varied symptoms of tachycardia, labile pulse, xerostomia, alopecia, dyspnea, polyneuritis, changes in vision and hearing and memory loss.[62,63] Recovery from this illness can be slow and take up to 1 year.[52] Mortality can range from 9 to 50% in hospitalized patients.[64]

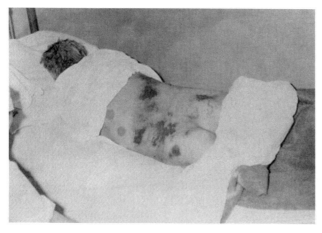

Figure 25-7 • Blotchy, cutaneous lesions over back and buttocks in a patient infected with Crimean-Congo hemorrhagic fever. (*Courtesy of the CDC.* https://phil.cdc.gov/Details.aspx?pid=2315.)

Diagnosis

Diagnosis is via PCR or viral culture. Antibodies for IgG/IgM will usually become positive after Day 7 of infection.[50,65] IgG levels remain positive for as long as 5 years, but IgM levels may decline a few months after infection to undetectable at 4 months in some cases.[50]

Treatment

Supportive care is key. Ribavirin can be used to treat severe cases of CCHF.[50,66]

REFERENCES

1. Bhatt S, Gething PW, Brady OJ, et al. The global distribution and burden of dengue. *Nature*. 2013;496(7446):504-507.
2. World Health Organization. *Dengue: Guidelines for Diagnosis, Treatment, Prevention and Control*. Geneva: World Health Organization; 2009:1-147.
3. Guzman M, Halstead S, Artsob H, et al. Dengue: a continuing global threat. *Nat Rev Microbiol*. 2010;8:S7-S16.
4. Simmons C, Farrar JJ, Van Vinh Chau N, et al. Current Concepts in Dengue. *N Engl J Med*. 2012;366:1423-1432.
5. Avirutnan P, Punyadee N, Noisakran S, et al. Vascular leakage in severe dengue virus infections: a potential role for the nonstructural viral protein NS1 and complement. *J Infect Dis*. 2006;193:1078-1088.
6. Vaughn DW, Green S, Kalayanarooj, et al. Dengue in the Early Febrile Phase: Viremia and Antibody Responses. *J Infect Dis*. 1997;176:322.
7. Burke DS, Nisalak A, Johnson DE, Scott RM. A Prospective Study of Dengue Infections in Bangkok. *Am J Trop Med Hyg*. 1988;38(1):172.
8. Sangkawibha N, Rojanasuphot S, Ahandrik S, et al. Risk factors in dengue shock syndrome: a prospective epidemiologic study in Rayong, Thailand. I. The 1980 outbreak. *Am J Epidemiol*. 1984;120(5):653.
9. Martina BE, Koraka P, Osterhaus AD. Dengue virus pathogenesis: an integrated view. *Clin Microbiol Rev*. 2009;22(4):564.
10. Gubler JD. Dengue and Dengue Hemorrhagic Fever. *Clin Microbiol Rev*. 1998;11(3):480-486.
11. Wilder Smith A, Ooi EE, Horstick O, Wills B. Dengue. *Lancet*. 2019;393:350-363.
12. US. Food and Drug Administration. https://www.fda.gov/news-events/press-announcements/first-fda-approved-vaccine-prevention-dengue-disease-endemic-regions. Updated May 1, 2019. Accessed November 1, 2020.
13. Schwartz O, Albert ML. Biology and pathogenesis of chikungunya virus. *Nat Rev Microbiol*. 2010;8:491-500.

14. Burt FJ, Chen W, Miner JJ, et al. Chikungunya virus: an update on the biology and pathogenesis of this emerging pathogen. *Lancet Infect Dis.* 2017;17(4):e107-e117.

15. Lindsey NP, Staples JE, Fischer M. Chikungunya Virus Disease among Travelers—United States, 2014–2016. *Am J Trop Med Hyg.* 2018;98(1):192-197.

16. Centers for Disease Control and Prevention. Notes from the field: chikungunya virus spreads in the Americas—Caribbean and South America, 2013–2014. *MMWR Morb Mortal Wkly Rep.* 2014;63:500-501.

17. Centers for Disease Control and Prevention. Chikungunya Virus in the United States. https://www.cdc.gov/chikungunya/geo/united-states.html. Updated June 4, 2020. Accessed January 27, 2021.

18. Weaver S, Lecuit M. Chikungunya Virus and the Global Spread of a Mosquito-Borne Disease. *N Engl J Med.* 2015;372:1231-1239.

19. Gérardin P, Barau G, Michault A, et al. Multidisciplinary prospective study of mother-to-child chikungunya virus infections on the island of La Réunion. *PLoS Med.* 2008;5(3):e60.

20. Panas MD, Ahola T, McInerney GM. The C-terminal repeat domains of nsP3 from the Old World alphaviruses bind directly to G3BP. *J Virol.* 2014;88:5888-5893.

21. World Health Organization. Guidelines for Prevention and control of Chikungunya fever. https://www.who.int/publications/i/item/guidclines-for-prevention-and-control-of-chikungunya-fever. Updated December 27, 2019. Accessed November 1, 2020.

22. Silva Jr JVJ, Ludwig-Begall LF, de Oliveira-Filho EF et al. A scoping review of Chikungunya virus infection: epidemiology, clinical characteristics, viral co-circulation complications and control. *Acta Tropica.* 2018;188:213-224.

23. Horarau JJ, Bandjee MCH, Trotot PK, et al. Persistent Chronic Inflammation and infection by Chikungunya arthritogenic alphavirus in spite of a robust host immune response. *J. Immunol.* 2010;184(10):5914-5927.

24. Sales GMPG. Treatment of Chikungunya Chronic Arthritis: A Systematic Review. *Rev Assoc Med Bras.* 2018;64(1):63-70.

25. Ribeiro AMBM, Pimentel CM, Guerra ACCG, Lima MRO. Physiotherapeutic approach on the late phase of chikungunya: a case report. *Rev Bras Saúde Matern Infant.* 2016;16(Suppl 1):S57-S62.

26. Suhrbier A. Rheumatic manifestations of chikungunya: emerging concepts and interventions. *Nat Rev Rheumatol.* 2019;15:597-611.

27. Josseran L, Paquet C, Zehgnoun A, et al. Chikungunya disease outbreak, Reunion Island. *Emerg Infect Dis.* 2006;12:1994-1995.

28. Staples JE, Barrett ADT, Wilder-Smith A, et al. Review of data and knowledge gaps regarding yellow fever vaccine-induced immunity and duration of protection. *NPJ Vaccines.* 2020;5(1):54.

29. Centers for Disease Control and Prevention. https://www.cdc.gov/global-health/newsroom/topics/yellowfever/index.html. Updated September 14, 2018. Accessed January 27, 2021.

30. Johansson MA, Arana-Vizcarrondo N, Biggerstaff BJ, Staples JE. Incubation Periods of Yellow Fever Virus. *Am J Trop Med Hyg.* 2010;83(1):183-188.

31. Monath T. Yellow Fever and Update. *Lancet. Infectious Diseases*. 2001;1:11-20.

32. Gardner CL, Ryman KD. Yellow Fever: A Reemerging Threat. *Clin Lab Med*. 2010;30(1):237-260.

33. Chung KM, Liszewski MK, Nybakken G, et al. West Nile virus nonstructural protein NS1 inhibits complement activation by binding the regulatory protein factor H. *Proc Natl Acad Sci U S A*. 2006;103(50):19111-19116.

34. Lindenbach BD, Rice CM. Molecular biology of flaviviruses. *Adv Virus Res*. 2003;59:23-61.

35. Johansson MA, Vasconcelos PF, Staples JE. The whole iceberg: estimating the incidence of yellow fever virus infection from the number of severe cases. *Trans R Soc Trop Med Hyg*. 2014;108(8):482-487.

36. Low JG, Ng JHJ, Ong EZ, et al. Phase 1 Trial of a Therapeutic Anti-Yellow Fever Virus Human Antibody. *N Engl J Med*. 2020;383:452-459.

37. Centers for Disease Control and Prevention. www.cdc.gov/yellowfever/vaccine/vaccine-recommendations.html. Updated December 18, 2020. Accessed January 27, 2021.

38. World Health Organization. Yellow Fever. https://www.who.int/ith/vaccines/yf/en/. Updated 2021. Accessed January 27, 2021.

39. Gershman MD, Staples JE. Chapter 4: Travel-Related Infectious Diseases. Centers for Disease Control and Prevention. wwwnc.cdc.gov/travel/yellow-book/2020/travel-related-infectious diseases/yellow-fever. Updated December 18, 2020. January 27, 2021.

40. Centers for Disease Control and Prevention. Lassa Fever. www.cdc.gov/vhf/lassa/index.html. Updated January 31, 2019. Accessed January 27, 2021.

41. Omeh DJ, Achinge GI, Echekwube PO. Lassa Fever in West Africa: A Clinical and Epidemiological Review. *JAMMR*. 2017;24(6):1-12.

42. Ogbu O, Ajuluchukwu E, Uneke CJ. Lassa fever in West African sub-region: An overview. *J Vect Borne Dis*. 2007;44:1-11.

43. McCormick JB, Webb PA, Krebs JW, Johnson KM, Smith ES. A prospective study of the epidemiology and ecology of Lassa fever. *J Infect Dis*. 1987;155(3):437-444.

44. Richmond JK, Baglole DJ. Lassa fever: epidemiology, clinical features, and social consequences. *BMJ*. 2003;327:1271-1275.

45. Yun NE, Walker DH. Pathogenesis of Lassa Fever. *Viruses*. 2012;4:2031-2048.

46. Cummins D, et al. Acute sensorineural deafness in Lassa fever. *JAMA*. 1990;264:2093-2096.

47. Hallam HJ, Hallam S, Rodriguez SE, et al. Baseline Mapping of Lassa Fever Virology, Epidemiology and Vaccine research and Development. *NPJ Vaccines*. 2018;3:11.

48. Bausch DG, Rollin PE, Demby AH, et al. Diagnosis and clinical virology of Lassa fever as evaluated by enzyme-linked immunosorbent assay, indirect fluorescent-antibody test, and virus isolation. *J Clin Microbiol*. 2000;38:2670-2677.

49. Appannanavar SB, Mishra B. An Update on Crimean Congo Hemorrhagic Fever. *J Glob Infect Dis*. 2011;3(3):285-292.

50. Ergönül O. Crimean-Congo haemorrhagic fever. *Lancet Infect Dis*. 2006;6:203.

51. www.who.int/news-room/fact-sheets/detail/crimean-congo-haemorrhagic-fever.

52. Shayan S, Bokaean M, Shahrivar MR, Chinikar S. Crimean-Congo Hemorrhagic Fever. *Lab Med.* Summer 2015;46:180-189.

53. Yolcu S, Kader C, Kayipmaz AE, Ozbay S, Erbay A. Knowledge levels regarding Crimean-Congo hemorrhagic fever among emergency healthcare workers in an endemic region. *J Clin Med Res.* 2014;6(3):197-204.

54. Celikbas AK, Dokuzoğuz B, Baykam N, et al. Crimean-Congo hemorrhagic fever among health care workers, Turkey. *Emerg Infect Dis.* 2014;20(3):477-479.

55. Izadi S, Holakouie-Naieni K, Majdzadeh S, et al. Seroprevalence of Crimean-Congo hemorrhagic fever in Sistan-va-Baluchestan province of Iran. *Jpn J Infect Dis.* 2006;59(5):326-328.

56. Maltezou HC, Andonova L, Andraghetti R, et al. Crimean- Congo hemorrhagic fever in Europe: current situation calls for preparedness. *Euro Surveill.* 2010;15(10):19504.

57. Mertens M, Schmidt K, Ozkul A, Groschup MH. The impact of Crimean-Congo hemorrhagic fever virus on public health. *Antiviral Res.* 2013;98(2):248-260.

58. Chinikar S, Persson S-M, Johansson M, et al. Genetic analysis of Crimean-Congo hemorrhagic fever virus in Iran. *J Med Virol.* 2004;73(3):404-411.

59. Papa A, Ma B, Kouidou S, Tang Q, Hang C, Antoniadis A. Genetic characterization of the M RNA segment of Crimean Congo hemorrhagic fever virus strains, China. *Emerg Infect Dis.* 2002;8(1):50-53.

60. Peyrefitte CN, Perret M, Garcia S, et al. Differential activation profiles of Crimean-Congo hemorrhagic fever virus- and Dugbe virus-infected antigen-presenting cells. *J Gen Virol.* 2010;91(1):189-198.

61. Erickson BR, Deyde V, Sanchez AJ, Vincent MJ, Nichol ST. N-linked glycosylation of Gn (but not Gc) is important for Crimean Congo hemorrhagic fever virus glycoprotein localization and transport. *Virology.* 2007;361(2):348-355.

62. Ergonul O, Tuncbilek S, Baykam N, Celikbas A, Dokuzoguz B. Evaluation of Serum Levels of Interleukin (IL)-6, IL-10, and tumor necrosis factor-alpha in patients with Crimean-Congo hemorrhagic fever. *J Infect Dis.* 2006;193:941-944.

63. Hoogstraal H. The epidemiology of tick borne Crimean-Congo hemorrhagic fever in Asia, Europe, and Africa. *J Med Entomol.* 1979;15:307-417.

64. www.cdc.gov/vhf/crimean-congo/symptoms/index.html.

65. Shepherd AJ, Swanepoel R, Leman PA. Antibody response in Crimean-Congo hemorrhagic fever. *Rev Infect Dis.* 1989;11:S801-S806.

66. Ergonul O, Celikbas A, Dokuzoguz B, Eren S, Baykam N, Esener H. The characteristics of Crimean-Congo hemorrhagic fever in a recent outbreak in Turkey and the impact of oral ribavirin therapy. *Clin Infect Dis.* 2004;39:284-287.

26 NIPAH, HENDRA, AND RIFT VALLEY FEVER VIRUSES

Jodi Galaydick, MD, MPH

▌INTRODUCTION

The possibility of zoonotic infections causing pandemics has been a concern for decades. Nipah virus (NiV), Hendra virus (HeV), and Rift Valley fever virus (RVFV) are all zoonotic infections that can cause encephalitis in humans, sometimes fatally. In this chapter we will discuss these viruses and their effects on humans along with proper infection control measures.

▌NIPAH VIRUS

Epidemiology and Risk Factors

The Nipah virus (NiV) causes a zoonotic infection which was first described in Sungai Nipah village in Malaysia in 1998[1] (Figure 26-1). Nipah virus is an enveloped single stranded RNA virus and is a part of the *Henipavirus* genus and *Paramyxoviridae* family. The virus ranges from 120 to 500 nm in diameter. The first outbreak occurred in Malaysia in 1999. NiV and HeV have only minor ultrastructural differences and have significant cross reactivity on serological tests.[2,3]

Both NiV and HeV are transmitted by specific fruit bats known as flying foxes, from the *Pteropus* genus. Flying foxes are endemic to Asia, China, Australia, some parts of Africa and the Pacific islands.[4] Infected bats shed NiV and HeV in their saliva, urine, semen, and excreta but are asymptomatic carriers. Infection in humans occurs through contact with flying fox urine, saliva, secretions or an intermediate host like pigs through contact with sick animals or animal products.[4]

Outbreaks of NiV have occurred in humans in Malaysia, Singapore, Bangladesh, India, and the Philippines. Outbreaks in Bangladesh and India appear to happen on an almost annual basis. The outbreaks in Malaysia and Singapore were thought to be through direct contact with NiV-infected pigs and their products. In the Malaysian and Singaporean

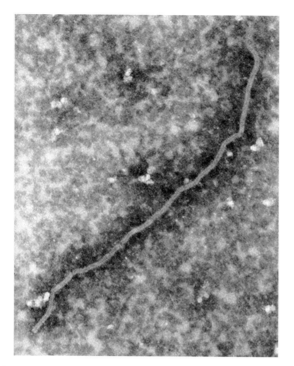

Figure 26-1 • Negative stain transmission electron microscopy of Nipah virus. (*Courtesy of the CDC.* https://phil.cdc.gov/Details.aspx?pid=8256.)

outbreaks 92% of infections were associated with pigs. Pigs likely become infected through ingestion of food contaminated by flying fox secretions. Dogs were also found to be infected during the Malaysian and Singaporean outbreaks and dogs dying on farms was found to be another risk factor.[5] Control of the outbreak led to culling over a million pigs followed by its disposal by deep burial and decontamination with quick lime, use of protective equipment when handling contaminated animal products, and banning animal trade during the outbreak.[2] Person-to-person transmission was not proven experimentally in the outbreaks in Malaysia or Singapore.

In the Bangladesh's and India's outbreaks there was no clear evidence of infection via pigs and it appeared that the outbreaks were seasonal.[2] Infections likely occurred through consumption of raw date palm sap or consumption of fruits contaminated by flying fox secretions. The outbreaks seemed to coincide with the sap harvesting (December–May).[6] There was strong evidence of person-to-person transmission found in the Bangladesh outbreaks. Transmission likely occurred via droplets.[7] India also saw a significant transmission of infections from person to person with transmission occurring in healthcare settings in some places.[8] The Philippines outbreak also occurred in 2014 which appeared to be related to horses and possible horse meat consumption. Seventeen cases were found. Person-to-person transmission was also noted in this outbreak.[9]

Pathogenesis

Infection with NiV occurs when the virus enters via the oronasal route. It is unclear where initial replication occurs, but postmortem studies show high levels of antigen in the lymphoid and respiratory tissues, likely the early sites of replication. The virus then enters the bloodstream and is followed by replication in the endothelium. The NiV primary infection involves the blood vessels in the form of vasculopathy and vasculitis resulting from perivascular cellular infiltration, inflammation, and necrosis. A high viremia likely results in cytokines and chemokines being released causing vascular damage.[10] The glycoprotein G of NiV binds to the cellular receptor Ephrin-B2 which is expressed on the endothelium and smooth muscle cells.[2]

Clinical Manifestations

The incubation period for NiV is 4 to 21 days; however, in some cases the incubation period may extend up to 4 months or more. Clinical manifestations can range from asymptomatic disease to severe acute encephalitis and respiratory failure which is highly fatal.[2] Typically, people have a short incubation period followed by fever, headache, and myalgia. Encephalitis symptoms occur typically in 1 week which consist of altered mental status, areflexia, hypotonia, segmental myoclonus, gaze palsy, and limb weakness. Patient typically will quickly deteriorate and fall into a coma followed by death in a few days.[2] Another clinical manifestation is respiratory disease which can also lead to increased morbidity and mortality. Respiratory involvement was more common in the outbreaks in Bangladesh and India. Respiratory symptoms could be cough, atypical pneumonia, and respiratory distress which could lead to respiratory failure and Acute respiratory distress syndrome (ARDS). A higher mortality was seen in Bangladesh and India than in Malaysia and Singapore.[2] Cardiac involvement has also been suggested as myocarditis in some literature.

Diagnosis

NiV can be diagnosed using multiple methods. The best for diagnosis is polymerase chain reaction (PCR) due to its high sensitivity and specificity.

The US Centers for Disease Control and Prevention (CDC) has developed a conventional PCR targeting the N gene; PCR can be used for tissue samples, swabs, CSF, and urine.[1] RT-PCR can be also be used for respiratory secretions, urine, and CSF and is also highly reliable. Immunochemistry may be used on tissue, typically the brain, lung, spleen, kidney, and lymph nodes. Viral culture can also be done but requires a BSL-4 laboratory. Typical specimens used are respiratory secretions, urine and CSF, other tissue specimens can also be used. Antibody testing with IgM and IgG can be useful. ELISA is the most commonly used test for serologic diagnosis. It is rapid, extremely sensitive, easy, and safe to use. IgM antibodies have been found in 50% of patients on Day 1 of illness while IgG antibodies are positive in 100% of patients after Day 18. IgG antibodies are positive for several months.[2] Detection of IgM in the serum or CSF can be useful for diagnosis; whereas detection of IgG can be used for surveillance and for identification of reservoir animals.[2] The gold standard test is a serum neutralization test for diagnosis, but this must be carried out in a BSL-4 laboratory since live virus is required to complete the test.

Treatment

Treatment is primarily supportive, in cases of severe coma or respiratory failure, mechanical ventilation along with intensive care management is required. Experimental treatment has been tried with Ribavirin; it has in vitro effectiveness but in human studies and animal models it has not been found to be effective. In the absence of effective therapy Ribavirin is used in India. Adult oral dosing typically is a 2000 mg loading dose, days 1–4 1000 mg q6h, and day 5–10 500 mg q6h. Dosing for children is weight based; loading dose 20 mg/kg, days 1–4 15 mg/kg q6h and days 5–10 7.5 mg/kg q6h. Intravenous dosing follows the same weight-based recommendations for adults and children. Other experimental drugs include favipiravir which has been shown to be useful in animal models and the use of human monoclonal antibodies targeting viral glycoproteins for post exposure prophylaxis is also being studied.[10] As of 2020, there are 13 vaccines in preclinical stages.

Prevention

Due to the human to human transmission infection control is of vital importance. Respiratory and fomite transmission means that isolation requires standard, contact, and droplet precautions. Personal protective equipment required would be gown, gloves, and surgical mask when caring for patients or handling contaminated products. Infection control practices for NIV may also require airborne precautions in certain circumstances such as aerosolizing procedures, in these cases a particle respirator such as an N95 mask or powered air purifying respirator (PAPR) should be worn along with gowns and gloves. It is unclear how long people are infected for but it is presumed to be 21 days and it is recommended patients remain in isolation for 21 days after confirmation of infection.[10] Research on NiV requires Biosafety Level 4 laboratory conditions which makes study difficult in resource-poor countries. Also, restriction of movement for sick animals and culling of infected animals during outbreaks have been used to decrease transmission. Disinfectants that will kill NiV include 2% domestic bleach solutions, 75% ethanol, quaternary ammonia, and 6% formulated hydrogen peroxide.[10] Dry heat and steam autoclave have also shown to kill NiV.[11]

Complications and Prognosis

In patients who survive, 20% have neurologic deficits that range from fatigue, focal neurologic deficits, and depression. There have been cases of relapsing or late onset NiV encephalitis.[12] NiV has a case fatality rate of 40 to 75% depending on the outbreak. This can vary based on the local capabilities for surveillance and clinical management.

▌HENDRA VIRUS

Epidemiology

The Hendra virus (HeV) belongs to the genus *Henipavirus* and *Paramyxoviridae* family and is also an enveloped single stranded RNA virus. Transmission electron microscope shows it to be 280 nm in diameter. It was first described in 1994 when it was first seen as a severe respiratory disease in horses resulting in 14 deaths from 21 infected horses; in this outbreak a trainer and a stable hand who both had close contact with sick horses were infected, the trainer unfortunately died.[13] Australia has seen regular outbreaks of HeV in horses and seven infections in humans have occurred between 1994 and 2013 with four people dying.[14] Horses and humans develop severe respiratory diseases.

The reservoir of HeV is the same as NiV which are fruit bats, specifically the flying fox. Horses likely become infected though contamination of horse feed, pasture or vegetation by bat urine/reproductive products of bats. Infection in humans appears to only occur via contact with infected secretions from sick horses, no human-to-human or bat-to-human transmission has been reported.[15] Outbreaks also appear to have a seasonal component to them with most outbreaks occurring in the months of June, July, August, and September.[15]

Pathogenesis

Incubation is usually 48 hours to 16 days in most of the cases but periods of incubation may extend up to 4 months or more. The exact mode of transmission is unknown but it is thought that infection occurs via contact or droplet transmission. In cases till date infection seemed to occur after direct contact with nasal or oral secretions and by other equine tissues and fluids, or by droplet transmission. Horses are considered to present the most risk to humans 72 hours prior to the onset of symptoms.[14] It is thought that replication may occur in the upper respiratory tract or nasopharynx. Viremia occurs rapidly after the onset of fever and signs of systemic illness develop after HeV replication begins to occur in other organs—pulmonary system, central nervous system.[16]

Clinical Manifestations

Symptoms include an influenza-like illness and respiratory symptoms, neurologic symptoms are also common. The first two human infections presented with a influenza-like illness and respiratory symptoms.[13] The third patient had mild meningoencephalitis originally; he recovered but 13 months later he developed seizures and severe encephalitis and died.[17] Two cases had occurred that had self-limiting influenza-like illness. Three cases had occurred who had influenza-like illness followed by encephalitis; one recovered, two died.[14]

Diagnosis

The initial signs and symptoms are non-specific, and the diagnosis is usually missed. Similar to NiV, diagnosis for HeV can be made via real time PCR from bodily fluids, antibody testing with ELISA, and cell viral culture.[14]

Treatment and Prevention

Currently there is no approved treatment for HeV infection. As with NiV, Ribavirin has been used with mixed results in patients with HeV, in some studies it has been shown to reduce viral load while others showed treatment with Ribavirin to be unsuccessful.[15,18] The strongest means of protection currently available is vaccination based on the G glycoprotein in horses which has been available since 2012 in Australia. Limiting horses' exposure to flying foxes has also been utilized. The use of human monoclonal antibodies after exposure is another area of study.[19]

Infection Control

Currently no human to human transmission has been reported but appropriate infection control practices should be enforced. The exact mode of transmission from horses is unknown but it is thought that infection occurs via contact or droplet transmission and in cases of aerosolizing procedures airborne transmission is of concern. Because of these factors, PPE is recommended for possible exposure to blood/bodily fluids include gloves, gown/overalls, rubber boots, eye protection, and fluid resistant mask, and any aerosol generating procedures would require a partial respirator or PAPR. Any animal showing signs or symptoms should be quarantined.

Although no human to human cases have been documented, but there is evidence of NiV transmission from human to human, and as both viruses are very similar there is the potential for similar transmission in the Hendra virus.[14] Disinfectants that will kill HeV include 2% domestic bleach solutions, 75% ethanol, quaternary ammonia, and 6% formulated hydrogen peroxide.[10] Dry heat and steam autoclave have also shown to kill HeV.[11]

Complications and Prognosis

With few human cases thus far understanding of post-infection complications is incomplete. There have been reported cases of relapsing encephalitis. The case fatality rate is high where of the seven human infections four people died.[18]

▌ RIFT VALLEY FEVER

Epidemiology

Rift Valley fever virus (RVFV) is a negative-sense RNA enveloped virus 80–120 nm in size and causes an acute viral hemorrhagic fever. It is a *Phlebovirus* in the *Phenuiviridae* family (formerly *Bunyaviridae*) (Figure 26-2). Rift Valley fever virus was first recognized in 1930 near Lake Naivasha in Rift Valley, Kenya, and now it is found in multiple African countries and the Arabian Peninsula.[20] The largest RVFV outbreak on record occurred in Egypt from 1977 to 1979 which resulted in 598

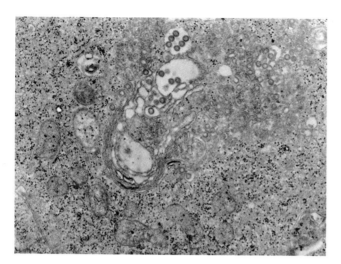

Figure 26-2 • Transmission electron microscopic image of Rift Valley Fever virus, depicted here as spherical shape viral particles. (*Courtesy of the CDC.* https://phil.cdc.gov/Details.aspx?pid=8242.)

deaths out of an estimated 200,000 cases.[21]. More recent outbreaks have occurred in 2008 in Sudan with 747 human cases and 230 deaths and in Niger and East Africa in 2016 with multiple deaths.[22] The first outbreak of RVFV outside the African continent occurred in 2000 in Saudi Arabia and in Yemen. In Saudi Arabia there were 123 deaths in 880 laboratory confirmed cases and in Yemen there were 166 deaths out of 1328 cases.[23] These outbreaks cause substantial animal death and result in significant socioeconomic consequences. The subsequent reduction in production has cost millions of dollars in economic loss.

The vectors in this disease appear to be mosquitoes, most commonly *Aedes* and *Culex* mosquitoes. Other arthropods have been shown to carry the disease, but it is unclear if they can transmit to humans. Mosquitoes transmit the disease to wildlife and livestock; sheep are more at risk than other species. Epidemics tend to occur during the rainy season due to increased population of mosquitoes. Because of the relationship between rainfall and changes in vegetation, outbreaks can sometimes be predicted.[20] The virus spread from female mosquitoes to their offspring through the eggs. In the eggs the virus remains viable for several years during dry conditions and the eggs will hatch when the rainy season arrives. Mosquitoes then spread the virus to wildlife, livestock, and to a lesser extent humans. Most human infections occur from handling of infected animals. Direct transfer between animals appears to be rare if not non-existent and younger animals seem to be more likely to succumb to disease than adults. Unlike animals most human infections are attributed to contact with infected tissues or fluids of infected animals and a small number come from mosquito bites. There has not been any documented evidence for direct human-to-human transmission even during epidemics and in hospital settings with suboptimal personal protective equipment.[24] Infection with RVFV has occurred in laboratories where workers appear to have been infected via aerosolization.[25] Vertical transmission in animals especially livestock is common, typically the first sign of an outbreak is large numbers of abortions in pregnant sheep termed "abortion storms" and experimental models have demonstrated that RVFV can directly infect human placental tissue.[26,27] In a rodent model vertical transmission occurred in both sick and asymptomatic rats, with pregnant animals being more prone to death than their non-pregnant counterparts but similar outcomes have not been seen in humans. The placenta in the rat model appeared to be a major site of replication.[28] In human population those more at risk of infection tend to be adults and those exposed to animals (herders).

Pathogenesis

Humans become infected with RVFV when infected mosquitoes bite and inoculate and the virus travels throughout the body via regional lymph nodes. Early viral replication occurs in lymph nodes resulting in viremia and spread via blood. Further replication occurs in the target organs which include the liver, spleen, and the brain.[29] Involvement of the liver can cause a fulminant hepatitis and abnormal coagulation leading to disseminated intravascular coagulopathy. Active viral replication in the brain can lead to necrotizing encephalitis. The virus has been demonstrated in the blood during the febrile period which is usually during the first 3–4 days, whereas neutralizing antibodies start to appear on the 4th day of symptoms.[30] RVFV encodes for several virulence factors, the most important is the NSs protein which helps the virus evade the host innate immune response.[30]

Clinical Manifestations

Most humans develop asymptomatic or mild disease. The incubation period is between 2 and 6 days. The typical presentation includes headache, fever, backache, and generalized muscle joint pain usually lasting between 4 and 7 days.[4,17,35,36] Less than 8–10% of symptomatic cases develop severe disease which is represented by ocular, hemorrhagic or neurologic symptoms. Morbidity and mortality vary from one outbreak to another. In recent outbreaks severe cases of RVFV may have represented up to 20% cases.[31] Risk factors for infection seem to be related to direct animal contact and slaughter. Adults seem to be more susceptible than children. Immunocompromised patients or patients with coinfections with other pathogens seem to lead to more severe disease. Viremic loads have been reported to correlate to more severe disease. Acute malaria co-occurrence was observed in severe forms and HIV-positive status was associated with a 75% case fatality rate in Tanzania in 2007. Schistosomal liver involvement and other bacterial and fungal infections were also seen in fatal cases.[32]

Severe Disease

- **Hepatitis, jaundice and hemorrhagic disease**—Hemorrhagic disease appears usually within 2 to 4 days after the onset of disease; the liver is the primary site of replication and is frequently involved early in severe disease. This can cause liver failure and jaundice in the first 3 weeks. Elevated liver enzymes and jaundice is associated with a higher mortality. A decrease in hemoglobin and platelets, along with other coagulation factors can lead to disseminated intravascular coagulation.[33] Thrombosis may also be seen with severe disease.[32] Hemorrhage may consist of melena hematemesis, petechial/purpuric rash, bleeding from the gums, nose, menorrhagia or bleeding from IV sites.[25,33] Patients with hemorrhagic fever also have a high fatality rate up to 65% and death usually occurs within a week or two.[32,33]

- **Ocular disease**—Ocular disease is another manifestation of severe disease, it occurs in 2–10% of infections.[32] Disease can be unilateral or bilateral. It can typically occur 1–3 weeks from onset of disease.[25] The most common lesions tend to be macular and paramacular retinitis. Symptoms include photophobia, reduced vision, and blind spots. Symptoms resolve spontaneously in 10 to 12 weeks but macular or paramacular scarring, vascular occlusions, and post-infection optic atrophy associated to the central scarring and can lead to decreased vision or blindness.[20,32]

- **Encephalitis and neurological disease**—Meningoencephalitis can occur 1 to 4 weeks after symptoms first appear. It may be mild or subclinical. Some cases of RVFV have had neurologic symptoms occur up to 60 days after the initial symptoms. Clinical features may be headache, focal neurologic deficit, rigor, neck rigidity, hyperreflexia, hypersalivation, choreiform movements, loss of memory, hallucinations, confusion, disorientation, vertigo, convulsions, ataxia, lethargy, decerebrate posturing, locked-in syndrome and coma.[20,25,33,34] Death in encephalitis is rare but neurological deficits may be severe and long-lasting.[20]

Diagnosis

Diagnosis in the acute stages of RVFV can be done via ELISA to detect IgM toward RVFV antigens.[35] Molecular methods such as RT-PCR can also be used to detect viral RNA which is highly sensitive and specific. The virus can also be isolated via cell culture from the blood during the febrile stage or from organ samples taken post-mortem.[20] Also, histopathological methods can be used in post-mortem examination of the liver for hepatic lesions. To evaluate for prior exposure to RVFV, viral neutralization assays are the gold standard and are highly sensitive and specific but must be done in specialized laboratory settings.

Treatment and Prevention

Most cases are asymptomatic and do not require treatment. For severe cases supportive care is the only treatment available. Ribavirin was used in the 2000 outbreak in Saudi Arabia but was stopped due to possible increase in neurologic disease.[20] Ribavirin and favipiravir have shown efficacy in rodent models.[25] Due to lack of antiviral treatment for RVFV, vaccination is of great interest. All species infected with RVFV are protected by long-lived neutralizing antibodies which can be detected within the first week post-infection.[20] Animal vaccinations are the primary mechanism to prevent disease in animals and thus transmission to humans. Different types of vaccines are available for use in animals. Inactivated vaccines have not been practical for use due to the need for multiple doses. A modified live vaccine (the Smithburn vaccine) is one of the oldest and most widely used vaccines for RVFV in Africa. The vaccine only requires a single dose but use in pregnant livestock has caused birth defects and abortions. The vaccine may also only provide limited protection in cattle.[25] There are several vaccines under development and being studied—MP-12 has shown encouraging results in laboratory trials in domesticated animals and the live attenuated Clone 13 vaccine was recently registered and used in South Africa.[25]

Infection Control

Standard precautions are required when managing patients with RVFV. Hand hygiene is a major component and one of the most effective methods to prevent transmission. A study of the 2000 Arabian Peninsula outbreak did not show significant nosocomial spread and concluded that standard precautions are sufficient for healthcare workers exposed to RVFV patients; this is in contrast with other viral hemorrhagic fevers such as Ebola.[24] The CDC recommends that standard contact and droplet precautions with eye protection should be used with hemorrhagic fever viruses. These would include gloves, gown, and goggles. In resource-poor countries outbreaks have been controlled with basic hygiene, barrier precautions, safe injection practices, and safe burial practices. Prevention of infection can be done by using gloves and protective clothing when doing high risk animal procedures such as assisting in birth or slaughter especially if the animal is sick. If aerosolizing procedures are performed a particle respirator or PAPR should be worn. Consumption of raw or undercooked meat, milk or animal blood, and slaughtering of sick animals for consumption should be avoided. Protection from mosquitoes using DEET, netting, and avoiding sleeping outside during an outbreak is a third method for prevention.[33] Mitigation during outbreaks includes larvicide measures at mosquito breeding sites, along with using DEET and netting. RVFV is inactivated at pH < 6.8, disinfectants such as calcium hypochlorite, sodium hypochlorite, acetic acid, lipid solvents, and detergents are effective.[36] Heat sterilization or boiling heat resistant products for 20 minutes will also kill RVFV.[11]

Complications and Prognosis

The majority of cases are asymptomatic or mild; however, a small percentage of around 8–10% develop severe symptoms. Post-infection complications could include blindness or decreased vision secondary to ocular disease. Neurological involvement can result in long lasting sequelae.

▌ REFERENCES

1. Chua KB. Nipah virus outbreak in Malaysia. *J Clin Virol*. 2003;26(3):265-75.
2. Aditi SM. Nipah virus infection: A review. *Epidemiol Infect*. 2019;147:e95.
3. Banerjee S, Gupta N, Kodan P, et al. Nipah virus disease: A rare and intractable disease. *Intractable Rare Dis Res*. 2019;8(1):1-8.
4. Singh RK, Dhama K, Chakraborty S, et al. Nipah virus: epidemiology, pathology, immunobiology and advances in diagnosis, vaccine designing and control strategies - a comprehensive review. *Vet Q*. 2019;39(1):26-55.
5. Parashar UD, Sunn LM, Ong F, et al. Case-control study of risk factors for human infection with a new zoonotic paramyxovirus, Nipah virus, during a 1998-1999 outbreak of severe encephalitis in Malaysia. *J Infect Dis*. 2000;181(5):1755-9.

6. Khan MS, Hossain J, Gurley ES, Nahar N, Sultana R, Luby SP. Use of infrared camera to understand bats' access to date palm sap: implications for preventing Nipah virus transmission. *Ecohealth*. 2010;7(4):517-25.

7. Homaira N, Rahman M, Hossain MJ, et al. Nipah virus outbreak with person-to-person transmission in a district of Bangladesh, 2007. *Epidemiol Infect*. 2010;138(11):1630-6.

8. Chadha MS, Comer JA, Lowe L, et al. Nipah virus-associated encephalitis outbreak, Siliguri, India. *Emerg Infect Dis*. 2006;12(2):235-40.

9. Ching PK, de los Reyes VC, Sucaldito MN, et al. Outbreak of henipavirus infection, Philippines, 2014. *Emerg Infect Dis*. 2015;21(2):328-31.

10. Biswas A. Clinical Management Protocol for Nipah Virus Disease. 2018.

11. Evers DL, Foweler CB, Mason JT, Blacksell SD. Laboratory Decontamination of HHS-listed and HHS/USDA Overlap Select Agents and Toxins. *Applied Biosafety*. 2013;18:59-72.

12. Sejvar JJ, Hossain J, Saha SK, et al. Long-term neurological and functional outcome in Nipah virus infection. *Ann Neurol*. 2007;62(3):235-42.

13. Selvey LA, Wells RM, McCormack JG, et al. Infection of humans and horses by a newly described morbillivirus. *Med J Aust*. 1995;162(12):642-5.

14. Hendra Virus Infection Prevention Advice. 2014.

15. Tulsiani SM, Graham GC, Moore PR, et al. Emerging tropical diseases in Australia. Part 5. Hendra virus. *Ann Trop Med Parasitol*. 2011;105(1).1-11.

16. Middleton D. Hendra virus. *Vet Clin North Am Equine Pract*. 2014;30(3):579-89.

17. O'Sullivan JD, Allworth AM, Paterson DL, et al. Fatal encephalitis due to novel paramyxovirus transmitted from horses. *Lancet*. 1997;349(9045):93-5.

18. Mahalingam S, Herrero LJ, Playford EG, et al. Hendra virus: an emerging paramyxovirus in Australia. *Lancet Infect Dis*. 2012;12(10):799-807.

19. Broder CC, Weir DL, Reid PA. Hendra virus and Nipah virus animal vaccines. *Vaccine*. 2016;34(30):3525-34.

20. Wright D, Kortekaas J, Bowden TA, Warimwe GM. Rift Valley fever: biology and epidemiology. *J Gen Virol*. 2019;100(8):1187-99.

21. Laughlin LW, Meegan JM, Strausbaugh LJ, Morens DM, Watten RH. Epidemic Rift Valley fever in Egypt: observations of the spectrum of human illness. *Trans R Soc Trop Med Hyg*. 1979;73(6):630-3.

22. Baba M, Masiga DK, Sang R, Villinger J. Has Rift Valley fever virus evolved with increasing severity in human populations in East Africa? *Emerg Microbes Infect*. 2016;5.e58.

23. Samy AM, Peterson AT, Hall M. Phylogeography of Rift Valley Fever Virus in Africa and the Arabian Peninsula. *PLoS Negl Trop Dis*. 2017;11(1):e0005226.

24. Al-Hamdan NA, Panackal AA, Al Bassam TH, et al. The Risk of Nosocomial Transmission of Rift Valley Fever. *PLoS Negl Trop Dis*. 2015;9(12):e0004314.

25. Rift Valley Fever. Centers for Disease Control and Prevention. https://www.cdc.gov/vhf/rvf/index.html. Updated February 25, 2020. Accessed October 10, 2020.

26. Adam I, Karsany MS. Case report: Rift Valley Fever with vertical transmission in a pregnant Sudanese woman. *J Med Virol*. 2008;80(5):929.

27. Arishi HM, Aqeel AY, Al Hazmi MM. Vertical transmission of fatal Rift Valley fever in a newborn. *Ann Trop Paediatr*. 2006;26(3):251-3.

28. McMillen CM, Hartman AL. Rift Valley fever in animals and humans: Current perspectives. *Antiviral Res*. 2018;156:29-37.

29. Smith DR, Steele KE, Shamblin J, et al. The pathogenesis of Rift Valley fever virus in the mouse model. *Virology*. 2010;407(2):256-67.

30. Ikegami T, Makino S. The pathogenesis of Rift Valley fever. *Viruses*. 2011;3(5):493-519.

31. Pepin M, avec la participation de la CR-MelIdVS. [Rift Valley fever]. *Med Mal Infect*. 2011;41(6):322-9.

32. Javelle E, Lesueur A, Pommier De Santi V, et al. The challenging management of Rift Valley Fever in humans: literature review of the clinical disease and algorithm proposal. *Annals of Clinical Microbiology and Antimicrobials*. 2020;19(1).

33. GUIDELINES ON RIFT VALLEY FEVER. June 22, 2018.

34. Javelle E, Lesueur A, Pommier de Santi V, et al. The challenging management of Rift Valley Fever in humans: literature review of the clinical disease and algorithm proposal. *Ann Clin Microbiol Antimicrob*. 2020;19(1):4.

35. Williams R, Ellis CE, Smith SJ, et al. Validation of an IgM antibody capture ELISA based on a recombinant nucleoprotein for identification of domestic ruminants infected with Rift Valley fever virus. *J Virol Methods*. 2011;177(2):140-6.

36. Kasye M, Teshome D, Abiye A, Eshetu A. A review on rift valley fever on animal, human health and its impact on live stock marketing. *Austin Virol and Retrovirology*. 2016;3(1):1020.

27 PEDIATRICS IN PANDEMICS

Katharine N. Clouser, MD, Saranga Agarwal, MD, and Karen Eigen, MD

INTRODUCTION

In a time of pandemic or crisis, providers are often called upon to care for patients who are not within their area of expertise. Providers may be called upon to care for patients who are older or younger than their usual specialty, which may be out of their comfort zone. Oftentimes, children can be a challenge for those trained in wartime or crisis medicine. Modern conflicts have been taking an increasing toll on civilians and children, and close coordination of care requires collaboration.[1]

Pandemics often pose their own challenges, as children may present differently, and may require specific treatment different from their adult counterparts. Each illness can pose its own challenge, but there are some overarching themes that can be applied to the care of the pediatric population.

GENERAL CONSIDERATIONS IN CHILDREN

For all infectious diseases, children are not simply to be thought of as small adults. Though some principles of initial stabilization can be applied from adults to children, there are specific things needed to appropriately care for children. The physiology can change across the spectrum of ages seen within the pediatric population. The American Academy of Pediatrics has a Disaster Preparedness Advisory Council, which has drafted documents to assist in the care of children. The lack of recognition of a child's special healthcare needs can lead to unneeded harm to them.[2] Pediatric populations also can have different presentations of illnesses that may be subtler than in their adult counterparts. Many pediatric illnesses present with fever and nonspecific symptoms such as fatigue and decreased oral intake, which can overlap with the initial symptoms of infectious pandemics. This provides for a diagnostic challenge, which should be recognized by clinicians prior to evaluating children.

Medications

The general approach to pediatric dosing is weight based. Medication that can be titrated to smaller doses is important. Often, standard formulations can result in overdosing in an infant or child. Dosing guidelines using weight-based dosing should be readily available to those caring for this population.

Understanding available routes is also important to the care of the patient. Not every child can swallow pills, and not every medication has a liquid form easily available. Optimal care during a pandemic requires people to be resourceful and have some knowledge of whether medications can be crushed and compounded into a liquid or used as a suppository.

Many medications do not currently have pediatric indications. Knowledge and rapid application of pathophysiology will be important in preparation for a pandemic. Stockpiles available to people from disaster preparedness organizations do not always have parity between children and adult needs.[2] Planning prior to an illness, using a model and thought that includes children will be important for optimal care of the pediatric population.

Equipment

In disaster preparedness, knowledge of the equipment available is important. Intravenous needles, nasogastric tubes, chest tubes, and similar medical equipment should be available to a provider in smaller sizes if they are expected to care for children. Papooses, or other devices to help keep an infant or young child still during a procedure should be available.

The ideal setup in a crisis situation should have pediatric specific areas. Rapid development of these field centers has been seen in disasters such as earthquakes and hurricanes.[3] Staff should be adequately trained in the use of the pediatric specific equipment and how the kits and tools may differ from that which they are used to. Ideally, these field areas will be staffed by appropriately trained staff members.

Personnel

When needed, access to pediatric providers can be important to the care of children in a pandemic. Their emotional, developmental, and physiological needs are different than in adults. Nurses and physicians comfortable with these differences do provide optimal care. When resources do not allow for this, consultation availability should be considered and planned for. In addition, recognition of the need to involve pediatricians in planning should be key when developing disaster response teams.

Education

A majority of pediatric care is provided in the outpatient arena. Communication between crisis providers and providers in the community is important. This includes two-way education about the illness or crisis, as well as situational awareness of what may be going on in the community. Schools may also need to be involved in planning, when responding to an illness requires a coordinated, public health response. Provision for routine care and vaccinations is also an important component of children's health, which supports healthy children who are often spared or less severely affected in many infectious pandemics.[2]

There are various models that have been used to educate providers who may not have expertise in a particular area on care of these patients. It can extend specialists and educate them for front line care delivery. Video training from specialists has been used to train providers in rural areas.[4] Depending on the resources available, this can be a method of education of care delivery. Utilization of age appropriate literature and availability of textbooks is also appropriate. Point of care applications can be downloaded to devices when internet access or other connections will be uncertain.

Extraction

In times of crisis, it is important to remember that planning for evacuation and extraction is important. Children can be separated from parents, which requires a coordinated effort for those caring for children. The separation can result in multiple challenges, including gathering an adequate history from a child, as well as dealing with the trauma that comes with being separated from family. Special consideration with trained personnel should be taken to care for these children.

Orphans

Sometimes underappreciated effect of infectious pandemics and other crises in children is parental death. When a large proportion of adults are ill or die from a particular event or infection, children can be left without parents or other caregivers. Planning for accommodations, food, and medical care will be important in any disaster planning and it will allow for children to remain to be taken care of.

▌PANDEMIC ILLNESSES

Severe Acute Respiratory Syndrome Coronavirus (SARS-CoV) And Middle East Respiratory Syndrome Coronavirus (MERS-CoV)

Epidemiology

These two viruses emerged in the 2000s, with SARS-CoV surfacing in 2002 and MERS-CoV in 2012. SARS-CoV was first seen in mainland China and MERS-CoV in Saudi Arabia.[5] Children were not heavily affected by the SARS-CoV virus. Various cases series were published, and it appeared that there were under 150 cases of pediatric SARS-CoV across the world. Countries affected seemed to be Canada, Hong Kong, Taiwan, and Singapore.[6] Younger children seemed to have a more favorable outcome, and there were no reported deaths. The median age of MERS-CoV was 50 at the height of the illness, but patients of all ages were reported.[7] Various case reports estimate that the infection rate in children was less than 1%, with no reported pediatric deaths.[8]

Presentation

In children, the most common presentation for SARS-CoV is fever, seen in 98% of patients. Cough, nausea, and vomiting are also commonly seen. Patients older than 12 years of age present more similarly to adults, with respiratory distress, radiographic abnormalities, and oxygen requirement. Dry, nonproductive cough is a common symptom. Older children are more likely to need intensive care than younger children.[6] Radiographic findings are usually consistent with pneumonia.[9]

MERS-CoV symptoms range from no symptoms to fever, cough, chills, sore throat, myalgia, and diarrhea. Children had less severe presentations in the initial outbreak in 2012, with some being asymptomatic, and laboratory values typically remained normal.[11]

Considerations in Children

There has not been much transmission from children to children or children to adults published within the literature, though data is limited. Restriction of children's normal activities does not appear needed for disease control.[9,10] Children appear to respond to treatments similar to adults, with steroids being a mainstay of treatment in these illnesses.[5,6]

Availability of pediatric-sized oxygen delivery devices would be important in disaster planning for these illnesses. Children over the age of 12 during these outbreaks are more likely to require oxygen, so with limited resources, adult sizes may be appropriate. Recognition of lower flow rates for comfort of pediatric patients is also important.

Severe Acute Respiratory Syndrome Coronavirus-2 (SARS-CoV-2)- COVID-19

Epidemiology

SARS-CoV-2 which emerged from China affected United States of America, India, and Brazil. The death rate worldwide for this virus is < 1%.[12] The rate of infection of children through July of 2020 was much lower than in adults, and their death and hospitalization were less frequent as well. In the pediatric population within the United States of America, for example, the hospitalization rate through July was 8 per 100,000 versus 164.5 per 100,000 in adults.[13] These numbers have been climbing, but children seem to continue to be less severely affected than adults, with 7.3% of infections in the United States being in those aged 0–17.[14] Children were not initially prioritized in the early testing. In much of the world, schools were shut down and normal childhood activities were limited, which may have impacted epidemiology in children.

Presentation

Clinical presentation in children and adults has some overlaps and some differences. The incubation period appears to be 2–14 days, with an average of 6 days.[15] Symptoms in children include fever, headache, cough, loss of taste or smell, sore throat, difficulty breathing, abdominal pain, nausea, vomiting, and diarrhea.[15] Many children present with non-specific symptoms that can mimic other illnesses. There is some evidence that up to 45% of children may be asymptomatic.[16] Children can progress to multi-organ failure and shock. In addition, many pediatric patients have developed coagulopathy and thrombus with this infection.[14]

In May 2020, guidance came from the Royal College of Paediatrics and Child Health regarding an inflammatory condition following infection with the SARS-CoV-2 virus.[17] The Centers for Disease Control and Prevention (CDC) in the United States of America came out with a case definition shortly thereafter. The clinical features include:

- An individual aged < 21 years presenting with fever for longer than 24 hours, laboratory evidence of inflammation, and evidence of clinically severe illness requiring hospitalization, with multisystem

($\geq$2) organ involvement (cardiac, renal, respiratory, hematologic, gastrointestinal, dermatologic or neurological); AND

- No alternative plausible diagnoses; AND
- Positive for current or recent SARS-CoV-2 infection by RT-PCR, serology, or antigen test; or exposure to a suspected or confirmed COVID-19 case within the 4 weeks prior to the onset of symptoms.[18]

The laboratory findings include C-reactive protein, ferritin, and D-dimer, which have been elevated in many described patients. Their end organ damage may be seen on laboratory or physical examination. Elevated neutrophils along with reduced lymphocytes and hypoalbuminemia have been seen and described frequently in the inflammatory condition.[19] The illness often presents after a primary SARS-CoV-2 infection, whether symptomatic or asymptomatic. At the date of publication, the time from infection to development of this condition is not known.

Considerations in Children

Children, though perhaps presenting less severely than adults, warrant planning and accommodations for care. Pediatric patients often require supportive care including intravenous fluids and oxygen support when being treated for acute COVID-19. The National Institutes of Health supports the use of dexamethasone treatment or other glucocorticoid treatment in the pediatric population for COVID-19 requiring mechanical ventilation.[20] Availability of pediatric preparations, or ability to dilute standard preparations safely will be important to care for children who may be infected by this virus.

Different treatment mechanisms have been discussed regarding treatment for Multi-System Inflammatory Syndrome in Children. A standardized treatment has not been published, but organizations have recommended intravenous immunoglobulin and steroid treatment for this illness.[21] As resources are frequently limited in pandemics, these medications may be important when gathering supplies and making medications available.

Influenza

Epidemiology

Influenza is a highly contagious respiratory illness that is caused by the influenza virus which contains a single-stranded negative-sense

RNA genome. There are four types of influenza (flu) viruses: A, B, C, and D. The influenza A and B viruses that routinely spread in humans are responsible for seasonal flu epidemics each year. Influenza viruses that have caused pandemics in the past have typically originated from animal influenza viruses that have mutated to infect humans.

Influenza A viruses are the only influenza viruses known to cause flu pandemics. The first and most severe pandemic in recent history, known as "Spanish influenza," occurred in 1918 and was caused by an H1N1 influenza A virus (IAV) strain. Approximately 500 million people were infected, and 50 million people died during this pandemic. The second pandemic, known as "Asian influenza," occurred in 1957 and was caused by an H2N2 IAV strain. The third pandemic, known as "Hong Kong flu," happened in 1968 and was caused by an H3N2 IAV strain. The second and third pandemics each resulted in approximately one million deaths worldwide. The fourth pandemic was caused by the H1N1 strain pdm09 virus, also known as the "novel influenza A virus," and resulted in 151,700–575,400 deaths worldwide from 2009 to 2010.[22–25]

Influenza A viruses are divided into subtypes based on two proteins on the surface of the virus: hemagglutinin (H) and neuraminidase (N). Of all the influenza viruses that routinely circulate and cause illness in people, influenza A(H3N2) viruses tend to change more rapidly, both genetically and antigenically resulting in reduced effectiveness of vaccines; this creates a challenge in antiviral therapy leading to outbreaks of seasonal epidemics.

Hospitalizations and deaths caused by influenza vary from one season to the next. The severity and outcomes are determined by various factors such as host immunity, age, sex, morbidities, and genetic variations. Worldwide, these annual epidemics are estimated to result in about 3 to 5 million cases of severe illness and about 290,000 to 650,000 respiratory deaths; 99% of deaths in children under 5 years of age are found in developing countries.[26]

Data for rates of hospitalization with laboratory-confirmed influenza are from the Influenza Hospitalization Surveillance Network (FluSurv-NET).[27] As per this data high risk groups include the elderly (over 65 years), pregnant women, young children who are 5 years old or younger, those who are immunocompromised or with other comorbidities, and since 2010 non-Hispanic Black persons had the highest flu-related hospitalization rates (68 per 100,000). As per the CDC, flu-related hospitalizations among children younger than 5 years old have ranged from 7,000 to 26,000 in the United States.

Presentation

The most common symptoms in children are fever, chills, runny nose, cough, and body ache and occasionally vomiting and diarrhea. The vast majority of children with no comorbidities recover from these symptoms in around 7 days without any need of hospitalization. The most common complications of flu are viral pneumonia and secondary bacterial pneumonia which can advance into acute respiratory distress syndrome and multi-organ failure without early recognition and appropriate management. Some of other complications are myocarditis, encephalitis, and myositis.

A majority of cases of human influenza are clinically diagnosed but can have overlap with other flu-like illness. Laboratory confirmation of influenza virus from nasopharyngeal secretions is commonly performed by detection of influenza-specific RNA by reverse transcriptase-polymerase chain reaction (RT-PCR). Rapid molecular assays are the preferred diagnostic tests because they can be done at the point of care, are highly accurate, and give quick results.

Special Considerations for Children

Treatment for the vast majority of patients who are not in a high-risk group, such as children, is supportive care by managing fever and assuring hydration. If there is clinical deterioration with complication of pneumonia or sepsis, hospitalization and early therapy with antiviral drugs is advised. Children less than 5 years will require respiratory support and close hemodynamic monitoring as they can go into shock and multi-organ failure.[28] Oseltamivir is a neuraminidase inhibitor which is an antiviral medication that blocks the viral neuraminidase enzyme and has activity against both influenza A and B viruses. It is US Food and Drug Administration-approved if presented within 48 hours of symptom onset and is given for a total of 5 days.

Plague

Epidemiology

Plague, which is also known as bubonic plague or Black Death, is a zoonotic infection caused by the transmission of the bacterium *Yersinia pestis*. It can be transmitted to humans via flea bites, handling the tissue or body fluids of plague-infected animals, aerosols, or contaminated food.[29,30] Plague primarily affects rodents but several other animal species including cats, rabbits, and camels can also become infected.[31,32] The bacterium has been shown to survive in soil, which serves as a reservoir, making eradication of the disease particularly challenging.[29] Many species of fleas can be vectors of plague, but the most commonly known is the oriental rat flea *Xenopsylla cheopis*. Transmission, though less common, can occur from person to person through respiratory droplets in the pneumonic form of the disease.[29]

The plague has been responsible for three major pandemics throughout history, each time causing extreme social and economic disruptions and millions of deaths.[30] The first plague pandemic, known as the plague of Justinian, originated in Egypt and Central Africa in 541 AD. It was carried via land and sea trade routes to Northern Africa and coastal cities along the Mediterranean, spreading throughout Europe as far north as Ireland. This was the first time the characteristic "buboes," described as painful swollen lymph nodes which turn black or necrotic, were recorded.[33]

The second major plague pandemic, known as The Black Death of 1347, was reported to have killed a quarter of the population in Europe and another 25 million people in Asia and Africa. In some major cities, more than half the population died.[33] The plague re-emerged for the third time in China and waxed and waned for 5 decades causing over 12 million deaths, the majority of which were in India.[33] There are still sporadic cases of plague today which are limited to sub-Saharan Africa, Asia, and the Americas, with about 1,000 cases per year occurring over the past 5 years. The most recent outbreaks have been reported in China, Madagascar, and the Democratic Republic of the Congo.[34] The first documented case of plague in the United States was in 1,900 and there have been just over 1,000 cases to date. Outbreaks were initially limited to populous port cities, but cases in the United States currently occur primarily in the rural west.

Plague has been recognized as a potential agent of bioterrorism and is identified by the CDC as a category A bioterrorism agent based on its ease of access, short incubation period, high mortality rate, and ease of dissemination through aerosolization and person-to-person transmission. Its role as a biological weapon in military conflicts has been documented throughout history and more recent attempts at mass production of aerosolized *Yersinia pestis* have been reported.[35–37]

Presentation

Plague exists in three clinical forms: bubonic plague, septicemic plague, and pneumonic plague. The clinical presentation depends upon the mode of infection. Bubonic plague is acquired from the bite of an infected flea and is the most common form of the disease. The classic "bubo" is a tender lymph node, located in the groin, axilla, head or neck, which becomes necrotic or suppurative. This is typically associated with a febrile flu-like syndrome which occurs 1–7 days after inoculation. The bacterium can disseminate to the blood, spleen, liver or lungs, resulting in septicemia.[32] Inhalation of the *Yersinia pestis* bacterium results in primary pneumonic plague. Individuals contract the disease either through inhalation of droplets spread by an infected person with pneumonic disease, a form of human-to-human transmission, or through hematogenous spread as a secondary complication of the bubonic form. Symptoms include cough with mucopurulent or bloody sputum, shortness of breath, and chest pain. Other rare forms of plague, such as cutaneous or gastrointestinal plague, have also been reported.[36] The mortality rate without treatment is 40–70% for bubonic plague and nearly 100% for the other forms of the disease.[35] The diagnosis of plague is based on epidemiology, symptomatology, and laboratory identification of *Yersinia pestis* either in culture or with antigen or serologic testing.[36] With the support of the World Health Organization (WHO), a laboratory validated rapid dipstick test is now widely used in Africa and South America.[34] The majority of human cases can be treated successfully with effective antibiotics according to the CDC's recommendation. Antibiotics and other supportive treatment initiated early in the course of the illness are associated with a more favorable outcome.[34]

Considerations in Children

Children of all ages are susceptible to plague, and cases have been documented throughout history, as well as in contemporary times.[38] According to the World Health Organization, over half of the reported plague cases in countries such as Madagascar, Democratic Republic of the Congo, and Peru—where plague is endemic—have occurred in populations under the age of 18 years.[39] Historians chronicle plagues from 1361 onward as "plagues of children."[39] Children are particularly vulnerable to infectious diseases and considerations must be taken with regard to treatment and containment of the disease in the pediatric population. Delays in diagnosis in children may be seen due to the overlap in symptoms of plague and other common pediatric infectious diseases. Although plague vaccines have been developed and used since the late 19th century and there have been encouraging recent advances in research and development, there is currently no licensed and readily available safe and effective vaccine for commercial use in children in the United States.[40] A live attenuated *Yersinia pestis* vaccine is used in Russia and China but requires yearly boosting.[41] There are currently as many as 17 vaccines in production.[42]

Children are also particularly vulnerable to plague, which can be used as a biological weapon, and vaccine development and use of effective prophylactic antibiotics could be protective.[43] Early antibiotics are the key to effective treatment due to the rapid progression of the disease. Recommended antibiotic treatment of plague in children are streptomycin, gentamicin, levofloxacin, ciprofloxacin, doxycycline, and chloramphenicol (for children > 2 years). Streptomycin and chloramphenicol are not widely available in the United States. Recommended medications for post-exposure prophylaxis (PEP) in children are doxycycline and ciprofloxacin, both are relatively contraindicated in young children.[44]

Tularemia

Epidemiology

Francisella tularensis is the infectious agent of tularemia. The pathogen has been listed as a potential bioterrorism agent, possibly developed during the Cold War. The disease appears to be seasonal, with the highest incidence in late spring, summer, and early autumn. The illness has been reported throughout the northern hemisphere but has not been seen in the southern hemisphere. Small and large outbreaks have been noted in many countries in North America and Europe. In the United States of America, the tick is the most important vector. Mosquitos have also been described as a vector in other countries. It has also been described in hares, prairie dogs, and mink. Humans are infected with the bacteria through arthropod bites, direct contact with infected animals or their tissues and fluids, by ingestion of contaminated water or food, or by inhalation of aerosols with infectious particles. The infectious aerosols can be weaponized.[45] Person-to-person transmission has not been shown to be a method of transmission.[46]

There is no available age-based data, but the illness has been seen in all ages. In the United States, there have been on average 143 cases per year. Two thirds of cases occur in males, and approximately 25% occur in children 1 to 14 years of age.[46]

Presentation

Typically, ulcerations of the glands starting with a maculopapular lesion at the entry site. The ulcers tend to present within glands and are slow healing, with tender lymphadenopathy that can drain. There is also a glandular variant, which has lymphadenopathy without ulcer. Less common symptoms include conjunctivitis and preauricular lymphadenopathy, vesicular skin lesions, high fever, and respiratory tularemia. Typically, respiratory tularemia has hilar adenopathy and dry cough, which is often seen with activities of aerosol release.[46] This may be the presentation in a weaponized form of the illness.

Considerations in Children

Due to the zoonotic nature of the illness, care with children is important to prevention. Protective clothing and insect repellents, along with removal of ticks is important in the control of this illness. Interaction with dead animals should be prevented in children. In the event of a large-scale illness (such as a bioterrorism attack), doxycycline or ciprofloxacin should be used, despite the warnings against these medications in younger children.[46]

Ebola

Epidemiology

Ebola first emerged in 1976 from both Sudan and what was at the time Zaire. It was thought to be native to East Africa, but bat migration has led to outbreaks in other areas. Outbreaks continued throughout the subsequent decades, with a notable outbreak in 2014. Children seemed to be less affected than adults, but some female children in certain countries seemed to have a higher risk.[47] In 2014–2016, approximately 20% of those in the four more affected African countries were children. Notably, children were most affected as an estimated 30,000 became orphans.[48]

Presentation

Like many other viral illnesses, Ebola can cause nonspecific symptoms. Patients will present with a 2–21-day history of contact with a person who was diagnosed with the illness. Generally, children will present with fever, weakness, decreased oral intake, vomiting, bleeding, and profuse watery diarrhea. Fever has been described in all cases. The degree of hemorrhage is related to the degree of the illness. Diagnosis is made by detection of the PCR from the Ebola antigen.[48]

Considerations in Children

There is no specific approved antiviral treatment for Ebola. Supportive care is the most important in the administration of patient care. In outbreak settings with limited resources, intravenous fluids used for adults can be used for children at smaller rates. In severe hemorrhage, blood products given at 10–15 mL/kg at a time can help to replace lost volume. Immunologic medications in investigative trials have not been adequately investigated in the pediatric population.

Dengue, Lassa Fever, Yellow Fever, Chikungunya, Crimean-Congo Hemorrhagic Fever

Epidemiology

Viral hemorrhagic fevers (VHF) are caused by single-stranded, enveloped RNA viruses with common features characterized by transmission via a vector to human and have a similar constellation of multisystem signs and symptoms such as clinically significant hemorrhage and marked thrombocytopenia. Humans are not the natural reservoir for any of these viruses and are infected when they come into contact with infected hosts, which occur widely in tropical and subtropical regions. Most common are Ebola, Crimean–Congo hemorrhagic fever (CCHF), Lassa fever, dengue, yellow fever, and Chikungunya. These viruses are classified as Biosafety Level 4 (BSL-4) pathogens and as such must be handled in special facilities designed to contain them safely.

Lassa Fever

Lassa virus is an arenavirus responsible for human cases of Lassa fever and spreads via contact with food or household items contaminated with rodent urine or feces. It may also be spread between humans through direct contact with the blood, urine, feces, or other bodily secretions of a person infected with Lassa fever. It is endemic in parts of West Africa including Sierra Leone, Liberia, Guinea, and Nigeria. An estimated 100,000 to 300,000 infections of Lassa fever occur annually, with approximately 10,000 deaths.[49,50] Though Lassa fever is not well studied in children, those under age 10 years are considered most vulnerable, with one study showing 15% sero-positivity for Lassa virus in that population in West Africa.[51] The first imported case of Lassa fever in more than 20 years occurred in New Jersey in 2004.

Crimean–Congo Hemorrhagic Fever (CCHF)

Crimean-Congo hemorrhagic fever is caused by *Nairovirus* found in Africa, parts of Eastern and southern Europe, Mediterranean, northwestern China, Central Asia, the Middle East, and the Indian subcontinent. Ixodid (hard) ticks are both a reservoir and a vector for the CCHF virus. Animal herders, livestock workers, and slaughterhouse workers in endemic areas are at risk of CCHF. Transmission to humans occurs through contact with infected ticks or from one infected human to another by contact with infectious blood or bodily fluids.

Dengue Fever

Dengue fever is caused by infection with 1 of the 4 serotypes of dengue virus, which is a Flavivirus transmitted by female mosquitoes mainly of the species *Aedes aegypti* and, to a lesser extent, *Ae. albopictus*. Dengue is widespread throughout the tropics. Severe dengue affects most Asian and Latin American countries and has become a leading cause of hospitalization and death among children and adults in these regions. Human-to-mosquito transmission can occur up to 2 days before clinical signs to 2 days after the fever has resolved. The number of dengue cases reported to WHO have increased dramatically over the last 2 decades, to over 4.2 million in 2019. Reported deaths between the year 2000 and 2015 increased from 960 to 4,032 and is endemic in more than 100 countries with Latin American countries, South-East Asia, and Western Pacific regions the most seriously affected, with Asia bearing ~70% of the global burden of disease.[52]

Yellow Fever

Yellow fever is caused by the yellow fever virus, which is the prototype member of the *Flavivirus* genus. The virus is endemic in regions of South America and Africa and is transmitted to humans via mosquitoes of the *Haemogogus* and *Aedes* genera. As per WHO around 200,000 cases of yellow fever occur annually in 47 countries, with 30,000 deaths per year. A recent modeling study estimated that yellow fever may infect up to 1.8 million individuals in Africa annually resulting in 180,000 cases and 78,000 deaths.[53] Infection affects the age group of 15 to 45 years, but young children are also equally vulnerable. Reports of yellow fever in the United States are rare, with the last outbreak reported in New Orleans in 1905. It was a rare cause of illness among returning travelers and between 1970 and 2002, nine cases of yellow fever were reported in unimmunized travelers from the United States and Europe.

Chikungunya Fever

Chikungunya fever is a self-remitting febrile viral illness that has been associated with frequent outbreaks in tropical countries in Africa and Southeast Asia. The term refers to the "stooped-over posture" as a consequence of severe chronic incapacitating arthralgia in adults. Chikungunya virus belongs to the Togaviridae family which is transmitted to humans through Aedes mosquitoes. Humans are the primary host of chikungunya virus during epidemic periods. As of 2017, about 1.8 million cases had been reported from 44 countries. Cases in US states occurred in travelers returning from the affected areas, whereas cases in US territories were all locally acquired in Puerto Rico. It is a notifiable disease to CDC since 2015. As of October 1, 2020, a total of 17 chikungunya virus disease cases with illness onset in 2020 have been reported to ArboNET from eight U.S. states.[54]

Presentation

Susceptibility to VHF in endemic regions is often highest for young children and the adults affected are frequently those who have the most occupational exposure. Disease manifestations range from asymptomatic to mild symptoms in over 80% of cases and include fever, cough, sore throat, abdomen pain, and myalgia. More severe cases result in nose bleeds, petechial rashes, hemorrhage, shock, and coma. Lassa fever has specific symptoms like deafness which can occur in 25% of patients who survive. Swollen baby syndrome with signs of edema, abdominal distention, and bleeding is a severe form of Lassa virus infection described in a case series from a Liberian hospital[55] and is transmitted from infected mothers. Severe dengue presents as dengue hemorrhagic fever and dengue shock syndrome which is caused by vascular permeability causing circulatory shock in children. A subset of severe dengue cases, hemophagocytic lymphohistiocytosis (HLH), is increasingly recognized in children. In Puerto Rico, 22 dengue HLH cases, including one death, were detected from 2008 to 2013.[56] Similarly, jaundice is distinct in yellow fever and severe cases can progress to shock and liver and renal failure. If patient with high suspicion of VHF has polyarthralgia and in severe cases neurological manifestations like meningoencephalitis, myelitis, Guillain-Barré syndrome, and cranial nerve palsies, then the diagnosis is more consistent with Chikungunya fever.

Considerations in Children

Pediatricians should consider VHF with a consistent clinical picture in any febrile child arriving from endemic countries after ruling out malaria and typhoid. Laboratory test shows leukopenia, thrombocytopenia, elevated transaminases, and coagulation abnormalities. Confirmation tests are reverse transcriptase polymerase chain reaction (RT-PCR) assay to detect RNA and antibody enzyme-linked immunosorbent assay (ELISA) which are done at specific reference labs after ensuring careful handling of highly infectious sample.[57]

Treatment is supportive and includes aggressive management of hypovolemia, electrolyte imbalances, and correcting coagulopathies. During shock, the patient will need an intensive care unit for respiratory and hemodynamic support. Blood, platelet, and plasma replacement therapy are often given in severe dengue and CCHF. The antiviral Ribavirin has been shown to be effective in lowering the mortality for adult patients if given early in the disease course of Lassa fever and CCHF, but no studies show its effectiveness in children.

Nipah Virus, Hendra Virus, and Rift Valley Fever

Epidemiology

There are a few different emerging viruses causing encephalitis. Nipah virus, a paramyxovirus was isolated in 1999 during an outbreak among the pig farmers in Malaysia and Singapore. This virus, though limited in numbers, was deadly with a 40–75% rate of death. In 2001, a different strain was isolated due to contaminated date palm sap and bat contact. This outbreak was also associated with nosocomial person-to-person transmission. Age greater than 45 seems to be a higher risk for death in this virus.[58] From 2001 to 2014, 37% of published cases were in patients under 14, but their illness did not seem to be as contagious as their adult counterparts.[59] Hendra virus, another paramyxovirus was isolated from outbreaks in Australia, and is related to Nipah virus. Only seven cases have been reported in humans. The flying fox is its reservoir.[60]

Rift Valley fever, caused by a bunyavirus, has caused outbreaks throughout the twenty-first century. Generally, epizootic outbreaks with large animal deaths lead to increased contact with humans and deceased animals. It primarily affects animals. Mosquitos seem to be a reservoir of this illness. No human-to-human transmission has been documented. Adults in outbreaks have been more affected than children, perhaps related to the increase in occupational exposure.[61]

Presentation

These viruses have a wide range of symptoms. Both Nipah and Hendra viruses present with encephalitis anywhere from 3 to 16 days following exposure. Symptoms include fever followed by drowsiness and altered mental status. The illnesses can progress to coma.[58,60] Rift Valley fever can be more indolent, with an initial phase of fever, weakness, and dizziness. It can progress to encephalitis, with seizures and confusion anywhere from 1 to 4 weeks post initial illness. This is a very rare presentation in less than 1% of infected patients.[61] Children have not had any special presentations described in the literature. It is not clear how many children have progressed to seizure and encephalitis.

Considerations in Children

All of the above pandemic causes of encephalitis are treated with supportive care only. Children may require special equipment as outlined in the initial part of this chapter. The key to treatment for these illnesses is prevention. For the mosquito and animal borne illnesses, protection of children needs to be taken into account. Keeping children away from deceased animals will help decrease exposure. Appropriate protection from mosquitos, using tenting and repellents is another mechanism for keeping the illness away from pediatric patients. In addition with the loss of livestock, food and money supply can impact children. Support to those who may be orphaned or displaced from parents will be important in planning.

Smallpox

Epidemiology

Smallpox, a devastating disease caused by the DNA orthopoxviruses *Variola major* and *Variola minor*, is the only infectious disease of humans that is considered to be completely eradicated. *Variola major* caused the more severe form of the disease. Several factors are believed to have contributed to the successful elimination of this disease from the human population, including the early development of effective vaccines and the fact that humans are its only natural reservoir. The epidemiologic origin of smallpox in unknown but it is believed to have existed for more than 3000 years. It is thought to date back to the Egyptian Empire around the 3rd century BCE (Before Common Era), based on smallpox-like rashes found on ancient mummies.[1] The spread of smallpox has been traced to the growth and spread of civilizations, global exploration, and expanding trade routes over the centuries.[62]

There was no known pharmacologic treatment of smallpox prior to its eradication through a massive global immunization campaign beginning in 1959. Attempts to prevent the disease in populations was practiced as early as 1000 BCE through a process referred to as variolization, where those not previously exposed to the virus were inoculated with material from smallpox lesions. Those exposed by this method then went on to develop a milder form of the disease with a much lower death rate. Early vaccination techniques began in 1796 with the cowpox virus, a Vaccinia orthopox virus which is antigenically similar to the Variola virus.[63] The last recorded case of smallpox was in 1977. On May 8, 1980, the 33rd World Health Assembly officially declared the world to be smallpox free.[64] Eradication of smallpox has been considered the biggest achievement in international public health.[65]

Presentation

Smallpox has been regarded as a devastating and disfiguring disease responsible for the deaths of millions of people throughout history. The virus was transmitted from person to person through respiratory droplets or aerosolization, or in some cases from physical contact with the infected person, contaminated clothing or bedding. It had an overall mortality rate of 30%, with variations among disease types, age groups, geographic location, and time period of outbreak. There was no known treatment and those who survived were left with terrible disfiguring and disabling scars or blindness. Symptoms of smallpox included high fever, fatigue, and severe back pain, with later development of the characteristic "pox" rash, which began on the face, forearms and hands and then spread to the rest of the body. The exact cause of death associated with smallpox is unknown, but there is believed to be multi-system organ failure associated with viremia or an uncontrolled cytotoxic immune response.[66]

Bioterrorism

Smallpox is thought of as one of the most dangerous of all potential biological weapons due to its easy storage capability, potential spread through aerosolization, delays in diagnosis, infectivity, and lack of established or clinically trialed treatments.[65] It qualifies as a high-priority category A bioterrorism agent by the CDC. Research labs at the CDC in the United States and the Russian State Centre for Research on Virology and Biotechnology are the only two laboratories in the world that are approved to have smallpox virus for research. Over the past 20 years, there have been several unproven allegations and reports of illegal stocks of the virus carried to rogue nations such as Iraq, Iran, North Korea, and France.[66] Concerns about smallpox as a biological weapon grew after September 2001 and the United States government established a nation-wide smallpox preparedness program. This involved the availability of post-exposure vaccinations, vaccinia immune globin (VIG) and antiviral medications.[62] The smallpox vaccine is protective if given within 3 days of smallpox exposure and stockpiles are held by the WHO headquarters in Switzerland, as well as in France, Germany, New Zealand, the United Kingdom, and the United States in the event of an outbreak due to a bioterrorism attack. There are currently three antiviral medications which may be useful in the event of a smallpox outbreak. Tecovirimat was approved by the FDA in 2018. Cidofovir and brincidofovir have demonstrated in vitro potency against DNA viruses and could be used for isolated cases or during an outbreak.[67]

Monkeypox

Epidemiology

Human monkeypox is a zoonotic infection caused by a DNA orthopox virus similar to Variola virus, the virus responsible for smallpox.[68] Unlike smallpox, a disease found only in humans, monkeypox virus (MPXV) infects many mammalian species. Its primary natural host reservoir is unknown, but the disease has been found most commonly in rodents. Monkeypox was first seen in 1958 in an outbreak among captive monkeys transported from Africa to Europe. The first case in humans was reported in 1970 in the Democratic Republic of the Congo, just 7 years prior to the global eradication of smallpox and is believed to coincide with waning smallpox immunity.[69] Transmission of the virus occurs when a person comes in contact with an infected animal through a bite or scratch, during preparation of bushmeat, or through indirect contact of lesions with a contaminated material. Person-to person-transmission is also possible through exposure to respiratory droplets or bodily fluids, accounting for some of the larger outbreaks in West and Central Africa.[68] There are two known groups (or clades) of monkeypox virus, the Central African clade and the West African clade. Symptoms of the Central African strain of the virus are believed to be more severe, with higher mortality rates and greater likelihood of person-to-person transmission.[70] The case fatality rate varies between 1 and 10% and is higher in HIV positive and immunocompromised populations.

Many factors are believed to contribute to the rising prevalence of monkeypox in the African continent.

Some of them are:

1. Discontinuation of the smallpox vaccine, which is thought to confer cross-protective immunity
2. Environmental factors associated with climate change, bringing animal and human hosts into closer proximity
3. Poverty causing increased interaction of humans with animal species through overcrowding, hunting, and the consumption of bushmeat
4. HIV/AIDS prevalence
5. Geopolitical and armed conflicts in disease area

The number of human monkeypox cases in Central and West Africa has increased exponentially over the past 20 years, although it is uncertain whether this is partially due to improved surveillance and reporting. An outbreak in the United States in 2003 was linked to a shipment of small mammals from Ghana which secondarily infected prairie dogs. There have also been cases reported in the United Kingdom and Israel associated with travel from Nigeria.[68]

Presentation

Symptoms of monkeypox are similar to that of smallpox, but they are generally milder and can mimic the clinical presentation of chickenpox and

other exanthematous infectious diseases.[68,70] Symptoms include a prodrome of fever, headache, swollen lymph nodes, and body aches followed
by the development of a rash which usually begins on the face and progresses to the rest of the body.[68,70] The illness typically lasts 2–4 weeks and
the incubation period can range from 6 to 21 days.[71] Complications contributing to higher mortality rates include secondary bacterial infections,
pneumonia, encephalitis, gastroenteritis, and dehydration.[68] Symptoms
are more severe and mortality rates are higher in patients who are younger
or immunocompromised. Diagnosis can be made based on clinical and
epidemiologic criteria. Laboratory diagnosis may be made using viral
culture, PCR (polymerase chain reaction) or serologic testing, but these
are generally not available in monkeypox endemic areas and specimens
require storage and shipping to remote labs. Serologic false positives are
possible for those previously exposed to the smallpox vaccine. There is
currently no proven safe and effective treatment for monkeypox. Potential
treatment options are similar to those developed for a potential smallpox
outbreak and include antiviral medications, smallpox vaccine, and vaccinia immunoglobin. Smallpox vaccine in not currently available to the
general public but trials amongst healthcare workers in endemic areas
with the third-generation smallpox vaccine, Imvamune, are currently in
process.[72]

Considerations in Children

The first reported case of monkeypox in 1970 was found in a 9-year-old
boy in the Democratic Republic of the Congo.[71] Children are particularly
susceptible to contracting the disease and are more vulnerable to complications resulting in increased mortality rates.[68,71] Infectious diseases are still
the leading cause of death among children under age 5 for a variety of
reasons. They have developing immune systems compared to adults and
greater likelihood of disease transmission due to increased hand-to-mouth
activity. In addition, they have a greater likelihood of exposure to pathogens via inhalation due to increased respiratory rates and alveolar uptake.[72]
Delays in diagnosis of monkeypox in children are likely because its presentation is similar to that of other common childhood diseases, such as chickenpox, impetigo or molluscum contagiosum. There are currently no widely
available recommended treatments for monkeypox and there have been no
clinical trials of established antiviral medications, such as cidofovir, in children. Smallpox vaccine has been shown to be protective against monkeypox if given within 2 weeks of exposure. Although the vaccine has been well
studied in children, pediatric patients are more likely to experience severe
adverse reactions such as encephalitis, especially those under 1 year old.[72]

REFERENCES

1. Samuel N, Epstein D, Oren A, et al. Severe pediatric war trauma: a military-civilian collaboration from retrieval to repatriation. *J Trauma Acute Care Surg.* 2021;90(1):e1-e6.

2. DISASTER PREPAREDNESS ADVISORY COUNCIL, COMMITTEE ON PEDIATRIC EMERGENCY MEDICINE. Ensuring the health of children in disasters. *Pediatrics.* 2015;136(5):e1407-e1417.

3. Burnweit C, Stylianos S. Disaster response in a pediatric field hospital: lessons learned in Haiti. *J Pediatr Surg.* 2011;46(6):1131-9.

4. Arora S, Thornton K, Murata G, et al. Outcomes of treatment for hepatitis C virus infection by primary care providers. *N Engl J Med.* 2011;364(23):2199-207.

5. de Wit E, van Doremalen N, Falzarano D, Munster VJ. SARS and MERS: recent insights into emerging coronaviruses. *Nat Rev Microbiol.* 2016;14(8):523-534.

6. Stockman LJ, Massoudi MS, Helfand R, et al. Severe acute respiratory syndrome in children. *Pediatr Infect Dis J.* 2007;26(1):68-74.

7. MERS Clinical Features. 2020, August 28. Available at https://www.cdc.gov/coronavirus/mers/clinical-features.html. Accessed October 13, 2020.

8. Al-Sehaibany FS. Middle East respiratory syndrome in children. Dental considerations. *Saudi Med J.* 2017;38(4):339-343.

9. MERS Clinical Features. 2020, August 28. Available at https://www.cdc.gov/coronavirus/mers/clinical-features.html. Accessed October 13, 2020.

10. SARS. 2005, May 03. Available at https://www.cdc.gov/sars/clinical/guidance.html. Accessed October 13, 2020.

11. Alfaraj SH, Al-Tawfiq JA, Altuwaijri TA, et al. Middle East respiratory syndrome coronavirus in pediatrics: a report of seven cases from Saudi Arabia. *Front Med.* 2019;13:126-130.

12. COVID-19 Map. 2020. Available at https://coronavirus.jhu.edu/map.html. Accessed February 2, 2021.

13. Hospitalization rates and characteristics of children aged 18 years hospitalized with laboratory-confirmed COVID-19 - COVID-NET, 14 States, March 1–July 25, 2020. Available at https://www.cdc.gov/mmwr/volumes/69/wr/mm6932e3.htm. Updated August 13, 2020. Accessed October 2020.

14. Information for Pediatric Healthcare Providers. n.d. Available at https://www.cdc.gov/coronavirus/2019-ncov/hcp/pediatric-hcp.html. Accessed October 2020.

15. CDC. COVID-19 Pandemic Planning Scenarios. Available at https://www.cdc.gov/coronavirus/2019-ncov/hcp/planning-scenarios.html#table-2.

16. Poline J, Gaschignard J, Leblanc C, et al. Systematic severe acute respiratory syndrome coronavirus 2 screening at hospital admission in children: a French prospective multicenter study. *Clin Infect Dis.* 2021;72(12):2215-2217.

17. Guidance: Paediatric multisystem inflammatory syndrome temporally associated with COVID-19. 2020, May 1. Available at https://www.rcpch.ac.uk/sites/default/files/2020-05/COVID-19-Paediatric-multisystem-%20inflammatory%20syndrome-20200501.pdf.

18. Information for Healthcare Providers about Multisystem Inflammatory Syndrome in Children (MIS-C). 2020, August 28. Available at https://www.cdc.gov/mis-c/hcp/. Accessed October 14, 2020.

19. Feldstein LR, Rose EB, Horwitz SM, Collins JP, et al. Overcoming COVID-19 Investigators - CDC COVID-19 Response Team. Multisystem Inflammatory Syndrome in U.S. Children and Adolescents. *N Engl J Med.* 2020;383(4):334-346.

20. COVID-19 Treatment Guidelines Panel. Coronavirus Disease 2019 (COVID-19) Treatment Guidelines. National Institutes of Health. Available at https://www.covid19treatmentguidelines.nih.gov/.

21. Henderson LA, Canna SW, Friedman KG, et al. American College of Rheumatology Clinical Guidance for Multisystem Inflammatory Syndrome in Children Associated with SARS-CoV-2 and Hyperinflammation in Pediatric COVID-19: Version 1. *Arthritis Rheumatol.* 2020;72(11):1791-1805.

22. Jordan D. The Deadliest Flu: The Complete Story of the Discovery and Reconstruction of the 1918 Pandemic Virus. Centers for Disease Control and Prevention, National Center for Immunization and Respiratory Diseases (NCIRD), December 17 (2019). Available at https://www.cdc.gov/flu/pandemic-resources/1918-pandemic-h1n1.html. Accessed March 19, 2020.

23. Glezen WP. Emerging infections: pandemic influenza. *Epidemiol Rev.* 1996;18:64-76.

24. Viboud C, Grais RF, Lafont BA, Miller MA, Simonsen L. Multinational impact of the 1968 Hong Kong influenza pandemic: evidence for a smoldering pandemic. *J Infect Dis.* 2005;192:233-48.

25. Garten RJ, Davis CT, Russell CA, et al. Antigenic and genetic characteristics of swine-origin 2009 A(H1N1) influenza viruses circulating in humans. *Science.* 2009;325:197-201.

26. Nair H, Brooks WA, Katz M, et al. Global burden of respiratory infections due to seasonal influenza in young children: a systematic review and meta-analysis. *Lancet.* 2011;378(9807):1917-30.

27. Rolfes MA, Foppa IM, Garg S, et al. Annual estimates of the burden of seasonal influenza in the United States: A tool for strengthening influenza surveillance and preparedness. *Influenza Other Respir Viruses.* 2018;12(1):132-137.

28. Gaitonde DY, Moore FC, Morgan MK. Influenza: diagnosis and treatment. *Am Fam Physician.* 2019;100(12):751-758.

29. Raoult D, Mouffok N, Bitam I, Piarroux R, Drancourt M. Plague: history and contemporary analysis. *J Infect.* 2013;66(1):18-26.

30. Zietz BP, Dunkelberg H. The history of the plague and the research on the causative agent *Yersinia pestis. Int J Hyg Environ Health.* 2004;207(2):165-78.

31. Cohn SK Jr. Epidemiology of the Black Death and successive waves of plague. *Med Hist Suppl.* 2008;(27):74-100.

32. Carniel E. Plague Today. *Med Hist Suppl.* 2008;(27):115-122.

33. Frith J. The History of Plague – Part 1. The Three Great Pandemics. https://jmvh.org/article/the-history-of-plague-part-1-the-three-great-pandemics/. Accessed December 1, 2020.

34. Plague. World Health Organization. https://www.who.int/health-topics/plague# tab=tab_1. Updated March 15, 2016. Accessed November 1, 2020.

35. Galy A, Loubet P, Peiffer-Smadja N, Yazdanpanah Y. La peste : mise au point et actualités [The plague: An overview and hot topics]. *Rev Med Interne*. 2018;39(11):863-868.

36. Yang R. Plague: recognition, treatment, and prevention. *J Clin Microbiol*. 2017; 56(1):e01519-e01517.

37. Riedel S. Plague: from natural disease to bioterrorism. *Proc (Bayl Univ Med Cent)*. 2005;18(2):116-124.

38. Mann JM, Shandler L, Cushing AH. Pediatric plague. *Pediatrics*. 1982;69(6): 762-767.

39. Andrianaivoarimanana V, Piola P, Wagner DM, Rakotomanana F, Maheriniaina V, Andrianalimanana S. Trends of human plague, Madagascar, 1998–2016. *Emerg Infect Dis*. 2019;25(2):220-228.

40. Sun W, Singh AK. Plague vaccine: recent progress and prospects. *Vaccines*. 2019;4(11).

41. Derbise A, Guillas C, Gerke C, Carniel E, Pizarro-Cerdà J, Demeure CE. Subcutaneous vaccination with a live attenuated Yersinia pseudotuberculosis plague vaccine. *Vaccine*. 2020;38(8):1888-1892.

42. Dillard RL, Juergens AL. Plague. 2020 Aug 10. In: StatPearls [Internet]. Treasure Island, FL: StatPearls Publishing; 2020.

43. aap.org/en-us/advocacy-and-policy/aap-health-initiatives/Children-and-Disasters/Pages/Biological-Terrorism-and-Agents.aspx.

44. Available at https://www.cdc.gov/plague/healthcare/clinicians.html.

45. WHO Guidelines on Tularemia.

46. American Academy of Pediatrics. Tularemia. In: Kimberlin DW, Brady MT, Jackson MA, Long SS, eds. *Red Book: 2018 Report of the Committee on Infectious Diseases*. American Academy of Pediatrics; 2018;861-864.

47. Olupot-Olupot P. Ebola in children: epidemiology, clinical features, diagnosis and outcomes. *Pediatr Infect Dis J*. 2015;34(3):314-6.

48. Ebola (Ebola Virus Disease). 2019, November 05. Available at https://www.cdc.gov/vhf/ebola/index.html. Accessed October, 2020.

49. McCormick JB. Lassa fever. In: Saluzzo JF, Dodet B, eds. *Emergence and Control of Rodent-Borne Viral Diseases*. Elsevier; 1999:177-195.

50. Kofman A, Choi MJ, Rollin PE. Lassa fever in travelers from West Africa, 1969–2016. *Emerg Infect Dis*. 2019;25(2):245-248.

51. Kernéis S, Koivogui L, Magassouba N, et al. Prevalence and risk factors of Lassa seropositivity in inhabitants of the forest region of Guinea: a cross-sectional study. *PLoS Negl Trop Dis*. 2009;3(11):e548. Erratum in: PLoS Negl Trop Dis. 2010;4(1).

52. Bhatt S, Gething PW, Brady OJ, et al. The global distribution and burden of dengue. *Nature*. 2013;496(7446):504-7.

53. Morens DM, Fauci AS. Dengue and hemorrhagic fever: a potential threat to public health in the United States. *JAMA*. 2008;299(2):214-6.

54. CDC. Chikungunya Virus Geographic Distribution 2020 provisional data for the United States. CDC. Available at https://www.cdc.gov/chikungunya/geo/united-states-2020.html.

55. Monson MH, Cole AK, Frame JD, Serwint JR, Alexander S, Jahrling PB. Pediatric Lassa fever: a review of 33 Liberian cases. *Am J Trop Med Hyg.* 1987;36(2):408-15.

56. Ellis EM, Sharp TM, Pérez-Padilla J, et al. Incidence and Risk Factors for Developing Dengue-Associated Hemophagocytic Lymphohistiocytosis in Puerto Rico, 2008–2013. *PLoS Negl Trop Dis.* 2016;10(8):e0004939.

57. Khan A, et al. Viral Hemorrhagic Fevers. Seminars in Pediatric Infectious Diseases. Philadelphia: WB Saunders Co., 1997;8(suppl 1):64-73.

58. Nipah Virus (NiV). 2014, March 20. Available at https://www.cdc.gov/vhf/nipah/index.html. Accessed October 2020.

59. Nikolay B, Salje H, Hossain MJ, et al. Transmission of Nipah Virus—14 Years of Investigations in Bangladesh. *N Engl J Med.* 2019;380(19):1804-1814.

60. Hendra Virus Disease. 2014, March 17. Available at https://www.cdc.gov/vhf/hendra/index.html. Accessed October 2020.

61. Rift Valley Fever. 2020, February 25. Available at https://www.cdc.gov/vhf/rvf/index.html. Accessed October 2020.

62. Available at www.cdc.gov/smallpox/history/history.html.

63. Jacobs BL, Langland JO, Kibler KV, Denzler KL, White, SD, Holecheck SA. Vaccinia virus vaccines: past, present and future. *Antiviral Research.* 2009;84(1):1-13.

64. Simpson K, Heymann D, Brown CS, et al. Human monkeypox – After 40 years, an unintended consequence of smallpox eradication. *Vaccine.* 2020;38(33):5077-5081.

65. Available at www.who.int/health-topics/smallpox.

66. Atkinson W, Hamborsky J, McIntyre L, Wolfe C. *Appendix Chapter on Smallpox – Epidemiology and Prevention of Vaccine-Preventable Diseases.* 10th ed. Atlanta: Centers for Disease Control and Prevention (CDC). 2007:281-306. Available at http://www.docsimmunize.org/immunize/cdcmanual/original/smallpox.pdf.

67. Lane JM, Summer L. Smallpox as a weapon for bioterrorism. Bioterrorism and Infectious Agents: A New Dilemma for the 21st Century. 2009;147-167.

68. Petersen E, Kantele A, Koopmans M, et al. Human monkeypox: epidemiologic and clinical characteristics, diagnosis, and prevention. *Infect Dis Clin North Am.* 2019;33(4):1027-1043.

69. Sklenovská N, Van Ranst M. Emergence of monkeypox as the most important orthopoxvirus infection in humans. *Front Public Health.* 2018;6:241.

70. Available at www.cdc.gov/poxvirus/monkeypox/transmission.html.

71. Petersen BW, Kabamba J, McCollum AM, et al. Vaccinating against monkeypox in the Democratic Republic of the Congo. *Antiviral Res.* 2019;162:171-177.

72. McFee RB, Leikin JB. *Toxico-Terrorism. Emergency Response and Clinical Approach to Chemical. Biological and Radiological Weapons.* New York, NY: McGraw Hill; 2008.

SECTION III
Crises in War and Natural Disasters

BIOTERRORISM 28

Ronaldo C. Go, MD

▌INTRODUCTION

Unlike epidemics or pandemics, in bioterrorism there is a deliberate act to cause harm. It can be distinguished by a point source outbreak with exposure to many people, uncommon infectious agent, and not endemic to the area.[1]

Biological weapons have been used throughout history. The first documented use was of tularemia-infected rams by the Hittites.[2] In the 4th century BC, Scythian archers used arrows dipped with decomposed cadavers of adders that contained *Clostridium perfringens* and *Clostridium tetani*.[3] In 1348, the Mongols used plague-ridden cadavers to besiege Caffa.[4] This technique was used by the Lithuanian army in 1422 and the Russian army against the Swedish army in Estonia in 1710.[5–8] Although ineffective compared to respiratory transmission, transmission of small pox via fomites was used by the Europeans to wipe out American Indians.[9–11] In 1797, Napoleon flooded Italian plains in hopes of spreading malaria. In 1863, Confederate soldiers sold clothes infected with small pox and yellow fever to Union soldiers.[6] In 1925, 108 nations signed "The Protocol for the Prohibition of the Use in War of Asphyxiating, Poisonous or other Gases, and of Bacteriological Methods of Warfare."[9–11]

During World War I, the Germans tried to infect their enemies with anthrax, *Pseudomonas pseudomallei*, cholera, and plague.[6] A Japanese program, Unit 731, inoculated prisoners of war with *Bacillus anthracis*, *Neisseria meningitides*, *Vibrio cholerae*, *Shigella*, and *Yersinia pestis*.[6] During World War II, the Germans experimented with *Rickettsia prowazekii*, Hepatitis A, and malaria on prisoners.[6–11] Americans and British experimented on Anthrax.[6] After World War II, the Americans experimented with *Aspergillus fumigatus*, *Bacillus subtilis var. globigii*, *Serratia marcescens*, *Francisella tularensis*, and *Coxiella Burnetti* in Fort Detrick, Maryland and other testing sites all over the country.[6–11] In 1972, the Convention on the "Prohibition of the Development,

Production, and Stockpiling of Bacteriological and Toxin Weapons and on their Destruction" or BTWC was developed although it did not provide guidelines for inspection, control of disarmament, and adherence to protocol.[6–11] In the United States, research efforts continued to develop countermeasures such as vaccines and antisera and the entire arsenal of biological weapons were destroyed by February 1973.

In 1979, there was an epidemic of Anthrax in Ekaterinburg, Russia from an accidental leak in a biological research facility.[6–11] During the first Persian Gulf War, there was concern for both biological and chemical warfare which prompted the United States and allied nations to prepare for such an attack during Operation Desert Shield.[6–11] In 1984, the Rajneeshee cult used *Salmonella typhimurium* in Oregon.[6–11] In 1995, the Aum Shinrikyo tried to release sarin in the Tokyo subway system and also tried Anthrax, botulinum toxin, and Ebola.[6–11] In June 2018, a Tunisian extremist living in Cologne, Germany was found to have produced ricin.[6–11]

SPECIFIC PATHOGENS

The Centers for Disease Control and Prevention (CDC) has stratified the pathogens based on their ease of dissemination, mortality rates, ability to cause public panic, and need for special preparedness into Categories A, B, and C (see Table 28-1).[12] Pathogens that are not described in the pandemic section will be discussed here.

Table 28-1 CDC PATHOGEN CATEGORIES		
Category A	**Category B**	**Category C**
• Anthrax	• Brucellosis	• Nipah Virus
• Botulism	• *Clostridium perfringens*	• Hanta Virus
• Plague	• Salmonella	
• Small Pox	• *E. coli* 0175:H7	
• Tularemia	• *Shigella*	
• Viral hemorrhagic fevers	• Glanders	
	• Melioidosis	
	• Psittacosis	
	• Q-Fever	
	• Ricin toxin	
	• Staphylococcal enterotoxin B	
	• Typhus fever	
	• Viral encephalitis	
	• *Vibrio cholerae*	
	• *Cryptosporidium parvum*	

Category A

Smallpox

Smallpox is caused by the Variola virus, a member of genus *Orthopoxvirus* (Figure 28-1). It was infecting 10–15 million a year and killed 300 million people in 20th century.[13,14] With the help of vaccination, it was declared eradicated in 1980.[13,14] Since then, the smallpox vaccine has not been used for decades, herd immunity is minimal, and the vaccine may be ineffective after onset of illness. There are currently only two smallpox repositories, the United States Centers for Disease Control and Prevention (CDC) in Atlanta, Georgia, and the State Research Center of Virology and Biotechnology (VECTOR) in Novosibirsk, Russia.[14,15] The possibility of an outbreak or synthesis de novo is real and antivirals, such as tecovirimat and brincidofovir, and modified vaccinia Ankara have been

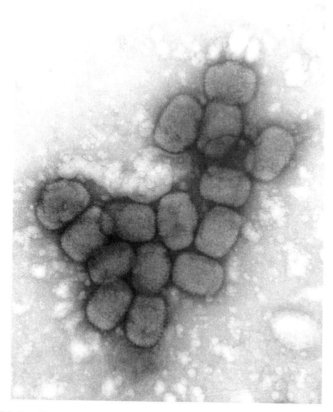

Figure 28-1 • Transmission electron microscope of a cluster of smallpox viruses. (*Courtesy of the CDC.* https://phil.cdc.gov/Details.aspx?pid=10144.)

developed.[16–18] The antivirals were developed from less deadly orthopox such as monkeypox and rabbitpox.[16–18]

The only known hosts are humans and the mode of transmission is face to face contact via infected oropharyngeal saliva, nasal or respiratory mucosa. The virus can linger on clothes, bedding or fomites.

Clinically, there is a 2–4 day prodromal stage of fever, malaise, headache, back pain, abdominal pain, and vomiting.[19] Fever may disappear and be followed by a maculopapular rash in centrifugal distribution. The rash is initially on the oral mucosa, face, hands, forearms and progresses toward the trunk[19] (Figure 28-2). The lesions progress from macules, to papules, and to pustular vesicles. From 8 to 14 days, the pustules form scabs and fall off 3–4 weeks later. They can leave scars. Patients are infectious from the onset of the rash until all scabs have detached. Two forms that are fatal even in vaccinated patients are hemorrhagic smallpox, which

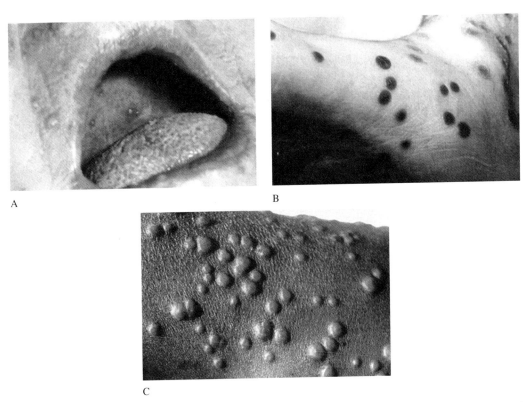

A

B

C

Figure 28-2 • A. Maculopapular vesicles on 3rd day of illness. (*Courtesy of the CDC.* https://phil.cdc.gov/ Details.aspx?pid=21632.) **B.** Modified variola major rash on medial and planter aspect of the foot. (*Courtesy of the CDC.* https://phil.cdc.gov/Details.aspx?pid=21635.) **C.** Maculopapular rash over neck and upper back of a patient on 5th day of illness. (*Courtesy of the CDC.* https://phil.cdc.gov/Details.aspx?pid=16056.)

is accompanied by hemorrhage into mucous membranes and malignant smallpox, which does not have a pustular stage.[19]

Diagnosis is based on immunofluorescence microscopy, negative stain electron microscopy, PCR, or detection of anti-smallpox antibodies through virus neutralization, hemagglutination inhibition, western blot, ELISA, or complement fixation. Treatment includes vaccination, which as per WHO, the replication-competent vaccinia vaccine ACAM2000 can be given 4 days into illness but contraindicated in pregnancy or patients who are immunocompromised, tecovirimat 600 mg PO BID × 14 days, and new vaccines Ankara and LC16m8.[16–18]

Monkeypox

From the same genus as smallpox, monkeypox is clinically similar and predominantly found in Central and West Africa.[19] Reservoirs are prairie dogs, squirrels, rats, and monkeys.[19,20] Human transmission is possible via exposure to infected body fluids, skin lesions, or recently contaminated objects[19] (Figure 28-3).

The incubation period can range from 5 to 21 days. Initially, it presents with fever, headaches, back pain, fatigue, and myalgias. Characteristic is the lymphadenopathy and rash that shortly follows fever.[21,22] The adenopathy can be firm, tender, and painful and often located in maxillary, cervical or inguinal regions.[22] The fever may decline 3 days after onset of rash.[22] The rash is more concentrated—in descending order—on the face, palms, soles, oral mucosa, genitalia, and conjunctivae. The rash also evolves from macules, to papules, vesicles, and pustules, and then crusts

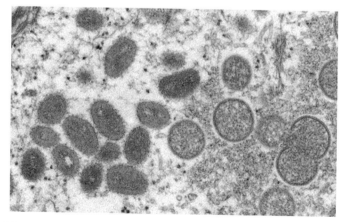

Figure 28-3 • Electron microscope of monkeypox viruses. (*Courtesy of the CDC.* https://phil.cdc.gov/Details.aspx?pid=22664.)

and falls off (Figure 28-4). It is self-limited, but complications include secondary infections, encephalitis, and blindness. Diagnosis is via viral culture, electron microscopy, immunohistochemistry, PCR, and anti-orthopoxvirus IgG.[23] Treatment includes cidofovir, CMX-001, ST-246, and the smallpox vaccines (ACAM2000, Ankara, and LC16m8).[24-26]

Anthrax

Bacillus anthracis is a non-motile spore forming, Gram-positive rod-shaped bacteria that causes the disease anthrax[27] (Figure 28-5). Even

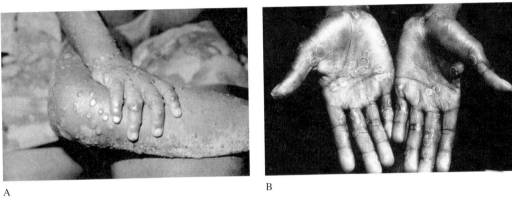

A   B

Figure 28-4 • A and B. Maculopapular monkeypox lesions that are similar to smallpox. (*Courtesy of the CDC.* https://phil.cdc.gov/Details.aspx?pid=2329 and https://phil.cdc.gov/Details.aspx?pid=12761.)

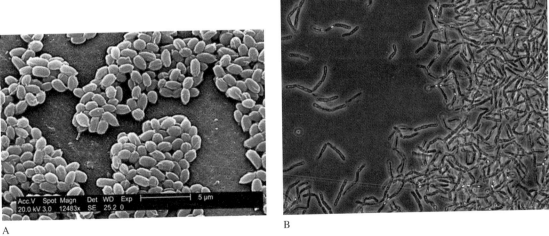

A   B

Figure 28-5 • A. Scanning electron microscope of *Bacillus anthracis*. (*Courtesy of the CDC.* https://phil.cdc.gov/Details.aspx?pid=10122.) **B.** Endospores under phase contrast microscopy. (*Courtesy of the CDC.* https://phil.cdc.gov/Details.aspx?pid=1893.)

with treatment, the mortality rate for cutaneous or injection is 28%, gastrointestinal > 40%, inhalation 45%, and meningeal nearly always fatal.[27–31] Once inside the host, the spores germinate or transport to lymph nodes. Toxins are produced within hours of germination. These toxins are edema toxin which is a combination of protective antigen and edema factor, and lethal toxin which is a combination of protective antigen and lethal factor.[27] This causes inhalation, cutaneous, gastrointestinal, and meningeal disease (Figure 28-6A–C). Hemorrhage and necrosis is found in mediastinal adenopathy and lungs.[21] Treatment begins with hemodynamic support and adjunct dexamethasone may be used due to

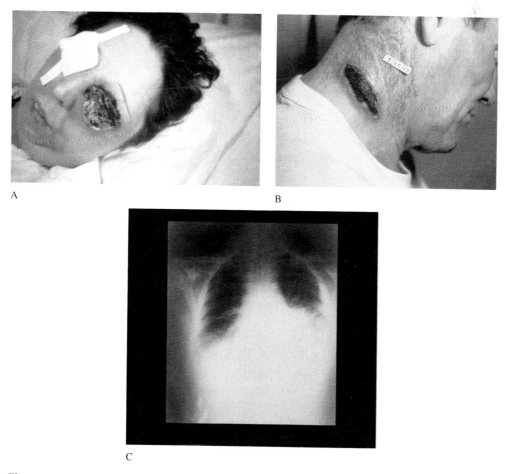

A

B

C

Figure 28-6 • A. Blackened eschar over infected left eye. (*Courtesy of the CDC.* https://phil.cdc.gov/Details.aspx?pid=4505.) **B.** Blacked eschar on patient's neck. (*Courtesy of the CDC.* https://phil.cdc.gov.Details.aspxpid=1934.) **C.** Chest radiograph of a widened mediastinum. (*Courtesy of the CDC.* https://phil.cdc.gov/Details.aspx?pid=1118.)

observational studies in cutaneous head and neck anthrax and meningeal anthrax.[26–28]

Antibiotic choice should be to treat the production of the toxin, decrease the potential for antimicrobial drug resistance, target meningeal involvement, and target latent spores.[27–33] For systemic disease with possible meningitis, ≥3 antimicrobial drugs are needed for >2 weeks. To reduce the production of exotoxin, protein synthesis inhibitors are needed such as linezolid > clindamycin > rifampin > chloramphenicol. Intravenous ciprofloxacin is the primary antibacterial drug. Meropenem is the second antimicrobial; and if unavailable, doripenem and imipenem/cilastatin can be used.

If meningeal involvement is ruled out, treatment should consist of ≥2 antimicrobial drugs, with ≥1 bactericidal activity and ≥ 1 should be a protein synthesis inhibitor.[27,32] This should be given for at least 2 weeks or until clinically stable; whichever is longer.

For cutaneous anthrax without systemic involvement with suspected bioterrorism, treatment is longer than a 7–10 day course of oral fluroquinolones or doxycycline due to inhaled spores.

Antitoxins inhibit the binding of PA to the anthrax toxin and translocation of LT and ET into cells.[27] Raxibacumab has not been tested for systemic anthrax but FDA approved for post-exposure prophylaxis PEP at a dose of 40 mg/kg.[27,34] Anthrax immune globulin is not FDA approved but can be given under investigational new drug protocol.[27,32]

Anthrax prevention requires the immediate use of ciprofloxacin, and doxycycline for > 18 years of age exposed to inhalation anthrax.[27,33] Levofloxacin is an alternative to ciprofloxacin. Anthrax vaccine adsorbed (AVA) should be given at diagnosis and repeated every 2 weeks for a total of three doses.

Botulism

Clostridium botulinum is a gram-positive motile rod (Figure 28-7). It has seven distinct toxins that block the acetylcholine transmission at the presynaptic motor-neuron terminal. Initially there is symmetrical cranial nerve palsies, followed by symmetrical flaccid paralysis. The symmetrical flaccid paralysis begins with muscles of the neck, shoulder, proximal and then distal upper extremities followed by proximal and distal lower extremities. Paralysis of diaphragm and accessory respiratory muscles occurs next. Deep tendon reflexes disappear. Constipation appears to be almost universal. Hypotension may occur.

There are several botulism-related syndromes. There is foodborne botulism, particularly when food is obtained in an anaerobic environment,

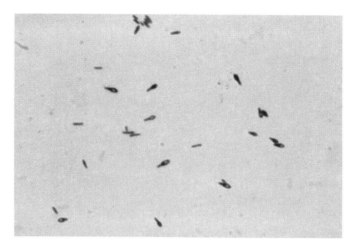

Figure 28-7 • *Clostridium botulinum* in gram-stained thioglycolate broth specimen. (*Courtesy of the CDC.* https://phil.cdc.gov/Details.aspx?pid=3870.)

with temperature of 70–110°F, pH < 4.5, and low salt and sugar content; infant botulism when normal bowel florae can't compete with *C. botulinum* and risk factor of honey; adult intestinal toxemia botulism where patients have anatomical or functional abnormalities or use of antimicrobials which allow the Clostridia species to flourish; wound botulism, particularly in IV drug use; and inhalation botulism.[35–51] Inhalation botulism is considered a possible biological threat. Symptoms develop within 12–36 hours regardless of exposure.

Diagnosis is confirmed with demonstration of *C. botulinum* or toxin in wound, gastric secretions or stool and serum samples. Treatment is supportive and anti-toxin. Ideally, antitoxin is given < 24 hours after symptom onset to neutralize still unbound toxin molecules.[52]

Category B

Brucellosis

Four species, *Brucellosis melitensis* (Figure 28-8), *B. abortus*, *B. suis*, and *B. canis* cause the disease brucellosis. Typical mode of transmission is consumption of unpasteurized dairy products; airborne transmission is possible in the context of bioterrorism. Once inside the human body, it is taken up by lymphocytes and transferred to regional lymph nodes and circulated throughout the body. The inoculation is from 2 to 4 weeks, but can be up to 5 months.[53–55]

Figure 28-8 • *Brucella melitensis* coccobacillus culture. (*Courtesy of the CDC.* https:// phil.cdc.gov/Details.aspx?pid=1901.)

Clinical presentations include constitutional symptoms such as fever but also with malodorous perspiration, lymphadenopathy, hepatospleno megaly, liver abscess, osteoartricular diseases such as peripheral arthritis, reactive arthritis, and sacroiliitis, particularly the lumbar spine, epididymo-orchitis, central nervous system complications such as meningitis, encephalitis, meningoencephalitis, brain abscess, and demyelinating syndromes, and endocarditis.[53,54]

Post-exposure prophylaxis (PEP) includes doxycycline 100 mg PO BID and rifampin 600 mg daily for 3 weeks. TMP-SMZ can be substituted for doxycycline or rifampin. Treatment consists of doxycycline 200 mg daily with rifampin 600–900 mg daily for 6 weeks or the alternative is replacement of rifampicin with 15 mg/kg streptomycin for the first 2–3 weeks.[53–55]

Clostridium Perfringens

Clostridium perfringens is a Gram-positive spore forming anaerobe that can create the epsilon toxin (ETX)[50] (Figure 28-9). It can naturally be found in soil, dust, litter, cadavers and digestive systems of healthy animals but can be used in biological warfare via aerosolization and ingestion.[56] Enterotoxin increases cell permeability, causing shock and death. Its aerosolized form is stable for up to 8 hours, and symptoms can appear from 1 to 12 hours from exposure.[56] Diagnosis is via 10^6 *C. perfringens* spores per gram of stool within 48 hours of symptoms or ELISA, classic

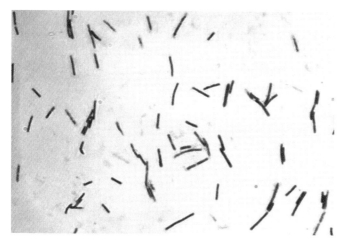

Figure 28-9 • Gram stained specimen of *clostridium perfringens* in Schaedler broth. (*Courtesy of the CDC.* https://phil.cdc.gov/Details.aspx?pid=2995.)

mouse assay, quantitation of ETX protein via mass spectrometry, latex agglutination test, and cytotoxic assay.[56] There may be hemolytic anemia, thrombocytopenia, hypoxia, cerebral edema, seizures, and elevated liver function tests. Treatment is supportive and formalin-inactivated vaccine and equine-derived antitoxin.[56–62]

Ricin Toxin

The castor plant *or Ricinus communis*, produces the toxin ricin. It can be injected, ingested, or inhaled. Ricin enters the cell through membrane-bound receptors and inhibits protein synthesis at the level of ribosome. Fifty percent of ricin can be inactivated at a temperature of 80°C for at least > 1 hour, or chlorine solutions.[63,64] Patients can progress to acute respiratory distress syndrome and death within 36–72 hours if inhaled, local muscle necrosis and adenopathy if injected, and nausea, vomiting, diarrhea, hematuria and renal failure if ingested. Diagnosis is via immunoassays. Treatment is supportive and exposure should prompt decontamination with soap and water.[65,66]

Staphylococcal Enterotoxin B

This is produced by *Staphylococcus aureus*, a Gram-positive bacterium that can exist in skin, mucosa, and even as a part of the normal respiratory tract flora in 20% of patients. It can enter humans through consumption, respiratory tract, and vaginal tract. It cannot be transmitted from person to person.[67,68] Symptoms are dependent on the route of entry. With inhalation, fevers occur within 3–12 hours followed by cough, acute respiratory distress syndrome, and multiorgan failure. Ingestion can lead to nausea, vomiting, diarrhea within 1–8 hours and without fever. Symptoms improve by 48 hours. Toxin can be detected via immunologic assays if within 12–24 hours from exposure. Treatment is supportive.

E. coli 0175:H7

Shiga toxin produced by *E. Coli* has a similar structure and function to Shiga toxins produced by *Shigella dystenteriae* type 1[69,70] (Figure 28-10). It causes an enterohemorrhagic diarrhea, which can later progress into hemolytic uremic syndrome (HUS). This is characterized by thrombocytopenia, hemolytic anemia, and renal failure.[71–73] Diagnosis is via selective culture or Shiga toxin testing via immunoassay or molecular technology. Treatment is supportive care and antibiotics are avoided.

Shigella

Shigella is a Gram-negative enterobacteriaceae that can result in watery to bloody diarrhea[74] (Figure 28-11). The bacteria enters enterally and enters host via M Cells. The bacteria induces phagocytosis via macrophages and leads to macrophage death and lysis of surrounding phagosome. Diagnosis is via culture and PCR. Treatment is ciprofloxacin or azithromycin.

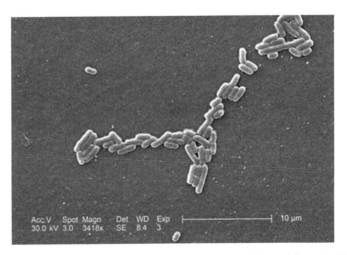

Figure 28-10 • Scanning electron microscopic image of *E. coli* bacteria 0157:H7. (*Courtesy of the CDC.* https://phil.cdc.gov/Details.aspx?pid=10070.)

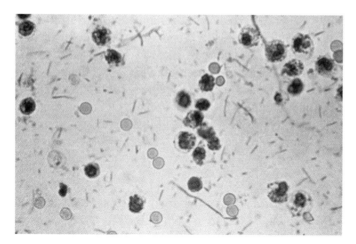

Figure 28-11 • Shigella bacterial in stool exudates. (*Courtesy of the CDC.* https://phil.cdc.gov/Details.aspx?pid=6659.)

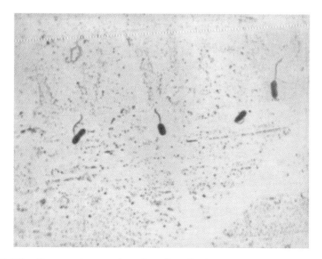

Figure 28-12 • Gram stain revealing flagellated *Vibrio cholerae*. (*Courtesy of the CDC.* https://phil.cdc.gov/Details.aspx?pid=23062.)

Vibrio Cholerae

Vibrio cholerae is a Gram-negative bacteria that can cause watery diarrhea which can lead to hypovolemic shock (Figure 28-12). Ingestion of 10^8 is required to induce symptomatic infection. Fever is absent and stool loss can be > 1 liter per hour.[75,76] Patients at risk for severe infection include those with blood type O and less acidic gastric pH. *V. cholerae* O1 or O139 serogroups excrete an exotoxin that induces fluid secretion in the small intestine, particularly jejunum.[75,76] Colonization is secondary to cholera toxin co-regulated pilus, which is a soluble hemagglutinin/Zn-metalloprotease that facilitates penetration; and flagella which moves the bacteria.[75,76] Diagnosis is via culture on thiosulfate-citrate-bile salts sucrose agar or taurocholate tellurite-gelatin, or dark field microscopy. If it is in endemic areas, diagnosis can be made clinically. Azithromycin or cirprofloxacin can be used for treatment in addition to fluid resuscitation and electrolyte replenishment. Vaccines are available for prevention.

Salmonella

Salmonella is a gram negative, non-spore forming flagellated facultative anaerobe (Figure 28-13). It is harbored in the intestinal tracts of humans and farm animals and transmitted via fecal and oral route.[77] A dose of 10^5 to 10^6 cells constitutes the infective dose and the bacteria targets enterocytes. The bacteria also exudes toxins: enterotoxin and cytotoxin. The enterotoxin induces fluid accumulation and cytotoxin inhibits protein synthesis, causing mucosal damage. The O antigen lipopolysaccharide influences the virulence; and length of chain determines virulence.[78–82] *Salmonella* also has virulence genes which are responsible for dissemination.[78–82] Diagnosis is via blood cultures, Widal test, enzyme-linked immunosorbent assay, and PCR. Treatment is via supportive care and 14-day course of antibiotics. If immunocompromised, a longer course of antibiotics might be necessary. Fluroquinolones (ciprofloxacin 400 mg IV

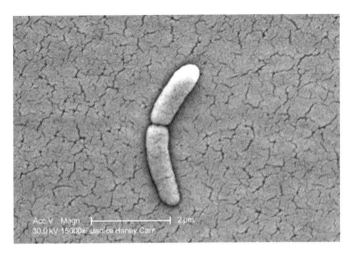

Figure 28-13 • Single Gram-negative *Salmonella typhimurium* at the process of cell division. (*Courtesy of the CDC.* https://phil.cdc.gov/Details.aspx?pid=10993.)

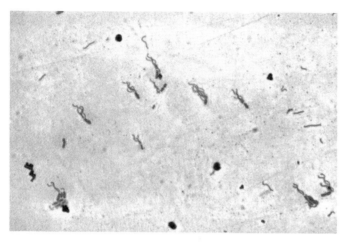

Figure 28-14 • Gram-negative flagellated *Burkholderia pseudomallei*. (*Courtesy of the CDC*. https://phil.cdc.gov/Details.aspx?pid=16985.)

twice a day or levofloxacin 500–750 mg IV daily), 3rd generation cephalosporins (ceftriaxone 1–2 g IV daily or cefotaxime 2 g IV every 8 hours), trimethoprim-sulfamethoxazole (8–10 mg/kg/day), or ampicillin (2 g IV every 4 hours). Vaccinations can be used to prevent infection.

Burkholderia

Burkholderia is a genus of Gram-negative bacteria that causes glanders (*Burkholderia mallei*) and melioidosis (*Burkholderia pseudomallei*)[83–85] (Figure 28-14). Human-to-human transmission occur via respiratory droplets and cutaneous secretions. There is a shorter incubation time if inhaled (1–2 days) compared to cutaneous transmission (up to 14 days). In addition to constitutional symptoms, inhalation exposure leads to pneumonia, necrosis, adenopathy, and dissemination from other organs. Cutaneous exposure leads to pustules and adenopathy and systemic dissemination between 1 and 4 weeks. Diagnosis is via cultures. Treatment is via 10–14 days of antibiotics followed by 3 months of oral therapy. Choice of antibiotics include carbapenems, ceftazidime, cefepime, azithromycin, clarithromycin, doxycycline, TMP/SMX, and gentamicin.[83–85]

Psittacosis

Chlamydia psittaci is an intracellular Gram-negative bacteria (Figure 28-15). Human illness is caused by inhalation of aerosols from urine or feces from infected birds. Incubation time is between 5 and 30 days.

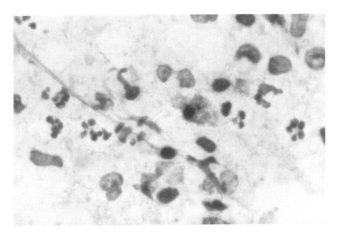

Figure 28-15 • Gram-negative *Chlamydophila psittaci.* (*Courtesy of the CDC.* https://phil.cdc.gov/Details.aspx?pid=15732.)

Symptoms include high fever, low pulse, cough, shortness of breath, rash, vomiting, abdominal pain, and diarrhea. It can have complications such as myocarditis, endocarditis, encephalitis, and acute respiratory distress syndrome (ARDS). Diagnosis is via culture, serologies via complement fixation, microimmunofluorescent antibody test, and monoclonal antibody techniques, and PCR. Treatment is a 10–14-day course of doxycycline 100 mg PO every 12 hours or tetracycline 500 mg PO every 6 hours.[86–88] Second line therapy includes erythromycin, azithromycin, chloramphenicol, and rifampin.

Q-Fever

Coxiella burnettii is a Gram-negative bacterium that causes Q fever (Figure 28-16). This is an intracellular bacterium and host cell is the macrophage. Cattle, goats, sheep, cats, rabbits, pigeons, dogs, and ticks are common reservoirs. In humans, inhalation of contaminated aerosols and consumption are common sources

Incubation time is 20 days and Q fever syndromes include acute Q fever, chronic Q fever, and post Q fever syndrome. Acute Q fever is marked by high grade fever, headache, myalgias, pneumonia, granulomatous hepatitis, maculopapular rash, pericarditis, myocarditis, meningitis, encephalitis, or acute acalculous cholecystitis.[89–95] Chronic Q fever affects the heart, bones, and liver such as endocarditis, aneurysms, osteomyelitis, pericardial effusion, pulmonary interstitial fibrosis, pseudotumor of lung, amyloidosis, and mixed cryoglobulinemia. Diagnosis

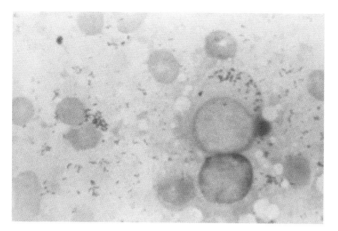

Figure 28-16 • Gram-negative *Coxiella burnetii*. (*Courtesy of the CDC*. https://phil.cdc. gov/Details.aspx?pid=19135.)

is difficult since cultures are negative. Patients may have elevated ESR, elevated aminotransferases, hyperglobulinemia, rheumatoid factor, and anemia. Confirmation of diagnosis is dependent on antibodies for phase I and phase II antigens and PCR. Treatment is warranted for symptomatic patients. Tetracycline, doxycycline, ofloxacin, and pefloxacin have been used.[89-95]

Cryptosporidiosis

Cryptosporidium parvum is a parasite that causes diarrhea (Figure 28-17). It is mainly transmitted through the fecal oral route although it can also be inhaled. It is typically self-limited, but in the immunocompromised, it can cause profuse chronic diarrhea, malabsorption, and inflammatory biliary disease leading to obstructive sclerosing cholangitis, papillary stenosis, and pancreatitis. Diagnosis is identification of oocytes in feces. Treatment is supportive and nitazoxanide in non-immunocompromised patients.[96-99]

Typhus Fever

This is caused by bacteria that is spread by fleas (murine typhus), chiggers (scrub typhus), and lice (epidemic typhus)[100] (Figure 28-18). Scrub typhus is predominantly from the Asia-Pacific region. Symptoms begin 7 days from exposure and include fever, chills, headaches, and altered mental status. Patients develop adenopathy, eschar, and rash. Laboratory

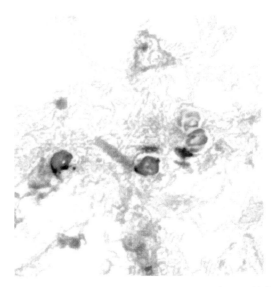

Figure 28-17 • *Cryptosporidium parvum* oocysts stained in acid-fast method and appear bright red. Oocysts contain sporozoites, which are the motile stage of the disease. (*Courtesy of the CDC*. https://phil.cdc.gov/Details.aspx?pid=7829.)

abnormalities include elevated liver function tests, hepatosplenomegaly, acute renal failure, acute respiratory failure, and encephalitis. Diagnosis is via serologic assays such as immunofluorescence assay, ELISA, and indirect immunoperoxidase assays. Murine typhus is caused by *Rickettsia typhi*.[100] Infection is via contact with flea species or inhalation. Symptoms begin 7–14 days after exposure and include myalgias, gastrointestinal symptoms, altered mental status, and cough. Much like scrub typhus, it can have elevated liver function tests, but also anemia, thrombocytopenia, leukopenia, and hyponatremia.[100] Rash occurs at the end of the first week and is a maculopapular eruption on the trunk and spreads peripherally; sparing palms and soles.[100] Diagnosis is via indirect immunofluorescence antibody, immunohistochemistry.[100] Epidemic typhus is from human louse and the bacteria is *R. prowazekii*. Infection can occur with contact or inhalation. Symptoms occur 8–16 days from exposure and consist of fever, headache, gastrointestinal symptoms, and altered mental status. Rash is similar to murine typhus. Treatment is ≥ 3-day course of doxycycline 100 mg PO twice a day and for children < 45 kg, 2.2 mg/kg body weight twice per day until the fever subsides or when there is clinical improvement.[100] Alternatives for scrub typhus include azithromycin, chloramphenicol or rifampin.[100]

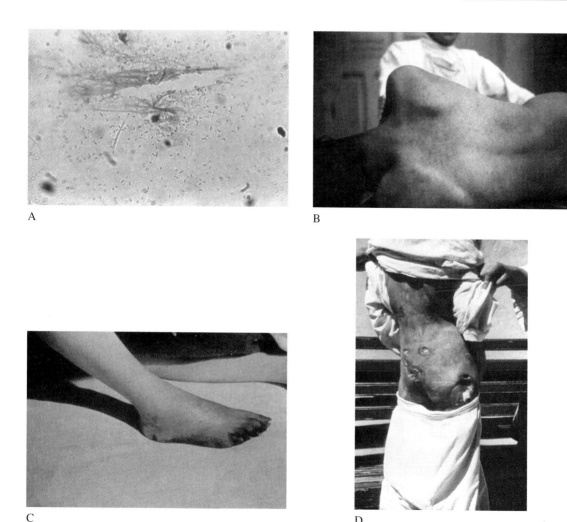

Figure 28-18 • A. Rickettis sp. In Gimenez-stained yolk sac smear. (*Courtesy of the CDC*. https://phil.cdc.gov/Details.aspx?pid=20205.) **B.** Maculopapular rash on chest. (*Courtesy of the CDC*. https://phil.cdc.gov/Details.aspx?pid=18838.) **C.** Typhus gangrene of right foot after typhus fever. (*Courtesy of the CDC*. https://phil.cdc.gov/Details.aspx?pid=18840.) **D.** Ulcerations of lower back and right hip due to typhus fever. (*Courtesy of the CDC*. https://phil.cdc.gov/Details.aspx?pid=18841.)

▌REFERENCES

1. Green MS, LeDuc J, Cohen D, Franz DR. Terrorism and health 2: Confronting the threat of bioterrorism: realities, challenges, and defensive strategies. *Lancet Infect Dis*. 2019;19:e2-e13.
2. Trevisatano SI. The 'Hittite plague' an epidemic of tularemia and the first record of biological warfare. *Med Hypotheses*. 2007;69:1371-1374.
3. Grmek MD. Les ruses de guerre dans l'Antiquité. *Rev Etud Grec*. 1979;92:141-163.

4. Wheelis M. Biological warfare at the 1346 siege of Caffa. *Emerg Infect Dis.* 2002 [serial online] Sep [date cited] Available at http://wwwnc.cdc.gov/eid/article/8/9/01-0536.htm. Accessed April 9, 2014.

5. Robertson AG, Robertson LJ. From asps to allegations: biological warfare in history. *Mil Med.* 1995;160:369-373.

6. Riedel SM. Biological warfare and bioterrorism: a historical review. *BUMC Proc.* 2004;17:400-406.

7. Poupart JA, Miller LA. History of biological warfare: catapults to capsomeres. *Ann N Y Acad Sci.* 1992;666:9-20.

8. Frischknecht F. The history of biological warfare human experimentation, modern nightmares and lone madmen in the twentieth century. *EMBO Rep.* 2003;4(suppl 1):S47-S52.

9. Christopher GW, Cieslak TJ, Pavlin JA, Eitzen EM. Biological warfare. A historical perspective. *JAMA.* 1997;278:412-417.

10. Henderson DA, Inglesby TV, Bartlett JG, et al. Smallpox as a biological weapon: medical and public health management. Working Group on Civilian Biodefense. *JAMA.* 1999;281:2127-2137.

11. Sipe CH. *The Indian Wars of Pennsylvania.* Harrisburg, PA: Telegraph Press; 1929.

12. Emergency Preparedness and Response. Centers of Disease Control and Prevention. Available at https://emergency.cdc.gov/bioterrorism/. Updated November 12, 2020. Accessed January 25, 2021.

13. World Health Organization. Smallpox: Eradicating an ancient scourge. World Health Organization. Available at http://www.who.int/about/bugs_drugs_smoke_chapter_1_smallpox.pdf. Updated May 27, 2018. Accessed January 1, 2021.

14. Inglesby T. Horsepox and the need for a new norm, more transparency, and stronger oversight for experiments that pose pandemic risks. *PLoS Pathog.* 2018;14(10):e1007129.

15. Centers for Disease Control and Prevention. CDC Media Statement on Newly Discovered Smallpox Specimens. Centers for Disease Control and Prevention. 2014 July 8. Available at https://www.cdc.gov/media/releases/2014/s0708-nih.html. Updated May 27, 2018. Accessed January 1, 2021.

16. Grosenbach DW, Honeychurch K, Rose EA, et al. Oral Tecovirimat for the treatment of smallpox. *N Engl J Med.* 2018;379:44-53.

17. Foster SA, Parker S, Lanier R. The role of brincidofovir in preparation of a potential smallpox outbreak. *Viruses.* 2017;9(11):320.

18. Pittman PR, Han M, Lee HS, et al. Phase 3 efficacy trial of modified vaccinia Ankara as a vaccine against small-pox. *N Engl J Med.* 2019;381(20):1897-1908.

19. World Health Organization. Available at https://www.who.int/csr/delibepidemics/annex3.pdf. Updated 2004. Accessed January 1, 2021.

20. World Health Organization. Available at https://www.who.int/news-room/factsheets/detail/monkeypox. Accessed January 1, 2021.

21. Reed K, Melski JW, Graham MB, et al. The detection of monkeypox in humans in the western hemisphere. *N Engl J Med.* 2004;350:342-350.

22. Sklenovska N, van Ranst M. Emergence of monkeypox as the most important orthopoxvirus infection in humans. *Front Public Health.* 2018;4(6):241.

23. McCollum AM, Damon IK. Human monkeypox. Emerging Infections. CID. January 15, 2014;58:260-267.

24. Kenner J, Cameron F, Empig C, Jobes DV, Gurwith M. LC16m8: An attenuated smallpox vaccine. *Vaccine*. 2006;24(47):7009-7022.

25. Eto A, Saito T, Yokote H, Kurane I, Kanatani Y. Recent advances in the study of live attenuated cell-cultured smallpox vaccine LC16m8. *Vaccine*. 2015;33(45):6106-6111.

26. Andrei G, Snoeck R. Cidofovir activity against poxvirus infections. *Viruses*. 2010;2:2803-2830.

27. Hendricks KA, Wright ME, Shadomy SV, et al. Centers for Disease Control and Prevention expert panel meetings on prevention and treatment of anthrax in adults. *Emerg Infect Dis*. 2014;20(2):e130687.

28. National Anthrax Outbreak Control Team An outbreak of anthrax among drug users in Scotland, December 2009 to December 2010. Glasgow (Scotland): Health Protection Scotland; 2011. [cited 2013 Nov 25]. Available at http://www.documents.hps.scot.nhs.uk/giz/anthrax-outbreak/anthrax-outbreak-report-2011-12.pdf.

29. Beatty ME, Ashford DA, Griffin PM, Tauxe RV, Sobel J. Gastrointestinal anthrax: review of the literature. *Arch Intern Med*. 2003;163:2527-31.

30. Barakat LA, Quentzel HL, Jernigan JA, Kirschke DL, Griffith K, Spear SM, et al. Fatal inhalational anthrax in a 94-year-old Connecticut woman. *JAMA*. 2002;287:863-8.

31. Sejvar JJ, Tenover FC, Stephens DS. Management of anthrax meningitis. *Lancet Infect Dis*. 2005;5:287-95.

32. Demirdag K, Ozden M, Saral Y, Kalkan A, Kilic SS, Ozdarendeli A. Cutaneous anthrax in adults: a review of 25 cases in the eastern Anatolian region of Turkey. *Infection*. 2003;31:327-30.

33. Tahernia AC. Treatment of anthrax in children. *Arch Dis Child*. 1967;42:181-2.

34. Migone TS, Subramanian GM, Zhong J, Healey LM, Corey A, Devalaraja M. Raxibacumab for the treatment of inhalational anthrax. *N Engl J Med*. 2009;361:135-44.

35. Sobel J. Botulism. *Clinical Infectious Disease*. 2005;31:1167-73.

36. International Commission on Microbiological Specifications for Foods. *Clostridium botulinum*. In: Micro-organisms in foods 5: characteristics of microbial pathogens. New York: Blackie Academic & Professional; 1996:68-111.

37. Shapiro R, Hatheway CL, Swerdlow DL. Botulism in the United States: a clinical and epidemiologic review. *Ann Intern Med*. 1998;129.

38. Gangarosa EA. Botulism in the US, 1899–1969. *Am J Epidemiol*. 1971;93:93-101.

39. Wainright RB, Heyward WL, Middaugh JP, Hatheway CL, Harpster AP, Bender TR. Food-borne botulism in Alaska, 1947–1985: epidemiology and clinical findings. *J Infect Dis*. 1988;157:1158-62.

40. Sobel J, Tucker N, McLaughlin J, Maslanka S. Foodborne botulism in the United States, 1990–2000. *Emerg Infect Dis*. 2004;10:1606-11.

41. Werner SB, Passaro DJ, McGee J, Schechter R, Vugia DJ. Wound botulism in California, 1951–1998: a recent epidemic in heroin injectors. *Clin Infect Dis*. 2000;31:1018-24.

42. Passaro DJ, Werner SB, McGee J, MacKenzie W, Vugia D. Wound botulism associated with black tar heroin among injecting drug users. *JAMA*. 1998;279:859-63.

43. Arnon S. Infant botulism. In: Feigen RD, Cherry JD, eds. *Textbook of Pediatric Infectious Diseases*. 4th ed. Philadelphia: WB Saunders; 1998:1570-7.

44. Spika JS, Shafer N, Hargrett-Bean N. Risk factors for infant botulism in the United States. *Am J Dis Child*. 1989;143:828-32.

45. Long S. Epidemiologic study of infant botulism in Pennsylvania: report of the infant botulism study group. *Pediatrics*. 1985;75:928-34.

46. Arnon SS, Midura TF, Clay SA, Wood RM, Chin J. Infant botulism: epidemiological, clinical, and laboratory aspects. *JAMA*. 1977;237:1946-51.

47. Chia JK, Clark JB, Ryan CA, Pollack M. Botulism in an adult associated with food-borne intestinal infection with *Clostridium botulinum. N Engl J Med*. 1986;315:239-54.

48. Arnon S. Botulism as an intestinal toxemia. In: Blaser MJ, Smith PD, Ravdin JI, Greenberg HB, Guerrant RL, ed. *Infections of the Gastrointestinal Tract*. New York: Raven Press; 1995:257-71.

49. Fenicia L, Franciosa G, Pourshaban M, Aureli P. Intestinal toxemia botulism in two young people, caused by Clostridium butyricum type E. *Clin Infect Dis*. 1999;29:1381-7.

50. Griffin PM, Hatheway CL, Rosenbaum RB, Sokolow R. Endogenous antibody production to botulinum toxin in an adult with intestinal colonization botulism and underlying Crohn's disease. *J Infect Dis*. 1997;175:633-7.

51. McCroskey L, Hatheway CL, Woodruff BA, Greenberg JA, Jurgenson P. Type F botulism due to neurotoxigenic Clostridium baratii from an unknown source in an adult. *J Clin Microbiol*. 1991;29:2618-20.

52. Chalk CH, Benstead TJ, Pound JD, Keezer MR. Medical treatment for botulism. *Cochrane Database Syst Rev*. 2019;4(4):CD008123.

53. Franco MP, Mulder M, Gilman RH, Smits HL. Human Brucellosis. *Lancet Infect Dis*. 2007;7:775-786.

54. Pappas G, Akritidis N, Nosilkowsvki M, Tsianos E. Brucellosis. *N Engl J Med*. 2005;352:2325-2336.

55. Traxler RM, Guerra MA, Morrow MG, et al. Review of Brucellosis Cases from Laboratory Exposures in the United States in 2008 to 2011 and Improved Strategies for Disease Prevention. *J Clin Microbiol*. 2013;51(9):3132-3136.

56. Barkely Brunett L. Clostridium prefingens toxin (epsilon toxin) attack. In: Ciottone GR, Anderson PD, eds. *Disaster Medicine, First Edition*. Maryland Heights: Mosby Inc; 2006:705.

57. Alves GG, Machado de Avila R A, Chavez-Olortegui CD, Lobato FC. *Clostridium perfringens* epsilon toxin: the third most potent bacterial toxin known. *Anaerobe*. 2014;30102-107.

58. McClain MS, Cover TL. Functional analysis of neutralizing antibodies against *Clostridium perfringens* epsilon toxin. *Infect Immun*. 2007;75(4):1785-1793.

59. Titball RW. *Clostridium perfringens* vaccines. *Vaccine*. 2009;27(suppl 4):D44-D47.

60. Paddle BM. Therapy and prophylaxis of inhaled biological toxins. *J Appl Toxicol*. 2003;23(3):139-170.

61. Shane AL, Mody RK, Crump JA, et al. 2017 Infectious Diseases Society of America Clinical Practice Guidelines for the Diagnosis and Management of Infectious Diarrhea. *Clinical Infectious Disease*. 2017;65(12):e45-e80.

62. Available at https://www.cdc.gov/foodsafety/diseases/clostridium-perfringens.html. Accessed September 19, 2020.

63. Darling RG, Woods JB. *Medical Management of Biological Casualties Handbook*. 5th ed. Fort Dtrick MD: US Army Medical Research Institute of Infectious Diseases; 2004:P80-91.

64. Madsen JM. Toxins as weapons of mass destruction. A comparison and contrast with biological warfare and chemical warfare agents. *Clin Lab Med*. 2001;21:593-605.

65. Ricin Toxin. Centers for Disease Control and Prevention. Available at https://www.cdc.gov/niosh/ershdb/emergencyresponsecard_29750002.html. Updated May 11, 2011. Accessed September 19, 2020.

66. Available at https://emergency.cdc.gov/agent/ricin/clinicians/treatment.asp. Updated April 8, 2018. Accessed September 19, 2020.

67. McKay DM. Bacterial superantigens: provocateurs of gut dysfunction and inflammation. *Trends Immunol*. 2001;22:497-501.

68. Foster TJ. Immune evasion by staphylococci. *Nat Rev Microbiol*. 2005;3: 948-58.

69. Heiman KE, Mody RK, Johnson SD, Griffin PM, Gould LH. *Escherichia coli* O157 Outbreaks in the United States, 2003–2012. *Emerg Infect Dis*. 2015;21(8):1293-1301.

70. Centers for Disease Control and Prevention. Recommendations for Diagnosis of Shiga Toxin-Producing Escherichia coli Infections by Clinical Laboratories. *MMWR*. 2009;58(No. RR-12):1-20.

71. Mead PS, Griffin PM. *Escherichia coli* O157:H7. *Lancet*. 1998;352:1207-12.

72. Rowe PC, Orrbine E, Lior H, et al. Risk of hemolytic uremic syndrome after sporadic *Escherichia coli* O157:H7 infection: results of a Canadian collaborative study. *J Pediatr*. 1998;132:777-82.

73. Slutsker L, Ries AA, Greene KD, Wells JG, Hutwagner L, Griffin PM. *Escherichia coli* O157:H7 diarrhea in the United States: clinical and epidemiologic features. *Ann Intern Med*. 1997;126:505-13.

74. Baker S, The HC. Recent insights into Shigella: A Major Contributor to the Global Diarrhoeal Disease Burden. *Current Opin Infect Dis*. 2018;31:449-454.

75. Clemens JD, Nair GB, Ahmed T, Qadri F, Holmgren J. Cholera. *Lancet*. 2017;390:1539-1549.

76. Weil AA, Ryan ET. Cholera: recent updates. *Curr Opin Infect Dis*. 2018;31:455-461.

77. Gut MA, Vaslijeic T, Yeager T, Donkor O. Salmonella infection – prevention and treatment by antibiotics and probiotic yeasts: a review. *Microbiology*. 2018;164:1327-1344.

78. Song J, Gao X, Galán JE. Structure and function of the Salmonella Typhi chimaeric A2B5 typhoid toxin. *Nature*. 2013;499:350-354.

79. Chopra AK, Huang JH, Xu X, et al. Role of Salmonella enterotoxin in overall virulence of the organism. *Microb Pathog*. 1999;27:155-171.

80. Chong A, Lee S, Yang YA, Song J. The role of typhoid Toxin in Salmonella Typhi virulence. *Yale J Biol Med*. 2017;90:283-290.

81. Nakano M, Yamasaki E, Ichinose A, et al. Salmonella enterotoxin (Stn) regulates membrane composition and integrity. *Dis Model Mech*. 2012;5:515-521.

82. Ibarra JA, Steele-Mortimer O. Salmonella virulence factors that modulate intracellular survival. *Cellular Microbiology*. 2009;11:1579-1586.

83. Available at https://www.centerforhealthsecurity.org/resources/fact-sheets/pdfs/glanders_melodosis.pdf.

84. *Textbook of Military Medicine: Medical Aspects of Chemical and Biological Warfare*. Chapters 6–7. Washington, DC: Office of the Surgeon General at TMM Publications; 2007. Available at http://www.bordeninstitute.army.mil//published_volumes/biological_warfare/biological.html.

85. Currie B. Burkholderia pseudomallei and Burkholderia mallei: Melioidosis and glanders. Chapter 218. In: *Principles and Practice of Infectious Diseases*. Churchill Livingston; 2004.

86. Nieuwenhuizen AA, Dijkstra F, Notermans DW, van der Hoek W. Laboratory for case finding in human psittacosis outbreaks: a systemic review. *BMC Infectious Diseases*. 2018;18:442.

87. Hogerwerf L, De Gier B, Baan B, Van der Hoek W. Chlamydia psittaci (psittacosis) as a cause of community-acquired pneumonia: a systematic review and meta-analysis. *Epidemiol Infect*. 2017;145:3096-3105.

88. Beeckman DSA, Vanrompay DCG. Zoonotic chlamydophila psittaci infections from a clinical perspective. *Clin Microbiol Infect*. 2009;15:11-17.

89. Eldin C, Melenotte C, Mediannikov O, et al. From Q fever to Coxiella burnetii infection: a paradigm change. *Clin Microbiol Rev*. 30:115-190.

90. Raoult D, Tissot-Dupont H, Foucault C, et al. Q fever 1985–1998: clinical and epidemiologic features of 1383 infections. *Medicine (Baltimore)*. 2000;79(2):109-23.

91. Foucault C, Lepidi H, Poujet-Abadie JF, et al. Q fever and lymphadenopathy: report of four new cases and review. *Eur J Clin Microbiol Infect Dis*. 2004;23:759-64.

92. Fournier PE, Raoult D. Comparison of PCR and serology assays for early diagnosis of acute Q fever. *J Clin Microbiol*. 2003;41(11):5094-8.

93. Foucault C, Lepidi H, Poujet-Abadie JF, et al. Q fever and lymphadenopathy: report of four new cases and review. *Eur J Clin Microbiol Infect Dis*. 2004;23:759-64.

94. Fournier PE, Raoult D. Comparison of PCR and serology assays for early diagnosis of acute Q fever. *J Clin Microbiol*. 2003;41(11):5094-8.

95. Raoult D, Tissot-Dupont H. Q fever. *Infect Dis Clin N Am*. 2008;22:505-514.

96. Innes EA, Chalmers RM, Wells B, Pawlowic MC. A One Health Approach to Tackle Cryptosporidiosis. *Trends in Parasitology*. 2020;36(3):290-303.

97. Gibson AR, Striepen B. Quick guide: cryptosporidium. *Current Biology Magazine*. 2018:R187-R207.

98. Gerace E, Presti VDML, Biondo C. Cryptosporidium infection: epidemiology, pathogenesis, and differential diagnosis. *Eur J Microbiol Immunol*. 2019;9(4):119-123.

99. Parasites – Cryptosporidium. Center for Disease Control and Prevention. Available at https://www.cdc.gov/parasites/crypto/treatment.html. Updated August 16, 2017. Accessed September 29, 2020.

100. Typhus fevers. Centers for Disease Control and Prevention. Available at https://www.cdc.gov/typhus/healthcare-providers/index.html. Updated August 2, 2019. Accessed October 3, 2020.

29 CHEMICAL WARFARE

Abdulrahman Elabor, MD, Nikhita Gadi, MD, Marianne Minock, MSN, APN-C, Andre Sotelo, MD, and Ronaldo C. Go, MD

▌ INTRODUCTION

Chemical weapons have been used since the Middle Ages, though it took industrial advancements in the 19th century to make their mass production and deployment possible.[1] Chlorine, phosgene, sulfur mustard, and lewisite caused 100,000 deaths and 1.2 million casualties in World War I.[2] Hydrogen cyanide was used in World War II.[1] Agent Orange was used in the Vietnam War.[1] Sarin was used in the Tokyo subway, causing 5,500 casualties and 12 deaths. An Iraqi nerve gas attack in Halabja killed 5,000 civilians.[3]

There are 70 different chemicals that can be used in chemical warfare which may elicit a common response.[1] Multi-Threat Medical Countermeasure (MTMC) is based on the premise that the body's response to any toxic chemical involves a common underlying biochemical signal pathway.[4] MTMC drugs can target this common pathway and thus protect against various chemical agents. This pathway is the inflammatory pathway and involves proteases, inflammatory cytokines such as tumor necrosis factor (TNF), interleukin-1, interleukin-8, platelet activating factor, N-methyl-d-aspartate glutamate receptors, acethylcholine, substance P and poly (ADP-ribose) polymerase. However, there is still no specific drug to empirically treat any chemical attack; thus the approach would be specific to one chemical agent. Nerve agents, vesicants, psychomimetics, and riot controlling agents will be discussed here.

▌ NERVE AGENTS

Nerve agents are a class of chemical warfare agents that act through the irreversible inhibition of acetylcholinesterase via phosphorylation at cholinergic and central nervous system (CNS) synapses (Table 29-1). This process leads to the accumulation of acetylcholine in the central and peripheral nervous systems, with a host of autonomic symptoms that may

Table 29-1	AGENTS THAT CAN BE INHALED OR ABSORBED THROUGH THE SKIN			
Chemical Agent	**Characteristics**	**Clinical Features**	**Level of PPE**	**Decontamination**
Nerve Gas	Clear, colorless to pale or dark amber liquid.	Most toxic chemical warfare agent; can cause death within minutes.	Level A protective suit with a self-contained breathing apparatus.	Solution of detergent and cold or warm water (pH value between 8 and 10.5) with soft brushes.
Sulfur Mustard	Oily liquid ranging in color from colorless to yellow or brown; garlic or mustard odor.	Delayed onset; signs and symptoms of cholinergic toxicity.	Level A protective suit with a self-contained breathing apparatus.	Solution of detergent and cold or warm water (pH value between 8 and 10.5) with soft brushes.
Nitrogen Mustard	Colorless to pale yellow oily liquid. May be odorless, or have a fishy or fruity odor.	Onset of pain and other symptoms is delayed as the more immediate changes occur at a cellular level.	Level A protective suit with a self-contained breathing apparatus.	Solution of detergent and cold or warm water (pH value between 8 and 10.5) with soft brushes.
Phosgene oxime	Colorless, crystalline solid or yellowish-brown liquid.	Redness and hives (wheals & urticaria) upon contact; penetrates garments and rubber.	Level A protective suit with a self-contained breathing apparatus.	Solution of detergent and cold or warm water (pH value between 8 and 10.5) with soft brushes.
Lewisite	Oily liquid with a range of colors from colorless to violet-black, green, or amber.	Immediate burning pain and irritation from exposure to liquid or vapor with early tissue destruction.	Level A protective suit with a self-contained breathing apparatus.	Solution of detergent and cold or warm water (pH value between 8 and 10.5) with soft brushes.

ultimately lead to death. Nerve agents are, for the most part, colorless and tasteless liquids with high volatility that easily transform into vapor and aerosol forms, hence the common term, "nerve gases." Owing to their liposolubility and hydrosolubility, these agents are absorbed quickly through the eyes, skin, and respiratory tract.

There are two major groups of nerve agents. The G-series nerve agents, which derive their name from their original synthesis by German scientists, are highly volatile and aerosolized through dispersal devices and explosive blasts. They include the following agents: Tabun (GA): colorless to brownish; faintly fruity odor; Sarin (GB): colorless and odorless in its pure form; may be brownish and have a mustard-like smell in its impure form; Soman (GD): yellowish to brown color; has a camphor-like odor; and Cyclosarin (GF): colorless; sweet, musty odor.

The V-series nerve agents are second-generation agents, also known as persistent agents because they do not degrade or wash away easily. The etymology of the "V-series" is unclear, but they were developed in the United Kingdom. V-series nerve agents persist on clothes and other surfaces for prolonged periods, and their consistency is similar to that of oil; therefore, the contact hazard is primarily dermal. The most common V-series agents are known more commonly by their code names: VX, VE, VG, VM.[5]

Other nerve agents include Novichok agents and carbamates, which are sometimes grouped as third- and fourth-generation agents, respectively.

Routes of Exposure

Nerve agents are easily absorbed through inhalation via the respiratory tract and mucocutaneous contact via the skin and eyes. Ingestion is rare, though these compounds can be absorbed through the gastrointestinal (GI) tract.

Clinical Manifestations

While dependent on the route (dermal or inhalation) and concentration of exposure, the clinical presentation of nerve agents is, for the most part, reminiscent of a cholinergic crisis. Due to inhibition of receptors at the muscarinic junction, symptoms include miosis, blurry vision, lacrimation, salivation, rhinorrhea, bronchoconstriction, bradycardia, hypotension, cramping, abdominal pain, vomiting, diarrhea, and urinary and fecal incontinence. Inhibition of receptors at the nicotinic junctions found on the skin and skeletal muscles can cause diaphoresis, fasciculations, and, ultimately, muscular weakness with flaccid paralysis. Furthermore, seizures, ataxia, slurred speech, and respiratory depression can occur through the inhibition of CNS cholinergic receptors. Percutaneous absorption is slower than inhalation; therefore, the onset of symptoms with dermal exposure may be delayed, with localized signs presenting themselves before more systemic signs occur as absorption continues. With inhalation, the onset of symptoms is more rapid, with ocular and respiratory symptoms initially predominating. High concentrations of inhaled nerve agents may lead to a rapid loss of consciousness. Death through asphyxiation, respiratory failure, or cardiac arrest can occur within minutes.

Diagnosis

The diagnosis is mainly based on clinical presentation and history of exposure to suspected compounds. The effects of nerve agents can be estimated by measuring the percent reduction in red blood cell (RBC) cholinesterase. It is not sensitive and may not correlate with the severity of illness. The interpretations of such tests depend on the specific laboratory reference intervals, which are wide, variable, and difficult to interpret without a baseline.[1]

Treatment

Due to the risk of cross-contamination, the first step in the treatment is for healthcare workers to protect themselves with appropriate personal protective equipment (PPE). Proper equipment is imperative for emergency and healthcare personnel responding to affected victims and involves using fully encapsulated suits impervious to vapor and liquid chemical penetration with a self-contained breathing apparatus (Level A PPE).

Immediate decontamination is the most critical step following nerve agent exposure. Decontamination involves extricating the patient from the contaminated environment and removing all clothing, followed by extensive rinsing with room-temperature water. Using hot water or scrubbing materials may lead to greater absorption into the skin, and the use of diluted bleach solutions is no longer favored. Contaminated clothing and belongings should be sealed and double-bagged. Initial decontamination should be performed near the exposure site and before transportation to decrease further exposure.

Supportive Care

Supportive care for patients follows the universally accepted algorithm to ensure adequate airway, ventilation, and circulation. Commonly used measures include fluid resuscitation, use of bronchodilators, and adequate oxygenation. If intubation and mechanical ventilation is required, using depolarizing paralytic agents such as succinylcholine may lead to long-lasting paralytic effects, as nerve agents prolong their duration. Benzodiazepines such as diazepam and midazolam can effectively manage seizures and myoclonic jerks.

Specific Treatment

Specific therapies are similar to those used for organophosphate poisoning to counter cholinergic effects. Atropine sulfate blocks the muscarinic effects of nerve agents (i.e., nausea, vomiting, diarrhea, bradycardia, bronchorrhea, and bronchoconstriction). However, it does not affect nicotinic receptors and, therefore, does not reverse paralysis. The routine dose of atropine used is 2 mg intravenously every 2 to 5 minutes for mild to moderate symptoms in adults and 0.02 mg/kg in children. More severe symptoms may require higher doses.

Oxime compounds bind competitively to the phosphate moiety of the nerve agent, allowing the reactivation of acetylcholinesterase. Their effectiveness depends on the particular nerve agent used. Pralidoxime is the most commonly used drug: adult dosing is 30 mg/kg IV over 15 to 30 minutes.[6]

Prognosis

Over the long-term, survivors may suffer chronic neurological damage and psychiatric effects. Symptoms such as blurry vision, fatigue, memory decline, irritability, vocal hoarseness, palpitations, and insomnia are common.

▌VESICANTS

Vesicants are also known as blister agents due to their ability to induce painful vesicular blisters on the skin, typical of severe chemical burns. They are absorbed quickly through the eyes, lungs, and skin. The blistering agents include lewisite, nitrogen mustard, phosgene oxime, and sulfur mustard. The type of vesicant, amount of exposure, and route of exposure all influence the onset and severity of symptoms.[7]

Sulfur Mustards (H, HD, HT, HL, and HQ)

Commonly known as mustard gases, sulfur mustards are naturally colorless and viscous liquids at room temperature. However, they become yellowish-brown and release an odor reminiscent of the mustard plant when used in their impure form as warfare agents, hence the name. They may be deployed as liquid droplets from artillery shells, bombs, and rockets or sprayed from warplanes.

Mustard gases function mainly as incapacitating agents because their immediate fatality is low. At the cellular level, their mechanism of action involves deoxyribonucleic acid (DNA) alkylation and cross-linking, which prevent mitosis and lead to damaged DNA and apoptosis. These properties eventually result in mutagenic and carcinogenic effects.

Clinical Manifestations

The nocive effects of mustard gases are typically delayed, with symptoms occurring within 24 hours of exposure. Upon tactile exposure, victims develop generalized pruritus and skin irritation, followed by large blisters over areas of the skin exposed to the agent. First- and second-degree burns can be seen depending on the level of contamination. The liposolubility of mustard gases enhances their rapid cutaneous absorption, hence these effects. With ocular exposure, eye and mucosal pain with conjunctivitis, corneal ulceration, and keratitis develop. Irritation of the airways is commonplace upon inhalation and leads to bronchiolar hemorrhage. Mustard gases have a degree of cholinergic activity, explaining some gastrointestinal effects such as nausea and vomiting, although these symptoms are usually mild.

Treatment

Due to the lack of immediate effects, victims may be unaware of exposure, and decontamination may not happen immediately. Extended contamination leads to increased absorption and more extensive tissue damage. In addition to decontamination with large water volumes, medical management involves comprehensive support and symptomatic relief measures. Systemic analgesics, antipruritic agents, and intravenous volume resuscitation should be liberally used.

Denuded skin areas should be cleansed with sterile solutions or water with soap. Petrolatum and topical antimicrobial agents work well as protective ointments, and topical lotions such as calamine and menthol soothe skin irritation. The use of topical ocular protection, ophthalmic antibiotic ointments, and anticholinergic eye drops can reduce the incidence of infection and synechiae formation.[8]

Additionally, atropine can counter cholinergic effects such as nausea and vomiting. Bronchodilators may be helpful in cases of bronchospasm, and steroids may be considered to reduce airway edema. Close monitoring of patients' respiratory status is necessary, as intubation may need to be performed before laryngospasm and edema lead to complications.

Nitrogen Mustards (HN1, HN2, and HN3)

Nitrogen mustards are non-specific DNA alkylating agents synthesized in the 1930s. Though initially formulated for chemical warfare, they later became the first chemotherapeutic agents for cancer due to their strong cytotoxic effects. They have never been used in warfare.

Lewisite

Lewisite is an organoarsenic compound specially developed for use in warfare and considered an alternative to sulfur mustards. Given its higher density, it tends to settle in low-lying areas. It can persist for prolonged periods in the environment due to its high volatility and low freezing point. Lewisite can also penetrate clothing and latex rubber gloves. Upon contact with skin, it causes immediate irritation, burning pain, and pruritus, followed by a rash with large, fluid-filled blisters presenting within hours. Unlike mustard agents, irritation from lewisite is immediate but may not fully manifest until at least 12 hours after exposure.

Clinical Manifestations

"Lewisite shock" is from increased capillary permeability. Lewisite inhalation can lead to pulmonary edema, pneumonitis, and respiratory failure. Ocular exposure can cause lacrimation, conjunctivitis, periorbital edema, and blepharospasm, while globe perforation and blindness occur in the most severe cases. Compared to lewisite's vaporized formulation, its liquid formulation is associated with a more rapid onset of effects. Chronic exposure can lead to arsenic poisoning, as lewisite is frequently compounded with arsenic. Arsenic itself is categorized as a respiratory carcinogen.[8]

Treatment

Medical management primarily takes place through supportive care, with early decontamination being of utmost importance. Bleach (hypochlorite) may have neutralizing effects. British anti-Lewisite (BAL, also known as dimercaprol) was explicitly developed as an antidote to lewisite. It acts as a chelating agent that binds to the arsenic moiety to decrease its systemic effects and is now used in medicine as a chelating agent for other heavy metals.[8]

Phosgene Oxime (CX)

Clinical manifestations

Phosgene causes immediate corrosive skin and soft tissue damage upon contact, resulting in blanching erythema, wheal-like skin lesions, and intense pruritus. Skin scarring and necrotic eschars may develop days or weeks after exposure. Phosgene oxime can exist in vapor or liquid forms, both of which are extremely irritating. When inhaled, it irritates the eyes and airways and may cause pulmonary edema. There are no distinctive laboratory findings to confirm exposure.

Treatment
Decontamination with large volumes of water and symptomatic relief measures are the standard treatments. Though frequently grouped with vesicant chemical warfare agents, phosgene oxime is not a true vesicant, as it does not induce blisters.

Phosgene oxime is an urticant or nettle agent that causes immediate corrosive skin and soft tissue damage upon contact, resulting in blanching erythema, wheal-like skin lesions, and intense pruritus. Skin scarring and necrotic eschars may develop days or weeks after exposure. Phosgene oxime can exist in vapor or liquid forms, both of which are extremely irritating. When inhaled, it irritates the eyes and airways and may cause pulmonary edema. There are no distinctive laboratory findings to confirm exposure. Decontamination with large volumes of water and symptomatic relief measures are the standard treatments. Though frequently grouped with vesicant chemical warfare agents, phosgene oxime is not a true vesicant, as it does not induce blisters.

▌PSYCHOTOMIMETIC AGENTS

Psychotomimetic agents are a class of drugs that induce symptoms of psychosis in a dose dependent manner. Common manifestations of these agents include hallucinations and delusions in normal individuals. The onset of such symptoms after administration of these drugs is referred to as psychotomimesis.

The historical timeline of these agents is equally interesting as utility of these agents was recognized in variable social and academic circumstances. Naturally occurring hallucinogens have been used globally to attain altered level of cognitive states for religious and spiritual purposes. Today, such practices are tailored toward recreational use of these agents. Conversely, psychotomimetic agents were once considered wonder drugs for their stabilizing effects in treating various psychiatric illness including depression, anxiety, and alcoholism. Common categories of psychotomimetic agents used today include: hallucinogens, deliriogenics, and stimulants[9,10] (Table 29-2).

Evidently, the category of psychotomimetic agents comprises a variety of drugs and drug classes. Recognizing this level of diversity is crucial

Table 29-2   CHARACTERISTICS OF PSYCHOTOMIMETIC AGENTS

Psychotomimetic Agents	Subclass/mechanism	Clinical Manifestations
Hallucinogens 1) Phencyclidine (PCP) 2) Lysergic acid diethylamide (LSD) 3) N,N-dimethyltryptamine (DMT) 4) Ayahuasca 5) Mescaline 6) Psilocin and Psylocibin ("magic mushroom") 7) 3,4-methylenedioxy-methamphetamine (MDMA) 8) Ketamine 9) Dextromethorphan (DXM) 10) Cannabinoids 11) Salvinorin A 12) Antimuscarinic xenobiotics	1–6: classic hallucinogens or psychedelics 7: Mixed serotonin and dopamine reuptake inhibitors (entactogens) 8–9: NMDA antagonist (dissociative anesthetics) 10–12: Atypicals	- Neurocognitive effects (changes in perception, distortion in time, euphoria, synesthesia, visual illusions and visual distortions, dissociation from reality) - Sympathomimetic affects (mydriasis, tachycardia, hypertension, hyperthermia) - Gastrointestinal manifestations: nausea, vomiting, diarrhea - LSD, MDMA are common causes of serotonin syndrome - PCP common to cause destructive and violent behavior, nystagmus, incoordination
Deliriogenics 1) Atropine, datura, dicyclomine 2) Benzodiazepines (zolpidem, diazepam, lorazepam, zolpidem) 3) Fentanyl, hydrocodone, codeine, morphine, hydromorphine, Neurontin, gabapentin 4) Cimetidine, famotidine, ranitidine	1) Anticholinergic agents 2) Hypnosedatives 3) Analgesics (opioid and non-opioid) 4) Histamine receptor antagonists	- Fluctuating consciousness - Shifting attention span - Disorientation - Illusion - Hallucinations
Stimulants 1) Amphetamine 2) Dextroamphetamine 3) Methylphenidate	1–2: promote release of dopamine, norepinephrine, and serotonin and inhibit function of monamine oxidase 3: Inhibit phosphodiesterase enzymes, increasing intracellular cyclinc adenosine monophosphate. Block adenosine receptors and increase movement of extracellular calcium	- Autonomic hyperactivity (hypertension, palpitations, syncope, arrhythmia, tremors, angina) - CNS symptoms (insomnia, weakness, dizziness, confusion, mydriasis) - Teratogenic, cause developmental delays, metabolites distributed in breast milk (avoid in pregnancy and lactation) - other effects: diarrhea, constipation, nausea, vomiting, blurry vision, and anorexia

(Continued

Treatment of Toxicity	Complications
Behavioral: place in calm environment, physical restraints First line Agent: Benzodiazepines Second line: sedatives Adjunctive Treatment: Neuroleptics (haloperidol) for persistent psychosis Antiemetics for nausea and vomiting * Serotonin syndrome antidote: cyproheptadine * No specific antidote exists for hallucinogens	Cardiac Arrhythmias, cardiovascular collapse, traumatic injuries Unwanted neuropscychiatric effects including fear of death, frank psychosis, dysphoria, frightening imagery, impaired judgment
1) Physiostigmine and donepezil (cholinesterase inhibitors) 2) Flumazenil 3) Narcan, supportive care 4) Decontamination with gastric lavage or activated charcoal, discontinuation of drug, supportive care	1) Cutaneous vasodilation, anhidrosis, anhidrotic hyperthermia, nonreactive mydriasis, delirium, urinary retention 2) CNS depression, respiratory depression, ataxia, slurred speech, myosis, nystagmus 3) Serotonin toxicity, acute amnesia, QRS prolongation and arrhythmias, QT prolongation, miosis 4) CNS depression, hypotension, bradycardia
Supportive care	Primary findings: severe hyperpyrexia, severe hyponatremia, cardiovascular arrhythmias Secondary conditions: rhabdomyolysis, disseminated intravascular coagulation, GI bleeding, hepatic necrosis Chronic use: increased risk of vasculitis, neuropsyciatric abnormalities, cardiomyopathy

as it helps explain the variable nature in pathogenesis of such agents. The pharmacology of these agents is extensive and invariably confusing. Broadly speaking, different classes of psychotomimetic agents induce remarkable differences in the type of psychosis seen. The neurobiology of each drug type is variable involving complex interactions with numerous neurotransmitters including serotonin (5-HT), dopamine, and glutamate. Some drugs cause profound cognitive deficits associated with gross disorientation causing what is commonly referred to as "organic psychosis" or "dementia." Others induce a variable degree of hallucinations or alterations of consciousness. The exact mechanism of inducing hallucinations is unknown but most drugs in this class share a common ability to bind to 5-HT2A receptors in neocortical pyramidal cells.[11,12] The degree of drugs encompassing hallucinogens is vast and can be further divided into four common subtypes: psychedelics, entactogens, dissociatives, and atypicals.

Deliriogenics also comprises a vast class of various drug types. The most common drug known to cause delirium particularly in the elderly involves toxicity of anti-cholinergics and hypnosedatives. Common examples include atropine and dicyclomine for the former and benzodiazepines such as diazepam or lorazepam for the latter. Anticholinergic agents competitively inhibit binding of the neurotransmitter, acetylcholine, targeting either muscarinic acetylcholine receptors (AChR) or less commonly nicotinic acetylcholine receptors. There are five subtypes of muscarinic receptors, M1–M5. All five are found on nerve endings in the central nervous system: M1 AChRs are found on secretory glands, M2 AChRs are found in cardiac tissue, M3 AChRs are found in smooth muscle and in secretory glands. Various G protein receptors are composed of both types of receptors, muscarinic and nicotinic.[8] Symptom manifestation upon activation of these receptors is described in the next section. Analgesics such as fentanyl/morphine and histamine receptor antagonists such as cimetidine can also cause delirium when ingested in toxic amounts.

Stimulants including amphetamine and dextroamphetamine are frequently used for management of a common psychiatric condition prevalent in today's society—attention deficit hyperactivity disorder.[11]

Clinical Manifestations

The clinical manifestations of each category of these agents are broad. Hallucinogens, also known as psychedelics, induce profound changes in perception altering the experience of time and space. Patients who are under the influence of hallucinogenic agents exhibit a wide array of behaviors that fluctuate between a state of euphoria and that of agitation and at times aggression. Drugs that induce delirium, or deliriogenics drugs, should be suspected with acute or sub-acute deterioration in behavior and cognition. The features of delirium were once described by Hippocrates as "phrenitis," a transient mental disorder associated with a disturbance in perception, mood, and wit.[14] Deliriogenics can also induce visual hallucinations, in addition to persecutory or grandiose delusions.

The etiology of delirium is multifactorial; however, excessive use of anticholinergic agents is perhaps the leading cause of drug-induced delirium and drug induced memory disorders. Anticholinergic toxicity commonly manifests in a series of symptoms recognized by the mnemonic "blind as a bat, mad as a hatter, red as a beet, hot as a hare, and dry as a bone," with symptom manifestations of mydriasis, delirium, hyperthermia, with dry and flushed skin. Symptoms of delirium typically involve memory and cognitive impairment as noted above. Additional symptoms include dry eyes, constipation, difficulty swallowing, decreased sweating, and urinary retention.[14] Though it is useful to recognize these common adverse effects of anticholinergic toxicity, it is most important to know that many other drugs have anticholinergic properties inducing the same level of symptoms. Such examples include antidepressants, anti-muscarinics, antipsychotics, antispasmodics, and all opioids.[14] Additionally, overuse of benzodiazepines can lead to respiratory depression, which may require invasive life saving procedures including mechanical ventilation and intubation to maintain adequate oxygenation. Overdose or benzodiazepine toxicity can also cause CNS depression leading to coma, which may not always be reversible.[15] Histamine receptor antagonists, such as loratidine or cimetidine, are less common types of drugs that are known to induce delirium. The most notable quality of these agents is that they are readily available over the counter, rendering it easy for a person of any age to misuse this drug. In addition to inducing delirium, overuse of this particular drug class can cause bradycardia, diarrhea, flushing of skin, low blood pressure, difficulty breathing, and somnolence.[15,16]

Amphetamines typically increase the overall effect of neurotransmitter activity of dopamine, norepinephrine, and serotonin. This invariably places one in a state of euphoria but can also enhance symptoms of autonomic hyperactivity. Other common adverse effects particularly when taken in excessive amounts include insomnia, weakness, tremors, and may even contribute to anorexia commonly seen in young adolescent women. Amphetamines are also noted to be teratogenic and should be avoided during pregnancy and lactation.[11,15]

Treatment

Some psychedelic agents have been utilized in recent times for treatment of cluster headaches, substance use disorders, end-of-life anxiety, obsessive-compulsive disorder, and depression. Use of enactogens, specifically MDMA, has been show to have therapeutic benefits in post-traumatic stress disorder (PTSD) and in evaluation for treatment of social anxiety in adults with autism spectrum disorders. Dissociatives are typically used for anesthesia and substance use disorders. Atypical hallucinogens such as salvinorin A or cannabinoids have shown therapeutic benefit in treating chronic neuropathic or cancer related pain, nausea, and vomiting due to chemotherapy. Despite the various subtypes of hallucinogenic agents, they exhibit a distinct similarity in their ability to cause profound changes in consciousness, affecting acute changes in somatic, perceptual, and cognitive processes. Overuse of psychotomimetic agents, commonly seen with recreational use of hallucinogens and deliriogenics manifest in different presentations of drug toxicity, as summarized in Table 29-2.[9,11,15]

Given that almost all hallucinogens act on 5-HT2A receptors, symptoms related to over-activation of these receptors can cause a potentially life threatening condition called serotonin syndrome (toxicity). This is often seen with high therapeutic medication use, inadvertent interactions with other drug classes (i.e., selective serotonin reuptake inhibitors or SSRIs, lithium, meperidine, tryptophan, and monoamine oxidase inhibitors), intentional self-poisoning or abuse of common psychedelics including LSD or MDMA. Clinical findings often include alterations in mental status, autonomic hyperactivity (i.e., restlessness, tachycardia, diaphoresis, and hyperthermia), and neuromuscular hyperactivity manifesting as tremors, muscle rigidity, myoclonus, and hyperreflexia.

Two neuropsychiatric signs that are particular for this condition include hyperreflexia and clonus as well as rigidity most pronounced to the lower extremities. Treatment of serotonin syndrome depends on severity of illness and is often multifactorial. Five principles are central to appropriate management and include the following: discontinuation of all serotoninergic agents, supportive care and normalizing of vital signs, sedation with benzodiazepines, administration of serotonin antagonists, and assessment for need to resume serotonergic agents after resolution of symptoms. Mild cases can be treated with supportive care and use of benzodiazepines such as lorazepam or diazepam to treat autonomic hyperactivity. Moderate to severe cases will require an aggressive form of therapy and may even require the serotonin antagonist known as cyproheptadine. If benzodiazepines and supportive therapy fail to treat symptoms, antidotal therapy with cyproheptadine, a histamine-1 receptor antagonist, is utilized. Other antidotes include antipsychotic agents with 5-HT2A-antagonist activity such as olanzapine and chlorpromazine, but efficacy remains unproven.[16,17]

Clinical manifestations and treatment of toxicity with deliriogenics again depend on which subclass of drugs are used, summarized for reference in Table 29-2. Degree of toxicity often dictates approach to management, which is a common approach to treating all drug toxicities. Supportive care measures and discontinuation of drugs are utilized in most cases with an initial approach to stabilize airway, breathing status, and circulation. It is crucial to note that specific antidotes for severe toxicity are utilized for four common deliriogenic drug types. The antidotes are as follows: physiostigmine for anticholinergic toxicity, flumazenil for benzodiazepine toxicity, gastric lavage and activated charcoal for histamine antagonist toxicity, and naloxone (or narcan) for acute opioid intoxication.[11] Amongst these treatment forms, it is imperative to carefully dose and administer naloxone as excessively high doses can lead to opioid withdrawal.[14,15]

Complications

Complications of drug toxicity are invariably dependent on drug type and subclass as they release different neurotransmitters. Severe vital sign abnormalities are uncommon findings of hallucinogens and more common findings of stimulants. This does not preclude the fact that changes in autonomic behavior do occur when using hallucinogens and deliriogenics. Severe toxicity with use of hallucinogens can cause hyperthermia with psychomotor agitation. Complications of severe hyperthermia, which coincidentally is a common manifestation of all psychotomimetic agents, can lead to rhabdomyolysis, renal failure, hepatic injury, disseminated intravascular coagulation, and multi-organ failure. Additional unwanted complications of hallucinogen toxicity include extensive neuropsychiatric effects. A peculiar neuropsychiatric finding known as synesthesia or blinding of the senses is seen with hallucinogens where users report hearing colors or seeing sounds. Recreational use of hallucinogens is sought after to experience positive neuropsychiatric effects such as heightened perception of sensation, euphoria, and a perception of being a passive observer of events or being outside of one's body. However, toxic use can lead to unwanted effects including persistent psychosis, dysphoria, frightening imagery which may severely impact one's judgment and even lead to death.

Complications of toxicity involving overuse of deliriogenics and stimulants are equally vast. Given that the subtypes of deliriogenics have drastically different mechanism of action, clinical manifestations and complications of toxicity are difficult to summarize. Common cardiovascular complications include cardiac arrhythmias, de pointes, vacuities, and cardiomyopathy. CNS and respiratory depression with benzodiazepine toxicity can require urgent need of mechanical ventilation and intubation. Chronic use of stimulants can lead to extensive cardiovascular abnormalities including myocardial infarction and cardiomyopathy with severe neuropsychiatric manifestations. It remains unclear if chronic exposure to all psychotomimetic agents can lead to irreversible neuropsychiatric damage as drug-induced schizophrenia and persistent psychosis continue to remain two of the most dreadful conditions induced by such agents.

▌RIOT CONTROLLING AGENTS

Riot controlling agents are designed to temporarily incapacitate individuals by causing irritation to the eyes and respiratory tract. Riot controlling agents are also known as "harassing" or "controlling agents," or "tear gases." Today, these agents are commonly used by law enforcement personnel and civilians for crowd disturbances as well as personal self-protection. There are three main agents: chloroacetophenone, ortho-chlorobenzylidene malononitrile, and oleoresin capsicum. The utility of these agents includes their rapid onset, limited duration, and high safety ratio.[18]

In 1869, chloroacetophenone was developed as the first chemical riot controlling agent. Chloroacetophenone was the most widely used riot control agent during WWI, however by the end of WWI, it was replaced by ortho-chlorobenzylidene malononitrile. This is due to ortho-chlorobenzylidene malononitrile having greater potency with the added benefit of lower toxicity. Finally, in the 1980s, ortho-chlorobenzylidene malononitrile was replaced by oleoresin capsicum, commonly known as pepper spray, for law enforcement use. This was due to the rapid effect and least toxicity. Oleoresin capsicum would further become commercially available as pepper spray.[18,19]

After the Cold War, at the International Chemical Weapons Convention, incapacitating agents including riot control agents were banned. However, the United States does not recognize riot control agents as chemical warfare agents. As such, the United States considers them legal for use by civilians, police, and military. Finally, the World Health Organization recognizes the use of riot control agents for both civil and hostile purposes.[20–23]

Chloroacetophenone, ortho-chlorobenzylidene malononitrile, and oleoresin capsicum are typically deployed as gaseous micro-particle clouds or as liquid sprays with additives of propellants and nonaqueous solvents. The typical sites of exposure and portal of entry include ocular, dermal, ingestion, and inhalation. Though the mechanism of action is not well understood, it is suggested that chloroacetophenone and ortho-chlorobenzylidene malononitrile are SN_2-alkylating agents, which inhibit lactate dehydrogenase, glutamic dehydrogenase, and pyruvic decarboxylase. Inhibition of these enzymes will lead to changes in cellular metabolism and subsequently cell injury.[13] The cellular injury is transient as there is rapid reactivation of the enzymes after the exposure is removed. The rapid reactivation of the enzymes allows for the toxic effects to cease after the exposure has ended.

Oleoresin capsicum is a "Capsaicin" containing compound. Capsaicin is a natural alkaloid found in chilies. Oleoresin capsicum's toxic effects occur through the alkaloid compound binding to transient receptor potential channels in the body leading to massive release of Substance P. Substance P in turn is a neuropeptide that signals the brain when there is extreme pain and inflammation.[20] The severity of the symptoms corresponds to the amount of exposure, time, and preexisting conditions.[23]

Clinical Manifestations

Chloroacetophenone, ortho-chlorobenzylidene malononitrile, and oleoresin capsicum present with similar signs and symptoms. Symptom severity is dictated by amount, concentration, and length of exposure to the agent. Symptom onset begins rapidly. Typically, symptoms occur within 20–30 seconds after exposure to the agent. Classic clinical manifestations involve ocular, respiratory, and dermatological disturbances. Usual symptoms include ocular lacrimation and irritation, nasal rhinorrhea and burning, and oropharynx irritation and burning. Respiratory symptoms include coughing, wheezing, chest tightness, and dyspnea. Additionally, variations in skin irritation from burning to itching is common.

Diagnosis

Exposure to riot control agents is diagnosed by patient presentation and clinical history. Patients will typically present with history of exposure to offending agent, pain, and tearing of the eyes. Laboratory studies are generally not needed unless in prolonged exposure or unclear diagnosis. In which case, diagnostic testing should include arterial blood gas, chest x-ray, slit lamp exam, and electrocardiogram. Physical exam findings on ophthalmic examination would reveal normal pupils with increased lacrimation. The oropharynx and nasopharynx may be erythematous with increased oral secretions and rhinorrhea present. Respiratory findings typically resolve prior to arrival but can include coughing, stridor, and wheezing. Finally, dermatological findings include skin erythema, edema, and vesicle formation.

Treatment

Classically, medical management for exposure to chloroacetophenone, ortho-chlorobenzylidene malononitrile, and oleoresin capsicum is directed toward resolution of exposure, decontamination, and symptom management. There is no available antidote for exposure to these agents. Most common exposures occur through the eyes, skin, and respiratory tract. Eyes should be thoroughly flushed with water or saline. Respiratory symptoms typically resolve with removal of agent and access to fresh air. If symptoms persist, provide the patient with humidified oxygen. Additionally, if the patient presents with stridor, consider racemic epinephrine. Bronchospasms and wheezing can be treated with Beta 2 agonists.

Exposure to riot control agents can present with various severities of dermal injury. Initial skin irritation and burning should be treated with copious washing of the skin with water or soapy water. Usual exposure-induced contact dermatitis resolves within a few hours after exposure has ended. Further treatment of dermatitis includes flushing the skin thoroughly with colloid solutions and dermatology consult. If vesicles or blisters are present, they should remain undisturbed. After prolonged exposure, more severe dermatitis and 2nd degree burns may be present.[21,24]

Complications

There are very few complications associated with exposure to riot control agents. These complications are generally related to the mechanism of delivery and length of exposure. Specifically, mechanism of delivery contributes heavily to the injuries and mortality associated with riot control agents. Projectile deployment of these agents has been associated with increased injuries including ocular globe rupture, blindness, traumatic brain injuries, functional loss of limb, and death. Additionally, life threatening, and long-term health effects were noted with exposures in confided or enclosed spaces.

Clinical complications include latent respiratory and dermatological complications. Classically, latent symptoms can be seen 1–2 weeks post exposure. Latent respiratory complications include persistent reactive airway disease, acute or chronic tracheobronchitis, laryngeal obstruction, and potential respiratory arrest. Latent dermatological findings included allergic contact dermatitis and blistering rash.[24,25]

▌ REFERENCES

1. Ganesan K, Raza SK, Vijayaraghavan R. Chemical Warfare agents. *J Pharm Bioallied Sci.* 2010;2(3):166-178.

2. Riley B. The toxicology and treatment of injuries from chemical warfare agents. *Curr Anaesth Crit Care.* 2003;14:149.

3. Smart JK. History of chemical and biological warfare: An American perspective. In: Sidell FR, Takafuji ET, Franz DR, eds. *Medical Aspects of Chemical and Biological Warfare.* Washington, DC: Office of the Surgeon General; 1997:15.

4. Cowan FM, Broomfield CA, Stojiljkovic MP, Smith WJ. A review of multi-threat medical countermeasures against chemical warfare and terrorism. *Mil Med.* 2004;169:850-853.

5. CDC Nerve Agents Emergency Preparedness & Response. Emergency.cdc.gov. Available at https://emergency.cdc.gov/agent/nerve/. Published 2020. Accessed October 1, 2020.

6. CBRNE - Nerve Agents, G-series - Tabun, Sarin, Soman: Practice Essentials, Pathophysiology, Epidemiology. Emedicine.medscape.com. Available at https://emedicine.medscape.com/article/831648-overview. Published 2020. Accessed October 1, 2020.

7. VESICANTS. Fas.org. Available at https://fas.org/nuke/guide/usa/doctrine/army/mmcch/Vesicant.htm. Published 2020. Accessed October 1, 2020.

8. Chapter 8 VESICANTS. Available at https://ke.army.mil/borderninstitute/published_volumes/chemwarfare/CH8_Pgs259–310.pdf. Accessed October 1, 2020.

9. Nicholas DE. Psychedelics. *Pharmacol Rev.* 2016;68(2):264-355.

10. Stimulants (Psychomotor Stimulants). Goodtherapy.org. https://www.goodtherapy.org/drugs/stimulants.html. Accessed October 8, 2020.

11. Fantegrossi WE, Murnane KS, Reissig CJ. The behavioral pharmacology of hallucinogens. *Biochem Pharmacol.* 2008;75:17.

12. Garcia-Romeu A, Kersgard B, Addy PH. Clinical applications of hallucinogens: a review. *Exp Clin Psychopharmacol.* 2016;24(4):229-268.

13. Carlson AB, Kraus GP. Physiology, Cholinergic Receptors. In: StatPearls. StatPearls Publishing; 2020.

14. United Nations Office on Drugs and Crime (UNODC). World Drug Report 2012. Available at https://www.unodc.org/documents/data-and-analysis/WDR2012/WDR_2012_web_small.pdf. Accessed October 8, 2020.

15. Consroe PF. Treatment of acute hallucinogenic drug toxicity: specific pharmacological intervention. *Am J Health Syst Pharm.* 1973;30(1):80-84.

16. Canan F, Korkmaz U, Kocer E, et al. Serotonin syndrome with paroxetine overdose: a case report. *Prim Care Companion J Clin Psychiatry.* 2008;10:165.

17. Fugate JE, White RD, Rabinstein AA. Serotonin syndrome after therapeutic hypothermia for cardiac arrest: a case series. *Resuscitation.* 2014;85:774.

18. Schep LJ, Slaughter RJ, McBride DI. Riot control agents: the tear gases CN, CS and OC–a medical review. *J R Army Med Corps.* 2015;161(2):94-99.

19. Hurst G, ed. Medical management of chemical casualties handbook. ProQuest Ebook Central. 2015. Available at https://ebookcentral-proquest-com.proxy.library.upenn.edu. Accessed September 19, 2020.

20. Public Health Response to Biological and Chemical Weapons WHO Guidance 2004. Available at https://www.who.int/csr/delibepidemics/biochemguide/en/#:~:text=The%20Public%20health%20response%20to%20biological%20and%20chemical,of%20biological%20and%20chemical%20agents%20that%20affect%20health. Updated 2004. Accessed October 15, 2020.

21. Tuorinsky SD, Sciuto AM. Medical aspects of chemical warfare. In: Tuorinsky SD, ed. *Textbooks of Military Medicine.* Washington, DC: Office of the Surgeon General; 2008:339-370.

22. Olajos EJ, Salem H. Riot control agents: pharmacology, toxicology, biochemistry and chemistry. *J Appl Toxicol.* 2001;21(5):355-391.

23. Haar RJ, Iacopino V, Ranadive N, Weiser SD, Dandu M. Health impacts of chemical irritants used for crowd control: a systematic review of the injuries and deaths caused by tear gas and pepper spray. *BMC Public Health.* 2017;17(1):831.

24. Dimitroglou Y, Rachiotis G, Hadjichristodoulou C. Exposure to the riot control agent CS and potential health effects: a systematic review of the evidence. *Int J Environ Res Public Health.* 2015;12(2):1397-1411.

25. Stopyra JP, Winslow JE 3rd, Johnson JC 3rd, Hill KD, Bozeman WP. Baby shampoo to relieve the discomfort of tear gas and pepper spray exposure: a randomized controlled trial. *West J Emerg Med.* 2018;19(2):294-300.

NATURAL DISASTERS, EVACUATION, AND CRITICAL CARE IN AUSTERE CONDITIONS

30

Ronaldo C. Go, MD

INTRODUCTION

Casualties from natural disasters can easily deplete available resources, and can cause issues with pre-existing healthcare systems.

TYPES OF INJURIES AFTER NATURAL DISASTERS

Natural disasters are classified as geophysical (earthquakes, volcano, dry mass movement such as landslide or avalanche), hydrologic (floods), meteorologic (storm, tornado), and climatologic (extremes in temperature).[1-5] Certain disasters can lead to predictable injuries and illness patterns.[5] Hurricane, a storm with winds > 74 mph, can cause traumatic injuries related to flying objects and wind pressure.[5] Tornado, a violent rotating column of air, can have craniocerebral injuries, crush injuries from falling structures, fractures which may be open, contusion, abrasions, soft tissue injuries, and sepsis.[5-7] Floods cause drowning and hypothermia.[5,7] Landslides, a downward movement of soil, lead to submersion or immersion injuries. Earthquakes, the sudden violent shaking of the ground, can lead to crush injuries, fractures, lacerations, and fire related injury such as burns or smoke inhalation. Tsunami, a high wave caused by underwater disturbance, can lead to trauma and drowning.[5] Forest fires can lead to burns, smoke inhalation injuries, hypovolemic shock, and sepsis. Heat waves can lead to heat exhaustion and heat stroke. On the opposite spectrum of temperature, winter storms can lead to automobile accidents with life threatening traumatic injuries, hypothermia, and carbon monoxide poisoning. Volcanoes can discharge air pollutants which can lead to new respiratory failure or exacerbation of pre-existing lung disease, conjunctivitis, arthralgias, burns, and cutaneous bullae.[5]

EVACUATION OF HOSPITAL DURING NATURAL DISASTER

Pre-Event ICU Evacuation planning should be in place as soon as possible.[1,2] Strategies should include shelter in place, partial evacuation, or early evacuation.[2] If possible, coordination with local government should be in place so there would be enough ground or flight support. Responders have suggested the following ICU-specific equipment: transport sleds (21%), oxygen tanks and respiratory therapy supplies (19%), flashlights (24%), portable ventilators and suctions (16%), and walkie-talkies (26%).[1] These ventilators should be able to support patients on current power and with adequate oxygenation.[2] Major stressors include lack of water, food, toilets, and concerns for family members.[1]

In time limited scenarios, patients who are less critical should be evacuated first to maximize the number of patients that can be moved out.[2] If there is adequate time, all critical care patients can be moved in parallel. Another approach would be to transfer similar patients together as a group; allowing the other facility to cluster resources.

Preparation of patient for evacuation involves stabilization, finishing diagnostic procedures, and addressing the physiologic changes during transportation.[2] Complete transfer of medical records, preferably electronically via the internet or with the patient using a USB flash drive and/or paper medical record, is key. Patient and supplies should be tracked.

ICU IN AUSTERE CONDITIONS

A make-shift ICU and/or ICU in austere conditions may rely on prognostic scores to help ration supplies, beds, and medical staff. Preventable deaths can be avoided by having a supervising intensivist on a 24-hour standby. Patients can be transferred from the hospital to mobile units and then to hotels and home quarantine depending on severity of symptoms.[3,4] Psychiatric and/or religious guidance is often needed.

Field hospitals, developed by military or civilian governments, are primarily developed for resuscitation and stabilization but also to treat pre-existing diseases and are ideal for austere conditions. They can evolve from a small 10-member crew such as the Small Portable Expeditionary Aeromedical Rapid Response (SPEARR) team, to a highly specialized 65 bed hospital with ICU capability[10] (see Table 30-1). Major limitations of field hospitals are their sustainability and capacity.[8–11]

Table 30-1 BASELINE SUPPLIES FOR SMALL PORTABLE EXPEDITIONARY AEROMEDICAL RAPID RESPONSE OR FIELD HOSPITAL	
Medications	
• Antibiotics	Amphotericin B, metronidazole, gentamicin, ceftriaxone, vancomycin, ampicillin/sulbactam, piperacillin/tazobactam, levofloxacin, cefazolin, acyclovir, bacitracin
• Pressors	Phenylephrine, norepinephrine, vasopressin, dopamine, dobutamine
• Antiarrhythmics and antihypertensives	Amiodarone, adenosine, lidocaine, metoprolol, Cardizem, Vasotec, nitroglycerine, clonidine, Cardene, verapamil, furosemide,
• Sedatives	Fentanyl, Haldol, acetaminophen, morphine, midazolam, lorazepam, ketorolac, succinylcholine, ketamine
• Antiplatelet and anticoagulation	Aspirin, heparin, warfarin, alteplase, tenecteplase
• Pulmonary	Methylprednisolone, prednisone, albuterol, ipratropium, acetylcysteine
• Gastro	Activated charcoal, pantoprazole, famotidine, Colace, senna, Miralax, lactulose
• Antidotes	Protaminine, naloxone, glucagon, flumazenil
• Renal	Kayexalate, patiromer, sodium zirconium, sodium bicarbonate, phosphate, potassium, magnesium, calcium, sodium tablets
• Endo	Lantus, insulin, d50
• ACLS	
• Tent	Alaska Structures Medical Shelter (tent system)
• Blood products	pRBC, FFP, whole blood, Factor VIIa, cryoprecipitate

(Continued)

Table 30-1   BASELINE SUPPLIES FOR SMALL PORTABLE EXPEDITIONARY AEROMEDICAL RAPID RESPONSE OR FIELD HOSPITAL (*CONTINUED*)

Medications	
• Electricity	MEP-7 electrical generator
• Laboratory	Expeditionary Medical System laboratory
• Oxygen	EDOCS 120B oxygen generator
• Diagnostics	Expeditionary Medical System radiology
• Mechanical ventilation	Impact 754 ventilator, Pulmonetics LTV 1000 ventilator
• Physiologic	Welch Allyn Propaq 206 EL physiologic monitor Zoll CCT monitor/defibrillator/external pacemaker Bronchoscope Ultrasound

EDOCS = Expeditionary Deployable Oxygen Concentration System.

Ultrasound

Ultrasound is portable and has been helpful in austere conditions in triage and troubleshooting.[12] The FAST examination, a 2–4 minute assessment mostly for trauma patients, can assess the pericardium, right upper quadrant, left upper quadrant, and pelvis around the bladder for free fluid after trauma, with a sensitivity of 83.3% and specificity of 99.7%.[13] It can also be used to detect pericardial effusion (sensitivity and specificity of 100%),[14] pneumothorax (88% sensitivity and 99% specificity),[15] long bone fractures (sensitivity of 97.5% and specificity of 95%),[16] detection of foreign body (sensitivity of 100% and specificity of 75%),[17] pulmonary edema (specificity of 97% and sensitivity of 89%),[18] and acute mountain sickness.

Blood Transfusions

Fresh whole blood (FWB) has full hemostatic function and can be stored at room temperature and used within 24 hours of collection or stored within 8 hours of collection, where it becomes stored whole blood (SWB). It can be stored for up to 21 days. Low titer (low anti-A and anti-B titers) group O WB is universal WB.[21–24] It has superior hemostasis compared to the 1:1:1 (platelet:plasma:RBC) which is recommended for damage control resuscitation.[24] Rh negative WB must be transfused to women < 50 years of age or unknown blood group to avoid alloimmunization.[24]

FWB can be obtained through a walking blood bank program.[24] Prescreening must be done for low titer group O WB. A caveat to this process is that it cannot screen for infectious diseases.

Renal Replacement Therapy

Peritoneal hemodialysis is a renal replacement therapy (RRT) that can be performed in areas with limited resources and no electricity. A flexible or rigid catheter is inserted via the Seldinger technique within an incision 2 cm below the umbilicus, directed caudal to the iliac fossa.[25] Contraindications include abdominal surgery, diaphragmatic injury, soft tissue infection and severe respiratory failure.[25]

Oxygen generators

Oxygen concentrators or oxygen generators are used to supply oxygen in makeshift or field hospitals. The three principles of oxygen generation technologies are cryogenic separation with liquefied oxygen; 2) molecular sieves using granular aluminosilicate material called zeolite, which absorbs nitrogen and leaves oxygen alone; and 3) electrochemical oxygen generation.[26]

Sterilization of Surgical Instruments

Boiling is highly unreliable and the three methods of decontamination are autoclave, dry heat, and chemical antiseptic.[27–29] The minimum standard has been the use of an enzymatic cleaner followed by antiseptics, such as formaldehyde, glutaraldehyde, and chlorhexidine.[29] Another approach is with vacuum sealing of chlorhexidine-scrubbed contaminated instruments with or without UVC irradiation. Chlorhexidine alone achieves a 99.5% reduction in colony forming units (CFU) and the addition of UVC causes 100% reduction.[27]

▌ REFERENCES

1. King M, Dorfman M, Einav S, Niven A, Kissoon N, Grissom C. Evacuation of intensive care units during disaster: learning from the hurricane sandy experience. *Disaster Med Public Health Prep.* 2016;10(1):20-27.

2. Christian MD, Devereaux AV, Dichter JR, et al. Introduction and executive summary: care of the critically ill and injured during pandemics and disasters: CHEST consensus statement. *Chest*. 2014;146(4 Suppl):8S-34S.

3. Kearns RD, Conlon KM, Matherly AF, et al. Guidelines for burn care under austere conditions: introduction to burn disaster, airway and ventilator management, and fluid resuscitation. *J Burn Care Res*. 2016;37(5):e427-39.

4. Lu X, Xu S. Intensive care for severe acute respiratory syndrome coronavirus 2 (SARS-CoV-2) in a makeshift ICU in Wuhan. *Crit Care*. 2020;24(1):199.

5. Hidalgo J, Baez AA. Natural Disasters. *Crit Care Clin*. 2019;35(4):591-607.

6. Cannon T. At risk: natural hazards, people vulnerability, and disaster. Paper presented at CENAT conference. Ticino, Switzerland, November 28–December 3, 2004.

7. Scott Z, Wooster K, Few R, et al. Monitoring and evaluating a disaster risk management capacity. *Disaster Prev Manag*. 2016;25(3):412-22.

8. Bell SA, Abir M, Choi H, Cooke C, Iwashyna T. All-cause hospital admissions among older adults after a natural disaster. *Ann Emerg Med*. 2018;71(6):746-754.e2.

9. Bell SA, Iwashyna TJ, Zhang X, Chen B, Davis MA. All-cause hospitalizations after large-scale hurricanes among older adults: A Self-Controlled Case Series Study. *Prehosp Disaster Med*. 2021;36(1):25-31.

10. Rice DH, Kotti G, Beninati W. Clinical review: critical care transport and austere critical care. *Crit Care*. 2008;12(2):207.

11. Grissom TE, Farmer JC. The provision of sophisticated critical care beyond the hospital: lessons from physiology and military experiences that apply to civil disaster medical response. *Crit Care Med*. 2005;33(1 Suppl):S13-21.

12. Russell TC, Crawford PF. Ultrasound in the austere environment: a review of the history, indications, and specifications. *Military Medicine*. 2013;178(1):21-28.

13. Rozycki GS, Ballard RB, Feliciano DV, Schmidt JA, Pennington SD. Surgeon-performed ultrasound for the assessment of truncal injuries: lessons learned from 1540 patients. *Ann Surg*. 1998;228(4):557-67.

14. Nelson BP, Chason K. Use of ultrasound by emergency medical services: a review. *Int J Emerg Med*. 2008;1(4):253-9.

15. Ding W, Shen Y, Yang J, He X, Zhang M. Diagnosis of pneumothorax by radiography and ultrasonography. *Chest*. 2011;140(4):859-66.

16. Heiner J, McArthur TJ. The ultrasound identification of simulated long bone fractures by prehospital providers. *Wilderness Environ Med*. 2010;21(2):137-40.

17. Illston BJ, Caudell MJ, Lyon ML, DiCarlo J, D'Zio R. Intra-articular sea urchin spine/foreign body evaluation: ultrasound versus fluoroscopy. *Wilderness Environ Med*. 2010;21:168.

18. Lichtenstein DA, Meziere GA. Relevance of lung ultrasound in the diagnosis of acute respiratory failure: the BLUE protocol. *Chest*. 2008;134;117-25.

19. Grathwohl KW, Venticinque SG. Organizational characteristics of the austere intensive care unit: the evolution of military trauma and critical care medicine; applications for civilian medical care systems. *Crit Care Med*. 2008 Jul;36 (7 Suppl):S275-83.

20. Geiling J, Burkle FM Jr, West TE, et al. Resource-poor settings: response, recovery, and research: care of the critically ill and injured during pandemics and disasters: CHEST consensus statement. *Chest*. 2014 Oct;146(4 Suppl):e168S-77S.

21. Katsura M, Matsushima K, Kitamura R, et al. The use of warm fresh whole blood transfusion in the austere setting: a civilian trauma experience. *J Trauma Acute Care Surg*. 2020;89(3):e28-e33.

22. Spinella PC, Perkins JG, Grathwohl KW, Beekley AC, Holcomb JB. Warm fresh whole blood is independently associated with improved survival for patients with combat-related traumatic injuries. *J Trauma*. 2009;66(4 Suppl):S69-76.

23. Spinella PC. Warm fresh whole blood transfusion for severe hemorrhage: U.S. military and potential civilian applications. *Crit Care Med*. 2008;36 (7 Suppl):S340-5.

24. Cap AP, Beckett A, Benov A, et al. Whole blood transfusion. *Mil Med*. 2018;183(suppl_2):44-51.

25. Gorbatkin C, Bass J, Finkelstein FO, Gorbatkin SM. Peritoneal dialysis in austere environments: an emergent approach to renal failure management. *West J Emerg Med*. 2018;19(3):548-556.

26. Available at https://apps.dtic.mil/dtic/tr/fulltext/u2/a581789.pdf. Accessed October 10, 2020.

27. Knox RW, Demons ST, Cunningham CW. A novel method to decontaminate surgical instruments for operational and austere environments. *Wilderness Environ Med*. 2015;26:509-513.

28. Available at https://jts.amedd.army.mil/assets/docs/cpgs/Prehospital_En_Route_CPGs/Austere_Resuscitative_Surgical_Care_30_Oct_2019_ID76.pdf. Accessed October 10, 2020.

29. World Health Organization, Best practice guidelines on emergency surgical care in disaster situations, WHO 2003. (info for procedures for sterility of instruments). Available at https://www.who.int/surgery/publications/BestPracticeGuidelinesonESCinDisasters.pdf. Published 2005. Accessed May 2019.

31 TRAUMATIC BRAIN INJURY

Ari M. Wachsman, MD

▌ INTRODUCTION

Traumatic brain injury is a major public health problem both in the developed and developing world. Its effects can be measured both in its costs to society and its effects on individual survivors and their families. Sustained effort on the part of researchers as well as clinicians, and major technological advances over the last 5 decades have improved survival from major head trauma and allowed more patients to achieve meaningful neurologic recovery, primarily through improvements in recognition, medical imaging, post-trauma monitoring, and surgical therapeutics.[1] Nevertheless, especially in the acute phase, the care of these patients is extremely resource intensive, highly complex, and is best served by a team of specialized clinicians in a dedicated neurocritical care unit. Management of traumatic brain injury (TBI) in a crisis situation—be it a mass casualty incident caused by a natural disaster, a terrorist attack, or any event which overwhelms a healthcare delivery system—adds an entirely different set of challenges to an already formidable problem.

▌ DEFINITIONS AND CLASSIFICATION BY SEVERITY

TBI is a heterogeneous entity with a variety of different potential manifestations depending on the mechanism of injury, as well as the magnitude, directionality, and type of extrinsic forces applied to the brain. The severity can be described as mild, moderate or severe. Criteria will depend on which of the numerous classification systems is being employed, and whether the determination is based on clinical or pathologic findings.

The CDC defines TBI as "disruption of normal function of the brain caused by a bump, blow, jolt, blast, or penetrating injury."[2] From a clinical standpoint, severity is based on the presence or absence of loss of consciousness; loss of memory, including both retrograde or post-traumatic amnesia; the presence or absence of accompanying neurologic deficits; and alteration of mental state following the injury, such as confusion, disorientation, slowed thinking, or difficulty concentrating. Mild TBI is characterized by preserved consciousness or loss of consciousness lasting less than 30 minutes, and normal CT or MR imaging of the brain. Loss of consciousness lasting 30 minutes to 24 hours comprises a moderate TBI, while loss of consciousness lasting more than 24 hours constitutes a severe TBI.[3]

In the prehospital or austere setting, severity of TBI has been based on injury severity scores, the most common of which worldwide is the Glasgow Coma Scale (GCS), which is a standardized and quickly and easily reproducible score based on the clinical exam. The GCS assigns a total number of points from 3 to 15 depending on the presence of spontaneous eye opening or the type of stimulation required to induce eye opening, with 1–4 possible points assigned; the degree of verbal responsiveness, with 1–5 possible points; and the type of spontaneous or evoked motor responses observed in the injured person, with 1–6 possible points. Minor TBI is described as GCS 13–15; a GCS of 9–12 is moderate, while 8 or less is severe.[4]

While classification based on GCS has some clear advantages, it is limited in several ways, most notably by the use of endotracheal intubation, sedation, or neuromuscular blockade, all of which may overstate the severity of a TBI, as well as poor inter-rater reliability and prognostic value[5]; that said, it remains a useful tool with nearly universal acceptance. Other clinical scoring systems such as the FOUR (Full Outline of UnResponsiveness) score attempt to improve inter-rater reliability by eliminating the verbal domain of the GCS and adding evaluation of respiration and brainstem reflexes, specifically pupillary, corneal and cough.[6] The FOUR score has been validated in several treatment settings as compared with the GCS,[7] and appears to have better sensitivity and specificity as well as positive predictive value in patients with altered level of consciousness,[8] but has yet to achieve the same level of acceptance as the GCS, which remains the standard for defining TBI severity in the acute setting.

EPIDEMIOLOGY

TBI is a massive public health problem, with an estimated 5.3 million people in the US, or approximately 2% of the population, living with a TBI-related disability,[9] and the incidence has increased significantly in recent years. In 2014, there were 2.87 million emergency department visits for TBI in the US, which is an increase of 54% from 2006;[10] over the same period, annual hospitalizations for TBI increased by 8% to 288,000, while deaths from TBI decreased by 6% to approximately 56,800, or about 155 deaths per day.[11]

TBI is a major cause of morbidity and mortality for military service members. Between 2000 and 2011, the incidence of TBI on the battlefield, especially from blast injuries, increased significantly due the common use of improvised explosive devices.[12] The true incidence of TBI is not known, as mild TBI in a combat or austere environment is highly under-reported.[13] Severe TBI is now the leading cause of death on the modern battlefield,[14] and in 2005 the Department of Defense referred TBI as the "signature wound of war in Iraq and Afghanistan".[15]

In certain types of crisis situations, such as an earthquake with collapse of multiple buildings, or a mass casualty incident involving a powerful explosion, conditions are similar to those encountered in a combat zone or an austere environment. As such, TBIs may be a common finding in patients seeking urgent medical attention, and numerous patients requiring urgent imaging and neurospecialist care may quickly overwhelm the local medical infrastructure.

CLINICAL AND PATHOPHYSIOLOGICAL ASPECTS OF TBI

Primary TBI

Primary TBI refers to the direct trauma to brain tissue and cerebral vasculature suffered at the moment of injury. Measures to mitigate primary TBI focus on prevention of injury and the use of protective equipment such as helmets or seat belts. The type of injury or injuries suffered will depend on the magnitude and vector of the forces applied to the head as the mechanism of injury. A direct blow to the head from a blunt projectile may cause skull fractures and/or contusion of the subjacent area to the impact site, along with coup-contrecoup injury of the brain regions opposite to the impact site as the brain rebounds off the inner table of the skull. A penetrating projectile will cause a different injury pattern, with injury of neuronal and vascular structures along the path of the missile, with or without diffuse axonal injury, while a blast injury will more commonly cause diffuse axonal injury and micro-hemorrhages throughout the brain.

According to the Monro-Kellie doctrine, the sum of the volumes of brain tissue, cerebrospinal fluid (CSF), and intracranial blood is constant.[16] Under normal conditions, the brain constitutes about 80% of the intracranial volume, arterial and venous blood about 10%, and cerebrospinal fluid the remaining 10%.[17] Within the closed box of the skull, an enlarging hematoma or infarct with edema will take up an increasingly larger volume of space and raise the intracranial pressure (ICP), unless available volume is increased. Rising ICP will compromise perfusion of the brain as blood entering the skull with a given mean arterial pressure (MAP) will have decreased flow with increasing resistance. The brain requires a given range of cerebral perfusion pressure, defined as MAP-ICP, in order to maintain adequate blood flow. Normal cerebral perfusion pressure (CPP) is about 60–80 mmHg in healthy subjects, and is maintained within that range despite fluctuations in MAP by means of vasoconstriction and vasodilatation at the arteriolar level.[18]

Below a certain threshold of CPP, typically about 45–50 mmHg,[19] cerebral blood flow will fall below the necessary minimum to prevent dysfunction due to ischemia. In terms of blood flow per volume of brain tissue, this corresponds to about 18–20 ml/100g/min, normal being 50–60 ml/100g/min.[20] If blood flow falls below 8 ml/100g/min, irreversible infarction of the ischemic tissue ensues within about an hour.[21] Total loss of global cerebral blood flow, as typically seen in cardiac arrest, can lead to some degree of permanent anoxic injury within 3–8 minutes of onset,[22] with worsening outcomes associated with more prolonged times prior to restoration of blood flow.[23]

Death often occurs early in severe primary TBI. A major factor raising mortality is bleeding resulting from traumatic injury to the arteries and/or veins of the brain, which portends a worse outcome.[24] Bleeding may be intra-parenchymal, epidural, subdural, subarachnoid and/or intraventricular, and typically more than one type of bleeding is present at any given time. Enlarging hematomas frequently cause herniation, or shifting of the intracranial contents. Compression of the delicate brain leads to irreversible tissue injury as well as compromise of the blood flow through adjacent vascular structures, leading to progressive arterial and venous infarctions within the first few hours of the injury, and compounding the injury to the brain. Bleeding into the ventricles of the brain with obstruction of CSF, or alternately compression of the tissue which compromises the flow of CSF, causes enlargement of the ventricles, which can be a major contributor to increasing pressure inside the skull.

Secondary TBI

Secondary TBI refers to a complex cascade of physiologic derangements set in motion at the time of the primary injury and lasting days to weeks afterward. Tissue damage and the body's response to it, including the pro-inflammatory activity of leukocytes, disorganized regulation of blood flow, abnormal release of neurotransmitters, generation of free radicals, and other factors cause a cascade of neuro-inflammation and thrombosis, further contributing to microvascular compromise and cell death.[25]

Swelling of the brain is a common manifestation of the secondary phase of TBI, and results from a number of different factors. Disruption of the blood-brain barrier (BBB) is frequently observed, leading to escape of water from the bloodstream into the extracellular milieu, in addition to plasma proteins and peripheral inflammatory cells. Resident immune cells, chiefly microglia, respond to injury to brain tissue with the release of pro-inflammatory cytokines that further contribute to BBB compromise.[26] A leaky BBB serves an important purpose in the immediate aftermath of TBI, as it allows for immune cells to migrate from the bloodstream to the injured tissue; however, it also contributes to worsening edema and a number of other maladaptive processes, some of which may be more dangerous than the initial injury itself.

Another salient aspect of secondary TBI is global or regional loss of cerebral pressure autoregulation, i.e. the process by which CPP is kept within physiologic parameters, leading to regions of vasodilation alongside regions of vasoconstriction and hypoperfusion, even though peripheral blood pressure is within normal range. Regions with insufficient blood supply due to vasoconstriction will be subject to ischemia and permanent injury due to infarction, while adjacent areas will be hyperemic and edematous, contributing to the decrease in compliance of the brain tissue and elevations in ICP.[27] Disordered cerebral blood flow is further exacerbated by the body's predisposition toward clotting after major trauma, including thrombosis of large vessels as well as the microvasculature, further compromising blood supply.

The brain's response to TBI is also characterized by massive release of excitatory neurotransmitters, chiefly glutamate, the primary excitatory neurotransmitter in the human brain. The unopposed activity of glutamate causes inappropriate energy consumption and worsening of mismatch between supply and demand. Energy failure is manifested by loss of function of transmembrane ion pumps as well as intracellular processes, ultimately culminating in apoptosis and death of the cell. Glutamate will also contribute to seizure activity, which constitutes a massive expenditure of energy with attendant consumption of available resources, and can cause tissue injury and cellular apoptosis due to calcium-induced excitotoxicity.[28]

Clinically, secondary TBI is marked by both local and global dysfunction as the processes set in motion by the primary injury continue to evolve. Dilated cerebral vasculature, focal contusions or confluent hemorrhages, obstructive hydrocephalus, and arterial and venous infarcts can all contribute to raised ICP. Through increased permeability of capillaries, there is progression of edema around areas of focal injury and hemorrhage. Mental status declines accordingly, and seizures are common. As regional and global cerebral blood supply is progressively compromised by increasing resistance to blood entering the skull, tissue ischemia and infarction ensues, which often leads to brain death unless treated aggressively.

Tertiary TBI

Tertiary TBI refers to the long-term sequelae of injury to the brain, much of whose pathophysiology is incompletely understood. Survivors of TBI suffer from a panoply of complaints including debilitating headache, personality change, impulsive or violent behavior, mood and attentional disorders, sleep-wake dysfunction, memory loss, slow cognitive tempo, among other major morbidities. The condition is frequently under-recognized and undertreated.[29] Tertiary TBI is a major cause of social and personal instability in survivors, as well as job loss, drug or alcohol abuse as self-medication, involvement of law enforcement and the judicial system, and the breakup of families. The attendant costs to society can be measured in the billions of dollars. Though a comprehensive discussion of tertiary injury is outside the scope of this chapter, it remains a major topic for future research.

STANDARD TREATMENT AND MONITORING OF TBI

The management of TBI in non-austere, non-crisis environments in developed countries depends on the prompt identification of the condition followed by specialized medical and surgical treatment according to evidence-based practices.

For the reasons alluded to above, diagnosis of TBI can be challenging, even in non-austere environments. The diagnosis of TBI devolves upon focused history taking, often through self-reporting, in addition to the clinical exam and medical imaging. History-taking is inherently problematic in patients with altered level of consciousness, and in those who are presently alert and oriented but may be amnestic to the traumatic event. In such patients the clinical exam assumes paramount importance. As previously mentioned, evaluation of patients with TBI will generally include an assessment of level of consciousness such as the GCS or FOUR score, as well as a comprehensive neurologic assessment aimed at identifying cranial nerve palsies and long-tract signs, i.e. focal or lateralizing sensorimotor dysfunction or ataxia.

Patients with decreased level of consciousness and focal neurological deficits are strongly suspected as having sustained a focal injury to the brain parenchyma such as a contusion or parenchymal hemorrhage and/or having an extra-axial hemorrhage, which may be subject to expansion and compression of the brain unless promptly evacuated. Until proven otherwise, these patients are considered to have severe TBI, and under normal circumstances will routinely receive a noncontrast CT of the brain and often the cervical spine. This commonplace radiologic test allows the care team to assess the severity of the primary injury and identify patients in need of urgent surgical intervention; for patients with a GCS of 14–15 and a negative preliminary CT reading, Livingston and colleagues calculated a negative predictive value of 99.7% for the need for subsequent neurosurgical intervention.[30] Depending on the results, patients may require transfer to a suitable neurocritical care unit or trauma ICU for close monitoring of the neurologic exam, serial imaging, and specialized care of the secondary injury as the patient hopefully stabilizes and recovers in the days and weeks to come. The CT may also demonstrate specific conditions such as unstable facial or skull base fractures which may change the approach to the patient. If the CT of the cervical spine or the clinical exam is suggestive, selected patients may also benefit from cervical vascular imaging such as CT angiography to assess for blunt cerebrovascular injury including dissection, pseudoaneurysm, or arterial transection.[31]

If an acute post-traumatic epidural or subdural hemorrhage is identified, any anticoagulant medications which the patient was taking must be reversed promptly, as the patient is at increased risk for rapid decompensation or death as the hemorrhage expands. As previously mentioned, an enlarging hematoma can cause death in two ways: either by causing herniation of brain tissue with compression and destruction of vital structures such as the brainstem or major arteries, or by raising ICP, compromising cerebral perfusion by decreasing the rate of blood flow into the increasingly pressurized cranial vault. These processes typically occur in tandem. If an extra-axial hemorrhage found on initial CT is felt to be acute and symptomatic, an emergent surgical intervention in the form of a craniotomy and evacuation or decompressive craniectomy is to be considered.[32] More commonly, a small hemorrhage is found but is believed not to be threatening the patient imminently, in which case the patient will usually be treated conservatively, and undergo repeat CT imaging after a short interval of time (usually 4–8 hours) to assess whether a visualized hematoma is increasing in size, suggesting active bleeding.[33]

ICP Monitoring

An invasive ICP monitoring device such as an external ventricular drain may be placed in patients at risk for deterioration, according to institutional policy. The Brain Trauma Foundation suggests placement of a transcranial monitoring device in the setting of GCS less than 9 with an abnormal CT, or GCS less than 9 with a normal CT if the patient is older than 40 and with abnormal posturing, with a CPP goal of 50–70 mmHg.[34] While some patients may be safely managed without placement of a monitor, ICP monitoring in appropriate patients significantly reduces mortality compared with patients with severe TBI who do not undergo monitoring,[35] and is essential for the traditional CPP-guided approach to neurologic resuscitation and support.

In the throes of secondary TBI, as cerebral edema worsens and abnormal vasomotor responses occur, the ICP may fluctuate widely and feature prolonged periods of elevation. Frequent or continuous ICP measurements is a critical part of the management of severe TBI. An external ventricular drain is considered the gold standard for ICP monitoring, as it not only allows for accurate real-time measurement of the ICP, but also affords the ability to drain off CSF and lower the ICP acutely in response to sudden elevations. In some situations a fiberoptic pressure monitor may be placed instead of an external ventricular drain, or alongside one, depending on the clinical context.[36]

Once an EVD has been placed, a follow-up CT of the head is usually done to confirm position and assess for post placement tract hemorrhage. It requires careful monitoring to ensure it does not become occluded by clot or tissue debris, the drain does not migrate out of position, and the patient is neither over- nor under-drained. Proper stewardship and best nursing practices are essential to avoid contamination of the CSF and subsequent ventriculitis or meningitis. To reduce the risk of infection, an EVD should be weaned and removed when it is no longer necessary to guide clinical decisions; the use of antibiotic coated EVDs may further reduce the risk.[37] Occasionally an EVD is used after TBI not only for pressure monitoring and CSF sampling, but as a conduit to introduce various medications, such as tPA to assist in lysis of intraventricular clot, or intrathecal antibiotics to treat intracranial infections. If a patient is unable to wean from the EVD over time, it will typically be internalized and converted to a ventriculoperitoneal (or alternately ventriculopleural or ventriculoatrial) shunt.

In order to ascertain whether the patient is maintaining optimal cerebral perfusion pressure, the ICP numbers generated by an external ventricular drain or fiberoptic strain catheter are only interpretable if the patient's blood pressure is known, so frequent BP measurement is crucial, optimally using an arterial line for beat-to-beat monitoring. The most detrimental effects on outcomes in hospitalized TBI patients are seen in the setting of hypoxia and hypotension, as well as hyperthermia.[38] As such, basic ICU care including hemodynamic monitoring, ventilator management driven by continuous bedside SpO_2, arterial blood gas sampling for monitoring of pH, pO_2 and PCO_2, and monitoring of real-time respiratory parameters, are paramount.

Carbon dioxide has a potent influence on cerebral arterial tone. While measurement of CO_2 is routine for any ICU patient, close monitoring of pCO_2 is particularly important for patients with elevated ICP, including those with severe TBI. Elevated pCO_2 causes vasodilatation which increases ICP as intracranial blood volume increases. Conversely, pCO_2 which is inappropriately low can cause vasoconstriction, potentially leading to worsening tissue ischemia and infarction. End-tidal capnography, usually measured in real time on a modern ICU ventilator through the use of an in-line cassette, is supplemented by periodic arterial or venous blood gas monitoring, as would be necessary in any patient on mechanical ventilation.[39]

Hyperthermia is common after severe TBI, occurring in up to 37% of patients, and is increasingly recognized as an independent risk factor for in-hospital mortality and poor outcomes as measured by Glasgow Coma Scale (GCS).[40] The specific mechanism for how hyperthermia exacerbates brain injury is not fully understood, but higher body temperature is clearly associated with intracranial hypertension and seizure propensity, among other factors. Hyperthermia may be seen in isolation or as a manifestation of paroxysmal sympathetic hyperactivity, or "neuro-storming", which typically includes hypertension, tachycardia, tachypnea, diaphoresis, and psychomotor agitation, and is commonly associated with increases in ICP. According to large retrospective analyses, patients with hyperthermia following a severe TBI have about a 1.5-fold risk of death compared with normothermic patients, and higher temperatures correlate with worse outcomes; induced hypothermia, however, has not been shown to be neuroprotective, and may increase mortality.[41] While neurogenic hyperthermia is a known complication of TBI, these patients are also subject to fevers due to infection, including bacterial cerebritis or meningoencephalitis, especially in the case of penetrating brain injuries, skull fractures which violate paranasal sinuses or the skull base, and CSF leaks. Empiric antibiotics and a focused search for a source of intracranial or systemic infection are frequent responses to fever in such patients. Given the high inflammatory burden and significant propensity for venous thrombosis, patients may also be assessed for deep vein thrombosis of the extremities and pulmonary embolism, as neurogenic hyperthermia is a diagnosis of exclusion.

Standard care for hyperthermic patients must include aggressive temperature control, both with pharmacologic interventions like acetaminophen and chilled intravenous or enteric solutions, and nonpharmacologic measures like the use of cooling blankets, dedicated electronic body surface cooling devices, or more invasive devices such as intravascular cooling catheters. Notably, shivering is a common problem in patients undergoing targeted temperature management, and can be refractory to standard measures such as deep sedation and counter warming of the extremities, at times becoming so severe as to require neuromuscular blockade with paralytic agents. In patients who have been sedated and paralyzed, relatively little can be discerned from the clinical exam, and the care team must rely on indirect assessments of the patient's neurologic status such as imaging and ICP trends.

Hyperosmolar therapy is often employed in severe TBI, either prophylactically or in response to elevations in ICP, in order to mitigate cerebral edema and improve cerebral oxygen delivery.[42] Its use requires frequent dose adjustments guided by serial monitoring of serum sodium and osmolality to stay in range. Available options for hyperosmolar therapy include hypertonic saline either by bolus or via continuous infusion, in concentrations ranging from 1.5% to 23.4%, most commonly between 2 and 3%; also 50/50 mixes of 3% sodium acetate and sodium chloride can be used instead, which reduces the incidence of hyperchloremic metabolic acidosis as compared to sodium chloride. In a patient with elevated intracranial pressure, a typical target for serum sodium would be 145–155 mEq/L and is typically monitored every six hours. In the event of severe refractory intracranial hypertension, a saturated saline solution of 23.4% concentration may be given in small volumes. Osmotic diuretics such as mannitol are also often used for rapid treatment of acutely raised intracranial pressure, though if other options exist, these are typically not used for more than 48 hours at a time due to the possibility of rebound edema upon discontinuation. Mannitol is most commonly encountered in the emergency room setting or in the ICU when hypertonic saline is insufficient to control an acute elevation in ICP.[43]

Sudden and unexplained increases in ICP may trigger an assessment for cerebral venous thrombosis. Patients with TBI have an increased risk of systemic venous thrombosis, as mentioned above, but also for intracranial venous thrombosis, which may involve large or small venous structures, and can be unilateral, bilateral or midline. This is most commonly noted affecting a dural venous sinus and is associated with an overlying skull fracture, but can also be due to direct injury to a cerebral venous structure, as seen in penetrating injuries of the brain. Venous thrombosis can also be seen in the context of compression of a vein or sinus by herniation of brain tissue with subsequent stagnancy of blood flow, or can arise post-operatively.[44] The ramifications of a venous thrombosis in the brain can be significant; as incoming blood enters brain capillaries but is unable to drain, oncotic pressure will drive water into the tissue. This interstitial edema will add to the cytotoxic edema already present and cause an increase in ICP. This is especially problematic when dealing with large venous sinuses, which subtend larger portions of the brain. Furthermore, as it worsens, the venous congestion may cause infarction and hemorrhage, which will further drive increases in intracranial volume and pressure. Cerebral venous thrombosis is an independent risk factor for in-hospital mortality and can be very difficult to diagnose.[45] Despite the likelihood of such patients to bleed intracranially, they may require treatment with systemic anticoagulation in the absence of any other contraindications. If this is ineffective or not feasible, selected patients may undergo direct infusion of thrombolytics into an occluded venous sinus using an end-vascular approach guided by real-time cerebral angiography; some may require surgical craniotomy and decompression.[46]

As the secondary injury progresses, some patients may require subacute surgical intervention to alleviate mass effect and restore adequate perfusion, such as decompressive hemicraniectomy, where a portion of the skull is removed to allow the brain to herniate externally rather than inward toward the midline. Occasionally, severe bihemispheric injury may require bilateral craniectomies. Craniotomy and evacuation of an intraparenchymal clot is relatively rare but may become necessary depending on a number of factors, such as whether it is causing uncal herniation or is rapidly expanding and likely to lead to further decompensation. These decisions are typically driven by changes in the neurologic exam, such as a newly dilated pupil, or autonomic fluctuations which trigger repeat CT scanning. Surgical decompression is more effective when performed promptly after identification of a herniation syndrome, and is obviously subject to timely availability of a consultant neurosurgeon, which is a necessary criterion for a designated Level I Trauma Center, as is a minimum annual volume of severely injured patients.[47]

CSF leaks are a common manifestation of both blunt and penetrating traumatic injuries, occurring in 10–30% of skull base fractures and 1–3% of all patients with closed TBI.[48] Isolated CSF rhinorrhea may resolve spontaneously in up to 60–70% of cases, but in the event of a large breach in the dura mater associated with skull fracture or penetrating injury, surgery may be required for primary repair.[49] Some patients with persistent leaks may require decompression of the CSF space using a lumbar drain, and potentially antibiotics to reduce the risk of bacterial meningitis, until the breach either heals spontaneously or is surgically repaired.[50] Many such patients present in a delayed fashion, as cerebral edema resolves and a previously occluded dural tear is revealed, or as hemorrhages are cleared by the body's normal process of healing. Positional headache which worsens on sitting up is classic for CSF leak and intracranial hypotension. The exact location of a dural tear may be elusive and require multiple neuroimaging studies before a diagnosis is reached. Treatment of such patients is often multidisciplinary, with input from specialists in neurosurgery, trauma, neurology, ENT, orthopedics, infectious disease, and interventional neuroradiology, among others.

Ancillary Monitoring Techniques

In addition to ICP monitoring and standard measurements of vital signs and blood gases, a number of specialized monitoring modalities exist which can provide further information to the clinician about the state of the brain. One salient and increasingly common monitoring tool is continuous video electroencephalography, or cVEEG. As previously discussed, seizures are common in this patient population, with an estimated incidence of 10%,[51] and while a convulsive seizure is often easy to diagnose, nonconvulsive status epilepticus may be clinically silent. As this is a condition of continuous and inappropriate energy expenditure in a milieu already characterized by inadequate energy supply, unremitting seizure activity can create demand ischemia, worsen calcium-induced excitotoxicity and potentiate brain cell death. EEG is also useful to detect areas of focal injury, such as in CVA, which may have lateralizing areas of slowing. Conversely, if the EEG is normal or has global physiologic state changes, it can be reassuring findings.

EEG is inherently limited by various factors, including the presence of confounding artifacts from muscle, eye movements, sweat, EKG artifact, or interference from any of the numerous types of electrical equipment present in a typical ICU room. Such artifacts may render the EEG uninterpretable or cause an inexperienced reader to diagnose seizures inappropriately. There may be constraints on standard electrode placement in the setting of surgical incisions or breaches in the skin caused by traumatic injury. A reliable EEG is also dependent on the proper technique of the EEG technologist in applying the electrodes, as well as the acumen of the interpreting physician. With this in mind, however, EEG is a useful tool in managing severe TBI, especially in an unconscious patient or one who has received neuromuscular blockade.

Automated pupillometry has become more commonplace over recent years.[52] This is typically a simple procedure performed by the bedside RN using a hand-held camera-based device powered by a rechargeable battery. While a general impression of the integrity of the pupillary reflex arc can often be obtained from simply shining a bright light into the eye, this may not be possible in all patients. Some patients may receive medications such as fentanyl infusions which cause pupillary constriction, and others may have sustained damage to the brain stem, optic or oculomotor nerve, or the globe itself which makes changes in pupillary diameter hard to quantify. An automated pupillometer allows for rapid assessment of pupillary size and responsivity down to a hundredth of a millimeter, and reduces inter-observer variability. Results can often be automatically populated into the electronic medical record and trended over time. It has been further reported that changes in the speed of pupillary constriction may precede ICP elevation events.[53] As a result, automated pupillometry is increasingly used in high-risk patients as part of a nurse's routine serial neurologic assessment (or "neuro-check").

To supplement these monitoring strategies, a neurosurgeon or neurointensivist may also be called upon to place another type of transcranial monitoring device, other than an ICP monitor. A broad array of devices can be found on the market, with varying degrees of acceptance and adoption by the neurotrauma community, as the benefit of using a given device must be weighed against potential complications such as infection, thrombosis or hemorrhage, and malposition. Available options include invasive brain tissue thermometers; cerebral parenchymal oximetry catheters, to measure oxygen saturation within the parenchyma surrounding the insertion site; brain perfusion catheters, which use thermodilution to provide measurements of blood flow in the region surrounding the catheter; and microdialysis probes, which aim to periodically measure byproducts of metabolism within the tissue and inform the clinician on the relationship between energy demand and supply, guiding changes in hemodynamics, ventilator settings, sedation, and further diagnostic measures.

Another less invasive option to measure intracranial oxygenation is a jugular bulb catheter, whereby an intravenous catheter may be placed under X-ray guidance with its tip above the facial vein, allowing for sampling of venous blood from the brain. Subtracting the venous saturation from the arterial oxygen saturation provides a measure of cerebral oxygen extraction, which can be trended over time. Carbon dioxide levels can also be measured. Such catheters may also be used for sampling of blood for lactate and pyruvate levels, and hence to monitor the dynamic metabolic demands of the brain. Jugular bulb catheters are relatively easy to place, though they are also subject to malposition; these catheters carry a risk of thrombosis, hemorrhage, and infection, but have a relatively benign safety profile.[54]

Transcranial Doppler, or TCD, uses focused ultrasound to assess the movement of blood within the arteries of the brain. Though most commonly used to monitor for vasospasm following aneurysmal subarachnoid hemorrhage, it is also used in some centers following TBI, primarily to monitor cerebral blood flow velocity and vascular bed resistance. Low diastolic blood flow velocity within the middle cerebral arteries, and/or high pulsatility index, are believed to signal hypoperfusion and increased resistance to forward flow.[55] Especially in conjunction with elevated ICP, non-reassuring TCD numbers may signal a clinician to raise the peripheral blood pressure or adjust medications to lower ICP. TCD is an attractive option because it is noninvasive; however, it also highly operator dependent, only provides measurements while it is being operated by a competent technologist, and not all patients have favorable acoustic windows for insonation.

More recently, near-infrared spectroscopy devices have been developed, which use near-infrared light to penetrate the skull and may be useful in assessing for oxyhemoglobin concentration and oxygen saturation of the cerebral cortex. These may be promising because they are noninvasive, standardized, provide continuous measurements, and have shown favorable correlation with invasive oximetry devices such as LiCox. However, these devices have yet to be widely validated. All of these modalities may have their place in a standardized monitoring setup alongside ICP monitoring as well as more widely accepted noninvasive monitors of brain function like automated pupillometry or continuous EEG.[56]

Some centers will more frequently employ invasive monitoring devices such as cerebral microdialysis or transcranial perfusion catheters compared with others, and protocols for hyperosmolar therapy or anticonvulsant may vary. Regardless of the specific monitoring protocol used, the optimal setting for the multidisciplinary management of a severe TBI is a dedicated neurocritical care unit or neurotrauma ICU. Protocols for monitoring and treatment should be standardized whenever possible and conform to evidence-based guidelines issued by relevant academic associations, such as the Brain Trauma Foundation and the Neurocritical Care Society. The field is rapidly changing, and adherence to such guidelines is critical for an institution's practices to remain up to date with the latest evidence and in line with the standard of care.

▌ ISSUES IMPACTING CARE IN CRISIS ENVIRONMENTS

As mentioned above, even in a developed country with a robust health-care system and the ready availability of tertiary and quaternary referral centers, an acute mass casualty incident will create conditions similar to a combat zone or other austere settings. In the immediate aftermath of an event such as a terrorist bombing or accidental explosion, or a natural disaster like an earthquake, roads may be impassable, delaying access of first responders to the site and prompt transport of victims to hospitals. Depending on the type of event, the hospitals themselves may not be operating. However, even if the infrastructure in a crisis zone is intact, a large volume of victims all seeking emergency care simultaneously can overwhelm any healthcare system. If the event occurs in or near a large metropolitan area in close proximity to multiple Level I (or equivalent) trauma centers, as occurred in the Boston Marathon bombings in 2013, the system may be able to absorb the demand, but this may not be the case in the event of a large mass casualty incident in a rural area.[57]

In austere, combat or crisis environments, specialized equipment may not be available and diagnostic equipment that requires power from the electrical grid may not be functional. Any specialized equipment used must be portable, must not require refrigeration or deionized water, and must be rugged enough to function despite fluctuations in temperature and humidity and the presence of sand, dirt or dust. Accordingly, depending on the nature of the event, CT scanners—the most essential imaging modality in diagnosing the severity of an injury to the brain—may not be available. CT scans are not only useful for diagnosis, but also triage; if CT is not available, triage is more complicated. Mobile CT scanners do exist, typically in the form of mobile stroke units mounted on truck or ambulance chassis, but at present are not ubiquitous and would depend on passable roads in order to access a disaster site.

As such, with regard to traumatic brain injury in particular, simply diagnosing the condition may present a major challenge in a crisis situation. As we have seen, the diagnosis of mild TBI is based on self-reporting and may be overlooked in a chaotic environment with multiple casualties. If there are no external signs of head injury, even a severe TBI in an unconscious patient with polytrauma may go completely unrecognized in the prehospital setting, only to be discovered following initial stabilization and transport when a neurologic assessment can be done or the victim undergoes a CT scan of the head when they arrive at a hospital capable of performing one.

The U.S. military, with its experience in treating such injuries and its history of involvement in disaster responses, has a five-tier classification for medical facilities when treating injured warfighters. Role 1 refers to immediate first aid provided by a buddy or combat medic; the only imaging typically available in this setting is point-of-care ultrasound. Role 2 describes a battalion aid station, which has access to ultrasound, standard X-ray, and at times fluoroscopy, though this would depend on the presence of a qualified technologist. Role 3 denotes a more advanced facility such as a combat support hospital or hospital ship, which features more advanced imaging and often includes CT scanners. Role 4 is a fully capable regional medical center, though usually not a trauma center, and Role 5 is a stateside hospital. It is the practice of the U.S. military to evacuate moderate and severe TBI patients to Role 4 or Role 5 facilities, and the concept of prompt evacuation would apply to brain-injured civilians in an austere environment as well.[58]

Beyond the diagnostic and triaging ability afforded by CT scans, treatment options in an austere environment are also limited. Only basic stabilization may be provided by a responding EMS crew, assuming conditions allow for access by an ambulance. Typically, most of the specialty medications used in a neurocritical care unit for management of TBI—hyperosmolar solutions for treatment of cerebral edema, most anticonvulsants, and various medications for sedation—will not be found outside of a hospital. Electronic IV pumps may not be available or functional depending on the type of disaster and the integrity of the electrical grid, meaning that gravity bags and pressure infusers might be the only options, and close titration of IV infusion rates may not be possible. As scarce as specialty medications and equipment might be in a crisis setting, the availability of neurosurgeons, neurointensivists, and other specially trained providers would be even more limited, as would their access to the disaster site.

Time is of the essence in severe acute TBI, especially in the setting of an expanding extra-axial hematoma. Some studies have suggested that in the event of an extradural hemorrhage, if hematoma evacuation can be accomplished within 90 minutes of onset of a herniation syndrome, favorable outcomes may be obtained in up to 78% of patients. If decompression is delayed, favorable outcomes fall to 33% within 4.5 hours. In an austere environment when resources are limited, it may not be feasbile to transport a patient for imaging within a reasonable time frame.

In the age before widely available CT scanning, emergency room physicians were typically trained in exploratory burr hole craniotomy for this very reason.[59-61] Several approaches to this procedure can be found in the literature. Once a patient develops a herniation syndrome such as a dilated pupil with declining mental status, the principle is to place a number of burr holes at strategic points in the calvarium in order to diagnose and potentially evacuate an extra-axial hematoma. Though in normal conditions such procedures are done in the operating room with power-driven craniotomes and other highly specialized equipment, as a life-saving measure this procedure can be undertaken with a standard cranial access kit using a hand-cranked twist drill and can be done without the use of electricity. As such it might be considered as a last resort but may allow for stabilization and survival to transfer to a higher level of care, when it becomes possible to do so.

RECOMMENDATIONS AND RATIONALE

The nature of the response to a crisis will depend in large part on the nature of the crisis itself, and the resources which may be brought to bear both acutely and in the days following. A crisis situation may be brought about by conditions as different as a pandemic which overwhelms healthcare infrastructure on a national level but spares vital infrastructure, or an earthquake and tsunami which cuts off basic utilities and makes roads impassable. It is therefore difficult to discuss all possible crisis situations as though they were monolithic. However, some basic underlying rules still apply.

First, victims of a mass casualty incident must be triaged appropriately in the field. Numerous triage scales are used throughout the world; the specific pre-hospital triage system which should be used has long been a matter of vigorous debate, and there is little consensus on the subject.[62] Regardless, some criteria must be used by EMS to identify those patients who are injured but stable, those who are critically ill and in need of urgent transport, and those who are beyond saving. It is the recommendation of the Brain Trauma Foundation that patients with a GCS of < 14 be transferred urgently to a trauma service with neurosurgery on-site wherever possible.[63] While this is a reasonable guideline under normal circumstances, this may not apply to crisis conditions where trauma centers are overwhelmed or rapid evacuation to said centers is not feasible. Patients who are conscious and interactive without focal neurologic deficits, though they may be drowsy or confused, may need to wait for transfer in favor of patients with more severe injury who are still salvageable. Conversely, if transport times are very prolonged, patients with major neurologic compromise or large penetrating head wounds may not qualify for evacuation due to the low expectation that they will survive.

Assuming EMS has access to the site, once TBI is identified, initial efforts in the field must focus on early resuscitation and stabilization. As discussed, outcomes worsen in the presence of sustained hypotension and hypoxemia, with secondary contributions by elevated intracranial pressure, uncontrolled seizures, and expansion of an extra-axial or intraparenchymal hemorrhage. Standard prehospital measures are crucial, with the need for fluids and/or vasopressors to maintain adequate BP and administration of oxygen or placement of an advanced airway with mechanical ventilation if necessary. Additional measures while waiting for transfer to a trauma center may include the administration of anti-epileptic drugs or benzodiazepines to suppress seizures, or drugs indicated for emergent mitigation of cerebral edema such as mannitol, both of which are subject to availability given a limited supply. ICP cannot be measured in the field, but sudden decline in mental status may suggest a rise in ICP and may warrant an attempt at hyperventilation, though again, induced hypocapnia can worsen outcomes and is usually a brief temporizing measure until more definitive measures such as surgical decompression or maximal medical therapy are available.[64]

If a patient can be transported to an emergency department without neurosurgery on site, standard initial pharmacotherapy such as anticonvulsants or mannitol would likely be available, as would advanced airway management. However, depending on the conditions imposed by a crisis situation, prompt transfer to a trauma center should be pursued. This is especially important if the patient has focal neurologic deficits and/or poor mental status which is otherwise not explained. In the event of a sudden decompensation suggesting an enlarging extra-axial bleed—decline in mental status with a dilated pupil and contralateral pathologic posturing—invasive procedures such as placement of ipsilateral exploratory burr holes may have a role. However, such measures should be considered only as a last-ditch effort to save the patient's life, and are subject to the availability of appropriately trained personnel.

In summary, TBI remains a major public health problem in developed countries, with a high level of morbidity and mortality despite advances in knowledge and therapeutics in recent years. Outcomes are improved with rapid transport of patients with severe TBI to designated trauma centers with trained and experienced staff, specialized equipment, and standardized management protocols. In the event of a disaster, delays in transport to appropriate centers are likely to increase mortality in such patients, and reduced availability of resources may affect triage decisions in the field. It is the responsibility of any mature healthcare system to have a detailed contingency plan in place—considering multiple possible disaster scenarios and taking into account the local and regional healthcare ecosystem—so that delays in transfer may be minimized, cooperation between EMS and various hospitals may be streamlined, and patients may be evenly distributed to appropriate centers whenever possible.

REFERENCES

1. Khellaf A, Khan DZ, Helmy A. Recent advances in traumatic brain injury. *J Neurol.* 2019;266(11):2878-2889.
2. Centers for Disease Control and Prevention. Traumatic brain injury in the United States: Fact Sheet [Internet]. CDC.gov.Atlanta (GA): CDC; [updated 2015 January 12]. 2015b. Available at http://www.cdc.gov/traumaticbraininjury/get_the_facts.html. Accessed September 1, 2020.
3. Dixon KJ. Pathophysiology of traumatic brain injury. *Phys Med Rehabil Clin N Am.* 2017;28(2):215-225.
4. Pavlovic D, Pekic S, Stojanovic M, Popovic V. Traumatic brain injury: neuropathological, neurocognitive and neurobehavioral sequelae. *Pituitary.* 2019;22(3):270-282.
5. Hawryluk GW, Manley GT. Classification of traumatic brain injury: past, present, and future. *Handb Clin Neurol.* 2015;127:15-21.
6. Nyam TE, Ao KH, Hung SY, Shen ML, Yu TC, Kuo JR. FOUR score predicts early outcome in patients after traumatic brain injury. *Neurocrit Care.* 2017;26(2):225-231.
7. Chen B, Grothe C, Schaller K. Validation of a new neurological score (FOUR Score) in the assessment of neurosurgical patients with severely impaired consciousness. *Acta Neurochir (Wien).* 2013;155(11):2133-9; discussion 2139.
8. Kasprowicz M, Burzynska M, Melcer T, Kübler A. A comparison of the Full Outline of UnResponsiveness (FOUR) score and Glasgow Coma Score (GCS) in predictive modelling in traumatic brain injury. *Br J Neurosurg.* 2016;30(2):211-20.
9. Faul M, Coronado V. Epidemiology of traumatic brain injury. *Handb Clin Neurol.* 2015;127:3-13.
10. Capizzi A, Woo J, Verduzco-Gutierrez M. Traumatic brain injury: an overview of epidemiology, pathophysiology, and medical management. *Med Clin North Am.* 2020;104(2):213-238.
11. Daugherty J, Waltzman D, Sarmiento K, Xu L. Traumatic brain injury-related deaths by race/ethnicity, sex, intent, and mechanism of injury — United States, 2000–2017. *MMWR Morb Mortal Wkly Rep.* 2019;68(46):1050-1056.
12. Ling G, Ecklund JM, Bandak FA. Brain injury from explosive blast: description and clinical management. *Handb Clin Neurol.* 2015;127:173-80.
13. Schmid KE, Tortella FC. The diagnosis of traumatic brain injury on the battlefield. *Front Neurol.* 2012;3:90.
14. Breeze J, Bowley DM, Harrisson SE, et al. Survival after traumatic brain injury improves with deployment of neurosurgeons: a comparison of US and UK military treatment facilities during the Iraq and Afghanistan conflicts. *J Neurol Neurosurg Psychiatry.* 2020;91(4):359-365.
15. Brundage JF, Taubman SB, Hunt DJ, Clark LL. Whither the "signature wounds of the war" after the war: estimates of incidence rates and proportions of TBI and PTSD diagnoses attributable to background risk, enhanced ascertainment, and active war zone service, active component, U.S. Armed Forces, 2003–2014. *MSMR.* 2015;22(2):2-11.

16. Wilson MH. Monro-Kellie 2.0: The dynamic vascular and venous patho-physiological components of intracranial pressure. *J Cereb Blood Flow Metab.* 2016;36(8):1338-50.

17. Neff S, Subramaniam RP. Monro-Kellie doctrine. *J Neurosurg.* 1996;85(6):1195.

18. Portella G, Cormio M, Citerio G, et al. Continuous cerebral compliance monitoring in severe head injury: its relationship with intracranial pressure and cerebral perfusion pressure. *Acta Neurochir (Wien).* 2005;147(7):707-13; discussion 713.

19. Nordström CH. Assessment of critical thresholds for cerebral perfusion pressure by performing bedside monitoring of cerebral energy metabolism. *Neurosurg Focus.* 2003;15(6):E5.

20. Bouma GJ, Muizelaar JP. Cerebral blood flow in severe clinical head injury. *New Horiz.* 1995;3(3):384-94.

21. Cold E. Cerebral blood flow in acute head injury: the regulation of cerebral blood flow and metabolism during the acute phase of head injury, and its significance of therapy. *Acta Neurochir Suppl (Wien).* 1990;49:2-64.

22. Weinberger LM, Gibbon MH, Gibbon JH Jr. Temporary arrest of the circulation to the central nervous system: pathologic effects. *Arch Neurol Psychiat.* 1940;43:961-986.

23. Tameem A, Krovvidi H. Cerebral physiology. *Continuing Education in Anesthesia Critical Care and Pain.* 2013;13(4): 113-118.

24. Fabbri A, Servadei F, Marchesini G, Stein SC, Vandelli A. Early predictors of unfavourable outcome in subjects with moderate head injury in the emergency department. *J Neurol Neurosurg Psychiatry.* 2008;79(5):567-73.

25. Kaur P, Sharma S. Recent advances in pathophysiology of traumatic brain injury. *Curr Neuropharmacol.* 2018;16(8):1224-1238.

26. Jha RM, Kochanek PM, Simard JM. Pathophysiology and treatment of cerebral edema in traumatic brain injury. *Neuropharmacology.* 2019;145(Pt B):230-246.

27. Armstead WM, Vavilala MS. Translational approach towards determining the role of cerebral autoregulation in outcome after traumatic brain injury. *Exp Neurol.* 2019;317:291-297.

28. Kinoshita K. Traumatic brain injury: pathophysiology for neurocritical care. *J Intensive Care.* 2016;4:29.

29. Bramlett HM, Dietrich WD. Long-term consequences of traumatic brain injury: current status of potential mechanisms of injury and neurological outcomes. *J Neurotrauma.* 2015;32(23):1834-1848.

30. Livingston DH, Lavery RF, Passannante MR, Skurnick JH, Baker S, Fabian TC, Fry DE, Malangoni MA. *Ann Surg.* 2000;232(1):126-32.

31. Rutman AM, Vranic JE, Mossa-Basha M. Imaging and management of blunt cerebrovascular injury. *Radiographics.* 2018;38(2):542-563.

32. Li LM, Kolias AG, Guilfoyle MR, et al. Outcome following evacuation of acute subdural haematomas: a comparison of craniotomy with decompressive craniectomy. *Acta Neurochir (Wien).* 2012;154(9):1555-61.

33. Bajsarowicz P, Prakash I, Lamoureux J, et al. Nonsurgical acute traumatic subdural hematoma: what is the risk? *J Neurosurg.* 2015;123(5):1176-83.

34. Talving P, Karamanos E, Teixeira PG, et al. Intracranial pressure monitoring in severe head injury: compliance with Brain Trauma Foundation guidelines and effect on outcomes: a prospective study. *J Neurosurg.* 2013;119(5):1248-54.

35. Shen L, Wang Z, Su Z, et al. Effects of intracranial pressure monitoring on mortality in patients with severe traumatic brain injury: A Meta-Analysis. *PLoS One.* 2016;11(12):e0168901.

36. Liu H, Wang W, Cheng F, et al. External ventricular drains versus intraparenchymal intracranial pressure monitors in traumatic brain injury: A Prospective Observational Study. *World Neurosurg.* 2015 May;83(5):794-800.

37. Fried HI, Nathan BR, Rowe AS, et al. The insertion and management of external ventricular drains: an evidence-based consensus statement: a statement for healthcare professionals from the Neurocritical Care Society. *Neurocrit Care.* 2016;24(1):61-81.

38. Vella MA, Crandall ML, Patel MB. Acute management of traumatic brain injury. *Surg Clin North Am.* 2017;97(5):1015-1030.

39. Wijayatilake DS, Jigajinni SV, Sherren PB. Traumatic brain injury: physiological targets for clinical practice in the prehospital setting and on the neuro-ICU. *Curr Opin Anaesthesiol.* 2015;28(5):517-24.

40. Li J, Jiang JY. Chinese head trauma data bank: effect of hyperthermia on the outcome of acute head trauma patients. *J Neurotrauma.* 2012;29(1):96-100.

41. Chen H, Wu F, Yang P, Shao J, Chen Q, Zheng R. A meta-analysis of the effects of therapeutic hypothermia in adult patients with traumatic brain injury. *Crit Care.* 2019;23(1):396.

42. Cook AM, Morgan Jones G, Hawryluk GWJ, et al. Guidelines for the acute treatment of cerebral edema in neurocritical care patients. *Neurocrit Care.* 2020;32(3):647-666.

43. Alnemari AM, Krafcik BM, Mansour TR, Gaudin D. A comparison of pharmacologic therapeutic agents used for the reduction of intracranial pressure after traumatic brain injury. *World Neurosurg.* 2017;106:509-528.

44. Netteland DF, Mejlænder-Evjensvold M, Skaga NO, Sandset EC, Aarhus M, Helseth E. Cerebral venous thrombosis in traumatic brain injury: a cause of secondary insults and added mortality. *J Neurosurg.* 2020:1-9.

45. Dobbs TD, Barber ZE, Squier WL, Green AL. Cerebral venous sinus thrombosis complicating traumatic head injury. *J Clin Neurosci.* 2012;19(7):1058-9.

46. Avanali R, Gopalakrishnan MS, Devi BI, Bhat DI, Shukla DP, Shanbhag NC. Role of decompressive craniectomy in the management of cerebral venous sinus thrombosis. *Front Neurol.* 2019;10:511.

47. Sugerman DE, Xu L, Pearson WS, Faul M. Patients with severe traumatic brain injury transferred to a Level I or II trauma center: United States, 2007 to 2009. *J Trauma Acute Care Surg.* 2012;73(6):1491-9.

48. Oh JW, Kim SH, Whang K. Traumatic cerebrospinal fluid leak: diagnosis and management. *Korean J Neurotrauma.* 2017;13(2):63-67.

49. Mourad M, Inman JC, Chan DM, Ducic Y. Contemporary trends in the management of posttraumatic cerebrospinal fluid leaks. *Craniomaxillofac Trauma Reconstr.* 2018;11(1):71-77.

50. Albu S, Florian IS, Bolboaca SD. The benefit of early lumbar drain insertion in reducing the length of CSF leak in traumatic rhinorrhea. *Clin Neurol Neurosurg.* 2016;142:43-47.

51. Kwon M, Lekoubou A, Bishu KG, Ovbiagele B. Association of seizure co-morbidity with early hospital readmission among traumatic brain injury patients. *Brain Inj.* 2020 Oct 14;34(12):1625-1629.

52. Lussier BL, Olson DM, Aiyagari V. Automated pupillometry in neurocritical care: research and practice. *Curr Neurol Neurosci Rep.* 2019;19(10):71.

53. Stevens AR, Su Z, Toman E, Belli A, Davies D. Optical pupillometry in traumatic brain injury: neurological pupil index and its relationship with intracranial pressure through significant event analysis. *Brain Inj.* 2019;33(8):1032-1038.

54. Coplin WM, O'Keefe GE, Grady MS, et al. Thrombotic, infectious, and procedural complications of the jugular bulb catheter in the intensive care unit. *Neurosurgery.* 1997;41(1):101–7; discussion 107-9.

55. Fatima N, Shuaib A, Chughtai TS, Ayyad A, Saqqur M. The role of transcranial doppler in traumatic brain injury: a systemic review and meta-analysis. *Asian J Neurosurg.* 2019;14(3):626-633.

56. Davies DJ, Su Z, Clancy MT, et al. Near-Infrared spectroscopy in the monitoring of adult traumatic brain injury: a review. *J Neurotrauma.* 2015;32(13):933-41.

57. Kellermann AL, Peleg K. Lessons from Boston. *N Engl J Med.* 2013 May 23;368(21):1956-7.

58. Grathwohl KW, Venticinque SG. Organizational characteristics of the austere intensive care unit: the evolution of military trauma and critical care medicine; applications for civilian medical care systems. *Critical Care Medicine.* July 2008;36(7): S275-S283.

59. Eaton J, Hanif AB, Mulima G, Kajombo C, Charles A. Outcomes following exploratory burr holes for traumatic brain injury in a resource poor setting. *World Neurosurg.* 2017;105:257-264.

60. Liu JT, Tyan YS, Lee YK, Wang JT. Emergency management of epidural haematoma through burr hole evacuation and drainage. A preliminary report. *Acta Neurochir (Wien).* 2006;148(3):313-7; discussion 317.

61. Andrews BT, Bederson JB, Pitts LH. Use of intraoperative ultrasonography to improve the diagnostic accuracy of exploratory burr holes in patients with traumatic tentorial herniation. *Neurosurgery.* 1989;24(3):345-7.

62. Jones N, White ML, Tofil N, et al. Randomized trial comparing two mass casualty triage systems (JumpSTART versus SALT) in a pediatric simulated mass casualty event. *Prehosp Emerg Care.* 2014;18(3):417-23.

63. Volovici V, Steyerberg EW, Cnossen MC, et al. Evolution of evidence and guideline recommendations for the medical management of severe traumatic brain injury. *J Neurotrauma.* 2019;36(22):3183-3189.

64. Marion DW, Firlik A, McLaughlin MR. Hyperventilation therapy for severe traumatic brain injury. *New Horiz.* 1995;3(3):439-47.

32 THORACIC TRAUMA

Avi Benov, MD and Aran N. Gilead, MD

▌ INTRODUCTION

Thoracic Trauma (TT) is a leading cause of severe injuries and fatalities and is the second leading cause of traumatic death after head trauma. Although the unique structural properties of the thoracic cage prevent many TT patients from sustaining fatal injuries, the presence of vital organs and all great vessels in the thorax lead to the high morbidity and mortality rate.[1,2]

Twelve injuries have been named the "Deadly Dozen" of TT. These comprise the "Lethal Six;" immediately life-threatening injuries that require immediate evaluation and treatment—airway obstruction, tension pneumothorax, massive hemothorax, pericardial tamponade, open pneumothorax, and flail chest. In contrast, the "Hidden Six" are potentially life-threatening injuries that warrant diagnosis and intervention but should not interfere with immediate care. These injuries are often diagnosed only with second-tier diagnostic imaging and include blunt aortic injury, tracheobronchial injury, myocardial contusion, pulmonary contusion, esophageal tear, and diaphragmatic injury.

Blunt injuries are the most common TT, and motor vehicle accidents are the most common injury mechanism, accounting for over 80% of all TT patients. Out of blunt injuries, rib fracture is the most common injury affecting 50% of blunt TT patients[3] with hemothorax being the second most common diagnosis found in 25% of cases, often combined with other injuries such as fractures and pneumothorax.

Intentional and violence-related injuries primarily cause penetrating TT, with an incidence rate that varies based on crime rates and the presence of violent conflicts. Penetrating TT accounts for 10% of all combat injuries and approximately 25% of casualties in modern armed conflicts. This chapter will review the management of major TT injuries and selected non-traumatic thoracic pathologies.

ANATOMY

The thorax consists of the chest wall and the thoracic viscera. The components of the chest wall are the rib cage, sternum, and spinal column. The posterior chest wall is reinforced with the scapulae and its muscles; the anterior chest wall includes the pectoralis major and minor muscles and the clavicles. The chest wall has a dual function: it facilitates the respiratory mechanism allowing ventilation and protects the thoracic viscera.

Neurovascular bundles run along the inferior aspect of every rib, supplying perfusion and innervation for the chest wall. The chest wall is covered with a parietal pleura on the internal aspect and the mediastinum. Visceral pleura covers the lungs. The pleural space is formed between the pleura; this potential space holds a small amount of physiologic fluid. Like trauma or infection, certain pathologic states may cause an accumulation of large volumes of air, blood, or fluid displacing the lung and causing compressive atelectasis. This volume can compress other adjacent organs such as the great vessels, heart, and diaphragm. The mediastinum is limited anteriorly by the sternum and posteriorly by the spinal column, positioned between the left and right hemithorax. It holds the heart and great vessels and the esophagus, trachea, thoracic duct, and several noticeable nerves. The heart lies in the mediastinum, is encased by the pericardium, and is responsible for blood circulation.

PNEUMOTHORAX AND PNEUMOMEDIASTINUM

A pneumothorax is the presence or accumulation of air in the pleural space. The mechanism in which this pathologic process occurs is the rupture of alveolar tissue due to various etiologies, and in rare cases, due to bronchial tear.[4] It is classified by the mechanism which caused it, where spontaneous pneumothorax (SP) is distinguished from traumatic and iatrogenic pneumothorax by the absence of a mechanical insult to the respiratory system.

SP in a patient with no known pulmonary disease (chronic or acute) is defined as primary SP (PSP). SP with an underlying pathology is considered secondary SP (SSP). Tension pneumothorax is a clinical diagnosis defined by pneumothorax's presence and signs of hemodynamic instability or shock.[5]

Pneumomediastinum is the presence of air in the mediastinum. It is also classified into spontaneous or secondary based on etiology. Pneumomediastinum is considered a benign disorder if the mediastinal air does not apply pressure against great vessels or the airway. Most patients diagnosed with pneumomediastinum require no treatment other than analgesia, but it is recommended to hospitalize them for at least 24 hours to ensure no significant injury has caused this condition, and its diagnosis was missed.[6,7]

Epidemiology and Etiologies

The annual incidence rate of PSP is 18 cases per 100,000 population, and the male to female ratio is estimated at 8:1. The majority of patients with PSP are young males (10 to 30 years old). Increased PSP risk has been described in patients with a thin habitus or a marfanoid appearance and cigarette smoking.

SSP is caused by many pulmonary disorders, most frequently by chronic obstructive pulmonary disease (COPD). Other etiologies include infectious diseases such as pneumocystis pneumonia and necrotizing pneumonia, interstitial lung diseases such as sarcoidosis and Langerhans cell histiocytosis, primary pulmonary malignancies, and pulmonary metastases. Iatrogenic pneumothorax can occur after interventions such as thoracocentesis, central venous catheter insertion, and transthoracic biopsy.

Diagnosis

Diagnosis is made by plain film chest radiograph or thoracic ultrasonography. The most sensitive modality for the diagnosis of pneumothorax is a computed tomography (CT). The widespread use of CT has led to the diagnosis of many small and clinically insignificant pneumothoraces, named occult pneumothorax. Diagnosing a tension pneumothorax requires immediate action and may be done based on physical examination and clinical assessment alone, without any diagnostic imaging studies.

Treatment

Once the diagnosis of a pneumothorax is confirmed, the clinician must choose the suitable treatment. The spectrum of possible interventions includes observation, needle aspiration, tube thoracostomy (chest tube), and surgical interventions such as video-assisted thoracoscopy (VATS) or a thoracotomy. Different factors to include are patient's current medical status, the medical team's expertise, available resources, and the proximity and availability of a level 1 trauma center. Small PSP in otherwise healthy young individuals with mild symptoms can be managed by observation only.[8] In contrast, an unstable patient with a traumatic pneumothorax must undergo immediate tube thoracostomy, and urgent thoracotomy should be considered if clinical goals are not met, or bronchial injury is suspected.

RIB FRACTURES

Rib fractures affect 10 to 15% of all trauma patients and can be caused by a wide range of mechanisms: motor vehicle accidents, falls, crush injuries, coughing, and violent assaults. Fractured ribs are associated with other critical injuries such as pulmonary contusions and pneumo-hemothorax.[9] The physician should rule out such thoracic injuries when diagnosing multiple rib fractures or high energy TT. Fractures of ribs 4–9 are the most common rib fractures. Fractures of ribs 1–3 are less common and may signify high energy trauma. Fractures of ribs 1–3 are associated with damage to adjacent structures like the subclavian artery or vein and brachial plexus. Rib fractures are disproportionately prevalent among older people due to osteoporosis and lower rib compliance. Minor trauma and falls in the elderly often result in multiple rib fractures or flail chest and should be suspected in even minor TT suffered by the elderly.

The most common presenting symptoms of rib fractures are focal pain and point tenderness, worsening any movement, including breathing. Physical examination may reveal ecchymosis, chest wall deformity, subcutaneous emphysema, or crepitus. In many cases, there will be no sign other than tenderness.[10]

Diagnosis of rib fractures can be made with a plain film radiograph of the chest or ribs, although its sensitivity is as low as 50%. Computed tomography (CT) has the highest sensitivity and specificity for rib fractures.[11] In addition to diagnosing fractures, thoracic CT scans can reveal other and potentially more severe injuries and should be performed when such injuries are suspected. The significant complications of rib fractures are pneumonia, acute respiratory distress syndrome (ARDS), and empyema in up to 48% of patients. The mortality rate of multiple rib fractures is also high, reaching 10% in adults and 22% in the elderly; this rate increases with every additional rib fracture.[12]

When working with limited resources, minor TT injuries causing a few rib fractures, and in the presence of a normal chest radiograph, it is reasonable to end the workup after associated injuries have been ruled out.

The therapeutic goal of isolated rib fractures is adequate pain control to restore respiratory mechanics. Adequate analgesia allows the patient to ventilate the entire vital capacity and remove bronchial secretions by coughing. Multiple rib fractures mandate aggressive analgesia. The use of epidural catheter analgesia, although controversial, is common for patients with multiple fractures, more so in trauma centers. Despite numerous studies, there are no evidence-based indications for the use of epidural analgesia.

FLAIL CHEST

Flail chest is defined as fractures of at least four adjacent ribs where each is fractured in at least two places. In essence, flail chest is the functional detachment of a segment of the chest wall that no longer functions in coordination with the respiratory effort or acts against it, i.e., paradoxical breathing.[13] Flail chest injury was present in 1.4% of all blunt TT patients in a large US-based cohort. Historical data reported a mortality rate of 20% and the need for mechanical ventilation in 60% of the cases. Recent reports of mortality rates are much lower. A study based on the National Trauma Databank shows an overall mortality rate of as low as 5.6% in patients with an isolated flail chest injury and mechanical ventilation was required in 29.8%. In the same study, 11.2% of patients with flail chest developed pneumonia, and 6.1% developed ARDS.[14]

The therapeutic goal is to maintain respiratory functions: ventilation, oxygenation, and removal of secretions. In the majority of cases, it is achieved by aggressive analgesia; nevertheless, mechanical ventilation is warranted in severe cases. Surgical fixation of ribs continues to be controversial, and flail chest remains one of the few accepted indications for this procedure.[15] Flail chest is an important diagnosis and warrants attention; it is a clinical marker for severe thoracic and extrathoracic injuries, and it is a predictor of secondary complications.

PULMONARY CONTUSION

Pulmonary contusion is a result of a mechanical insult to the parenchyma of the lung. Different injuries cause pulmonary contusions, such as blunt TT, penetrating TT, and blast injuries. The prevalence of these injuries differs in various scenarios, and so does the lead cause of pulmonary contusion. In wartime, most cases are caused by blast injuries, whereas traffic accidents and falls account for most peacetime cases. A pulmonary contusion occurs in 25–35% of all blunt TT patients and causes a 10–25% mortality rate. A review of cases of blast injuries from recent military deployments in Iraq and Afghanistan show that 7 to 11% of blast injury patients suffered a blast lung or pulmonary contusion, and only 44% of them survived to reach a medical facility. In these cases, 80% of the patients were mechanically ventilated.[16]

The clinical presentation of pulmonary contusion widely varies from asymptomatic to dyspnea and severe respiratory failure. Clinical and radiographic findings may appear hours and days post-injury. Severe cases will develop within hours, but minor contusions may develop as late as 48 hours after the insult. Plain film radiography is widely used for the diagnosis but is challenging to interpret because the coexisting thoracic injuries may obscure contusions. Another difficulty in imaging pulmonary contusions is the delay in appearance, normal radiographs obtained shortly after arrival do not rule out contusions and should be repeated with a 12-hour interval when clinically appropriate. CT scans have the highest sensitivity and specificity for pulmonary contusions and are used to evaluate the extent of the contusion and other coexisting injuries. Patients with contusions greater than 20% of the lung parenchyma are at a much higher risk for developing ARDS and pneumonia.

Blood gas analysis also contributes to the diagnosis, as contusions cause hypercapnia and hypoxemia by limiting ventilation and oxygenation.[17] The mainstay treatment of pulmonary contusions is supportive care for the prevention of complications. The therapy principles are prevention of atelectasis, pulmonary toilet, monitoring, avoiding barotrauma, and prevention of fluid overload. In selected cases, surgical fixation of a flail chest is warranted, and if all else fails, extra corporal oxygenation is used.

Pulmonary contusions usually heal over 5 to 7 days, but complications and inadequate treatment may deteriorate and delay the process resolution. The short-term complications of pulmonary contusions are ARDS and pneumonia, and the long-term complication is pulmonary fibrosis, which reduces respiratory volumes. Polytrauma patients are at much greater risk of developing complications (78% of patients) than patients with isolated contusion (17% of patients). A prospective study of blast lung injury survivors assessed their pulmonary function test and chest radiograph 1 year after the injury. All of the subjects had normal functions and a complete resolution on a chest radiograph.[18] The Murray score for acute lung injury (ALI) is easy to use and allows for a rapid assessment of ALI severity. It is based on four measurable parameters: Atelectasis, P to F ratio (PaO_2/FiO_2), Lung Compliance, and PEEP. The score ranges from 0 to 4, and scores above 2.5 represent severe ALI. In limited resources scenarios, this score may help allocate resources efficiently. When available, the Murray score is used for extracorporeal membrane oxygenation (ECMO) patient selection. Pulmonary contusion remains a challenging injury to assess and treat, consuming many valuable medical resources. ICU care, mechanical ventilation, and ECMO patient selection represent significant clinical challenge.[19]

BLUNT AORTIC INJURY (BAI)

BAI is the leading cause of death from blunt TT, and motor vehicle collisions (typically head-on collisions) are the leading cause of BAI, accounting for 80% of the cases. Motorcycle accidents, falls, crush injuries, and pedestrian vs. motor vehicle accidents account for the rest. Approximately 80% of the patients will die before arriving at a medical facility; the remaining 20% may suffer a life-threatening injury. In-hospital mortality is variable, estimated from 6 to 46% of patients in different reports. In all BAI cases, the injury mechanism is rapid deceleration, most commonly injuring the aortic isthmus, where the aorta transitions from the mobile aortic arch to the descending aorta, which is fixed to the chest wall.[20,21]

Since BAI is a rare injury, high energy accidents or falls should raise suspicion, considering that both signs and symptoms of BAI are not sensitive nor specific. Workup is guided as in all trauma cases by the advanced trauma life support algorithms, and priorities are no different. During the initial assessment, BAI signs can appear on Focused Assessment with Sonography for Trauma (FAST) or plain film, but these modalities' diagnostic value is limited. Diagnosis of BAI is made by thoracic CT angiography (CTA), which has a 100% sensitivity and allows for grading the BAI and planning of the repair when needed.

An estimated 30% of BAI patients that arrive at the hospital will die if left untreated. Treatment of BAI may be classified according to the intervention's urgency and the extent of the injury.[22] Minimal aortic injury, an ill-defined BAI (estimated at 10% of all BAI patients), is treated with beta blockade and antihypertensive drugs. Late intervention in these patients should be considered if a complication occurs. The remaining 90% of patients require intervention. The anatomical features of the BAI and coexisting injuries will determine the timing and type of intervention. Historically, an immediate intervention was preferred, and the repair was done by replacing the injured section with a synthetic graft via a left-sided thoracotomy. This approach required one-lung ventilation and clamping of the aorta. Despite technical advances and the use of bypass, the mortality rate remains high in such procedures. Later studies show that postoperative outcomes were better in delayed vs. immediate repair. It is now recommended to delay repair in stable hemodynamic patients.

The alternative intervention is endovascular repair. In this approach, an endovascular stent graft is placed in the aorta's injured section, excluding it from circulation. This procedure is done without the physiological insult of major surgery and general anesthesia, without ventilation, and minimal anticoagulation. Most current guidelines advocate delayed endovascular repair for all suitable candidates.

BLUNT CARDIAC INJURY (BCI)

BCI groups together a wide range of cardiac injuries caused by blunt TT, as its mechanism. The most common mechanism is a rapid deceleration from high impact motor vehicle collisions. Other mechanisms include falls, sports injuries, crush injuries, and combat injuries. The clinical range of BCI spans asymptomatic patients, symptomatic patients with transient and self-limiting arrhythmias, Commotio Cordis or cardiac arrest, and the heart's free wall rupture. BCI's incidence rate is hard to estimate because of the broad clinical range of these injuries, many of which are asymptomatic. The most common BCI is cardiac or myocardial contusion—the definition of which remains ambiguous and is considered a bruise of the myocardium.[23] Initial assessment and treatment of TT patients should follow the ATLS algorithm. Signs and symptoms of BCI are neither specific nor sensitive. Shock in a TT patient is hemorrhagic until ruled out, and cardiac tamponade and tension pneumothorax should also be ruled out during the primary survey. Due to the broad spectrum of BCIs, the presenting signs and symptoms vary accordingly.

The diagnosis of BCI is based on the physiologic effect of the injury, and it is commonly accepted to use both ECG and troponin I test to screen all patients with suspected BCI. Normal ECG and troponin I in a stable and healthy patient rule out BCI. No ECG abnormality is pathognomonic for BCI and can appear as tachycardia, new bundle branch block, or significant arrhythmia as well as ST changes. It may also be challenging to ascertain whether ECG abnormalities were caused by an acute coronary event that preceded the injury, an actual BCI, or a cardiac event caused by the physiologic burden of the trauma.[24] Most institutional guidelines recommend performing an echocardiogram on BCI patients with either an ECG abnormality or an elevated troponin test. Echocardiogram, whether transthoracic or transesophageal, demonstrates the heart and pericardium's anatomy and physiology and is widely accepted as the modality of choice to evaluate most BCIs. Routine workup of trauma patients includes chest radiography, CT scans, and FAST—all of which may assist with BCI diagnosis but will not be the studies of choice when BCI is suspected to rule out the diagnosis.[25]

▌PERICARDIAL EFFUSION

Pericardial effusion is the abnormal accumulation of fluid between the pericardium and the epicardium. Most sources consider up to 50 mL of pericardial fluid to be a physiologic amount. Various etiologies may cause pericardial effusion; among the most prevalent are malignancies, iatrogenic, and idiopathic. Blunt and penetrating TT may also cause either acute hemopericardium or sub-acute pericardial effusion. Pericardial effusion has a spectrum of clinical presentations ranging from mild dyspnea and pleuritic pain to obstructive shock; the onset of symptoms may be acute and severe or progressive and long-standing.[26]

A new pericardial effusion diagnosis can be elusive as signs and symptoms are nonspecific, and a high level of suspicion is required. Patients with known preexisting etiologies for pericardial effusion or cardiac tamponade, presenting with dyspnea and chest pain, warrant a rapid assessment. Even though the suspicion of pericardial effusion may rise by medical history, physical examination, chest X-ray, and ECG, the diagnosis is made by imaging the heart and pericardium by echocardiography computed tomography. Cardiac magnetic resonance imaging can accurately diagnose a pericardial effusion but is not usually required for this diagnosis.

The primary concern is assessing the patient's hemodynamic status. Hemodynamic instability or cardiac tamponade is a medical emergency and warrants urgent drainage of the pericardial sac. Stable patients should undergo a thorough workup to find the etiology of the effusion and provide appropriate treatment. Drainage of the effusion serves both diagnostic and therapeutic goals but has a low diagnostic yield and is not justified as a routine diagnostic procedure. Drainage is indicated in patients with suspected purulent pericardial effusion, patients with suspected malignant effusion, or patients with a large effusion with no exact etiology.

Drainage of a pericardial effusion can be made by either an open approach using a thoracic or abdominal incision or by a percutaneous pericardiocentesis. The drainage technique's choice is based on the clinical setting, physician preferences, and institutional guidelines.

Fast and efficient triage is the cornerstone of effective allocation of resources when these are scarce. Hemodynamically unstable patients should be diagnosed and treated expeditiously, while most patients with pericardial effusions can tolerate a delayed diagnosis and treatment.[27,28]

▌ESOPHAGEAL TRAUMA

Esophageal trauma is a rare injury with a high mortality rate. The incidence rate was reported to be less than 0.01% of trauma patients. Of all patients with esophageal trauma, the injury mechanism was gunshot wounds in 44.9%, stab wounds in 9.5%, and motor vehicle accidents in 18%. The overall mortality rate is estimated at 25% of patients. This is probably an underestimation as some of these patients die at the scene. Patients who survive the first 24 hours have a much lower mortality rate (7.5%), and the most significant mortality risk factor is the injury severity score (ISS).

The esophagus and its anatomic relation to adjacent structures explain the high mortality rate of esophageal trauma; any trauma that causes an esophageal tear has probably also damaged other cervical or thoracic organs.[29] The most common related injury is rib fractures, and other related injuries include pneumothorax, hemothorax, and various pulmonary and cardiac injuries.

The diagnosis of esophageal trauma is a clinical challenge, and the outcome of these patients is greatly affected by the time to diagnosis. Signs and symptoms of esophageal trauma are nonspecific, and most cases are in severely injured patients with distracting injuries. The most commonly used imaging studies in trauma are not sensitive or specific enough to diagnose esophageal injuries. Water-soluble contrast has a limited role in imaging esophageal tears, and barium esophagram is the study of choice in stable patients. Unstable patients should undergo endoscopy in the operating room. Untreated or underdiagnosed esophageal perforation will cause mediastinitis, empyema, and sepsis leading to poor outcomes and a high mortality rate.[30]

▌MEDIASTINITIS

Mediastinitis or acute infection of the mediastinum is a serious medical condition with a high mortality rate. The leading etiologies of mediastinitis are perforation of the esophagus or trachea followed by post sternotomy infection and descending oro-pharyngeal infection. The majority of esophageal perforations in developed countries are iatrogenic due to the wide use of endoscopy[31] Traumatic perforations of the aerodigestive tract are rare, and so is the incidence rate of traumatic mediastinitis.

Diagnosis of mediastinitis is based on clinical findings and imaging. Signs and symptoms are not specific and include chest pain, fever, and dyspnea. The imaging study of choice for stable patients is a barium-based contrast esophagram; endoscopy is chosen for patients who cannot swallow or are unstable. Once the diagnosis of mediastinitis is made, and the injury's anatomy has been understood, treatment can be planned. The principles of treating a perforation are:

1. Source control. The perforation must be controlled, and the leak of saliva into the mediastinum must be stopped.
2. Debridement. Necrotic mediastinal tissue must be removed to allow healing of the infection.
3. Supportive care. The patient must receive adequate antibiotic and antifungal treatment and sufficient fluids and nutrition either intravenously or through a jejunostomy.

The combination of a rare injury and high mortality rate requires a high level of suspicion and aggressive workup and treatment when deemed necessary.[32,33]

PENETRATING THORACIC TRAUMA (TT)

Although less common than blunt TT, penetrating TT has a higher mortality rate. A large majority of penetrating injuries are intentional, such as gunshot wounds and stab wounds. The prevalence of penetrating TT is challenging to estimate as it changes with time and region, with violence accounting for most of these injuries. Various types of violence cause different types of injuries. Since military conflicts were the leading cause of penetrating TT, military doctors gained expertise in treating these injuries and have developed the protocols and guidelines we now use.

During the First World War, the mortality rate of penetrating TT was as high as 56%, and it dropped to 3% in the Vietnam War some 50 years later. Recent military studies report that penetrating TT accounts for 10% of all injuries and 25% of combat mortality. Crime-related violence has different characteristics than military conflicts. Reports show variability in the prevalence of injuries. One large South African study reports that stab wounds account for 90% of all penetrating TT, and gunshot wounds the remaining 10%.[34]

In contrast, a study from Colombia reports that stab wounds account for 38%, and gunshot wounds account for 62% of the penetrating TT, whereas a large US study reports gunshot wounds account for 55% of all penetrating TT.[35] The overall mortality rate of penetrating TT varies and is hard to estimate. A longitudinal single-center study spanning 24 consecutive years reports 3049 patients with penetrating TT, from which the overall mortality rate is 2.8%. Subsets of injuries that are associated with a higher mortality rate are: cardiac injuries, thoracoabdominal injuries, and transaxial or transmediastinal injuries.[36]

Although vital organs occupy the entire thoracic cavity, the mediastinum holds an increased risk for a lethal penetrating injury. An area named the "cardiac box" or "the box" defines the area medial to the nipples, above the umbilicus, and below the sternal notch. From the dorsal aspect of the thorax, it is regarded as the area between the scapulae. All penetrating injuries to the box should raise a high level of suspicion for a cardiac, great vessel, tracheal, diaphragmatic, and esophageal injury or a combination of them.

Diagnosis

In the diagnosis, the initial assessment of all patients follows the ATLS algorithms. Specific interventions occur in the primary survey, such as thoracostomy or a resuscitative thoracotomy, when appropriate. The primary survey includes adjuncts such as chest X-ray, which is of great importance in diagnosing thoracic injuries. When the patient's clinical status allows, further studies are used based on the primary survey findings. Chest CT scans play a major role in developed countries; organ-specific studies such as echocardiography, bronchoscopy, or esophagoscopy are utilized when deemed necessary.

Treatment

Patients who are unstable during the primary survey generally go to the operating room for damage control surgery. The most common thoracic damage control surgery is via a thoracotomy. In selected cases, median sternotomy or other less common approaches are performed.[37] Stable patients proceed to a secondary survey and definitive treatment. Up to 90% of all penetrating TT patients will be treated with a chest tube only. Most lacerations of the lung and subsequent air leaks and bleeding will resolve without further intervention. Chest tubes are inserted to evacuate air and blood to prevent a tension pneumothorax and a retained hemothorax followed by an empyema.[38]

PENETRATING CARDIAC INJURY (PCI)

An estimated 80% of patients suffering a PCI will die before arriving at the hospital, and in-hospital mortality is also high. The right ventricle is the heart's most common injured structure due to its anterior location, followed by the left ventricle. Cardiac injuries may lead to cardiac tamponade or hemorrhagic shock, based on the nature of the injury and the pericardium's capacity to contain it. High mortality rates and unique surgical considerations turn the management of PCI into a complex surgical challenge. Treatment of PCI is surgical repair, and the preferred approach is dictated by the nature of the injury, the stability of the patient, and the availability of a cardiothoracic surgeon. Generally, for a stable patient with radiologic evidence of a PCI, a median sternotomy is the preferred approach as it allows access to all cardiac structures and a cardiac bypass. Other clinical scenarios may necessitate other surgical approaches, left anterolateral thoracotomy being the most common.[39]

OPEN PNEUMOTHORAX

Penetrating TT carries a high risk of causing an open or tension pneumothorax, two of the most common fatal violence-related injuries. An open pneumothorax, also known as an open sucking wound or a communicating pneumothorax, is caused by a chest wall defect equal to or greater than two-thirds of the tracheal diameter. In such extensive diameter injuries, the point of least resistance for air to enter the thoracic cavity is the chest wall defect rather than the trachea. This inflow may rapidly lead to respiratory and hemodynamic collapse. Diagnosis and treatment of an open pneumothorax should be made in the prehospital setting as it is an immediate life-threatening injury. The preferred initial treatment is placing a vented chest seal on the wound, stopping this dangerous process. When such a device is not available other non-vented seals can be used. Monitoring a patient with a non-vented chest seal is paramount, as a tension pneumothorax can rapidly evolve. Definitive treatment of an open pneumothorax should entail a thorough debridement of the wound and closure of the chest wall defect. Due to the extent of this injury and these patients' instability, this procedure is done urgently.[40]

TUBE THORACOSTOMY

Tube thoracostomy or chest tube insertion is the initial treatment for most TT patients. Ninety percent of these patients will not need any further intervention. Proper training will allow any physician to safely and timely perform this relatively simple procedure, reducing the risk of complications and increasing its safety.[41] A detailed description of chest tube insertion is beyond the scope of this chapter.

Before giving a brief overview of the steps of chest tube insertion, it is essential to understand a few fundamental principles:

1. **Environment**. The setting in which the procedure takes place will determine its difficulty. Even a seasoned surgeon may struggle with performing a prehospital chest tube insertion with poor lighting and in a physically uncomfortable position, whereas in near perfect conditions such as in an operating theater, a chest tube insertion can prove to be fast and straightforward even for a first-timer. A quiet environment with sufficient lighting, an adequate positioning of the patient, a comfortable posture of the physician, and exposure to a sterile field are of great importance for the procedure's success.

2. **Analgesia.** Adequate analgesia is essential for the insertion's success, patient well-being, and the physician performing the procedure. It is amplified in hemodynamically stable and alert patients. Any pleural intervention is painful, particularly a blunt intercostal dissection. Sufficient analgesia may be achieved with local anesthesia only, but many surgeons prefer to perform the insertion on sedated patients. Using a maximal dose of Lidocaine, and ensuring that all layers of the chest wall are anesthetized, will allow a successful insertion without the risks that come with sedation. Various intravenous analgesia such as tramadol or paracetamol can be used as needed.

3. **Location of the chest tube.** The "go-to" position of chest tube insertion is between the 4th and 5th intercostal space in the mid-axillary line. This location is the right choice for most patients. It is by no means the only or even the best choice of location for all patients requiring a chest tube. The Monaldi point at the 2nd intercostal space in the midclavicular line is used for apical or anterior pneumothoraces. Imaging-guided chest tube insertion can be done in any chest wall location if sufficient pleural space is visualized.

4. **Trocar insertion.** The use of trocars for the insertion of a chest tube is considered obsolete. It increases the risk of unintentional perforation of thoracic and abdominal organs and should not be used.[42]

CHEST TUBES

Chest tubes come in various sizes and designs, they serve the same purpose, but each has unique nuances. This brief overview will present some standard chest tubes, advantages, and disadvantages in different clinical scenarios.[43]

Large-Bore Straight Fenestrated Tubes

The most common chest tube size is 20F–32F. They are effective and easy to insert; they have a blunt tip that makes them safe to insert and less likely to lacerate the lung or other thoracic structures. They have a large internal diameter that allows the drainage of large volumes of air, fluid, or blood. The disadvantages of these large bore tubes are the relatively large incision and discomfort that they can cause. Large bore tubes are suitable for significant air leaks and hemothorax.

Pigtail Tubes

These small-bore (usually 10F–14F) tubes are very well suited for the drainage of air and pleural effusions of various etiologies. The main advantages are their accuracy and guided insertion with minimal tissue damage. The sharp tip of the tube can easily penetrate or puncture any thoracic or abdominal structure. The relatively small diameter may cause these small chest tubes to clog with blood if inserted for a hemothorax or be insufficient to drain large air leaks.

Foley Catheters

These readily available urethral catheters can replace conventional chest tubes when necessary, particularly in resource-limited scenarios. 18F–26F Foley catheters, whether made of latex or silicone, are inexpensive and effective.

Drain System

The simple and most common system is the water seal. Other systems include the Heimlich valve, a three-chamber seal, and a digital drain. It is recommended to prefer a commercially available water seal in a resource-limited setting when possible, but an improvised water seal can be used with good outcomes.[44]

▌THORACOTOMY

As discussed earlier, most patients with a penetrating Thoracic injury will require only a tube thoracostomy and supportive care. Thoracotomy, or the surgical opening of the rib cage, is needed in a subset of patients. Thoracotomies are classified according to their timing during treatment. Technical and anatomic aspects of this procedure are beyond the scope of this chapter. Thoracotomies should be performed only by trained physicians.[45]

Emergency Department Thoracotomy

Emergency department thoracotomy (EDT) is a resuscitative procedure reserved for patients *in extremis*. These are patients that have lost vital signs during treatment due to massive bleeding or a suspected cardiac tamponade. The goal of an EDT is limited to evacuate a cardiac tamponade, direct cardiac massage, control intrathoracic hemorrhage, or cross-clamp the aorta to control subdiaphragmatic hemorrhage. The prognosis of patients undergoing EDT is poor. After EDT, survival rates due to penetrating trauma were historically up to 10%, but recent studies report it to be as high as 26%. After EDT, the survival rate due to blunt TT was known to be 1–2% and is reported to reach 7% in more recent studies. Based on this procedure's low success rate, the surgeon's circumstances should play a key role in choosing when to perform an EDT. When performed with limited resources by an inexperienced team, it is a futile procedure that consumes valuable resources. In mass casualty events or when resources are scarce, EDT should be reserved for salvageable patients only.[46]

Urgent Thoracotomy

Patients suffering a massive hemothorax or massive air leak after tube thoracostomy should be taken to the OR for an urgent repair of the injured airway or vessel. Urgent thoracotomy is also indicated in unstable patients with a traumatic cardiac tamponade, and they should undergo urgent pericardiotomy. An intercostal artery injury often causes a massive hemothorax. Major vessel injury or cardiac laceration that is significant enough to cause a massive hemothorax tends to be fatal, and most patients will exsanguinate before arrival to a medical facility. The outcome of tracheal or bronchial tears depends on the injury site and the extent of the tear. Positive pressure ventilation is expected to worsen air leaks, and sufficient drainage will bridge the gap until the leak is controlled. Most tracheal and main bronchi injuries are best approached via a right-sided posterolateral thoracotomy and will present challenges such as surgical field intubation, cardiopulmonary bypass (CPB), or ECMO. Another indication for an urgent thoracotomy is an open sucking chest wound, as described earlier.

Early Thoracotomy

An indication for early thoracotomy, i.e., within 48 hours from injury is continued bleeding—significant hemothorax at the time of insertion of a chest tube (<1500 mL) that continues to bleed 500 mL of blood during the 1st hour *or* 200–300 mL of blood/hour for 2–3 hours after insertion.

After the initial drainage of a hemothorax, many bleeding sources can stop without further surgical intervention, and surgery can be avoided. Thoracotomy for hemostasis is reserved for patients who continue to bleed despite optimal drainage and resuscitation.

Late Thoracotomy

Indications for a late thoracotomy are surgical treatment for TT complications such as an empyema or a clotted hemothorax that did not resolve with tube thoracostomy. There are no absolute indications for surgical intervention, and if a surgical repair is needed, video-assisted thoracoscopy (VATS) is preferred in many cases when available.[47,48]

▍ REFERENCES

1. Locicero J, Mattox KL. Epidemiology of chest trauma. *Surg Clin North Am.* 1989;69(1):15-19.
2. Advanced Trauma Life Support for Doctors, Student Course Manual 10th Ed. American College of Surgeons Committee on Trauma 2018.
3. Platz JJ, Fabricant L, Norotsky M. Thoracic trauma: injuries, evaluation, and treatment. *Surg Clin North Am.* 2017;97(4):783-799.
4. Noppen M, De Keukeleire T. Pneumothorax. *Respiration.* 2008;76(2):121-127.
5. Lyra Rde M. Etiology of primary spontaneous pneumothorax. *J Bras Pneumol.* 2016;42(3):222-226.
6. Muckart DJJ, Hardcastle TC, Skinner DL. Pneumomediastinum and pneumopericardium following blunt thoracic trauma: much ado about nothing? *Eur J Trauma Emerg Surg.* 2019;45(5):927-931.
7. Iteen AJ, Bianchi W, Sharman T. Pneumomediastinum. In: *StatPearls.* Treasure Island, FL: StatPearls Publishing; May 19, 2020.
8. Brown SG, Ball EL, Perrin K. Conservative versus interventional treatment for spontaneous pneumothorax. *N Engl J Med.* 2020;382:405-15.
9. Witt CE, Bulger EM. Comprehensive approach to the management of the patient with multiple rib fractures: a review and introduction of a bundled rib fracture management protocol. *Trauma Surg. Acute Care Open.* 2017;2(1) :e000064. doi: 10.1136/tsaco-2016-000064
10. May L, Hillermann C, Patil S. Rib fracture management. *BJA Education.* 2016;16(1):26-32.
11. Shuaib W, Vijayasarathi A, Tiwana MH, Johnson J-O, Maddu KK, Khosa F. The diagnostic utility of rib series in assessing rib fractures. *Emerg. Radiol.* 2013;21(2):159-164.
12. Tignanelli CJ, Rix A, Napolitano LM, Hemmila MR, Ma S, Kummerfeld E. Association between adherence to evidence-based practices for treatment of patients with traumatic rib fractures and mortality rates among US trauma centers. *JAMA Network Open.* 2020;3(3) :e201316. doi: 10.1001/jamanetworkopen.2020

13. Dehghan N, De Mestral C, McKee M. Flail chest injuries: a review of outcomes and treatment practices from the National Trauma Data Bank. *J Trauma Acute Care Surg*. 2014;76(2):462-468.

14. Benjamin E, Recinos G, Aiolfi A, Inaba K, Demetriades D. Flail chest: less deadly than originally thought. *World J Surg*. 2018;42(12):3927-3931.

15. Beks RB, Peek J, Jong MBD, et al. Fixation of flail chest or multiple rib fractures: current evidence and how to proceed. A systematic review and meta-analysis. *Eur J Trauma Emerg Surg*. 2018;45(4):631-644.

16. Smith JE. The epidemiology of blast lung injury during recent military conflicts: a retrospective database review of cases presenting to deployed military hospitals, 2003–2009. *Philos Trans R Soc Lond B Biol Sci*. 2011;366(1562):291-294.

17. Ganie FA, Lone H, Lone GN, et al. Lung contusion: a clinico-pathological entity with unpredictable clinical course. *Bull Emerg Trauma*. 2013;1(1):7-16.

18. Hirshberg B, Oppenheim-Eden A, Pizov R, et al. Recovery from blast lung injury. *Chest*. 1999;116(6):1683-1688.

19. Miller PR, Croce MA, Bee TK, et al. ARDS after pulmonary contusion: accurate measurement of contusion volume identifies high-risk patients. *J Trauma Inj Infect Crit Care*. 2001;51(2):223-230.

20. Mouawad NJ, Paulisin J, Hofmeister S, Thomas MB. Blunt thoracic aortic injury – concepts and management. *J Cardiothorac Surg*. 2020;15(1).

21. Neschis DG, Scalea TM, Flinn WR, Griffith BP. Blunt Aortic Injury. *N Eng J Med*. 2008;359(16):1708-1716.

22. Fox N, Schwartz D, Salazar JH, et al. Evaluation and management of blunt traumatic aortic injury. *J Trauma Acute Care Surg*. 2015;78(1):136-146.

23. El-Menyar A, Thani HA, Zarour A, Latifi R. Understanding traumatic blunt cardiac injury. *Ann Card Anaesth*. 2012;15(4):287.

24. Marcolini EG, Keegan J. Blunt cardiac injury. *Emerg Med Clin North Am*. 2015;33(3):519-527.

25. Clancy K, Velopulos C, Bilaniuk JW, et al. Screening for blunt cardiac injury. *J Trauma Acute Care Surg*. 2012;73.

26. Adler Y, Charron P, Imazio M, et al. 2015 ESC guidelines for the diagnosis and management of pericardial diseases. *Rev Esp Cardiol (Engl Ed)*. 2015;68(12):1126.

27. Spodick DH. Acute cardiac tamponade. *N Engl J Med*. 2003;349(7):684-690.

28. Sagristà-Sauleda J, Mercé AS, Soler-Soler J. Diagnosis and management of pericardial effusion. *World J Cardiol*. 2011;3(5):135-143.

29. Gambhir S, Grigorian A, Swentek L, et al. Esophageal trauma: analysis of incidence, morbidity, and mortality. *Am Surg*. 2019;85(10):1134-1138.

30. Skipworth RJ, McBride OM, Kerssens JJ, Paterson-Brown S. Esophagogastric trauma in Scotland. *World J Surg*. 2012;36(8):1779-1784.

31. Bhatia FD, Inculet RI, Malthaner RA. Current concepts in the management of esophageal perforations: a twenty-seven year Canadian experience. *Ann Thorac Surg*. 2011;92(1):209-215.

32. Biancari F, D'Andrea V, Paone R, et al. Current treatment and outcome of esophageal perforations in adults: systematic review and meta-analysis of 75 studies. *World J Surg*. 2013;37(5):1051-1059.

33. Mureşan M, Mureşan S, Balmoş I, Sala D, Suciu B, Torok A. Sepsis in acute mediastinitis – a severe complication after oesophageal perforations. A Review of the Literature. *J Crit Care Med.* 2019;5(2):49-55.

34. Clarke DL, Quazi MA, Reddy K, Thomson SR. Emergency operation for penetrating thoracic trauma in a metropolitan surgical service in South Africa. *J Thorac Cardiovasc Surg.* 2011;142(3):563-568.

35. Isaza-Restrepo A, Bolívar-Sáenz DJ, Tarazona-Lara M, Tovar JR. Penetrating cardiac trauma: analysis of 240 cases from a hospital in Bogota, Colombia. *World J Emerg Surg.* 2017;12(1).

36. Mandal AK, Sanusi M. Penetrating chest wounds: 24 years experience. *World J Surg.* 2001;25(9):1145-1149.

37. Orlas CP, Herrera-Escobar JP, Zogg CK, et al. Chest trauma outcomes: public versus private Level I trauma centers. *World J Surg.* 2020;44(6):1824-1834.

38. Belmont PJ, Goodman GP, Zacchilli M, Posner M, Evans C, Owens BD. Incidence and epidemiology of combat injuries sustained during "The Surge" portion of Operation Iraqi Freedom by a US Army Brigade combat team. *J Trauma Inj Infect Crit Care.* 2010;68(1):2.

39. Gunay C, Cingoz F, Kuralay E, Demirkilic U, Tatar H. Surgical challenges for urgent approach in penetrating heart injuries. *Heart Surg Forum.* 2007;10(6): E473-E477.

40. Kotora JG, Henao J, Littlejohn LF, Kircher S. Vented chest seals for prevention of tension pneumothorax in a communicating pneumothorax. *J Emerg Med.* 2013;45(5):686-694.

41. Monaghan SF, Swan KG. Tube thoracostomy: the struggle to the "standard of care." *Ann Thorac Surg.* 2008;86(6):2019-2022.

42. Havelock T, Teoh R, Laws D, Gleeson F. Pleural procedures and thoracic ultrasound: British Thoracic Society pleural disease guideline 2010. *Thorax.* 2010;65(Suppl 2):i61-i76.

43. Filosso PL, Sandri A, Guerrera F, et al. When size matters: changing opinion in the management of pleural space-the rise of small-bore pleural catheters. *J Thorac Dis.* 2016;8(7):E503-E510.

44. Zisis C, Tsirgogianni K, Lazaridis G, et al. Chest drainage systems in use. *Ann Transl Med.* 2015;3(3):43.

45. Meredith JW, Hoth JJ. Thoracic trauma: when and how to intervene. *Surg Clin North Am.* 2007;87(1):95-118.

46. Seamon MJ, Haut ER, Van Arendonk K, et al. An evidence-based approach to patient selection for emergency department thoracotomy: A practice management guideline from the Eastern Association for the Surgery of Trauma. *J Trauma Acute Care Surg.* 2015;79(1):159-173.

47. Goodman M, Lewis J, Guitron J, Reed M, Pritts T, Starnes S. Video-assisted thoracoscopic surgery for acute thoracic trauma. *J Emerg Trauma Shock.* 2013;6(2):106-109.

48. Helling TS, Gyles NR, Eisenstein CL, Soracco CA. Complications following blunt and penetrating injuries in 216 victims of chest trauma requiring tube thoracostomy. *J Trauma Inj Infect Crit Care.* 1989;29(10):1367-1370.

ABDOMINAL TRAUMA 33

Jasmin Neal, MD and Matthew Giangola, MD

▌INTRODUCTION

Trauma, in its myriad patterns of injury, presents a constant battle not only within the patient but within the systems management of trauma care. Rightfully, the first priority is patient care—identifying those that need immediate invasive intervention, those that require further diagnostic information, and those that can be observed. The focus of this chapter will be abdominal trauma both from a tertiary center's perspective and within a resource-limited environment. One must stress the importance of adhering to the Advance Trauma Life Support (ATLS) and American College of Surgeons Committee on Trauma (ACS-COT) guidelines and principles.[1]

In all scenarios, the therapy provided will rise to the capability of the health system. In a system with abundant resources and staff, most if not all, standards at each level of care can be met easily. However, in crisis situations the allocation of staff is a priority as is the usage of supplies needed by them.[2] With a tiered response, a single credentialed specialist can guide those that are capable but unfamiliar with the nature of the inciting pathology/pandemic.[2] Supporting them are physician extenders and other providers who can care for the acutely injured or critically ill.

▌EPIDEMIOLOGY

Currently in the United States, motor vehicle collision (occupants and pedestrians struck by vehicles) is one of the most common mechanisms of injury in blunt abdominal trauma, comprising 80% of blunt injuries. Roughly 13% of these patients will have intraperitoneal injury. Large solid organs are the most commonly injured (spleen and liver); however, all the structures should be considered for injury when examining patients.[3,4] Penetrating abdominal trauma is on a decreasing trend across the country but is a significant source of mortality. Trauma is the leading cause of death in those younger than 45 and is still a significant cause of mortality in age groups above 45.[5]

▌TRIAGE AND MANAGEMENT

Penetrating injuries cause trauma via direct and indirect disruption of the traversed tissue. Blunt injury tends to be pressure against the retroperitoneal structures or shearing forces which then lead to vascular disruption and hollow viscus injury.[6] Simultaneous blunt and penetrating mechanisms can be combined during one event. The triage of this patient population is often related to the severity of the mechanism of injury and the presenting physiology/pathology of the victim. It is important to note that in order to effectively triage, no one single severity index, evaluation or factor can be recommended with Grade I evidence.[7] However, multiple studies focus on using a combined approach which can increase effective triage rates.[8,9] An experienced clinician's examination plus physiologic parameters can be used to effectively triage patients. The aim should be over-triaging when resources are plentiful and available. However, the tenets of ATLS—recognizing those that will succumb to their injuries no matter the timeliness of intervention from those that will benefit from rapid invasive treatment— are paramount to using limited resources most effectively.[10]

Only after the stabilization of circulation and airway and completion of primary survey can the assessment of the abdominal injury begin. If an obvious penetrating wound and/or unstable physiology is present, the patient should be considered for immediate operative exploration. Barring any actively exsanguinating injury (eviscerated organs/mesentery), the patient should be evaluated via a secondary survey noting the injury pattern and thus delineating the need for further work up. Multiple studies reveal that ruling out abdominal injury is increasingly difficult and the suspicion of injury must lead to radiologic evaluation in those that are otherwise stable.[11]

Imaging of the trauma patient may begin via focused assessment with sonography in trauma (FAST).[12,13] Using sonography, free fluid, free air or other injury can be evaluated quickly and can guide a clinician's management plan. If hemodynamically stable, further imaging via helical CT scan with intravenous contrast should be performed, extending from just above the diaphragm to below the pelvis. The sensitivity of a CT scan for trauma approaches > 95% for many pathologies but often will not show the exact pathology. Rather, it may show associated findings pointing toward an injury (free fluid, air, hematoma etc.).[14,15] It should be noted that controversy exists in the use of whole-body CT scans in the hemodynamically stable. In the resource-limited situation, it is reasonable to selectively scan patients with the appropriate admission and observation period.[16] Blunt injuries can occur to any intraabdominal organ as well as the retroperitoneal structures. Diagnostic peritoneal lavage (DPL) may have many drawbacks, but can be useful in resource-limited environments to rule-in abdominal hemorrhage. Solely relying on DPL has been discouraged in recent literature, deferring to bedside ultrasound and clinical suspicion. If local wound exploration at bedside shows peritoneal violation, which can be challenging to recognize, operative exploration is warranted. The trend in management of penetrating trauma in stable patients is reliable exams, allowing a window for transportation of patients to tertiary care for observation.[17]

Damage control resuscitation should be expedient.[18] Aggressive and immediate resuscitation should replace shed blood. Prediction of the need for a massive transfusion can be calculated using various methods but most focus on physiologic findings and mechanism of injury, such as the Assessment of Blood Consumption or ABC score.[19] This is optimally done with a ratio of 1:1:1 administration of packed red blood cells (PRBC), plasma, and platelets with an effort to reduce crystalloid volume.[20,21] If the ability to give whole blood can be afforded, this should be given immediately. Current studies reveal there may be a benefit to whole blood vs component resuscitation.[22] Fibrinogen repletion is also considered to be a new therapy which may help reduce the need for PRBCs, a limited commodity in limited-resource settings. Definitive endpoints of resuscitation are not universally accepted but one must restore circulating volume and fend off hypovolemic shock as soon as possible.[23] In fact, the evolution of the concept of permissive hypotension has made it a well-established approach to trauma care.[24] Commonly accepted goals are a systolic blood pressure of >90 mmHg,[25] normal mentation, and no requirement for vasopressor/fluid support. A mean arterial pressure goal of >50 to 65 mmHg are acceptable targets for permissive hypotension.[26] For critical care during resource limited situations, targeting these parameters is acceptable regardless of the abdominal injury. Traditionally, a hemoglobin count of 7 g/dL and a hematocrit level of 21% are the lower limits of acceptable parameters; however, the stability of these measurements over time predicts adequate response. Correcting perfusion to avoid acidosis is of clinical significance as well, i.e. maintaining a pH > 7.2 and correcting base deficit.[27] Often time, after acute hemorrhage, hemoglobin, as a measure of concentration, will not change and not reflect the volume of blood loss. After 4–6 units of packed red blood cells, if the above hemodynamic parameters are not met, the patient is considered unstable and labeled a non-responder. A transient responder is a patient who transiently meets these criteria but develops repeated symptoms of ongoing blood loss. Crystalloid fluids should be avoided in the acutely bleeding patient but can be initially given if resources are not available.[28] One should keep in mind that over-resuscitation can lead to worse outcomes.

If possible, tranexamic acid (TXA) may be given within 3 hours of the injury to combat fibrinolysis. Although civilian data differs from military research,[29] recommendations from multiple societies do advocate for an early use of TXA in select patients.[30] Coagulopathy should be reversed and reversal agents given if the patient has a history of anticoagulation use. Hypothermia should be prevented and reversed if present. A base deficit of 5 mEq/L is indicative of hypoperfusion and active acidosis. Attention should be toward the correction of the underlying cause of malperfusion. As an adjunct to common clinical parameters, bedside echocardiography can be performed to assess the intravascular volume.[31]

The expedient and voluminous resuscitative effort, along with traumatic inflammation, may lead to the development of abdominal compartment syndrome. In an effort to maintain normothermia, reverse coagulopathy, and reach ICU-level of care, once definitive hemostasis is achieved it is prudent to leave the abdomen "open" and exit the operating room. There are many approaches to increase the domain of the abdomen including but not limited to vacuum assisted devices, mesh bridges, penetrating towel clamps, and sterile intravenous bags.[32,33] In a resource-limited situation, definitive abdominal closure should not delay transfer.

ABDOMINAL COMPARTMENT SYNDROME

Should resuscitation continue in a nonoperative situation, abdominal compartment syndrome can be diagnosed by its deleterious effect on ventilation and perfusion. Elevated plateau pressures and hypercarbia are the result of increased resistance and loss of intrathoracic volume. Oliguria proceeding to anuria ensues due to the immense pressure placed on renal blood flow. Associated with that pressure is compression of the venous system and thus back pressure into the inflow of the intrabdominal visceral microcirculation. Hypotension from reduced preload may be seen as well. The diagnosis, supported by evidence from the Abdominal Compartment Society, is made when the intra-abdominal pressure as measured via the bladder is ≥ 20 mmHg. Therapies to decrease abdominal pressure may start at measured pressures of 12 mmHg using analgesics, sedation, stomach and bladder decompression and, if present, drainage of ascites/fluids from the abdomen. Once the physiologic sequelae of compartment syndrome are evident and a confirmed bladder pressure of ≥ 20 mmHg is present despite medical therapy, a decompressive laparotomy is recommended and the patient should undergo temporary abdominal closure. It is worth noting that even with the increased domain that temporary dressings provide, abdominal compartment pressures can still increase. If this should happen, the dressing should be removed.[34]

The intraabdominal pressure is measured via the bladder by connecting a transducing line to the side port of a Foley catheter. By instilling a volume of water (some institutions use 25 mL) into the bladder and clamping the drainage tube (blue clamp), a pressure can be transduced to the monitor (Figure 33-1). The same type of piezo-electric crystal apparatus (transducer) for arterial lines can be used for this measurement.

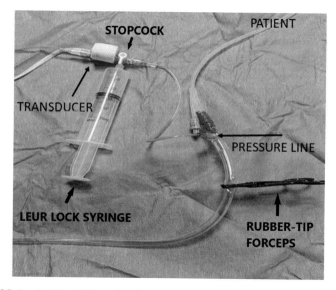

Figure 33-1 • A 500 ml Normal Saline (NS) bag is connected to the transducer. The transducer is connected to a pressure cable and adjusted to a 30 mmHg scale. The stopcock is turned off to the patient, the non-vented cap is removed and opened to atmosphere, the zero function is selected on the monitor. Then the stopcock is turned off to air, and the cap is replaced. Patient is placed supine with head of bed less than 20 degrees. The transducer is leveled off to iliac crest at mid-axillary line. The urinary drainage bag is clamped with rubber tip forceps. The stopcock is turned off the patient and opened to luer lock syringe and pressure transducer. Twenty five milliliter of NS is aspirated into a syringe by pulling a flush device on the transducer and pulling back on the luer lock syringe. The stopcock is turned off the pressure transducer set, opened to the patient and NS-filled luer lock syringe. Another 25 ml of NS is injected into the bladder. The clamp on urinary drainage bag is released to release air from the catheter since it will dampen pressure reading. Re-clamp and wait 30–60 seconds after instillation prior to measuring intraabdominal pressure. The stopcock is turned off to the luer lock syringe and opened to the transducer and patient. Abdominal pressure at end of expiration is measured.

❚ ZONES OF ABDOMINAL TRAUMA

The location of the injury can dictate when or if to intervene. Classically, penetrating trauma within the abdomen can be grouped into Zones I, II or III. In brief, Zone I incorporates the great vessels of the midline retroperitoneum—the aorta and vena cava and their immediate branches. Zone II includes the upper lateral retroperitoneal space, encompassing the renal blood supply and kidneys. Zone III consists of the pelvic retroperitoneum. All expanding hematomas due to penetrating injuries must be explored due to the likelihood of active bleeding. In blunt trauma, nonexpanding hematomas should be observed as venous injury is more likely in this pattern of injury. Most protocols published by major societies agree that a combination of early intervention, damage control surgery, and transfer to a trauma center are of utmost importance. The availability of interventional radiology, trauma surgeons, and ICU staff to care for the injured patient is paramount to the successful treatment of the severely injured patient.[35]

Splenic Trauma

One of the most commonly injured structures in blunt abdominal trauma is the spleen. The patient response will guide the surgeon toward prudent management as preservation of the spleen is preferable. In the hemodynamically stable patient, observation is prudent regardless of the grade of injury.[36] Grades I–V of solid organ injury are useful to predict the failure rate of non-operative management, but should not be a sole indication in operative decision making.

AAST Splenic Injury Grading:[37]

Grade I – subcapsular hematoma < 10% of surface area, parenchymal laceration < 1 cm in depth, capsular tear

Grade II – Subcapsular hematoma 10–50% of surface area, intraparenchymal hematoma < 5 cm, laceration 1–3 cm not involving the parenchymal vessels

Grade III – Subcapsular hematoma > 50%, intraparenchymal hematoma > 5 cm, ruptured hematoma, laceration > 3 cm involving trabecular vessels

Grade IV – Laceration of segmental or hilar vessels, greater than 25% devascularization of spleen

Grade V – Shattered spleen, devascularized spleen

The World Society of Emergency Surgery (WSES) recommends non-operative therapy for all splenic trauma, regardless of grade, provided the patient is hemodynamically stable. The work up for Grade III or greater should include angiography and investigation for pseudoaneurysm or extravasation of contrast. If resources allow, angioembolization is preferred for the transient responder. If unstable, operative therapy is recommended. It should be stressed that observing high grade injuries requires the resources to closely monitor the patient. Transfer to a level 1 trauma center is recommended if resources are scarce and the patient is stable for transportation. In rural or resource-limited areas (no follow-up possible, no interventional radiology for embolization), operative intervention can be more aggressive. Delayed splenic rupture or vascular pseudoaneurysm/fistula should be of long-term consideration. Post-splenectomy vaccination should be considered in those embolized or rendered asplenic.

Liver Trauma

Multiple modes of injury are capable of damaging the liver and due to its relatively large size, it is prone to injury from both penetrating and blunt mechanisms. Hepatic trauma is largely nonoperative with < 15% of patients requiring operative therapy. Most patients become stabilized via observation and/or angiography and embolization. The same principles of ATLS are used to initially evaluate a patient and those that are taken to the operating room should have failed resuscitation and/or are in immediate life-threatening hemorrhagic shock.

Grading of liver injury as defined by the AAST is as follows:[36]

Grade I – subcapsular hematoma < 10% of surface area. Parenchymal laceration < 1 cm
Grade II – Subcapsular hematoma 10–50% of surface area. Intraparenchymal hematoma < 10 cm, parenchymal laceration 1–3 cm deep and < 10 cm in length
Grade III – Subcapsular hematoma > 50% of surface area, ruptured subcapsular/parenchymal hematoma. Intraparenchymal hematoma > 10 cm. Laceration > 3 cm deep and/or any vessel injury
Grade IV – Parenchymal disruption 25–75% of a hepatic lobe. Active bleeding into the peritoneum
Grade V – Parenchymal disruption > 75% of a hepatic lobe. Vena cava injury and/or ventral major vein

Patients who exhibit hemodynamic stability and have no other associated injury requiring operative therapy may be closely monitored without abdominal exploration. It should be noted that hepatic injury is associated with further traumatic injury, such as a splenic laceration or a hollow viscus injury. Those with low grade injury but with peritonitis should still be explored. Liver hemostasis can be performed at that time if needed while repairing the concurrent injury. Penetrating injuries of the right upper quadrant with sufficient imaging can be managed non-operatively if there is no obvious contrast extravasation into the peritoneum or any Grade V injury. Interventional radiology consultation for embolization is the mainstay of treatment for those than can be resuscitated. Early investigation of lower grade injury via angiography and subsequent embolization portends the greatest benefit and success of observation. Damage control laparotomy with liver packing can undergo embolization if the injury is too difficult to control via operative maneuvers.

In resource-limited settings where observation or interventional radiology is unavailable, a more aggressive approach to hemostasis may be appropriate via direct cautery, coagulation, ligation and/or packing. The WSES recommends that if a patient was found hemodynamically stable and no new symptoms and signs, they can be managed nonoperatively. Transportation to a tertiary center once stable is recommended due to the downstream complications of vascular injury of the liver (abscess, necrosis, liver failure, biliary fistula, inadvertent bowel ischemia, etc.).

Renal Trauma

Similar to splenic and hepatic trauma, renal trauma is usually nonoperative unless vascular disruption and hemodynamic instability are present. At the time of laparotomy, if a pulsatile or expanding Zone II hematoma is found, vascular control and exploration should be carried out. If a renal vessel laceration is found, hemostasis can be achieved through ligation and nephrectomy provided there is a normal contralateral kidney. If there is no contralateral kidney, arterial repair (arteriorrhaphy, vein patch, reimplantation) is recommended. Nearly all Zone II blunt injuries should be observed if the patient is stable and there are no concerning hematoma features on laparotomy. As a tenet of trauma care, once stabilized, the patient should be transferred to a tertiary care facility for further evaluation. If hematuria is present as the only symptom, a CT angiogram/pyelogram with a renal protocol should still be ordered to detect collecting system injuries. Below, the AAST grading system of renal trauma is outlined.[36]

Grade I – Contusion: microscopic or gross hematuria, urologic studies normal. Hematoma: subcapsular, nonexpanding hematoma without parenchymal laceration

Grade II – Hematoma: nonexpanding perirenal hematoma confined to renal retroperitoneum. Laceration: laceration < 1 cm depth of renal cortex without urinary extravasation

Grade III – Laceration: laceration > 1 cm depth of renal cortex without collecting system rupture or urinary extravasation

Grade IV – Laceration: parenchymal laceration extending through the renal cortex, medulla, and collecting system (urine extravasation). Vascular: main renal artery or vein injury with contained hemorrhage.

Grade V – Laceration: completely shattered kidney. Vascular: avulsion of renal hilum or thrombosis that devascularizes the kidney.

In a resource-limited setting, it is prudent to monitor all Grades I–III blunt injuries. Debate continues regarding IV through V, but the availability of angioembolization should dictate how aggressively one can address the high-grade injuries. If unavailable and there is normal contralateral kidney function, one may opt for early intervention (surgical hemostasis, nephrectomy).

Trauma to the Great Vessels

Regarding location of the injury, the aorta is usually divided into three zones. The first zone is between the diaphragm and the superior mesenteric artery (SMA). The second zone includes the SMA to the renal vasculature. The third zone comprises the renal artery to the aortic bifurcation. Injuries in the upper portion of the aorta should be exposed via left medial visceral rotation. The mid and lower portion of the aorta can be exposed through the base of the transverse mesocolon. The iliac arteries can be exposed through the pelvic retroperitoneum.

The approach to great vessel injury is dictated by the stability of the patient. All attempts at proximal control via aortic cross clamping, resuscitative endovascular occlusion of the aorta (REBOA), direct compression, or vessel looping should be carried out.[38] Distal control is important but should not delay inflow control. Using vascular or non-crushing clamps, direct repair is often possible with small to medium defects within named vessels. Mesenteric vessels should also be considered for immediate repair prior to transfer.[39] Using interposition grafts such as the saphenous vein, femoral vein, or prosthetic grafts are all possible given the size of the defect. It is paramount to have prepped and draped the patient to their knees in order to harvest the appropriate graft if needed.

Efforts to control a contained aortic rupture or aneurysm via endoscopic routes should be reserved for resource-replete settings when hemodynamic stability is achieved.[40] Blunt aortic injury requires maintaining the normotension and pain control prior to transfer to a tertiary care center. Intrathoracic injuries are far more common than abdominal blunt injuries.

Inferior vena cava (IVC) injuries, particularly the retrohepatic IVC, are difficult injuries to repair. A right medial visceral rotation is required to view the infrahepatic IVC. Direct repair is possible through this vantage point. An atriocaval shunt using a chest tube is described in the literature and likely requires cardiac surgery capability/experience and immediate transfer to a tertiary care facility.

Blunt Pelvic Trauma

One of the most feared aspects of pelvic hemorrhage is the inability to obtain rapid and definitive hemostasis. In a resource-limited situation, pelvic binders are recommended provided they are placed correctly. Preperitoneal packing as well as "thumbtacking" can compress actively bleeding vessels and plexuses.[41] Literature regarding the utility of resuscitative endovascular balloon occlusion of the aorta (REBOA) is controversial but may spare the patient a thoracotomy.[42,43] If given the time with a known destination for definitive control, this may be entertained for transient hemostasis or partial occlusion. Once resuscitated and stable, transfer to a tertiary care facility is warranted. Angioembolization is the mainstay of therapy as well as reducing the size of the pelvic vault.[44] Operative correction of fractures and stabilization can then be pursued with greater resource availability. Along with bony injury and vessel laceration, intra-abdominal organ injury should be suspected in major trauma.[45,46] The bladder, hollow viscus organs, and other structures may also be compromised given the nature of the mechanical force.

Intestinal Trauma

Direct injury to the gastrointestinal tract can occur via blunt or penetrating mechanisms. Often, penetrating injuries are explored, Blunt injury on hollow viscus organs are more difficult to diagnose.[47] The mechanism of injury can tip one off to the possibility of injury, such as a motor vehicle accident as bowel injury is more prevalent via this mechanism.[48] Suspicion of a bowel injury can be elevated due to a positive FAST scan, peritonitis or CT scan findings of free fluid, mesenteric disruption or oral contrast extravasation.[49] Delayed injury can occur from contained vessel disruption leading to eventual ischemia or stricture of the downstream organ, classically referred to as a bucket handle injury.[50]

With respect to resource-limited settings, it is prudent to explore patients with concerning findings for a perforated viscus. The first priority is hemorrhage control and stability. If active bleeding is occurring from the other sites, intestinal perforations can be controlled with clamps or linear staplers. If the patient is stable, formal repair is indicated at that time, either through direct repair or segmental resection. In the small and large intestines, if < 50% of the circumference is injured, direct repair is possible; however, if a larger injury is incurred resection and anastomosis is advisable. Duodenal trauma is managed conservatively, avoiding the need for a "trauma Whipple" if the patient is stable. Stomach injuries can usually be directly repaired, but if a significant portion is devascularized, a wedge resection or partial gastrectomy may be needed. If injured, the rectum can be repaired primarily.[51] Extraperitoneal rectum/anal trauma will respond to diversion. In a resource-limited environment, a low threshold for diversion is acceptable although newer literature shows the relative safety of primary repair of colon and rectal injuries.[52] Like all anastomotic procedures, the patient should not be in extremis and should have few barriers to recovery before making the decision to restore continuity.

▌ CONCLUSION

Abdominal trauma, whether blunt or penetrating, mandates evaluation. Given the availability of resources, staff, and time, there exists a capacity to aid the injured. The guidelines of ATLS triaging and treatment should be reviewed and adhered to as closely as possible given these factors. In crisis situations, stabilization and transfer are of the utmost importance. If those goals cannot be achieved, stabilizing or definitive management may be needed to be completed at the initial site of presentation—stability of the patient dictates their needs. Close monitoring of abdominal injuries is needed in the above outlined situations and those that require intensive care should be transferred to a tertiary or quaternary center. Hemostasis and resuscitation are both key to improving outcomes in this patient population. STOP THE BLEED, ACLS and basic cardiopulmonary resuscitation classes are recommended requirements for those treating patients in such an acute environment. With continued research into the modalities of investigation of abdominal trauma as well as resuscitation, these guidelines will change but the underlying principle of triage and immediate care continues to be the greatest weapon against traumatic injury.

REFERENCES

1. Available at https://www.facs.org/quality-programs/trauma/atls. Accessed September 30, 2020.

2. Giangola M, Siskind S, Faliks B, et al. Applying triage principles of mass casualty events to the SARS-CoV-2 pandemic: From the perspective of the acute care surgeons at Long Island Jewish Medical Center in the COVID epicenter of the United States. *Surgery*. 2020;168(3):408-410.

3. Nishijima DK, Simel DL, Wisner DH, Holmes JF. Does this adult patient have a blunt intra-abdominal injury? *JAMA*. 2012;307(14):1517-1527.

4. Shackford SR, Mackersie RC, Holbrook TL, et al. The Epidemiology of Traumatic Death: A Population-Based Analysis. *Arch Surg*. 1993;128(5):571-575.

5. Available at https://www.cdc.gov/injury/wisqars/LeadingCauses.html. Accessed September 30, 2020.

6. Poplin GS, McMurry TL, Forman JL, et al. Nature and etiology of hollow-organ abdominal injuries in frontal crashes. *Accid Anal Prev*. 2015;78:51-57.

7. Lerner EB. Studies evaluating current field triage: 1966-2005. *Prehosp Emerg Care*. 2006;10(3):303-306.

8. Nishijima DK, Simel DL, Wisner DH, Holmes JF. Does this adult patient have a blunt intra-abdominal injury? *JAMA*. 2012;307(14):1517-1527.

9. Rowell SE, Barbosa RR, Holcomb JB, Fox EE, Barton CA, Schreiber MA. The focused assessment with sonography in trauma (FAST) in hypotensive injured patients frequently fails to identify the need for laparotomy: a multi-institutional pragmatic study. *Trauma Surg Acute Care Open*. 2019;4(1):e000207.

10. American College of Surgeons. Committee on Trauma. Advanced Trauma Life Support: ATLS Student Course Manual Chapter 1. American College of Surgeons, 2012.

11. Roberts GJ, Jacobson LE, Amaral MM, et al. Cross-sectional imaging of the torso reveals occult injuries in asymptomatic blunt trauma patients. *World J Emerg Surg*. 2020 Jan 9;15:5.

12. Ng AK, Simons RK, Torreggiani WC, Ho SG, Kirkpatrick AW, Brown DR. Intra-abdominal free fluid without solid organ injury in blunt abdominal trauma: an indication for laparotomy. *J Trauma*. 2002;52(6):1134-1140.

13. Schwed AC, Wagenaar A, Reppert AE, et al. Trust the FAST: Confirmation that the FAST Exam is Highly Specific for Intra-Abdominal Hemorrhage in over 1,200 Patients with Pelvic Fractures. *J Trauma Acute Care Surg*. 2021;90(1):137-142.

14. Shyu JY, Khurana B, Soto JA, Biffl WL, et al. American College of Radiology ACR Appropriateness Criteria®Major Blunt Trauma. 2019. Available at https://acsearch.acr.org/list?_ga=2.257911307.100882265.1601430538-1131491739.1601430538. Accessed September 30, 2020.

15. Van Vugt R, Keus F, Kool D, Deunk J, Edwards M. Selective computed tomography (CT) versus routine thoracoabdominal CT for high-energy blunt-trauma patients. *Cochrane Database Syst Rev*. 2013;2013(12):CD009743.

16. Caputo ND, Stahmer C, Lim G, Shah K. Whole-body computed tomographic scanning leads to better survival as opposed to selective scanning in trauma

patients: a systematic review and meta-analysis. *J Trauma Acute Care Surg.* 2014;77(4):534-539.

17. Sander A, Spence R, Ellsmere J, et al. Penetrating abdominal trauma in the era of selective conservatism: a prospective cohort study in a level 1 trauma center. *Eur J Trauma Emerg Surg.* 2020. Online ahead of print.

18. Cannon JW, Khan MA, Raja AS, et al. Damage control resuscitation in patients with severe traumatic hemorrhage. *J Trauma Acute Care Surg.* 2017;82(3):605-617. doi:10.1097/TA.0000000000001333.

19. Nunez TC, Voskresensky IV, Dossett LA, et al. Early Prediction of Massive Transfusion in Trauma: Simple as ABC (Assessment of Blood Consumption)? *J Trauma.* 2009;66(2):346-352.

20. Woolley T, Thompson P, Kirkman E, et al. Trauma Hemostasis and Oxygenation Research Network position paper on the role of hypotensive resuscitation as part of remote damage control resuscitation. *J Trauma Acute Care Surg.* 2018;84(6S Suppl 1):S3-S13.

21. Holcomb JB, Tilley BC, Baraniuk S, et al. PROPPR Study Group. Transfusion of plasma, platelets, and red blood cells in a 1:1:1 vs a 1:1:2 ratio and mortality in patients with severe trauma: the PROPPR randomized clinical trial. *JAMA.* 2015;313(5):471-482.

22. Pivalizza EG, Stephens CT, Sridhar S, et al. Whole Blood for Resuscitation in Adult Civilian Trauma in 2017: A Narrative Review. *Anesth Analg.* 2018;127(1):157-162.

23. Connelly CR, Schreiber MA. Endpoints in resuscitation. *Curr Opin Crit Care.* 2015;21(6):512-9.

24. Morrison CA, Carrick MM, Norman MA, et al. Hypotensive Resuscitation Strategy Reduces Transfusion Requirements and Severe Postoperative Coagulopathy in Trauma Patients With Hemorrhagic Shock: Preliminary Results of a Randomized Controlled Trial. *J Trauma.* 2011;70(3):652-663.

25. Available at https://www.cdc.gov/mmwr/preview/mmwrhtml/rr6101a1.htm. Accessed November 16, 2020.

26. Morrison CA, Carrick MM, Norman MA, et al. Hypotensive Resuscitation Strategy Reduces Transfusion Requirements and Severe Postoperative Coagulopathy in Trauma Patients With Hemorrhagic Shock: Preliminary Results of a Randomized Controlled Trial. *J Trauma.* 2011;70(3):652-663.

27. Mitra B, et al. Trauma patients with the 'triad of death'. *Emerg Med J.* 2012;29(8):622-625.

28. Kwan I, Bunn F, Chinnock P, Roberts I. Timing and volume of fluid administration for patients with bleeding. *Cochrane Database Syst Rev.* 2014;2014(3):CD002245.

29. Dixon A, Emigh B, Spitz K, et al. Does tranexamic acid really work in an urban US level I trauma center? A single level 1 trauma center's experience. *Am J Surg.* 2019;218(6):1110-1113.

30. Roberts I, Shakur H, Coats T, et al. The CRASH-2 trial: a randomised controlled trial and economic evaluation of the effects of tranexamic acid on death, vascular occlusive events and transfusion requirement in bleeding trauma patients. *Health Technol Assess.* 2013;17(10):1-79.

31. Ferrada P, Evans D, Wolfe L, et al. Findings of a randomized controlled trial using limited transthoracic echocardiogram (LTTE) as a hemodynamic monitoring tool in the trauma bay. *J Trauma Acute Care Surg.* 2014;76(1):31-37; discussion 37-38.

32. Coccolini F, Roberts D, Ansaloni L, et al. The open abdomen in trauma and non-trauma patients: WSES guidelines. *World J Emerg Surg*. 2018;13:7:1-16.

33. Nemec HM, Benjamin Christie D, Montgomery A, Vaughn DM. Wittmann Patch: Superior Closure for the Open Abdomen. *Am Surg*. 2020;86(8):981-984.

34. Available at http://www.wsacs.org/foam-resources/education/algorithms.html. Accessed September 30, 2020.

35. Available at https://www.east.org/education/practice-management-guidelines/triage-of-the-trauma-patient. Accessed September 30, 2020.

36. Stassen NA, Bhullar I, Cheng JD, et al. Selective nonoperative management of blunt splenic injury: An Eastern Association for the Surgery of Trauma practice management guideline. *J Trauma Acute Care Surg*. 2012; 73(5):S294-S300.

37. Available at https://www.aast.org/resources-detail/injury-scoring-scale#spleen. Accessed September 30, 2020.

38. Daskal Y, Hershkovitz Y, Peleg K, et al. Potential resuscitative endovascular balloon occlusion of aorta candidates: defining the potential need using the National Trauma Registry. *ANZ J Surg*. 2020;90(4):477-480.

39. Evans S, Talbot E, Hellenthal N, Monie D, Campbell P, Cooper S. Mesenteric Vascular Injury in Trauma: an NTDB study. *Ann Vasc Surg*. 2021;70:542-548.

40. D'alessio I, Domanin M, Bissacco D, et al. Thoracic endovascular aortic repair for traumatic aortic injuries: insight from literature and practical recommendations. *J Cardiovasc Surg (Torino)*. 2020;61(6):681-696.

41. Mikdad S, van Erp IAM, Moheb ME, et al. Pre-peritoneal pelvic packing for early hemorrhage control reduces mortality compared to resuscitative endovascular balloon occlusion of the aorta in severe blunt pelvic trauma patients: A nationwide analysis. *Injury*. 2020;51(8):1834-1839.

42. Coccolini F, Ceresoli M, McGreevy DT, et al. Aortic balloon occlusion (REBOA) in pelvic ring injuries: preliminary results of the ABO Trauma Registry. *Updates Surg*. 2020;72(2):527-536.

43. Vella MA, Dumas RP, DuBose J, et al. Intraoperative REBOA: an analysis of the American Association for the Surgery of Trauma AORTA registry. *Trauma Surg Acute Care Open*. 2019;4(1):e000340.

44. Cullinane DC, Schiller HJ, Zielinski MD, et al. Eastern Association for the Surgery of Trauma Practice Management Guidelines for Hemorrhage in Pelvic Fracture—Update and Systematic Review. *J Trauma*. 2011;71(6):1850-1868.

45. Tanizaki S, Maeda S, Ishida H, Yamamoto T, Yoshikawa J. Clinical characteristics of external iliac artery branch injury in pelvic trauma. *Am J Emerg Med*. 2017;35(11):1636-1638.

46. Figler BD, Hoffler CE, Reisman W, Carney KJ, Moore T, Feliciano D, Master V. Multi-disciplinary update on pelvic fracture associated bladder and urethral injuries. *Injury*. 2012;43(8):1242-9. Erratum in: Injury. 2013;44(12):1967.

47. Fakhry SM, Watts DD, Luchette FA; EAST Multi-Institutional Hollow Viscus Injury Research Group. Current diagnostic approaches lack sensitivity in the diagnosis of perforated blunt small bowel injury: analysis from 275,557 trauma admissions from the EAST multi-institutional HVI trial. *J Trauma*. 2003;54(2):295-306.

48. Watts DD, Fakhry SM; EAST Multi-Institutional Hollow Viscus Injury Research Group. Incidence of hollow viscus injury in blunt trauma: an analysis from 275,557 trauma admissions from the East multi-institutional trial. *J Trauma.* 2003;54(2):289-294. *J Trauma.* 2003;54(4):749.

49. Atri M, Hanson JM, Grinblat L, Brofman N, Chughtai T, Tomlinson G. Surgically important bowel and/or mesenteric injury in blunt trauma: accuracy of multidetector CT for evaluation. *Radiology.* 2008;249(2):524-533.

50. Extein JE, Allen BC, Shapiro ML, Jaffe TA. CT findings of traumatic bucket-handle mesenteric injuries. *Am J Roentgenol.* 2017;209(6):W360-W364.

51. Demetriades D, Murray JA, Chan L, Ordoñez C, Bowley D, et al. Committee on Multicenter Clinical Trials. American Association for the Surgery of Trauma. Penetrating colon injuries requiring resection: diversion or primary anastomosis? An AAST prospective multicenter study. *J Trauma.* 2001;50(5):765-775.

52. Maxwell RA, Fabian TC. Current management of colon trauma. *World J Surg.* 2003;27(6).

34 ORTHOPEDIC TRAUMA

Adam Gitlin, MD

▌INTRODUCTION

Orthopedic and musculoskeletal injuries comprise a substantial part of disaster scenarios. Treatment requires a coordinated approach between medical professionals and local emergency management officials. It involves safe extraction of patients from life-threatening environments with transfer to an associated treatment facility. This can range from a triage facility up to a tertiary care center, depending on the number of patients affected and the available facilities and resources that are functioning at the time of the incident.[1]

Initial Assessment

Initial presentation and management of the trauma patient with orthopedic injuries begins with a thorough assessment of life-threatening conditions. Evaluation of airway, breathing, and acute bleeding emergencies allow for prompt recognition of critical injuries. Assessment and treatment via advanced cardiac life support and advanced trauma life support protocols enable the care teams to appropriately risk stratify and triage patients according to the needs for care. A team-based approach allows for appropriate division of responsibilities. The patient's airway and breathing should be assessed first. Once performed, a thorough head-to-toe assessment should be carried out to evaluate for any injury, deformity or pain location. For fluid resuscitation, the patient should receive two large-bore IV access points. Once care has been established and patients initially stabilized, specific treatment can be implemented.

A thorough secondary survey should be performed by the treatment team once the patient is initially stabilized. The extremities should be examined for any deformity. Each extremity should be physically palpated and noted for tenderness and evidence of pain. The color and condition of the skin should be noted, and any areas of soft tissue disruption or bleeding should be treated with saline irrigation and bandaging. The chest wall and shoulders should be palpated with the patient performing deep inspiration and exhalation to examine for chest wall injuries. The pelvis should be compressed and distracted from the level of the iliac wing to examine for crepitus and motion, which may indicate underlying fracture. The patient should be asked to move each extremity and neurovascular status should be assessed for sensation, movement, and pulses.

Once the secondary survey has been completed, diagnostic imaging should be ordered. Radiographs of the affected areas should be obtained, starting with a single view chest and pelvis as per standard trauma protocols. The affected extremity should be examined above and below the area of injury to evaluate for bony or ligamentous injury. In the setting of an open fracture, IV antibiotics and tetanus toxoid should be administered, and resuscitation of the patient should continue while the treatment plan is being developed.

▌OPEN FRACTURES

Open fractures can be a potentially devastating injury that can result in excessive hemorrhage and life-threatening infection, sepsis, and potentially amputation. Open fractures result when a fracture, including bone, hematoma, and soft tissue becomes exposed to the outside environment. Disruptions in the integrity of the skin overlaying an injury can lead to introduction of bacteria and foreign material into the internal milieu. Inoculation of the soft tissue and osseous structures with foreign debris and bacteria may also occur. This can lead to difficult-to-treat infections with increased risk for development of osteomyelitis and worsening chances of systemic infection.

Typically, long bone fractures are the most common, with tibial shaft fractures the most common presentation. Lower extremity fractures are more common than those in the upper extremity. The increasing prevalence of bicycle and motorcycle transportation across the world has resulted in increasing rates of fractures involving the femur, knee, and proximal tibia (Figure 34-1A–D).

There are two main variations of open fractures that may be encountered in disaster and crisis scenarios. "Inside-out" injuries are more characteristic of lower energy mechanisms that result in smaller soft tissue injuries. Typically, there is less gross contamination and these open injuries are the result of lower-energy falls and low-velocity injuries. Higher energy injuries are commonly associated with high-speed motor vehicle collisions, gunshot wounds and projectiles, crush injuries, and

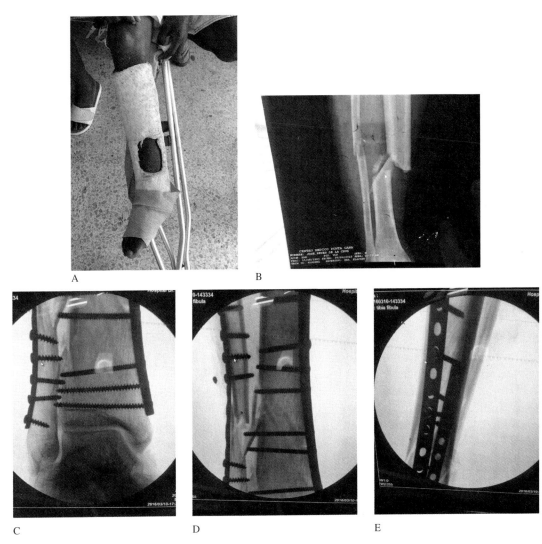

Figure 34-1 • A–E. A patient in a public hospital previously treated nonoperatively (A) for open tibia and fibula shaft fractures as a result of poor access to orthopedic care, with radiographs showing displaced fractures with nonunion. This patient was ultimately treated with surgery during a surgical mission trip (C–E). (From the archives of the author, Adam Gitlin, MD.)

compartment syndrome. These injuries are much more likely to have severe disruption to the soft tissues and skin with increased gross and microscopic contamination.

Early classification of open fractures was done based on the size of the open wound. Early treatment by Gustilo and Anderson emphasized prompt surgical debridement and closure, which led to the classification scheme that now bears their names.[2,3] Type I fractures involve disruption of less than 1 cm to the skin. Type II fractures involve traumatic disruptions from 1 to 10 cm. Type IIIA fractures involve traumatic disruptions greater than 10 cm, with Type IIIB requiring tissue flap coverage and Type IIIC involving vascular injury requiring surgical repair.[4]

Patients with open fractures will present with pain, deformity, and bleeding from the disruption of soft tissues at the site of the injury. They will complain of inability to move the extremity and possible alteration in sensation. Open fractures may also be seen in conjunction with other traumatic injuries and care must be taken to ensure that open fracture does not become a distracting injury. Advanced trauma life support protocols must be adhered to. Once the patient has been stabilized, radiographs of the injured extremity should be obtained. After the injury has been recognized, prompt administration of antibiotics is paramount and has been shown to be the most important factor in reducing infection risk. The open wound should be irrigated to decrease the burden of foreign debris prior to the reduction of the fracture. The injury should then be reduced and immobilized in a splint. Once the patient has been stabilized, surgical treatment can be undertaken.

Antibiotic treatment is initiated with a first-generation cephalosporin. More severe injuries treatment should include an aminoglycoside. Gross contamination involving organic material, such as farm-related injuries, should be treated with the addition of penicillin. Waterborne injuries should include fluoroquinolones as part of antibiotic coverage.

Surgical treatment focuses mainly on two aspects—debridement of nonviable tissue and the method of fixation. Nonviable tissue should be excised as it could become a nidus for infection. Irrigation with normal saline aids in the debridement of both macro and micro contamination. Recent studies have shown no difference in the use of high-pressure and low-pressure irrigation systems[5] and the use of any detergents or antibiotic solution has not been shown to add any benefit. Preferred treatment is normal saline irrigation.

Even in non-crisis scenarios, use of external fixation has been found to be a satisfactory temporizing measure and even for the method of definitive treatment for both closed and open fractures. External fixation allows for bone and soft tissue stabilization while managing debridement of open wounds and other life-threatening injuries that may have been sustained (Figure 34-2).

External fixators have been used traditionally for lower extremity injuries, with joint-spanning constructs used for articular injuries of the knee and ankle. For ankle, distal tibia, and foot injuries, a joint-spanning construct has been used that incorporates two half-pins into the tibia and one

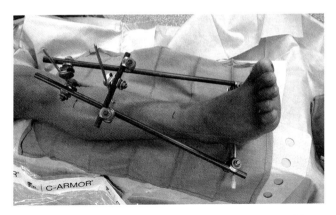

Figure 34-2 • An ankle-spanning external fixator for treatment of lower extremity orthopedic injuries. (From the archives of the author, Adam Gitlin, MD.)

full pin transfixing the calcaneus. Other half pin constructs may be added for midfoot and forefoot injuries. For injuries involving the distal femur or proximal tibia, a joint-spanning configuration is constructed from two half-pins placed into the femoral shaft and two half-pins in the tibia. For femoral shaft and tibial shaft fractures not requiring joint-spanning techniques, pins may be placed from anterior to posterior or in the coronal plane to allow for a "traveling" or "monorail" construct (Figure 34-3).

External fixators have been used to treat upper extremity injuries. Injuries involving the wrist or elbow joints can be treated both temporarily and definitively using joint-spanning frames that allow for soft-tissue stabilization and fracture alignment. For elbow-spanning fixators, two half-pins are placed into the proximal ulna from the lateral side and two pins are placed into the distal humerus. It is important to directly visualize placement of the pins through open approaches on the distal humerus to avoid injury to the radial nerve. For wrist-spanning constructs, two half-pins are placed into the second metacarpal just radial to the dorsal midline and two pins into the radial shaft. These also must be placed using direct visualization to avoid tendon injury.

Treatment duration in external fixators is dependent on multiple factors. External fixation, in most times, is considered a temporary treatment until the patient is able to undergo definitive fixation based on soft tissue characteristics. In non-disaster scenarios, external fixators will typically be used for 1 to 4 four weeks until the patient's skin and soft tissues are amenable to undergoing surgery. In crisis management, an external fixator can serve as definitive treatment for stabilization of orthopedic injuries. Typical treatment in external fixators can last anywhere from 6–12 weeks provided that the pin-bone-soft tissue interface is maintained. Pin site

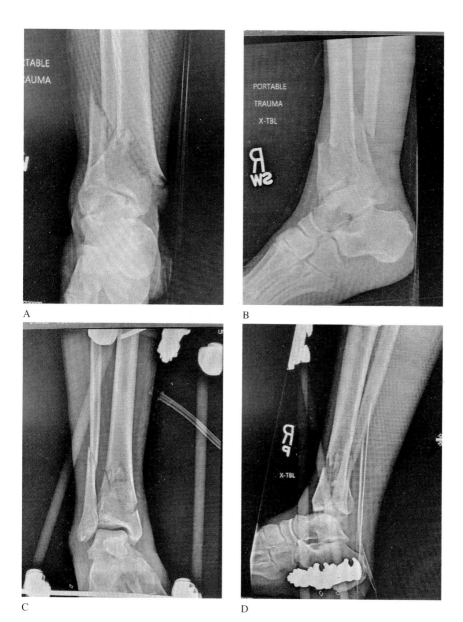

Figure 34-3 • A–D. A patient presented with open fractures of the distal tibia and fibula with preoperative radiographs (A and B) showing the displaced fractures followed by radiographs showing restoration of anatomic alignment after undergoing surgical debridement along with reduction and placement of external fixation (C and D). (From the archives of the author, Adam Gitlin, MD.)

skin care becomes important as non-disaster rates of pin site infections are extremely variable.[6]

The standard of care for almost all open fractures remains prompt antibiotic administration, followed by thorough debridement with placement of internal fixation and closure. Repeat debridement may be required until the soft tissues are amenable to placement of definitive implants. Soft tissue closure can be performed primarily or with the aid of rotational soft tissue flap coverage and skin grafting. Definitive treatment can be performed with the use of external fixation. Previous emphasis on early debridement with external fixation, followed by soft tissue coverage and secondary bone healing showed up to an 80% return to normal function.[7]

Another treatment method more common in developing countries is the use of skeletal traction. In patients with lower extremity fractures, treatment with skeletal traction and bed rest for 4–6 weeks has been shown to proceed to bony union.[7] However, treatment in this manner can lead to malalignment and nonunion and, given current capabilities, should be reserved for more extreme circumstances.

COMPARTMENT SYNDROME

Compartment syndrome is a devastating diagnosis that can lead to substantial morbidity and limb loss. Typical of traumatic scenarios, compartment syndrome can result from crush injuries, vascular compromise and reperfusion injury, polytrauma, and other conditions that result in compromised perfusion to extremities.

Compartment syndrome is a condition of the microvascular anatomy that results in loss of perfusion to the soft tissues. Within the extremity, muscle tissue, nerves, and blood vessels are contained within thick fascial compartments. Injury to the soft tissues results in edema and localized swelling. This loss of perfusion can lead to tissue ischemia and eventual tissue death and necrosis if not fully restored in an urgent manner.[8]

Awareness of the anatomy of both the upper and lower extremities is critical for accurate assessment, diagnosis, and treatment. The upper extremity is divided into two main fascial compartments and the lower extremity into four separate compartments. The forearm is divided into the dorsal and volar compartments. The lower extremity, typically the leg, is divided into four—the anterior, lateral, deep, and superficial posterior compartments. With exception of the deep posterior compartment, the compartments of the leg are superficial and readily accessible with superficial incisions. The deep posterior compartment only becomes superficial in the distal half of the leg. The most common cause of compartment syndrome in the leg is tibia fractures, with distal radius fractures being the most common cause of upper extremity compartment syndrome. Due to their location, the deep posterior and anterior compartments are more commonly affected in the leg. Care must be taken that the deep posterior compartment be sufficiently exposed and released when surgical treatment is undertaken, as this may be missed in certain scenarios.

Compartment syndrome is diagnosed by its clinical presentation and symptoms. Patients will experience pain "out of proportion" to their clinical examination. Pain medication requirements quickly and progressively increase as the patient's condition deteriorates. Patients will commonly present as "feeling restless" or unable to find a comfortable position, and will have a "sense of impending doom." Over time, patients will complain of decreased sensation and paresthesias in the extremity, decreased motor control and strength (paralysis), pallor (poikilothermia), and eventual loss of pulse. Physical exam findings will show a tense, swollen extremity and patients will experience substantial pain with passive stretch of the fingers or toes. The extremity may be warm to touch, but prolonged injury will lead to decreased temperature of the extremity corresponding to the lack of tissue perfusion. Once a patient has experienced loss of pulses, substantial tissue damage has already occurred and the patient has a high risk for tissue necrosis, limb loss, and subsequent amputation. Sensation loss and paralysis, both indicative of nerve damage, can set in as soon as 1 hour after injury and onset of ischemia to the extremity.

Radiographic imaging is of low utility in the diagnosis and treatment of compartment syndrome but can be obtained to rule out underlying fracture. Use of CT imaging can show soft tissue swelling but is nondiagnostic. CT angiography should only be used in the diagnosis of vascular causes for the compartment syndrome, such as major thrombus or transection of vascular structures that would require surgical management. MRI would only be beneficial in the diagnosis of missed compartment syndrome and muscle necrosis.

While compartment syndrome is a clinical diagnosis, tissue pressure monitoring can be employed as an adjunctive method for diagnosis. Patients who are intubated, obtunded or otherwise cannot undergo a reliable clinical examination may benefit from this diagnostic therapy. This is performed by using either a prefabricated system with an electronic gauge and hypodermic needle or can be fashioned using arterial blood pressure monitoring equipment. Absolute compartment pressures greater than 40 mmHg has been the classic teaching for diagnosis and treatment of extremity compartment syndrome. More recently, the difference in tissue perfusion pressure, otherwise known as pulse pressure, has been adopted as a mainstay in diagnosis and management. This compares the compartment pressure to the patient's diastolic blood pressure, where a difference of less than 30 mmHg is considered positive for compartment syndrome and should be managed appropriately. Care must be taken with technique regarding tissue pressure checks. It is advised that at least 5 cm be given between a site of injury and the location for the compartment check, as localized swelling and edema can falsely elevate pressure values. Multiple compartment checks can be performed but should be in variable locations to reduce the risk of post-procedure elevation in tissue pressure values. Compartment pressure checks and monitoring have been shown to also have wide variability, with studies showing that one-time measurements do not necessarily confirm compartment syndrome and subsequent need to proceed with fasciotomy. Many of these patients, while presenting with elevated compartment measurements, recovered without adverse effect. In more common practice, elevated compartment pressure checks typically lead to a low threshold for proceeding with fasciotomy.

Treatment is paramount on early recognition and diagnosis. Medical treatments consisting of induction of hypothermia, anticoagulation, and corticosteroid therapy have been shown in animal laboratory studies to potentially aid in increasing ischemia tolerance in muscle tissue, but disrupted perfusion limits their effectiveness. Hypothermia may show clinical benefit in a similar scenario as it does with cardiac ischemia. Surgical treatment for extremity compartment syndrome consists of fasciotomy of the affected compartment in the operating room. Compartment release allows the expansion of soft tissues and relieves the pressure on the microvasculature, enabling restoration of perfusion. Compartment release of the lower extremity is typically performed with a two-incision approach, with the lateral and anterior compartments being released from the lateral side of the lower extremity and the superficial and deep posterior compartments from the medial side. Surgeons may also opt for a four-compartment release from the lateral side alone and this may be advantageous in limiting the amount of soft tissue exposed in a hostile environment. Early definitive treatment with fasciotomy has been shown to improve outcomes with limb salvage.

Outcomes regarding limb salvage and compartment syndrome are dependent on timing of treatment. Recognition and treatment within 6 hours will provide variable outcomes, but treatment within 8 hours or greater will lean toward dismal outcomes as tissue necrosis has typically set in by this point. Reperfusion of an ischemic limb at this point will likely lead to edema and myonecrosis, which would still warrant fasciotomy.

Treatment for delayed or missed compartment syndrome is focused acutely on the systemic sequelae of myonecrosis. The intravascular release of myoglobin can lead to acute kidney injury and rhabdomyolysis. Close monitoring of kidney function and hydration is usually sufficient in aiding clearance of myoglobin and other metabolic byproducts. Delayed release of compartments is usually advised against, as late release of compartments exposes necrotic tissue to the outside environment and can become a nidus for infection. While function is compromised, patients can be managed acutely for the medical complications after the injury and be staged for definitive salvage treatments and potential amputation at a future date.

Management of compartment syndrome in disaster scenarios presents with its own challenges. Lack of access to an immediately available operating room and clean environment for post-surgical management can lead to complications related to hemorrhage and infection. Acute presentation of compartment syndrome can be treated with acute fasciotomy along with the addition of treatment of the orthopedic or vascular injury that accompanies it. Prolonged delay in recognition or treatment may be best treated nonoperatively in the acute setting, ensuring stabilization of the patient and treatment with definitive corrective surgery or amputation in a more stabilized manner. Nonviable muscle and soft tissue present as an increased risk for infection and may be better definitively treated with debridement or amputation in a future setting. In crisis and disaster scenarios, treatment of life-threatening injuries takes precedence. The difficulties in treatment of crush injuries and compartment syndrome could lead to life-threatening infection and increased risk of acute surgical management. It is up to the discretion of the treating team, after careful evaluation of resources, whether to proceed with acute surgical management or delay acute treatment, both of which may ultimately result in amputation.

For lower extremity compartment syndrome, four compartment fasciotomies done either through two incisions or a single lateral incision can be performed at the discretion of the surgeon. Immediate primary closure of the incisions at this time is advised against as it may lead to recurrence of the compartment syndrome. Coverage with wet-to-dry dressings, occlusive dressings or negative-pressure therapy wound dressings may be performed at the discretion of the treating surgeon. There are several published wound closure techniques and commercial devices available for use. Ultimately, the patient may require repeat procedures for debridement and staged wound closure. Skin graft coverage may be necessary and is usually well tolerated, but consideration must be given to increased risk of infection and morbidity to the skin graft donor site.

Thromboembolic Phenomenon

Thromboembolic phenomenon continues to play an adversarial role in the treatment of the trauma patient. Both venous thromboembolism and fat embolism can affect patients during the entirety of the injury, from the initial to the recovery phases at both the macrovascular and microvascular levels.

Venous thromboembolism (VTE) occurs due to disruption in the classic Virchow's triad, where venous stasis, injury to the endothelium, and hypercoagulability lead to the development of thrombi in the venous system. These thrombi can then mobilize from the endothelium to distant parts of the body where obstruction can lead to occlusion of downstream flow. In the trauma patient, this additionally manifests as a result of direct trauma to the vasculature, decreased mobility due to injury and pain, and increased propensity for hypercoagulable state due to inflammatory cascades.

The greatest propensity for this occurs at the level of the lungs which can lead to hypoxia and respiratory distress. In rare cases, thrombi can bypass the pulmonary tree and result in neurological sequelae. Treatment consists of supplemental oxygen and systemic therapeutic anticoagulation with conversion to either oral or subcutaneous agents. Diagnostic studies such as CT-guided angiography can be performed to identify vascular filling defects. Nuclear medicine scans may be of low yield in regard to reliability and availability in unstable environments.

Identifying at-risk patients can be challenging and risk factor scores have been developed with varying levels of utility and success.[9] Despite best prevention practices including prophylactic treatment, patients continue to develop VTE. Patients in disaster environments may be at even a greater risk.

Fat embolism presents its own challenge as it is primarily associated with trauma and orthopedic patients. Fat embolism results from intravascular mobilization of fat into peripheral or pulmonary circulation.[10] Traditionally it is associated with long-bone fractures, orthopedic procedures, and traumatic injuries, although the incidence is 0.17%.[10]

In addition to functioning as a mechanical obstruction, fat emboli also trigger the intravascular release of lipase, breaking down fat globules into free fatty acids and glycerol. These free fatty acids become toxic to endothelial cells, triggering an inflammatory cascade and prothrombic states. Severe cases can lead to sequestration of platelets and clotting factors, leading to disseminated intravascular coagulation.

The classic presentation is a triad of a petechial rash affecting the upper half of the body, respiratory distress, and neurologic changes that can affect the patient within 24–72 hours after the trauma. Severe cases require cardiovascular support including ventilation. At this point, there are no specific criteria or lab markers that support the definitive diagnosis of fat embolism syndrome, but radiologic studies can support the diagnostic picture. Chest radiographs can show bilateral diffuse or patchy opacities, but these may be nonspecific and can be confused with ARDS, pulmonary edema or infection. High-resolution CT can be more specific and may show ground glass opacities and consolidation with interlobular thickening. Treatment is mainly supportive with supplemental oxygen and respiratory support to support pulmonary function and IV fluids to support hemodynamics. Chemoprophylaxis has not been shown to be of any benefit.

Timing of surgery and stabilization of fractures has been shown to affect the rate of fat embolism syndrome in trauma patients. Patients who initially present in extremis and are not stable for early appropriate care are taken for stabilization and "damage control" procedures to provide provisional stabilization of fractures. Once patients are stabilized, they are able to return for definitive treatment. It has been thought that intramedullary reaming for intramedullary fixation of long bone fractures places increased risk on patients for fat embolism syndrome, though this has not been shown in the literature. Prompt timing for treatment of long bone fractures in trauma patients has been the best indicator for reduction of embolic events.

CLINICAL PRACTICE

Clinical duties and responsibilities can be started once a thorough assessment of patients and resources has been undertaken. Utilization of mass-casualty protocols aid with the triaging of patients who require immediate care. There are multiple triage systems in utilization across the world, all with the purpose of designating the most seriously injured patients that would benefit from emergent or prompt treatment. Patients with acute life-threatening injuries would take priority for emergent evaluation and treatment. Patients with time-urgent injuries such as open fractures would benefit from immediate non-OR based therapies such as local irrigation and immobilization in splints prior to undergoing external fixation. For patients with signs and symptoms of compartment syndrome, how long those signs and symptoms have been present and the timeline since the injury need to be taken into account. This aids in determining which patient need to proceed immediately for compartment releases or those that should be staged for delayed treatment. Patients with closed fractures should be immobilized in splints and taken to the OR when time and space allow. With closed fractures that meet operative criteria, priority should be given to those with long bone fractures such as in the femur and tibia.

SPECIAL CONSIDERATIONS

Orthopedic trauma has its foundation during times of conflict and natural disasters. Wartime injuries suffered by both military and civilian populations have provided ample opportunity for the development of new treatment methods and technologies. Wars also bring both the civilian and military populations together when both become casualties. War zones should be treated as hostile environments. The safety of the patient and surgical team becomes a key factor, with damage-control strategies implemented and prompt evacuation to safer environments. Temporizing procedures, such as external fixation, can be reliably performed with minimal risk regarding infection.[11]

In the past, biological threats have typically been listed in conjunction with mass casualty scenarios as a substantial part of the population can be affected in a short period of time. Past biological attacks have included local events such as nerve agents and local disease transmission, such as the sarin nerve gas attacks in Japan and anthrax in the United States, respectively. The increased social interaction and ease of travel have made pandemics a more recent and particularly devastating threat. The impact of the SARS-CoV-2 pandemic in 2020 greatly impacted how daily medical care was delivered. Treatment of the orthopedic trauma patient was impacted in multiple ways. While social distancing measures and gatherings reduced the number of everyday interactions, trauma centers did not see the corresponding drop in numbers that would be expected. Patients still presented with orthopedic and traumatic injuries and presented with both symptomatic and asymptomatic infections. Precautions and protocols were developed for care of trauma patients in the setting of COVID infections.

At our institution, all patients requiring operative treatment would be tested preoperatively for the purposes of risk stratification and identifying patients at risk for post-operative pulmonary complications.[12,13] In addition, perioperative risk becomes elevated for the surgical and anesthesia staff due to potential exposure and additional protective measures would be implemented. Patient isolation during the perioperative period would be increased and non-sterile equipment would be covered with plastic wrap to prevent local contamination. Surgical staff and the treatment team would don personal protective gear consisting of N95 masks, eye protection, and surgical gowns. The use of PAPR, or powered-air purifying respirators, would be utilized by the anesthesia team to provide protection during intubation and extubation. After treatment was completed, the OR room would be terminally cleaned by housekeeping staff in preparation for any following case. Treatment of the COVID-positive patient continues to evolve as more is learned regarding the long-term physiologic effects of infection.

REFERENCES

1. Pollak AN, Born CT, Kamal RN, Adashi EY. Update on disaster preparedness and progress in disaster relief. *J Am Acad Orthop Surg*. 2012;20(supp 1):S54-S58.
2. Bhandari M, The Flow Investigators. A trial of wound irrigation in the initial management of open fracture wounds. *N Engl J Med*. 2015;373:2629-2641.
3. Gustilo RB, Anderson JT. Prevention of infection in the treatment of one thousand and twenty-five open fractures of long bones: Retrospective and prospective analyses. *J Bone Joint Surg Am*. 1976;58:453-458.
4. Halvorson JJ, Anz A, Langfitt M, Deonanan JK, Scott A, Teasdall RD, Carroll EA. Vascular injury associated with extremity trauma: initial diagnosis and management. *J Am Acad Orthop Surg*. 2011;19:495-504.
5. Bhandari M, Jeray KJ, Petrisor BA, et al. A trial of wound irrigation in the initial management of open fracture wounds. *NEJM*. 2015;373:2629-2641.
6. Moroni A, Vannini F, Mosca M, Giannini S. Techniques to avoid pin loosening and infection in external fixation. *J Orthop Trauma*. 2002;16(3):189-195.
7. Gosselin RA, Mock CN, Joshipura M, et al. The challenges of orthopaedic trauma care in the developing world. Skeletal Trauma. 5th ed. Saunders; 2014.
8. Mauffrey C, Hak DJ, Martin MP III. Compartment Syndrome – a guide to diagnosis and management. Switzerland: Spring Open Access Publication; 2019.
9. Dashe J, Parisien RL, Pina M, De Giacomo AF, Tornetta P III. Is the Caprini score predictive of venothromboembolism events in orthopaedic fracture patients? *J Orthop Trauma*. 2019;33(6):269-275.
10. Rothberg DL, Makarewich CA. Fat embolism and fat embolism syndrome. *J Am Acad Orthop Surg*. 2019;27:e346-e355.
11. Galvin JW, Dannenbaum JH IV, Tubb CC, Poepping, TP, Grassbaugh JA, Arrington ED. Infection rate of intramedullary nailing in closed fractures of the femoral diaphysis after temporizing external fixation in an austere environment. *J Orthop Trauma*. 2015;29(9):e316-e320.
12. COVIDSurg Collaborative. Mortality and pulmonary complications in patients undergoing surgery with perioperative SARS-CoV-2 infection: an international cohort study. *Lancet*. 2020;396:27-38.
13. Clement ND, Hall AJ, Makaram NS, et al. IMPACT-Restart: the influence of COVID-19 on postoperative mortality and risk factors associated with SARS-CoV-2 infection after orthopaedic and trauma surgery. *Bone Joint J*. 2020;102-B(12):1774-1781.

35 BURNS

Kailash Kapadia, MD, Haripriya Ayyala, MD,
Michael Marano, MD, and Edward S. Lee, MD

▌ INTRODUCTION

Burn management continues to be a crucial part of trauma and critical care as severe burn injuries are encountered within the United States and globally. Burn management has evolved and advanced treatment modalities are utilized by countries with adequate resources. The American Burn Association (ABA) publishes updated guidelines periodically with these innovations to promote optimal burn care.

The recent pandemic resulted in the reallocation of resources and continues to put a strain on healthcare systems nationally and globally. Fortunately, the ABA has published protocols for crises or disasters which have potential for a significant number of burn injuries and a shortage in resources. Additionally, there are guidelines established by burn surgeons and healthcare workers who have worked in war zones where burn care also had to be performed under the constraints of limited resources. In this chapter, we will review the fundamentals of burn management and then focus on the guidelines for burn management in special conditions such as in a crisis.

▌ EPIDEMIOLOGY

The ABA reports annual data showing approximately 486,000 burn injuries requiring medical treatment, 40,000 hospitalizations, and about 200 admissions per year in each of the 128 burn centers nationally.[1] Per 2015 data, the survival rate for hospital admissions is 96.8%.[1] While this data looks promising, this is representing a developed nation with specialized burn care centers and resources that can accommodate the number of burn injuries seen. The World Health Organization (WHO) provides international data that shows approximately 11 million burn injuries requiring medical treatment in 2004; with a higher incidence of burn injuries in underdeveloped and developing countries than developed countries.[2]

Burn injuries have a higher mortality rate in these countries and they often lead to temporary or permanent disability in survivors.[2] Moreover, it is found globally that burn injuries correlate with the socioeconomic status; there is a higher incidence of burn injuries in people of low or middle socioeconomic status than high socioeconomic status.[2] These facts portray the unequal burden of burn disease globally and the need for further development of burn care in low resource conditions.

TYPES OF BURNS

The types of burns recorded at admission are categorized into thermal and non-thermal injuries. Most burn injuries are found to occur while at home.[1,2] Thermal injuries comprise fire or flame burns, scald burns from contact with hot liquids, and contact burns from touching hot objects. The ABA data demonstrates each of these incidences per year (Figure 35-1). This chapter will primarily focus on the assessment and management of thermal injuries as they constitute 86% of burn admissions nationally.[1] Non-thermal injuries constitute the remaining 14% of burn admissions (Figure 35-1). These comprise of electrical burns, chemical burns, frostbite, radiation, inhalation injuries only, skin diseases, and other types of unspecified burns.[1]

TYPES OF BURN INJURIES

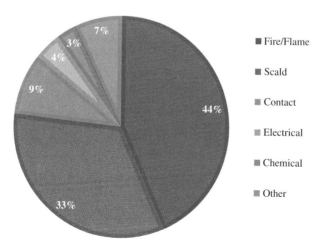

Figure 35-1 • Types of Burn Injuries

▌PATHOGENESIS

Burn injuries initially affect the integumentary system followed by other body systems when there are deeper injuries due to the extent of burn and its systemic effects.

Local Injury

Thermal injuries are often assessed through the extent of injury to the integumentary system which serves as a barrier between the external and internal environment. The skin has two layers, the epidermis and dermis, followed by subcutaneous tissue. The dermis consists of two layers—papillary and reticular dermis. The layers injured will determine the depth of burn or the degree of burn (Table 35-1). First degree burns are superficial burns that have only damaged the epidermis. Second degree burns are further subcategorized into: superficial—damage to the papillary dermis only, and deep—damage to the papillary dermis and part of the reticular dermis. Third degree burns have damaged the epidermis, full thickness of the dermis, and possible damage to underlying subcutaneous fat and

Table 35-1 DEGREE OF BURN		
Degree of Burn	**Layers Involved**	**Description**
First Degree (Superficial)	Epidermis only	• Dry • Erythematous • No blisters • Painful
Second Degree (Superficial)	Papillary Dermis only	• Wet • pink or red • blisters • painful
Second Degree (Deep)	Papillary & Partial Reticular Dermis	• Dry • mottled pink and white • may have open blisters • variable sensation
Third Degree	Epidermis & Full-thickness Dermis	• Dry • leathery, charred brown-black, or waxy white • nonblanching • insensate

muscle. The degree of burn is subject to change after initial assessment of the patient. This phenomenon is explained by the local zones of injury.[3] There are three zones of injury: zone of coagulation, zone of stasis, and zone of hyperemia. The zone of coagulation is usually the tissue most directly affected by the burn that has undergone necrosis or is no longer viable. Surrounding the zone of coagulation is the zone of stasis, which is the tissue with reversible damage, which can either be preserved with adequate resuscitation or be lost depending on how the burn injury progresses. Outside the zone of stasis is the zone of hyperemia which is redness of viable tissue resulting from the local adjacent injury.

Systemic Response

The metabolic responses to injury comprises both the classic hormonal response (catecholamines, cortisol, insulin, glucagon) and the systemic inflammatory response (SIRS) that eventually leads via capillary leak to burn shock. Furthermore, the systemic circulatory and pulmonary vasoconstriction leads to decreased perfusion, oxygenation, and nutrient delivery to tissues and decreased excretion of waste products from tissues. This combination of systemic response increases the risk of end organ failure. Further assessment, monitoring, and management of this systemic response will be discussed in the next section under nonoperative management of burns.

NONOPERATIVE MANAGEMENT

Assessment

Depending on severity of the burn injury and the context of patient presentation the ATLS protocol should be followed. Evaluation of airway, breathing, and circulation is a top priority followed by examining the patient for any burns, fractures, and internal injuries. The initial assessment will also include inquiry of the source of burn, duration of burn, and where the patient was at the time of injury. This is followed by a formal physical assessment of the burn itself. A burn patient's prognosis and mortality are predicted utilizing the Baux score which has been revised in the last decade (Table 35-2)—it is calculated from patient age, percent total body surface area burned, and the presence or absence of an inhalation injury.[4]

The calculation of %TBSA, or body surface area with second and/or third degree burns, is of great importance in determining patient's survival and in guiding the initial resuscitation and management of the patient.

Table 35-2 REVISED BAUX SCORE		
Formula	Score	% Mortality
Age + %TBSA + (17*n)	99	25
No Inhalation injury, n = 0	113	50
Inhalation Injury, n = 1	127	75
	200	100

There are various methods of calculating %TBSA; some are widely used for their ease and some are newer methods that attempt to improve accuracy and reliability. The "rule of nines" is the method most popularly used and taught in the medical field. Each body area is assigned a percentage that is divisible by nine. In general, it is 9% for the head, 36% for the torso, 9% for each upper extremity, and 18% for each lower extremity. Each of these areas is further split into halves and quarters to assist calculation; the remaining 1% is for the groin.[5] The rule of palms, as the name suggests, is when the size of the patient's palm is utilized to estimate %TBSA. The palm is estimated to be 1% TBSA though error often occurs from not knowing whether to include the fingers and thumb as "palmar surface area or not." A recent study found a palm without fingers and thumb is 0.5% TBSA and adding the digits increases this to 0.8% TBSA.[6] While this can be utilized as a quick alternative way to assess small burns, it can be time consuming and inaccurate for large burns. In literature the Lund and Browder chart is quoted as the gold standard assessment for %TBSA. It is a chart with preassigned percentages for all the body parts that are categorized by each small area to minimize user-dependent differences in calculations. It is comparable to the rule of nines though it is also found to be time consuming.[6] The emergence of new technology has resulted in laser dopplers which can be utilized within 48 hours of burn injury to 5 days after the burn to assess %TBSA. Laser doppler %TBSA calculation accuracy was found to be 90–97% in comparison to clinical calculation accuracy using the above methods at 53–71%.[7] A disadvantage of this method of evaluation is its high cost which further depletes resources during crises and pandemics.

Special Considerations

There are special considerations to keep in mind for burns in certain locations and/or of nonthermal nature such as electrical and chemical burns.

With regard to location, the face, the extremities, and the torso should be evaluated serially. For facial burns, the things to consider are airway patency, corneal injuries, and most importantly inhalation injury as this will require further treatment and work up. For extremities and torso, the concern is for any circumferential burns which can cause compartment syndrome and require fasciotomies. For electrical burns, again compartment syndrome in the extremities is a concern as well as monitoring cardiac and renal functions since these injuries could be much deeper than perceived. Electrical injury patients also need early and ongoing evaluation for myoglobinuria that may eventuate in acute kidney injury (AKI). It is treated with aggressive isotonic crystalloid resuscitation until the urine clears. For chemical burns, alkalis cause liquefactive necrosis which raises concern for deeper injuries with time whereas acids cause coagulative necrosis and limit the depth of penetration.[8] Some chemicals have antidotes that should be known and utilized to clean the burn area to neutralize the chemical and prevent further injury to tissue.

Criteria for Transfer to Burn Center

The criteria for transfer to burn care center obtained from the ABA (Table 35-3) is crucial for every hospital to understand and act upon in a timely fashion. However, these criteria will change in times of crisis management which will be covered in the section on burn management in special conditions.

Resuscitation

The Parkland formula is widely used over the years to determine the amount of resuscitative fluids for a new burn patient. Within the first 24–48 hours it is crucial to have adequate resuscitation. The Parkland formula is: 4 mL × %TBSA × body weight in kilograms. Once calculated, the first half is given over the first 8 hours from the time of burn injury and the second half over the next 16 hours. There are other formulas as well which try to refine this fluid requirement as over resuscitation and under resuscitation both have physiological consequences. Under resuscitation can lead to deepening of the burns and low tissue perfusion and over resuscitation can lead to pulmonary edema and worsening of the patient's respiratory status. Adequate resuscitation of the patient is evaluated by clinical examination and tracking certain parameters which include vital signs, urine output, and lab values. During this phase many use a mean arterial pressure (MAP) goal of greater than 60 mmHg to ensure tissue perfusion.[9] Urine output for an average adult should be in

Table 35-3	CRITERIA FOR TRANSFER TO BURN CENTER
1	Partial-thickness burn >10% TBSA
2	Burn to face, hands, feet, genitalia, perineum, or major joints
3	Third degree burns
4	Electrical burns
5	Chemical burns
6	Burn with inhalation injury
7	Burn patient with comorbidities that can complicate burn management
8	Burn injury itself is greatest risk of morbidity/mortality more so than other injuries
9	Pediatric burns in non-pediatric hospitals
10	Burn patient requiring special social, emotional, rehabilitative assistance

the 30–50 mL/hour rate—this will show adequate kidney perfusion and function.[9] After the initial resuscitative phase, the fluid status can also be tracked with daily weights. For those with larger burns and extensive fluid needs, physicians may also choose to use colloids such as albumin to keep tissue perfusion intact. The assessment of when to use crystalloids versus colloids for resuscitation or to utilize therapeutic plasma exchange is outside the scope of this chapter.

Inhalation Injury

A thermal burn with a concomitant inhalation injury affects patient survival and prognosis as discussed previously with the Baux score. This is due to the different aspects of inhalation injuries which correspond to respiratory and systemic effects. A burn patient with an inhalation injury should be considered for immediate or urgent care to address possible carbon monoxide poisoning, upper airway thermal burns and/or inhalation of combustion products. Carbon monoxide poisoning can be tested by ordering a laboratory measurement of carboxyhemoglobin level. While the gold standard for treatment of carbon monoxide poisoning is hyperbaric oxygen chamber, these patients usually come to burn centers due to the critical nature of their burn injuries.[9] For upper airway thermal burns, the main consideration is determining the need to intubate the patient. At the scene of incident, one may follow a set ATLS guidelines for intubation. In the hospital, if the patient is able to support their own airway, the additional indications for intubation are: direct visualization of pharyngeal burns with laryngoscopy, swelling below the vocal cords, and/or carbonaceous sputum.[9] The inhalation of toxic combustion products will also result in further injury to the lungs as well as systemic imbalance. If there is concurrent cyanide toxicity it can be treated with hydroxocobalamin.[9] The other products of combustion are the ones that cause lower airway injury leading to acute respiratory distress syndrome and pneumonitis which have to be managed appropriately.

Wound Care

Burn wound care is performed daily in designated hydrotherapy rooms in burn care centers. In this section we will discuss different topical agents that can be utilized for burn dressings. When the skin barrier is damaged by a burn injury, the first microbials to enter the wound will be skin flora and as time passes these wounds come in contact with other microbials such as gut and respiratory flora which can lead to wound infections. Topical agents attempt to fight these microbials that can otherwise aggregate in the wounds of these patients who are already in an immunocompromised state from their burn injuries. The topical agents can be categorized into silver-based agents, antibiotic ointments, antiseptic solutions, and others such as mafenide acetate and antifungals[10] (Table 35-4). The most popular topical agents are silver sulfadiazine and mafenide acetate.

Pain Management

Burn injuries can be very painful as they combine pain from thermal injury, local inflammation, as well as heightened anxiety. The types of pain that require treatment are categorized into background, procedural, and breakthrough pain.[11] Background pain is the resting pain generated from the injury itself. This is generally treated with long-acting pain medications which can be non-steroidal anti-inflammatory drugs in the outpatient setting and morphine for inpatient and/or ventilated patients. Those with chronic drug use can also benefit from being on methadone. Procedural pain is defined as pain from the additional activities of dressing change which entails cleaning and debridement of the wounds. Prior to hydrotherapy the patients are pre-medicated with short-acting narcotics as well as anxiolytics. Breakthrough pain is as the name suggests, pain experienced due to a break in background pain coverage and is caused by

Table 35-4 TOPICAL AGENTS FOR BURN WOUNDS		
Category	**Topical Agent**	**Properties/Side Effects**
Silver-based	Silver nitrate solution	• Poor eschar penetration • Multiple dressing changes
	Silver sulfadiazine	• Poor eschar penetration • Short-acting • Impedes wound healing • Transient leukopenia
	Silver-releasing dressings	• Sustained release of silver • Long-acting • Fewer dressing changes
Antibiotic ointments	Bacitracin	• Gram-positive coverage
	Polymixin B sulfate	• Gram-negative coverage (Pseudomonas) • Nephrotoxicity/ neurotoxicity
	Mupirocin	• Gram-positive coverage (MRSA)
Antiseptic solutions	Dakin's solution (0.25%)	• Short-acting • Multiple dressing changes • Deep/chronically infected wounds
	Acetic acid	• Deep/chronically infected wounds
Other	Mafenide acetate	• Penetrates eschar • Impedes wound healing • Metabolic acidosis/ compensatory hyperventilation
	Nystatin	• Fungal coverage

Source: Cartotto R. Topical antimicrobial agents for pediatric burns. *Burns & Trauma*. 2017;5:33.[10]

exertion, acute event, or any other stressors. This is treated with short- or long-acting narcotics or acetaminophen depending on the situation.

Rehabilitation

Physical therapy is an important part of patient care even when they are on ventilators, especially for extremity burns that involve joint surfaces as well as facial burns that involve the neck. Prolonged immobilization of joints and extremities leads to stiffness which despite restoration of the skin layer can result in poor function when these patients recover. These patients can develop burn contractures which can be debilitating if they are not regularly mobilizing these areas.

Nutrition

Burn patients are in a hypermetabolic and catabolic state for a prolonged period and their nutritional needs exceed baseline caloric needs. The goal is to start enteral nutrition as soon as possible; this needs to be high in protein and carbohydrate and low in fat. While albumin is a poor indicator of nutritional status, one can track the trend of pre-albumin and CRP levels. There are different formulas for calculating burn patients' caloric needs such as the Curreri formula and the Harris-Benedict equation. Having a nutritionist involved in burn patient care to monitor supplementation and nutritional status would be highly beneficial as they can also adjust the formula type based on the patient's individual needs. Due to systemic effects these patients can also be insulin resistant and they are often started on an insulin drip with a target glucose range of 100–180.[9]

Systemic Antibiotics

During the initial resuscitation phase burn patients can commonly spike fevers. During the first 72 hours the fever is expected and considered non-infectious, therefore typically no cultures are drawn. The use of systemic antibiotics is contraindicated without an identified source of infection such as positive blood culture even though these patients have a high risk of infection.[12] Patients with severe burn injuries can be on ventilators for prolonged periods of time and will often have positive sputum cultures. Once again this should be treated with antibiotics only if the patient's condition deteriorates and/or is in septic shock.

Prophylaxis

Deep vein thrombosis (DVT) prophylaxis and gastrointestinal (GI) prophylaxis are needed. In theory, these patients are in a hypercoagulable state from their injury and under prolonged immobilization when they are ventilated.[9] They are treated with proton pump inhibitors (PPIs) to prevent Curling's ulcers which can occur from low perfusion or ischemia of the gastric mucosa.

OPERATIVE MANAGEMENT

Operative management of burn patients is categorized into acute or early phase burn reconstruction and chronic or late phase burn reconstruction. Early interventions involve preparing or temporizing the wound whereas late interventions are for ultimate wound closure and to restore pre-burn form and function. This section will serve as a brief introduction to these operative interventions.

Early Phase Burn Reconstruction

For deep second degree or third degree burns that require excision, the decision to be made is whether to excise early or to delay. Many support early excision to decrease the risk of infection and further necrosis of the tissue. Those who decide to delay excision do it mainly to determine whether certain deep burns will recover on their own and therefore decrease the %TBSA that requires excision. After excision the fresh wound must be covered with temporary or permanent grafts (Table 35-5). Temporary grafts are utilized when the patient is unable to receive permanent grafts at that time. These grafts are not incorporated into the wound bed; they eventually slough off and have to be replaced by permanent grafts. Traditionally, permanent grafts have been autografts such as split-thickness or full-thickness skin grafts using the patient's own tissue. Recently, there have been technological advances that have created other options for permanent grafting; these are potentially costly but involve a smaller donor site.[13]

Late Phase Burn Reconstruction

Late phase burn reconstruction entails surgeries that will revise the deformity or dysfunction resulting from the burn injury. This can entail scar excision followed by local tissue rearrangement or skin grafting with a full-thickness skin graft to minimize scar contracture. Another option for areas with scar contracture such as the hand, neck, and joint spaces would be scar release with Z-plasties with or without skin grafts. Ultimately, for larger areas requiring revision and coverage, one can perform local, regional, or free flap-based reconstruction. In times of crisis and disaster the focus remains on preventing patient mortality and these interventions can later be utilized to improve the patient's appearance and functionality.

Table 35-5	GRAFTS FOR BURN WOUND COVERAGE	
Category	**Graft Type**	**Properties/Characteristics**
Temporary Grafts	Allograft	• Donor skin graft from same specie • Immune rejection – remove before final grafting
	Xenograft	• Donor skin graft from different specie • Immune rejection, potential scarring • Cheaper in cost
Permanent Autograft	Skin graft	• Split-thickness versus full-thickness • Large donor site
	Cultured epidermal autograft	• Patient cells culture in lab (delay) • Fragile – no dermal cells • Small donor site
	Non-cultured cell-based therapy	• Patient cells prepared intraoperatively (immediate) • Applied over STSG • Small donor site
Permanent Skin Substitutes	Dermal substitutes	• Improve granulation tissue formation • Decrease contracture • Thinner skin graft
	Acellular dermal matrix	• Allow dermal regeneration • Cover with skin graft

Source: Kogan S, Halsey J, Agag RL. Biologics in acute burn injury. *Annals of Plastic Surgery.* 2019;83(1):26–33.[13]

BURN MANAGEMENT IN SPECIAL CONDITIONS

Burn Management in Crisis

While we have the traditional criteria for burn center transfer, the transfer and referrals during a crisis or disaster are different. The focus shifts from providing high quality burn care to a few patients to being able to save as many lives as possible. In order to understand how to respond to an event or disaster it is crucial to be able to differentiate by severity of the event. A mass casualty event is one where there are a great number of casualties but enough rescue teams and supplies to manage the event.[14] Contrastingly, a disaster is one where there are a great number of casualties as well as destruction of infrastructure or resources to address these casualties. In such cases, the resources have to be brought in from elsewhere or the patients have to be transported to places where there are adequate resources.

Mass Casualty Incidents

In the northeast region there were certain mass casualty incidents (MCI) that brought to light the need for coordination and guidelines during such events that would allow for timely triage and management of multiple burn patients. During the 9/11 disaster in New York City, a high and potentially overwhelming volume of burn victims based on jet fuel burning and tens of thousands of people in those buildings was anticipated. However, most of the people trapped in the buildings died and the few who survived with burn injuries could not leave Manhattan because of shutdowns in transportation and communications. At the time, there was a burn bed capacity of 120 locally and there were 39 burn victims reported. On initial triage only 28% were sent to a burn center and afterward only two thirds of the victims were transferred to the two burn centers nearby for care.[15]

Burn Bed Capacity

To further understand the above-mentioned events, it is important to define the terminology. MCIs or disasters have the potential to result in multiple burn injuries which then require a rapid assessment of burn bed capacity locally, regionally, and nationally. Burn bed capacity entails a calculation of the number of burn centers, beds, surgeons, support staff, operating rooms, and supplies.[14] There is the actual capacity which is the maximum number of patients to be accommodated during a non-crisis period and the surge capacity during disaster and crisis. Per ABA, surge capacity is when burn centers accommodate 50% more than their actual capacity. At the time of an MCI or disaster it is important to know what the burn bed capacity is in order to appropriately triage the victims. Currently, the northeast region has a telephone bed census program that has collected data on regional bed availability at any given time to further assist the triage process during crisis or disaster.[16]

Triage Protocols

This brings us to a discussion of triage and what it means for burn crisis. During MCIs, triage is an ongoing process to allocate patients into appropriate categories by determining the acuity of care needed. Per ABA, the first triage is at the scene or in the emergency room of the first hospital to where the patient is taken. The second triage is utilized to determine referral to a burn center. For burn triage, the categories are Immediate, Urgent, Delayed, and Expectant which are universally color coded into red, yellow, green, and gray respectively.[14] The age and %TBSA are of top priority when triaging patients into different categories. Triage protocols ideally also take into consideration of supply and demand, which means assessing burn bed capacity and the number of casualties.

From a burn patient's initial triage to them receiving appropriate care at either a hospital or burn care center is a process that must be streamlined during crisis events. The initial transport from the scene to the hospital must consider factors such as need for intubation, warm fluids, warming blankets, as well as other urgent needs to temporize the patient's condition until they reach the hospital. The hospitals themselves can be categorized into first, second, and third line based on the distance and as well as resource availability. Immediate and urgent patients should be prioritized for first or second line hospitals and delayed category patients to the third line.[14] Based on transport availability at the time, expectant or deceased patients would be low priority as the goal is to save as many lives as possible. As opposed to the standing criteria for referral to a burn center, during a time of crisis, hospitals are encouraged to look at the survival grid published by the ABA in order to determine which burn patients should be referred to a burn center (Figure 35-2).[17] This translates to prioritizing patients with severe yet survivable burn injuries whose lives can potentially be saved by specialized burn care. Patients with minimal to moderate injuries can either be managed as outpatients or by the receiving hospital. Most importantly, patients with nonsurvivable burns should not be referred to a burn care center as that will consume resources that could otherwise save another patient's life.

Triage decision table of benefit-to-resource ratio based on patient age and total burn size

Age/ years	Burn size (percent TBSA)									
	0–10	11–20	21–30	31–40	41–50	51–60	61–70	71–80	81–90	91+
0–1.99	High	High	Medium	Medium	Medium	Medium	Low	Low	Low	Expectant
2–4.99	Outpatient	High	High	Medium	Medium	Medium	Medium	Low	Low	Low
5–19.9	Outpatient	High	High	High	Medium	Medium	Medium	Medium	Medium	Low
20–29.9	Outpatient	High	High	High	Medium	Medium	Medium	Medium	Low	Low
30–39.9	Outpatient	High	High	Medium	Medium	Medium	Medium	Medium	Low	Low
40–49.9	Outpatient	High	High	Medium	Medium	Medium	Medium	Low	Low	Low
50–59.9	Outpatient	High	High	Medium	Medium	Medium	Low	Low	Expectant	Expectant
60–69.9	High	High	Medium	Medium	Medium	Low	Low	Low	Expectant	Expectant
70+	High	Medium	Medium	Low	Low	Expectant	Expectant	Expectant	Expectant	Expectant

This table is based on national data on survival and length of stay.

Figure 35-2 • American Burn Association Survival Grid. (Used, with permission, from ABA Board of Trustees, Committee on Organization and Delivery of Burn Care: Disaster Management and the ABA Plan. *J Burn Care Res.* 2005;26(2):102-106.)

▌ BURN MANAGEMENT IN DISASTER AND AUSTERE CONDITIONS

Thus far we have discussed the standard of care in burn centers in the United States and how to respond in a crisis where there are adequate resources. In resource-poor countries where there are austere conditions or when there is a disaster, there is an imbalance in supply and demand. In such times, modifications are needed in order to manage burn injuries and save patients' lives. The research on burn care under austere conditions has mainly stemmed from burn injuries sustained and managed in war zones.

Resuscitation and Ventilation

In critical and severe burn patients, the initial resuscitation and ventilation are crucial to patient survival. During austere conditions there can be a shortage of equipment needed for intravenous lines or lack of staff to administer the intravenous fluids. In patients with up to 40% TBSA the alternatives that can be considered are oral rehydration therapy or reduced osmolarity oral solution.[18] Oral rehydration therapy is oral administration of fluids with electrolyte and glucose. Another consideration would be rectal infusion therapy where one can administer up to 400 mL per hour through the rectum.[19] Additionally, a ventilator triage team can be established which would consist of healthcare workers whose expertise and function are to solely evaluate the airway and respiratory needs of each patient.[20] The recommendation is to recognize which patients require airway protection with oxygen versus having true ventilation needs. Those who only need airway protection can be managed without being placed on a ventilator.[18]

Wound Care

The goals of burn wound care have been the same for centuries and regardless of whether it takes place in a resource-rich or resource-poor environment, these goals remain unchanged. These goals are evaluation of the wound, preventing infection, and timely intervention for ultimate wound closure. Evaluation of the wound remains the same in austere conditions—assessment of degree of burn and %TBSA. Preventing infections is done through daily dressing changes which allows for inspection, debridement, and cleaning. Ultimately, wound closure is a process that may be delayed depending on availability of other resources. In lieu of hydrotherapy rooms which may not be possible under austere conditions one should still find a designated area where dressing changes can be performed regularly and this area should be kept clean for this purpose.[21] The specialized wound care and nursing staff that participates in dressing change in the United States may not be sustainable in austere conditions and therefore the family members of the burn victim can be involved in the care.[21]

Typically, during dressing change the antimicrobial agents utilized are silver sulfadiazine or mafenide acetate. While these should still be prioritized, in austere conditions there are guidelines on alternative antimicrobials that can be used. If the lack of antimicrobials is also met with a lack of staff and resources for daily dressing changes one can consider silver-releasing dressings on burn wounds which can theoretically be kept in place for several days.[22] This can also be utilized in outpatient care where the family is not able to perform daily dressing changes. The exception would be heavily infected wounds for which the dressing would have to be changed daily in order to monitor the progression of the wound and clean it regularly. Another option would be soaking a non-adhesive gauze dressing in either aqueous mafenide or dilute Dakin's solution and apply it over the wound as a wet to dry dressing.[21] With this type of dressing there would ideally be multiple dressing changes in one day to aid the process of mechanical debridement which can be more labor intensive. Another alternative that has been known to be used as a home remedy is application of honey which carries antimicrobial properties and would also require daily dressing change.

Pain Management

In a regular setting the pain goal has been to medicate in order to achieve pain scores of 2–3/10. In austere conditions and disaster settings when there is a shortage in pain medications, the acceptable pain score can be raised to 6–8/10 for burn patients.[23] In such situations intravenous pain medications are reserved for procedural pain and there is wider use of oral or intramuscular injections for background and breakthrough pain.[23] Other options include utilizing regional anesthesia for procedures or considering cannabis for pain control.[23] There should be a designated personnel who is able to keep an active log of the amount and type of analgesics available along with the requirement of the existing burn patients in order to allocate appropriately.

Rehabilitation

The rehabilitation of these patients that is addressed by physical and occupational therapists in our burn centers will mainly fall onto the family members in austere conditions. The presence of family members who can position the patient and go through exercises will play a large role in the patient's recovery. It may be beneficial to have easily teachable exercises or stretching routines for families to perform with the patient while at the hospital and when at home.

Nutrition

The nutritional status of a burn patient correlates with their ability to heal and recover from burn wounds. Based on severity of burn wounds one can determine who will be able to manage with oral intake versus those who require enteral feeds. Patients with 10–20% TBSA can ideally increase their oral intake. Those with insufficient oral intake or high %TBSA burns can be considered for enteral feeds. When formulas are in scarce supply one may consider creating their own tube feeds by blending locally available nutrient rich foods.[23]

OPERATIVE MANAGEMENT

Once again, the goal of wound care is wound closure which can be expedited and accomplished by excision and grafting. When this process is delayed there is a higher risk of contamination and infection in the open wounds. At such times subeschar clysis can be employed where IV antibiotics are injected below the eschar into the tissue.[24] In infected wounds this can be done to avoid sepsis from wound bacteria being released into the bloodstream during excision.[21]

Furthermore, operative procedures require more forethought and planning in resource-poor areas. The surgeon must anticipate the equipment and blood products needed and ensure their availability as their absence can result in a mortality. Team communication is also of great importance as everyone present should be aware of the patient's needs and the order of events. The %TBSA that can be excised and/or the length of surgery will both be limited by the team's own experience as well as blood supply available. In austere conditions it is recommended to limit to 20% TBSA and/or 2 hours of surgery.[21] Another way to overcome low blood supply and inexperience is to perform fascial excisions as opposed to tangential excisions which will expedite surgical time and limit blood loss. If possible, a tourniquet should be used for all extremity excisions.

BURN MANAGEMENT DURING THE COVID-19 PANDEMIC

Burn Center Experiences

During the pandemic there was a reallocation of resources as well as staff since there were a great number of patients on ventilators requiring intensive critical unit (ICU) level care. The burn care center staff were well trained and equipped to work in an ICU setting and as such were optimal staff for reallocation.[25] Burn ICU beds and Burn step down beds were occupied by COVID patients and other ICU transfers, thereby blocking burn admissions. Any burn transfer from another institution had to be approved by a central command center because there were numerous intubated patients in other hospital wards (ED, same day surgery, OR, Peds ICU) that took precedence over outside burn admits. There was also a reduced operating room (OR) availability and OR staff availability. Only certain surgeries were prioritized to minimize the risk of spreading COVID-19 and to conserve blood products. Along with our own burn center, there have been reports of increase in burn admissions during the pandemic.[26] Despite this increase there was a change in management, in cases where early excision may have been a consideration it was delayed when possible in order to first test the patient for COVID-19.[27] Ventilated patients were consistently being reevaluated and taken off the ventilator as soon as permissible due to a shortage of ventilators available regionally for those deteriorating from COVID-19.

There was also variability in burn admissions as patients who would have generally been admitted to monitor, undergo hydrotherapy, and later decide whether operative intervention would be needed were being discharged home with instructions for wound care at home. Additionally, telemedicine became instituted as outpatient clinics were also closed. There was an increase in this type of outpatient care and patients were readmitted later after COVID testing became more routine. Admission was granted only to COVID negative patients.

Protection of Healthcare Workers During Burn Management

Burn management entails certain high-risk scenarios for healthcare workers secondary to the nature of care being provided. During the pandemic certain protective measures were taken to ensure the safety of workers. When severe burn patients come to the hospital it is important to establish central access as they may require large amounts of resuscitation.[28] As this is done immediately, it is unlikely that the provider would know the patient's COVID-19 status and hence full personal protective equipment (PPE) must be utilized.[27] A similar precaution is true for emergent endotracheal intubation and tracheostomy.[28] This would be a very high-risk scenario as there would be exposure to respiratory droplets as well. While wound care management and dressing changes are normally done daily, during the pandemic the dressing changes were extended to every 2–3 days in order to limit exposure. Taking a patient of unknown COVID-19 status was dangerous to staff and others so patients were tested multiple times prior to surgery and all elective surgeries were canceled.[27] Certain burn centers created a separate ward with patients who were both COVID positive and had burns—this was necessary because usually the same staff in the unit takes care of all the patients and therefore would be putting the patients without COVID at risk if they interacted with both.[27] The literature is still limited as we are still in the middle of the pandemic. However, we hope this chapter brings to light the history of burn management as well as alternatives for optimal management when there are limitations in resources.

▌CONCLUSION

In this new age of innovation there have been many advancements that have allowed physicians to optimize patient care. It is crucial to understand the fundamental principles of burn management in order to manage burn care under special conditions. Awareness of alternative management strategies and crisis or disaster protocols can help physicians save more patient lives when there is a constraint on resources or a surge of burn victims. The current pandemic further emphasizes the importance of understanding these principles as it has affected the healthcare system globally.

▎ REFERENCES

1. "Burn Incidence Fact Sheet." American Burn Association, American Burn Association, 8 May 2017, ameriburn.org/who-we-are/media/burn-incidence-fact-sheet/.
2. "Burns." World Health Organization, World Health Organization, 6 Mar. 2018, www.who.int/news-room/fact-sheets/detail/burns.
3. Kaddoura I, Abu-Sittah G, Ibrahim A, et al. Burn injury: review of pathophysiology and therapeutic modalities in major burns. *Ann Burns Fire Disasters.* 2017;30(2):95-102.
4. Osler T, Glance LG, Hosmer DW. Simplified estimates of the probability of death after burn injuries: extending and updating the baux score. *J Trauma.* 2010;68(3):690-697.
5. Moore RA, Waheed A, Burns B. Rule of Nines. In: StatPearls. edn. Treasure Island, FL: StatPearls Publishing; 2020.
6. Thom D. Appraising current methods for preclinical calculation of burn size - a pre-hospital perspective. *Burns.* 2017;43(1):127-136.
7. Zuo KJ, Medina A, Tredget EE. Important developments in burn care. *Plast Reconstr Surg.* 2017;139(1):120e-138e.
8. Friedstat J, Brown DA, Levi B. Chemical, electrical, and radiation injuries. *Clin Plast Surg.* 2017;44(3):657-669.
9. Mosier M, Gibran N. Management of the patient with thermal injuries. In: Scientific American Surgery. edn. 2016.
10. Cartotto R. Topical antimicrobial agents for pediatric burns. *Burns Trauma.* 2017;5:33.
11. Griggs C, Goverman J, Bittner EA, et al. Sedation and pain management in burn patients. *Clin Plast Surg.* 2017;44(3):535-540.
12. Yoshino Y, Ohtsuka M, Kawaguchi M, et al. The wound/burn guidelines - 6: guidelines for the management of burns. *J Dermatol.* 2016;43(9):989-1010.
13. Kogan S, Halsey J, Agag RL. Biologics in acute burn injury. *Ann Plast Surg.* 2019;83(1):26-33.
14. Haller HL, Wurzer P, Peterlik C, et al. Burn management in disasters and humanitarian crises. In: Total Burn Care. edn.: Elsevier Health Sciences; 2018:36-54.
15. Yurt RW, Bessey PQ, Bauer GJ, et al. A regional burn center's response to a disaster: September 11, 2001, and the days beyond. *J Burn Care Rehabil.* 2005;26(2):117-124.
16. Conlon KM, Bell R, Lee RA, Marano M. Determining immediate burn bed availability to support regional disaster response. *J Burn Care Res.* 2019;40(6):832-837.

17. ABA Board of Trustees; Committee on Organization and Delivery of Burn Care: Disaster Management and the ABA Plan. *J Burn Care Rehabil*. 2005;26(2):102-106.

18. Kearns RD, Conlon KM, Matherly AF, et al. Guidelines for burn care under austere conditions: introduction to burn disaster, airway and ventilator management, and fluid resuscitation. *J Burn Care Res*. 2016;37(5):e427-e439.

19. Tremayne V. Emergency rectal infusion of fluid in rural or remote settings. *Emerg Nurse*. 2010;17(9):26-28; quiz 29.

20. Hick JL, O'Laughlin DT. Concept of operations for triage of mechanical ventilation in an epidemic. *Acad Emerg Med*. 2006;13(2):223-229.

21. Cancio LC, Barillo DJ, Kearns RD, et al. Guidelines for burn care under austere conditions: surgical and nonsurgical wound management. *J Burn Care Res*. 2017;38(4):203-214.

22. Aurora A, Beasy A, Rizzo JA, et al. The use of a silver-nylon dressing during evacuation of military burn casualties. *J Burn Care Res*. 2018;39(4):593-597.

23. Young AW, Graves C, Kowalske KJ, et al. Guideline for burn care under austere conditions: special care topics. *J Burn Care Res*. 2017;38(2):e497-e509.

24. Barillo D, Brisim M. Pediatric burns in war environments. *Pediatric Burns*. 2012:477-483.

25. Barret JP, Chong SJ, Depetris N, et al. Burn center function during the COVID-19 pandemic: An international multi-center report of strategy and experience. *Burns*. 2020;46(5):1021-1035.

26. Williams FN, Nizamani R, Chrisco L, et al. Increased burn center admissions during COVID-19 pandemic. *J Burn Care Res*. 2020.

27. Saha S, Kumar A, Dash S, et al. Managing burns during COVID-19 outbreak. *J Burn Care Res*. 2020;41(5):1033-1036.

28. Huang Z, Zhuang D, Xiong B, et al. Occupational exposure to SARS-CoV-2 in burns treatment during the COVID-19 epidemic: Specific diagnosis and treatment protocol. *Biomed Pharmacother*. 2020;127:110176.

INHALATION INJURIES 36

Bar Cohen, MD, Shaul Gelikas, MD, MBA, and Avi Benov, MD, MHA

▌INTRODUCTION

Inhalation injury is a broad term that includes pulmonary exposure to a wide range of chemicals in various forms, including smoke, gases, vapors, fumes, aerosols, or dust.[1,2] Toxic chemical exposure can be a consequence of an industrial disaster, occupational exposure, recreational mishap, natural catastrophe, chemical warfare, or acts of terrorism.[3] The consequences of such exposure include direct injury to the upper respiratory tract and lung parenchyma, as well as systemic toxicity. The manifestation and severity of such injuries depend upon chemical characteristics (e.g., solubility, particle size, composition, etc.), the amount of toxic compound or compounds inhaled, and patient characteristics (e.g., age, premorbid conditions, etc.).

Inhalation injury can be classified according to cause: asphyxiants, choline esterase inhibitors, respiratory tract irritants, and vesicants (further elaborated in Table 36-1).[3] Chemical inhalation injury may be accompanied by thermal injury, as often happens with smoke inhalation.

Real-time identification of specific chemicals is difficult and many a times not feasible. Symptom onset and progression may be latent but are typically rapid, and the window for effective therapy is often narrow. Therefore, prompt, empirical therapy of casualties suffering from inhalation injury is required. Ending the exposure by evacuation and decontamination is invaluable in treating such casualties. Extrication of casualties from a contaminated zone is best performed by emergency personnel using adequate protective gear. Importantly, when a traumatic injury is suspected (i.e., following an explosion or a terror attack), emergency medical personnel should treat life-threatening situations according to trauma care guidelines.

This chapter presents an overview of some of the leading agents that are involved in inhalation injuries. It will discuss their history, epidemiology, properties, clinical manifestation, treatments, and long-term effects.

Table 36-1	CLASSIFICATION OF INHALED CHEMICALS
Class	**Agents**
Asphyxiants	Simple: methane, propane, nitrogen, carbon dioxide
	Chemical: carbon monoxide, cyanide, hydrogen sulfide
Cholinesterase Inhibitors	Organic phosphorus pesticides, carbamate pesticides
	Nerve agents: sarin, VX, soman, tabun
Respiratory Tract Irritants	Chlorine, phosgene, ammonia, bromine, hydrochloric acid, sulfuric acid, chloramines, tear gas
Vesicants	Sulfur mustard

▌SMOKE INHALATION

Smoke inhalation is one of the most commonly encountered inhalation injuries. It involves the exposure of a casualty's respiratory system to toxic chemicals released during material combustion and, not necessarily, to direct heat that causes thermal injury. Common toxic compounds that are found in smoke include carbon monoxide, ammonia, carbon dioxide, hydrogen cyanide, aldehydes, sulfur dioxides, and nitrogen dioxide.[1] In the United States, fire departments responded to a total of 1,291,500 fires that resulted in approximately 3,700 fatalities and 16,600 injured casualties in 2019.[4] Respiratory failure remains the leading cause of death from fire injuries, and smoke inhalation injuries affect up to one-third of all burn injury victims.[1]

The upper respiratory tract is more prone to thermal injury, whereas chemical toxins may cause damage to the airways, the alveoli, or both. This damage causes increased mucous production, edema, denudation of epithelium and mucosal ulceration, and hemorrhage. These can result in the obstruction of airflow, and pseudomembrane formation in the trachea or bronchi can cause organizing pneumonia. The widespread alveolar-capillary leak can deteriorate to acute respiratory distress syndrome (ARDS).[1]

Upper airway injury, usually caused by thermal injury, manifests as erythema, ulceration, and edema.[5] Face or neck burns may result in anatomic distortion which can compromise airway management. Chemicals in smoke usually cause tracheobronchial injury. Prominent symptoms are persistent coughing and/or wheezing, soot-containing secretions, hypoventilation, erythema, hyperemia, and increased pulmonary shunting due to lobar collapse or atelectasis. Smoke inhalation stimulates vasomotor and sensory nerves in the tracheobronchial area to release neuropeptides that induce an inflammatory response causing bronchoconstriction, increased vascular permeability, and vasodilation which contribute to the ventilation-perfusion mismatch. Injury to the lung parenchyma is typically more delayed and characterized by atelectasis and alveolar collapse, resulting in impaired oxygenation. Massive fibrin deposition also contributes to the ventilation-perfusion mismatch.

Blast Injury

There may be an accompanying blast injury associated with smoke inhalation from burns caused by explosion.[6] It might be primary, where the rapid alternations of compression and decompression can cause air and fat embolisms, pleural tearing, and other contusions and perforations in hollow organs, or secondary where a patient is thrown against a rigid surface or objects hit the patient.[6]

Approach

After thorough history taking, the physical examination must include looking for facial burns. There may be accessory muscle usage, tachypnea, cyanosis, stridor, nasal and oral soot, voice changes, singed facial hair, and wheezing. Evaluation should include pulse oximetry, chest radiographs, complete blood count (CBC), arterial blood gas, and a complete metabolic panel. Since loss of airway patency can develop over time, it is important to know the risk factors associated with a high likelihood of airway intubation. These include absence of airway protection, smoke inhalation injury or blast injury, stridor, face, neck or upper airway injury, burn surface area > 50%, and ingestion of hot liquid.[6]

Some patients are intubated early. Nasal intubation may be preferred over oral intubation. If the burns are > 15% TBSA, it may affect the metabolism of many drugs, such as muscle relaxant, therefore are avoided. This may be an issue since there is a hyperkalemic response in burns and succinylcholine is avoided. Bronchoscopy has been suggested to improve mortality and decrease the duration of mechanical ventilation and ICU stay.[7] It has also been used for prognostication via inhalation grading system.[7] Endorf and Gamelli found that patients with severe inhalation injury (grades 3–4) via initial bronchoscopy evaluation had worse outcomes than those with lower scores (grades 0 or 1)[7,8] (Table 36-2). Radiologist Scores (RADS) (Table 36-3) with the AIS improves composite end-point from 8.3 to 12.7.[9]

Table 36-2 ABBREVIATED INJURY SCORE		
Grade	**Class**	**Description**
0	No injury	Absence of carbonaceous deposits, erythema, edema, bronchorrhea, or obstruction
1	Mild	Minor or patchy areas of erythema, carbonaceous deposits, bronchorrhea, or bronchial obstruction
2	Moderate	Moderate areas of erythema, carbonaceous deposits, bronchorrhea, or bronchial obstruction
3	Severe	Severe inflammation with friability, copious carbonaceous deposits, or bronchial obstruction
4	Massive	Mucosal sloughing, necrosis, endoluminal obstruction

Table 36-3 RADIOLOGIST'S SCORE FOR INHALATION INJURY[9]	
Finding	**Score**
Normal	0
Increased Interstitial Markings	1
Ground Glass Opacification	2
Consolidation	3

Source: Endorf FW, Gamelli RL. Inhalation injury, pulmonary perturbations, and fluid resuscitation. *J Burn Care Res.* 2007;28(1):80-83.[9]

Other treatments sometimes provided to treat smoke inhalation are nebulized N-acetylcysteine (intended to decrease airway secretions), bronchodilators, or nebulized heparin (reduces the inflammatory response and fibrin cast formation). The American Burn Association recommends mixing the following: 3 mL of N-acetylcysteine (20% aerosolized solution), 1 mL of aerosolized heparin (10,000 unit(s)/mL) and 0.5 mL of albuterol sulfate (2.5 mg/0.5mL) together and given every 4 hours for 7 days post-inhalation injury and continued after extubation.[10-13]

Carbon Monoxide

Carbon monoxide inhalation may accompany inhalation injury; CO displaces oxygen from hemoglobin, forming carboxyhemoglobin (COHb) and binding to cytochrome c oxidase.[9] There is a shift of the oxygen dissociation curve to the left and leads to decreased oxygen delivery.[9] Complications include neurologic, hematologic, and cardiac. Diagnosis is dependent on CO-oximetry. Treatment involves 100% oxygen which lowers COHb half-life in 45 minutes or hyperbaric oxygen which lowers COHb half-life in 20 minutes.[9]

Cyanide

Cyanide is found in many molecular forms; it can occur as a solid, liquid or gas and is found in natural and manufactured sources. Exposure can occur through ingestion, inhalation or contact and, can be acute, sub-acute or chronic.[14] Hydrogen cyanide is released during the combustion of synthetic and natural materials. Cyanide from fire smoke is probably the most common cause of acute cyanide poisoning in developed countries.[15] However, intentional exposure to cyanide has occurred in suicides, attempted genocides, and wars and seems increasingly likely to result from terrorist activities.[16] It is believed to have caused more than one million deaths in Nazi gas chambers at Auschwitz, Buchenwald, and Majdanek. It has also been used as a chemical weapon by various governments. In 1978, it was used in a mass suicide led by Jim Jones of the People's Temple in Guyana and resulted in 913 deaths.[17,18]

It is not uncommon for humans to be exposed to cyanide daily from cyanogenic foods and human-made sources such as cigarette smoke. Fortunately, the concentration of CN from these sources is very low, and our body has endogenous mechanisms to detoxify it. Our endogenous cyanide detoxification mechanisms are easily overwhelmed during significant exposures, and this causes the morbidity and mortality associated with cyanide poisoning.[19] The cyanide ion, having a high affinity for metalloproteins, inhibits about 40 enzyme systems. In the mitochondria, cyanide reversibly binds ferric iron in cytochrome oxidase a3, inhibiting oxidative phosphorylation, leading to a cellular shift from aerobic to anaerobic metabolism, depletion of intracellular adenosine triphosphate, and lactic acidosis. Organs with a high demand for oxygen, such as the brain and heart, are the most susceptible to cyanide poisoning.[20-22] Since cyanide is a small lipid-soluble molecule, distribution and penetration of cyanide into cells is rapid.[23] Exposure to high concentrations of cyanide can result in death within seconds to minutes.

Cyanide poisoning is initially manifested as transient hyperpnea and tachycardia accompanied by headache, dizziness, palpitations, and nausea/vomiting. Patients become anxious, confused, and giddy. These manifestations are vague and relatively nonspecific and often mimic anxiety.[24–26] Thus, diagnosis often is missed in the absence of a reasonable index of suspicion. A rapid indicator is a visualization of equally red retinal arteries and veins. Poor oxygen extraction leads to abnormally increased oxygen in the venous supply and a more notable red color.[24–26] Similarly, it is useful to check both venous and arterial blood gases for supranormal venous oxygen content or "arterialization" of venous blood.[24–26]

The most prominent laboratory finding in cyanide toxicity is a profound high anion gap metabolic acidosis with dramatically elevated lactate concentrations. Cyanide tests are not readily available and often require a few days for the results to be available.[24–26] Later symptoms of acute cyanide poisoning reflect neurological, respiratory, and cardiovascular depression from the inability to compensate for tissue hypoxia.[24–26] Victims experience loss of consciousness progressing to coma, with fixed dilated pupils, hemodynamic compromise, arrhythmias, seizures, apnea, cardiac arrest, and finally, death.[26] Long-term cognitive deficits and neuropsychiatric problems have been reported.[24]

Patients with suspected inhalation exposure should first undergo decontamination by being evacuated from the contaminated area and having the affected clothing removed.[24] Airway management should be addressed initially. Supplemental oxygen is a crucial part of supportive care. Assisted ventilation is needed if the patient is unconscious or the airway seems compromised. The use of hyperbaric oxygen for cyanide toxicity is controversial.[19] Unlike poisons for which no specific antidote is available, cyanide has several antidotes with differing action mechanisms and diverse toxicological and clinical profiles. To date, few attempts have been made to evaluate the clinical profiles of the cyanide antidotes relative to each other or a hypothetical gold standard, and the international medical community lacks consensus about the antidote or antidotes with the best risk-benefit ratio.[22]

In the USA, a 3-drug antidote consisting of nitrites, thiosulfate, and hydroxocobalamin are currently being used, with most physicians tending to use hydroxocobalamin. The three-drug antidote kit has been the first defense line in treating cyanide poisoning in the U.S.A. for decades. The kit consists of three drugs: amyl nitrite, sodium nitrite, and sodium thiosulfate, which are used sequentially to obtain a synergistic effect. Nitrites reduce blood cyanide by forming methemoglobin, to which cyanide binds with higher affinity. Early studies with the nitrite thiosulfate combination found that patients were responsive to therapy up to 2.5 hours after cyanide exposure.[24] Significant side effects such as vasodilatation and hypotension are seen during treatment. These effects can be problematic, especially if compounded by coingestants or pre-existing medical conditions. It is recommended to avoid nitrites in smoke inhalation victims with concomitant carbon monoxide poisoning. The methemoglobin formation disrupted oxygen delivery to the cells and increased mortality in an animal model.[21] Intravenously administered sodium thiosulfate, which has a putative mechanism of action complementary to sodium nitrite, confers additional antidotal efficacy.[23]

Hydroxocobalamin works by an entirely different mechanism. It is an endogenous vitamin B12 precursor that binds cyanide to form cyanocobalamin, excreted in the urine. Animal models have demonstrated that hydroxocobalamin is an effective antidote against lethal doses of cyanide. It has a rapid onset of action as it dissolves into the different tissue compartments almost immediately when administered by infusion. Hydroxocobalamin does not interfere with tissue oxygenation and seems to be an appropriate antidote for empiric treatment of smoke inhalation. Side effects are the skin and urine turning red, urticarial eczema, and seldom anaphylactic shock.[21,26]

COMPLICATIONS

Complications associated with inhalation injury include pneumonia, airway obstruction from edema (which can peak 24 hours post-burn) or delayed consequence such as tracheomalacia, subglottic stenosis, or innominate fistula, endobronchial polyps, neck contractures, and tracheal stenosis.[8]

REFERENCES

1. Shubert J, Sandeep S. Inhalation Injury. StatPearls. Published 2020. Available at https://www.ncbi.nlm.nih.gov/books/NBK513261/. Accessed November 13, 2020.
2. Gorguner M, Akgun M. Acute inhalation injury/akut inhalasyon hasari. *Eurasian J Med.* 2010;42(1):28-35.
3. Kales SN, Christiani DC. Acute chemical emergencies. *N Engl J Med.* 2004;350(8):800-8.
4. Evarts B, Ahrens M. Fire loss in the United States.; 2020. Available at https://www.nfpa.org/News-and-Research/Data-research-and-tools/US-Fire-Problem/Fire-loss-in-the-United-States. Accessed October 13, 2020.
5. Sheridan RL. Fire-related inhalation injury. *N Engl J Med.* 2016;375(5).
6. Gregoretti C, Decaroli D, Stella M, et al. Management of blast and inhalation injury. *Breathe.* 2007;3(4):365-375.

7. Available at http://www.surgicalcriticalcare.net/Guidelines/Burn%20 Inhalation%20Injury%202019.pdf. Accessed September 11, 2020.

8. Walker PF, Buehner MF, Wood LA, et al. Diagnosis and management of inhalation injury: an updated review. *Crit Care*. 2015;19:351.

9. Endorf FW, Gamelli RL. Inhalation injury, pulmonary perturbations, and fluid resuscitation. *J Burn Care Res*. 2007;28(1):80-3.

10. Oh JS, Chung KK, Allen A, et al. Admission chest CT complements fiberoptic bronchoscopy in prediction of adverse outcomes in thermally injured patients. *J Burn Care Res*. 2012;33(4):532-8.

11. McIntire AM, Harris SA, Whitten JA, et al. Outcomes following the use of nebulized heparin for inhalation injury (HIHI study). *J Burn Care Res*. 2017; 38:45-52.

12. Miller AC. Influence of nebulized unfractionated heparin and N-acetylcysteine in acute lung injury after smoke inhalation injury. *J Burn Care Res*. 2009; 30:249-256.

13. Juschten J, Tuinman PR, Juffermans NP, et al. Nebulized anticoagulants in lung injury in critically ill patients: an updated systematic review of preclinical and clinical studies. *Ann Transl Med*. 2017;5:444.

14. Huzar TF, George T, Cross JM. Carbon monoxide and cyanide toxicity: Etiology, pathophysiology and treatment in inhalation injury. *Expert Rev Respir Med*. 2013;7(2):159-70.

15. Anseeuw K, Delvau N, Burillo-Putze G, et al. Cyanide poisoning by fire smoke inhalation: A European expert consensus. *Eur J Emerg Med*. 2013;20(1):2-9.

16. Eckstein M. Cyanide as a chemical terrorism weapon. *JEMS*. 2004;29(8):suppl 22-31.

17. Shepherd G, Velez LI. Role of hydroxocobalamin in acute cyanide poisoning. *Ann Pharmacother*. 2008;42(5):661-9.

18. Lawson-Smith P, Jansen EC, Hyldegaard O. Cyanide intoxication as part of smoke inhalation - a review on diagnosis and treatment from the emergency perspective. *Scand J Trauma Resusc Emerg Med*. 2011;19:14.

19. Gracia R, Shepherd G. Cyanide poisoning and its treatment. *Pharmacotherapy*. 2004;24(10):1358-65.

20. Peters CG, Mundy JVB, Rayner PR. Acute cyanide poisoning: The treatment of a suicide attempt. *Anaesthesia*. 1982;37(5):582-6.

21. Borgohain R, Singh AK, Radhakrishna H, Chalapathi Rao V, Mohandas S. Delayed onset generalised dystonia after cyanide poisoning. *Clin Neurol Neurosurg*. 1995;97(3):213-5.

22. Hamel J. A review of acute cyanide poisoning with a treatment update. *Crit Care Nurse*. 2011;31(1):72-81; quiz 82.

23. Hall AH, Saiers J, Baud F. Which cyanide antidote? *Crit Rev Toxicol*. 2009;39(7):541-52.

24. Baskin SI, Horowitz AM, Nealley EW. The antidotal action of sodium nitrite and sodium thiosulfate against cyanide poisoning. *J Clin Pharmacol*. 1992;32(4):368-75.

25. Moore SJ, Norris JC, Walsh DA, Hume AS. Antidotal use of methemoglobin forming cyanide antagonists in concurrent carbon monoxide/cyanide intoxication. *J Pharmacol Exp Ther*. 1987;242(1):70-3.
26. Hall AH, Dart R, Bogdan G. Sodium thiosulfate or hydroxocobalamin for the empiric treatment of cyanide poisoning? *Ann Emerg Med*. 2007;49(6):806-13.

37 IMMERSION, SUBMERSION, AND CRUSH INJURIES

Aminat Ibikunle, MD, Anna C. Go, MD, Christina Hajicharalambous, DO, and Chinwe Ogedegbe, MD, MPH

INTRODUCTION

Immersion, submersion, and crush injuries are related to conditions where the body is consumed by a medium, which may be liquid, semi-solid, or solid. Immersion injuries occur when the head is above the surface of the medium whereas submersion injuries refer to the body and head below the surface of the medium. Death due to liquid medium can be from asphyxia, laryngospasm, aspiration, surfactant failure, hemolysis due to hemodilution, hypothermia, and infection. In semi-solid or solid medium, death can be related to hypoxia, direct trauma to vital organs and/or crush injuries with rhabdomyolysis and electrolyte disturbances.

EPIDEMIOLOGY

Death rates vary by country, medium, and context. In 2016, there were an estimated 320,000 annual drowning mortalities worldwide, which accounted for 75% of deaths from floods.[1] In South Korea from 1990 to 2008, drowning (60.3%) caused the greatest number of deaths followed by landslide (19.7%), and structural collapse (10.1%).[2] In Utah, United States, avalanche fatalities were secondary to asphyxia.[3] During the eruption of Mount St. Helen in Washington, upper and lower airway injuries were the most common causes of death.[4] In Uganda, landslides caused more death than floods.[5] In Mali, mine landslides is an occupational hazard.[6] A large number of patients can easily overwhelm the available relief channels.[7]

Earthquakes have been associated with crush injures: Armenia in 1988 had 25,000 deaths with 600 crush injuries; Kobe, Japan in 1995 had 5,000 deaths with 372 crush injures; Turkey in 1999 had > 17,000 deaths with 639 crush injuries; Taiwan in 1999 had 2,405 deaths with 52 crush injuries; India had 20,023 deaths with 35 crush injuries; Algeria 2,266 deaths with 20 crush injuries; Iraq had 26,000 deaths with 124 crush injuries; and Pakistan had > 80,000 deaths with 118 crush injuries.[8]

PATHOPHYSIOLOGY

Cold immersion injury results in impaired circulatory control, direct microcirculatory damage with microvascular thrombosis and endothelial damage, and reperfusion injury.[9,10] In warm water immersion injury, there is hyperhydration that allows water to travel in between the layers of skin if immersed > 72 hours.[11]

In immersion or submersion injuries related to landslide, sand and air can penetrate into the sinuses and subcutaneous tissues.[12]

In submersion injuries caused by liquid, the resultant aspiration of liquid and/or reflex laryngospasm can lead to hypoxia. Saltwater aspiration results in intrapulmonary shunting, while freshwater aspiration results in more washout of surfactant with both types ultimately causing profound hypoxia from decreased lung compliance, micro-atelectasis, and decreased lung volume.[13]

Most patients who present with submersion injuries have multi-organ dysfunction as a result of prolonged hypoxia. Clinical presentation may vary from cough, mild dyspnea and tachypnea to respiratory failure. Physical exam findings of rales, rhonchi, or wheezing are not uncommon. Fluid aspiration can result in varying degrees of hypoxemia which often produces noncardiogenic pulmonary edema and can lead to acute respiratory distress syndrome (ARDS). A wide array of cardiac arrhythmias may occur secondary to hypothermia, acidemia or hypoxia and treatment efforts should be geared toward reversing these. Significant hypoxia leading to central nervous system depression or permanent brain injury should also be considered. Hematologic and electrolyte abnormalities are usually rare and never life threatening;[13,14] however, coagulopathy may occur in the setting of prolonged hypothermia. Renal failure commonly occurs as a result of myoglobinuria or acute tubular necrosis from hypotension or hypoxia, but about 80% of drowning victims have resolution within 10 days.[13]

The temperature, extent, and duration of exposure can have varying clinical manifestations. There are four stages to nonfreezing cold injury: (1) loss of sensation; (2) discoloration to pale blue with delayed capillary refill, after being removed from the cold environment and until after rewarming; (3) hyperemia with bounding pulses but delayed capillary refill and hyperalgesia that can last for 6–10 weeks; and (4) appears normal but very sensitive to cold and hyperhidrosis. For warm water immersion injury, after immersion in water at 15–32°C for 72 hours, the extremities might be painful, white, and have mild swelling. In tropical immersion of the foot, there will be burning pain and swelling, and it appears red and tender with demarcation of the footwear. Lymphadenopathy maybe present.

In crush injuries, impaired renal perfusion is secondary to obstruction of myoglobin and uric acid and clinical manifestations related to hyperkalemia and hypocalcemia.[8]

TREATMENT

Prehospital

Immediate resuscitative efforts should occur once the victim is rescued onto a flat surface. The ABCs (Airway, Breathing, and Circulation) should always be assessed first and if deemed necessary initiation of high-quality cardiopulmonary resuscitation is the most important factor influencing survival and successful outcomes.[15] Ventilatory efforts with a bag-valve-mask should be initiated for those who are unresponsive and do not have an adequate spontaneous respiratory effort. If the victim is breathing spontaneously, oxygenation is critically important so a high flow nonrebreather mask should be applied. Endotracheal intubation can be considered as part of the pre-hospital phase; indications include a PaO_2 to < 60 or an oxygen saturation < 90%, despite administration of supplemental oxygen. If trauma is suspected, cervical spine immobilization should be performed.[16,17]

For crush injuries, early fluid resuscitation is important once the patient is extricated.[8] Resuscitation with 1 liter per hour (10–15 mL/kg/hr) while the patient is under the rubble followed by hypotonic saline after rescue.[8] Sodium bicarbonate (50 meq) can be added to each second or third liter to maintain urinary pH > 6.5 and if urinary flow > 20 mL per hour, 50 mL of 20 percent mannitol (1–2 g per kg per day at a rate of 5 g per hour) can be added to each liter of infusate to decrease compartmental pressure.[8]

Inpatient

Medical management of the submersion victim should occur in a monitored setting with targeted prevention and treatment of complications. Neurologic status, respiratory status, and core temperature should immediately be evaluated and treatment interventions initiated.

Continuous cardiac monitoring, pulse oximetry, frequent neurologic reassessments should be performed on all patients. Drug screen is ordered if concomitant drug intoxication is suspected. ECG is necessary to assess arrhythmias secondary to hypothermia and hypoxemia including sinus tachycardia, sinus bradycardia, atrial fibrillation, and ventricular fibrillation. Hypothermia patients are very prone to dysrhythmias, even with mild disturbance experienced during patient transfer and should always be on a cardiac monitor. Chest radiograph or computed tomography can be obtained to evaluate the extent of injury; but it is important to note that results can vary from normal to localized, perihilar or diffuse pulmonary edema and cannot predict severity of illness, prognosis or subsequent development of ARDS. Depending on clinical picture such as in the case of trauma, other imaging studies may need to be obtained.

Victims who present with hypothermia (core body temperature < 35°C) should have passive and active warming initiated. ECG variations range from Osborne (J) wave as an indicator of hypothermia to life threatening ventricular fibrillation. Cessation of resuscitative efforts should only occur after the patient is warmed to at least 32°C. Other indications for code cessation include severely hypothermic < 32°C with serum potassium level > 12 mmol/L as together these are associated with incompatibility with life.[12]

Cold Water Injuries

For inpatient management of extremities with non-freezing cold water injuries, limbs should be elevated about the level of the heart and kept open to air and loosely dressed. During the hyperemic stage, pain control via cooling with fat in a cool room may be helpful along with administration of amitriptyline 50–100 mg PO at bedtime or gabapentin. Although fever is common and does not necessarily indicate infection, concomitant cellulitis is not rare and should be treated empirically with antibiotics.

Warm Immersion Injuries

For warm water immersion injuries, extremities are kept dry for 2–3 days, with bed rest and elevation of foot. Improvement might take up to 10–12 days.

Inpatient management includes addressing possible electrolyte abnormalities, pulmonary complications like ARDS, and cardiac and renal complications, for example severe dysrhythmias and acute tubular necrosis. Coagulopathies and hemolysis are uncommon and more linked with unaddressed hypothermia. Early neurologic compromise such as increased intracranial pressure and decreasing Glasgow Coma Scale (GCS) should be addressed in the inpatient setting, as these problems often lead to significant long-term morbidity and mortality.[18] The specific mechanisms leading to these include ongoing cerebral ischemia, cerebral edema, hypoxemia, fluid and electrolyte imbalances, acidosis, and seizure activity. Therapeutic hypothermia and extracorporeal membrane oxygenation (ECMO) can also be considered in severe cases.[19]

Crush Injuries

Hyperkalemia and hypocalcemia can occur and serial measurements are necessary in the first few days. Hospitals should also anticipate the need for renal replacement therapy and surgical fasciotomy, particularly if compartment pressure > 35 mmHg.[8]

PROGNOSIS

Drowning victims who are asymptomatic or mildly symptomatic can be monitored for 4–6 hours in the ED. There is no need for additional lab tests or imaging. If there is no clinical deterioration, vitals are normal, and the physical exam remains normal, patients can be discharged home. Victims who required pre-hospital or ED resuscitation should be admitted to the intensive care unit for continuous cardiopulmonary and frequent neurologic monitoring. Most show rapid improvement within the first 24 hours. Those who did not require Cardiopulmonary resuscitation (CPR) at the scene or in the ED are expected to have full recovery within 48 hours. Those who required CPR have a poor prognosis especially if there was a prolonged downtime (> 30 minutes).[20]

Prognostication is important in terms of allocation of resources and counseling for family members. Duration of submersion can predict risk of death: 0–5 minutes have 10% risk of death; 6–10 minutes have 56% risk of death; 11–25 minutes have 88% risk of death; and > 25 minutes have 100% risk of death.[21] Other poor prognostic factors include > 10 minutes to effective basic life support, resuscitation duration > 25 minutes, age > 14 years, GCS < 5, and arterial blood gas pH < 7.1.[22–32]

REFERENCES

1. Drowning. World Health Organization. Available at https://www.who.int/news-room/fact-sheets/detail/drowning. Published February 3, 2020. Accessed December 2, 2020.
2. Jang JY, Myung HN. Causes of death and demographic characteristics of victims of meteorological disasters in Korea from 1990 to 2008. *Health.* 2011;10(82):1-9.
3. McIntosh SE, Grissom CK, Olivares CR, Kim HS, Tremper B. Cause of death in avalanche fatalities. *Wilderness Environ Med.* 2007;18:293-297.
4. Baxter PJ, Ing R, Falk H, et al. Mount St Helens eruptions, May 18 to June 12, 1980. An overview of acute health impact. *JAMA.* 1981;246(22):2585-2589.
5. Agrawal S, Gorkhovich Y, Doocy S. Risk factors for mortality in landslide and flood-affected populations in Uganda. *Am J Disaster Med.* 2013;8(2):113-122.

6. Mangané M, Almeimoune A, Diop TM, et al. Aspects Epidemiocliniques des Traumatismes au Cours de L'Orpaillage Traditionnel au Service D'Accueil des Urgences du CHU Gabriel Toure de Bamako [Epidemiological scope of traditional gold panning with trauma in emergency service at Gabriel Touré teaching hospital]. *Mali Med.* 2018;33(2):5-8. French.

7. Pereira BMT, Morales W, Cardoso RG, Fiorelli R, Fraga GP, Briggs SM. Lessons learned from a landslide catastrophe in Rio de Jeneiro, Brazil. 2013;8(4):253-258.

8. Sever MS, Vanholder R, Lameire N. Management of crush-related injuries after disasters. *N Engl J Med.* 2006;354:1052-1063.

9. Collier T, Patel A, Rinaldi R. Hypothermia-induced peripheral polyneuropathy after an episode of drowning. *PM R.* 2012;4(3):230-3.

10. Loseth S, Bagenholm A, Torbergsen T, Stalberg E. Peripheral neuropathy caused by severe hypothermia. *Clin Neurophysiol.* 2013;124(5):1019.

11. Allen AM, Tapin D. Tropical immersion foot. *Lancet.* 1073;2(7830):1185.

12. Langdon S, Johnson A, Sharma R. Debris flow syndrome: injuries and outcomes after the Montecito debris flow. *Am Surg.* 2019;85(10):1094-1098.

13. Alpert JJ, Guyer B, Spyker DA. Submersion Injury. In: *Symposium on Injuries and Injury Prevention.* Philadelphia, PA: Saunders; 1985:113-125.

14. Quan L, Mack CD, Schiff MA. Association of water temperature and submersion duration and drowning outcome. *Resuscitation.* 2014;85:790.

15. Olshaker JS. Submersion. *Emerg Med Clin North Am.* 2004 May;22(2):357-67, viii.

16. Schmidt AC, Sempsrott JR, Hawkins SC, et al. Wilderness Medical Society Practice Guidelines for the Prevention and Treatment of Drowning. *Wilderness Environ Med.* 2016;27:236.

17. Tobin JM, Ramos WD, Pu Y, et al. Bystander CPR is associated with improved neurologically favourable survival in cardiac arrest following drowning. *Resuscitation.* 2017;115:39-43.

18. Cline D, Ma OJ, Meckler GD, et al. Chapter 209: Hypothermia. In: *Tintinalli's Emergency Medicine: A Comprehensive Study Guide.* New York, NY: McGraw-Hill Education; 2020.

19. Guenther U, Varelmann D, Putensen C, Wrigge H. Extended therapeutic hypothermia for several days during extracorporeal membrane-oxygenation after drowning and cardiac arrest: Two cases of survival with no neurological sequelae. *Resuscitation.* 2009;80:379.

20. Cline D, Ma OJ, Meckler GD, et al. Chapter 215: Drowning. In: *Tintinalli's Emergency Medicine: A Comprehensive Study Guide.* New York, NY: McGraw-Hill Education; 2020.

21. Szpilman D, Bierens JJLM, Handley AJ, Orlowski JP. Drowning. *N Engl J Med.* May 21, 2012;366:2102-2110.

22. Quan L, Mack CD, Schiff MA. Association of water temperature and submersion duration and drowning outcome. *Resuscitation.* 2014;85:790.

23. Bierens JJ, van der Velde EA, van Berkel M, van Zanten JJ. Submersion in The Netherlands: prognostic indicators and results of resuscitation. *Ann Emerg Med.* 1990;19:1390.

24. Orlowski JP. Prognostic factors in pediatric cases of drowning and near-drowning. *JACEP*. 1979;8:176.

25. Biggart MJ, Bohn DJ. Effect of hypothermia and cardiac arrest on outcome of near-drowning accidents in children. *J Pediatr*. 1990;117:179.

26. Dean JM, Kaufman ND. Prognostic indicators in pediatric near-drowning: the Glasgow coma scale. *Crit Care Med*. 1981;9:536.

27. Lavelle JM, Shaw KN. Near drowning: is emergency department cardiopulmonary resuscitation or intensive care unit cerebral resuscitation indicated? *Crit Care Med*. 1993;21:368.

28. Levin DL, Morriss FC, Toro LO, et al. Drowning and near-drowning. *Pediatr Clin North Am*. 1993;40:321.

29. Quan L, Wentz KR, Gore EJ, Copass MK. Outcome and predictors of outcome in pediatric submersion victims receiving prehospital care in King County, Washington. *Pediatrics*. 1990;86:586.

30. Suominen P, Baillie C, Korpela R, et al. Impact of age, submersion time and water temperature on outcome in near-drowning. *Resuscitation*. 2002;52:247.

31. Habib DM, Tecklenburg FW, Webb SA, et al. Prediction of childhood drowning and near-drowning morbidity and mortality. *Pediatr Emerg Care*. 1996;12:255.

32. Quan L, Bierens JJ, Lis R, et al. Predicting outcome of drowning at the scene: A systematic review and meta-analyses. *Resuscitation*. 2016;104:63.

Index

Note: Page references followed by "f" denote figures and "t" denote tables.

A

AABIP. *See* American Association for Bronchology and Interventional Pulmonology
AACN. *See* American Association of Critical Care Nurses
AAMI. *See* Association of Advancement Instrumentation
AASLD. *See* American Association for the Study of Liver Diseases
Abbreviated injury score, 698t
Abdominal compartment syndrome, 231, 648–649
Abdominal trauma
  blunt, 645–646
  blunt pelvic trauma, 654
  computed tomography of, 646
  damage control resuscitation for, 647
  epidemiology of, 645
  great vessels, 653–654
  intestines, 654–655
  liver, 651–652
  management of, 646–647
  motor vehicle accidents as cause of, 645
  overview of, 645
  packed red blood cells for, 647
  penetrating, 645–646
  renal, 652–653
  spleen, 650–651
  summary of, 655
  tranexamic acid after, 648
  triage of, 646–647
  zones of, 650–655
ABO incompatibility, 111
Abscess, 150t
Acalabrutinib, 43
ACEI. *See* Angiotensin-converting enzyme inhibitors
Acetaminophen, 316t
Acetylcysteine, 182
Acidosis
  metabolic, 232
  vasopressors and, 137

ACS. *See* Abdominal compartment syndrome
ACS-COT. *See* American College of Surgeons Committee on Trauma
ACTH. *See* Adrenocorticotropic hormone
Activated charcoal, 103
Activated prothrombin complex concentrate, 102
Acute adrenal insufficiency, 140
Acute coronary syndrome, 266t
Acute hemolytic transfusion reaction, 111
Acute ischemic strokes, 96
Acute kidney injury
  complications of, 232
  in COVID-1P patients, 253
  definition of, 228
  dialytic treatment of, 233–236
  electrical burns and, 679
  epidemiology of, 230
  etiology of, 230–231
  fluid overload in, 232–233
  myoglobinuria and, 679
  nondialytic management of, 231–233
  overview of, 228–230
  pathophysiology of, 230–231
  renal replacement therapy for. *See* Renal replacement therapy
  risk factors for, 228
  staging of, 229t
  summary of, 240
Acute Kidney Injury Network, 228, 230
Acute lung injury
  description of, 181
  diagnosis of, 209
  incidence of, 210
  Murray score for, 631
  pulmonary contusions as cause of, 631
Acute myocardial infarction, 141
Acute normovolemic hemodilution, 113
Acute respiratory distress syndrome
  American-European Consensus Conference definition of, 209

Acute respiratory distress syndrome
    (*Cont.*)
  Berlin Definition of, 209, 210t
  continuous positive airway pressure
      for, 211
  COVID-19–associated, 407, 426
  definition of, 206, 208–209, 210t
  description of, 10, 14, 93, 181
  epidemiology of, 209–210
  expiratory positive airway pressure
      for, 211
  exudative phase of, 207–208
  fibrotic phase of, 208
  fluid aspiration as cause of, 705
  high flow nasal cannula for, 210–212
  history of, 208–209
  hypoxemia in
      description of, 206–207, 207f
      refractory, 216–218
      shunt physiology and, 218
  mechanical ventilation for
      driving pressure, 213–214
      extubation, 215–216
      indications for, 210–211
      initial settings, 212–213, 213t
      intubation for, 212
      modes of, 216–217
      open lung ventilation, 217–218
      positive end expiratory pressure,
          209, 213–214
      pressure limited mode, 216–217
      readiness testing, 216
      recruitment maneuvers, 217
      refractory hypoxemia, 216–218
      tidal volume adjustments, 214, 215t
      titrated settings, 213–214, 214t
      weaning, 215–216
  mild, 211
  noninvasive support in
      description of, 210–212
      epoprostenol, 222
      extracorporeal membrane
          oxygenation, 219–220
      fluid management, 222–223
      glucocorticoids, 223
      inhaled vasodilators, 221–222
      neuromuscular blocking agents,
          220–221
      proning, 218–219
  noninvasive ventilation for, 210–211
  pathogenesis of, 207–208, 208t
  proliferative phase of, 208
  prone positioning for, 218–219
  pulmonary contusions as cause of, 631
  refractory hypoxemia in, 216–218
  in SARS patients, 386
  summary of, 223–224
  V/Q mismatch in, 218
Acute respiratory infections, 125
Acute right heart syndrome, 142
Acute stress disorder, 344
Acute stress reactions, 364
Adenosine diphosphate, 40
Adenosine monophosphate, 40
Adenosine triphosphate, 39–40
ADH. *See* Antidiuretic hormone
Adjustment disorder, 347–348
ADP. *See* Adenosine diphosphate
Adrenal insufficiency
  acute, 140
  shock caused by, 139–140, 148, 150
  treatment of, 148, 150
Adrenocorticotropic hormone, 197
Advance Trauma Life Support, 645, 655
Ad26.ZEBOV/MVA-BN-Filo vaccine,
    486t, 488
Aedes aegypti, 495, 496f, 499, 539
Aedes albopictus, 499, 539
Aerosol-generating procedures, 416
Aerosolized delivery, of medications
    nebulizer for, 180–181
    pressure meter dosing inhaler for,
        180, 181t
Agent Orange, 578
Agitation, 327–333
Agoraphobia, 342
AHTR. *See* Acute hemolytic
    transfusion reaction
AI. *See* Artificial intelligence
Airborne precautions, 72
Airway pressure release ventilation, 177
AKI. *See* Acute kidney injury
AKIN. *See* Acute Kidney Injury
    Network
Albumin, 131t, 132
ALI. *See* Acute lung injury
Alpha-1 adrenergic receptors, 135
American Academy of Pediatrics
    Disaster Preparedness Advisory
    Council, 526

American Association for Bronchology and Interventional Pulmonology, 187

American Association for the Study of Liver Diseases, 249

American Association of Critical Care Nurses, 23

American Burn Association, 674

American College of Surgeons Committee on Trauma, 645

American Geriatrics Society, 301, 302t

AMP. *See* Adenosine monophosphate

Amphetamines, 589

Analgesia
recommended therapies for, 163–170, 164t–165t
therapeutic options for, 162–170

Analgesics. *See also specific analgesic*
routes of administration, 170
shortage of, 162–163

Andexanet alfa, 102

Anemia
in critically ill patients, 105, 115
phlebotomy as cause of, 115

Angiotensin converting enzyme-2, 196, 404–405

Angiotensin converting enzyme-2 receptors, 195

Angiotensin-converting enzyme inhibitors, 44

Angiotensin receptor blocker, 44

Angiotensin II, 136

ANH. *See* Acute normovolemic hemodilution

Anthrax, 554, 558f–559f, 558–560

Anticholinergic agents, 588

Anticholinergic toxicity, 328t

Anticoagulation therapy
COVID-19 treated with, 103, 421–422
pulmonary embolism treated with, 100
sepsis treated with, 103
thrombosis prevention using, 306

Anticonvulsants, 316t

Antidepressants, 316t, 346

Antidiuretic hormone, 136

Antigen testing, for SARS-CoV2, 411, 426

Antihistamines, 315

Antipsychotics, 166t, 174–175, 331–332, 348

Antivirals, for influenza virus, 446–449, 448t

Anxiety, 339–340

Anxiety disorders
in children, 339t, 339–343
treatment of, 343, 344t, 346t

Aorta, blunt injury to, 632–633

APCC. *See* Activated prothrombin complex concentrate

Apophysomyces trapeziformis, 122

APRV. *See* Airway pressure release ventilation

ARB. *See* Angiotensin receptor blocker

Arbidol, 44–45

ARDS. *See* Acute respiratory distress syndrome

Arenaviruses, 96

ARIs. *See* Acute respiratory infections

Arterial blood gases, 9

Artificial intelligence, 42–43

"Asian flu," 436t, 437, 532

Aspergillus fumigatus, 553

Aspirin, 103–104

Association of Advancement Instrumentation, 84

AstraZeneca vaccine, 425t

ATLS. *See* Advance Trauma Life Support

Atoltivimab, maftivimab, and odesivimab-ebgn, 485, 486t

ATP. *See* Adenosine triphosphate

Atracurium, 175, 176t

Atropine sulfate, 582

Autoclaves, for mask recycling, 81–82

Automated peritoneal dialysis, 235

Automated pupillometry, 616

Avalanches, 704

Avian influenza
blood transfusions in, 109t
treatment of, 447

Azithromycin, 45

B

Bacillus anthracis, 553, 558, 558f

Bacillus Calmette Guerin, 46

Bacillus subtilis var. globigii, 553

Background pain, 681

Bacterial pneumonia, 444

Bag valve mask, 13
BAI. *See* Blunt aortic injury
Balanced crystalloid fluids, 129–130
Baloxavir, 447, 448t
Bamlanivimab, 420
Baricitinib, 45–46
Baux score, 677, 678t
BBB. *See* Blood-brain barrier
BCG. *See* Bacillus Calmette Guerin
BCI. *See* Blunt cardiac injury
Benzodiazepines, 10
  in children, 344t
  sedation uses of, 170–171
Beta-1 adrenergic receptors, 135
Bicarbonate, 130
Bioreactance, 147
Biosafety, 71, 72t
Bioterrorism agents/pathogens, 74t–75t,
    554t, 554–571
  anthrax, 554, 558f–559f, 558–560
  botulism, 560–561, 561f
  brucellosis, 561–562, 562t
  Burkholderia, 567, 567f
  Clostridium perfringens, 562–563,
    563f
  Coxiella burnetii, 568–569, 569f
  cryptosporidiosis, 569, 570f
  E. coli 0175:H7, 564, 564f
  history of, 553–554
  monkeypox, 557f–558f, 557–558
  plague for, 534, 536
  psittacosis, 567–568, 568f
  Q fever, 568–569, 569f
  ricin toxin, 563
  Salmonella, 566f, 566–567
  Shigella, 564, 565f
  smallpox for, 543, 555–557, 556f–557f
  staphylococcal enterotoxin B,
    563–564
  typhus fever, 569–570, 571f
  Vibrio cholerae, 565f, 565–566
Bipolar disorder, 346–347
Bisacodyl, 167t
Bitrex™, 79
Black Death of 1347, 462, 533–534
Bleach solution, 85
Bleeding, blood transfusions for,
    106–107
Blister agents, 582–585
Blood-brain barrier, 608

Blood draws, 115
Blood transfusions. *See* Transfusion(s)
Blood work, in COVID-19 protocol,
    9–10
Blunt aortic injury, 632–633, 653
Blunt cardiac injury, 633–634
Blunt trauma
  abdominal, 645–646
  pelvis, 654
  thoracic. *See* Thoracic trauma, blunt
BNT152b2 vaccine, 425, 425t
Botulism, 560–561, 561f
Braden Scale, 308
Breakthrough pain, 681–682
Breath stacking, 221
Breathing circuits, 179
British anti-Lewisite, 584
Bronchodilators, 12
  aerosolized, 181–182
Bronchoscopy, 187
Brucellosis, 561–562, 562f
Brucellosis melitensis, 561, 562f
Bruton tyrosine kinase inhibitor, 43
Buboes, 465, 465f, 534
Bubonic plague, 464–465, 465f, 533–535
Buckle handle injury, 654
Bunyaviruses, 96
Bupropion, 347
Burkholderia, 567, 567f
Burn(s)
  American Burn Association
    guidelines for, 674
  antibiotic prophylaxis for, 683
  assessment of, 677–678
  Baux score for, 677, 678t
  bed capacity for, 686–687
  blood transfusions for, 108
  burn center transfer criteria, 679, 680t
  in COVID-19, 691–692
  in crisis situations, 686
  deep vein thrombosis prophylaxis in,
    683
  degree of, 676t, 676–677
  in disasters, 688–689
  electrical, 679
  epidemiology of, 674–675
  facial, 679
  first-degree, 676, 676t
  fluid resuscitation for, 679–680,
    688–689

Burn(s) (*Cont.*)
  healthcare worker protection during
    management of, 692
  inhalation injury from, 680–681
  local injury, 676–677
  in mass casualty incidents, 686
  nonoperative management of,
    677–683
  nutrition for, 683, 690
  operative management of, 684, 685t,
    690–691
  pain management in, 681–682, 690
  Parkland formula for, 679
  pathogenesis of, 676–677
  reconstructive surgery for, 684, 685t
  rehabilitation for, 682–683, 690
  second-degree, 676, 676t
  skin grafts for, 684, 685t
  survival table for, 688t
  systemic response to, 677
  third-degree, 676t, 676–677
  total body surface area calculations
    in, 677–678
  triage protocols for, 687
  types of, 675, 675f
  venovenous extracorporeal
    membrane oxygenation for, 287
  volcanic eruptions as cause of, 123
  wound care for, 681, 682t, 689–690
Burn care center, 679, 680t
Burnout, 335
Burr hole craniotomy, 619–620
BVM. *See* Bag valve mask

C
CABG. *See* Coronary artery bypass
    grafting
Calcineurin, 47
CAM. *See* Confusion Assessment
    Method
Cannabinoids, 348, 590
Carbon monoxide inhalation injury, 699
Carbon monoxide poisoning, 680
Carboxyhemoglobin, 699
Cardiac contusion, 633
Cardiac tamponade, 142–143, 143f, 151
Cardiogenic shock
  intra-aortic balloon pump for, 152
  pathogenesis of, 140–142
  treatment of, 152

  venoarterial extracorporeal
    membrane oxygenation for, 261
Cardiomyopathy
  decompensated, 266t
  hypertrophic, 141
  shock caused by, 140–141
Cardiopulmonary resuscitation, 31
Cardiovascular system, 407–408
Care transitions, in older adults,
    317–318
Care Transitions Intervention, 318
Casirivimab/imdevimab, 420
Catecholamines, 133t–134t
Cathepsin G, 92
Catheter-directed thrombolysis, 151
CBT. *See* Cognitive behavioral therapy
CCHF. *See* Crimean-Congo
    hemorrhagic fever
CCL2, 38t
CCL3, 38t
CCL4, 38t
CDT. *See* Catheter-directed
    thrombolysis
Cellulitis, 149t
Center for Medicare and Medicaid
    Services, 28, 254
Central cannulation, 261
Central nervous system, 407
Centre of Research on the
    Epidemiology of Disasters, 122
Cerebral perfusion pressure, 607, 611
Cerebral venous thrombosis, 613
Cerebrospinal fluid leaks, 614–615
Chart by exception, 28
Chemical restraints, 307–308
Chemical weapons/warfare
  blister agents, 582–583
  history of, 578
  lewisite, 584
  multi-threat medical countermeasure
    for, 578
  mustard gases, 582–583
  nerve agents, 578–582, 579t
  nitrogen mustards, 584
  phosgene oxime, 584–585
  psychotomimetic agents. *See*
    Psychotomimetic agents
  riot controlling agents, 592–595
  sulfur mustards, 582–583
  vesicants, 582–585

Chemokines, 35–36, 38t
Chest computed tomography, for
    COVID-19, 413, 414f
Chest tubes, for thoracic trauma,
    639–640
Chest wall, 627
Chest x-rays, for COVID-19, 412–413,
    413f, 414t
Chikungunya fever, 73t, 539
Chikungunya virus, 499–501, 500f, 539
Children. *See* Pediatric patients
Chlamydia psittaci, 567
Chloramphenicol, for plague, 467t, 468
Chlorhexidine, 601
Chloroacetophenone, 592–594
Chloroquine and hydrochloroquine, 47
Cholangitis, 150t
Cholecystitis, 150t
Cholera, 565f, 565–566
Ciprofloxacin
    plague treated with, 468t
    tularemia treated with, 476
Cisatracurium, 175, 176t
Clinical trials, 313
Clonidine, 173, 332–333
Closed fractures, 671–672
Clostridium botulinum, 560–561, 561f
Clostridium perfringens, 553, 562–563,
    563f
Clostridium tetani, 553
CMS. *See* Center for Medicare and
    Medicaid Services
Co-ventilation, 177
Co-venting, 13
Coagulation cascade, 90
Coagulation system
    COVID-19–related abnormalities of,
        95, 95t
    description of, 90
Coagulopathy
    Ebola virus as cause of, 481, 485
    SARS-CoV2 as cause of, 95
    sepsis-associated, 103
    trauma-induced, 104, 114
CODE bags, 16
Cognitive behavioral therapy, 343, 345
Cold immersion injuries, 705, 707
Colloids
    albumin, 131t, 132
    shock treated with, 128, 131t, 148

volume-sparing effect of, 130
Combat settings
    orthopedic trauma in, 672
    penetrating thoracic trauma in, 626
    pulmonary contusions in, 630
    traumatic brain injury in, 606
Community acquired pneumonia, 149t
Compartment syndrome, 666–671
Complement system, 40
Computational-based repurposing, 42
Computed tomography
    abdominal trauma evaluations, 646
    chest, for COVID-19, 413, 414f
    compartment syndrome evaluations,
        667
    pneumothorax evaluations, 628
    rib fracture evaluations, 629
    traumatic brain injury evaluations,
        610
Confusion Assessment Method, 304
Conjunctivitis, influenza virus-related,
    455–456
Constipation
    in mechanically ventilated patients,
        166, 167t–168t
    in older adults, 315
    opioids as cause of, 166, 167t–168t
Contact precautions, 72
Continuous ambulatory peritoneal
    dialysis, 235
Continuous blood pressure monitoring,
    14–15
Continuous positive airway pressure,
    12, 211
Continuous renal replacement therapy,
    233–234, 238t, 239
Continuous sedation, 171
Continuous video
    electroencephalography, 615
Convalescent plasma
    for COVID-19, 108, 110, 250t,
        391–392, 420
    for MERS-CoV, 393
    for 1918 influenza pandemic, 449
Coping
    categories of, 370–371
    definition of, 370
    strategies for, 371–377
"Corona phobia," 341
Coronary artery bypass grafting, 152

Coronavirus disease 2019. *See*
   COVID-19
Coronaviruses, 381
Corticosteroids, 316t
   COVID-19 treated with, 47–48, 421
   Middle East Respiratory Syndrome-
      CoV treated with, 393
   SARS-CoV1 treated with, 390–391
Corticotrophin-releasing hormone,
   196
Cortisol, 140
Coup-contrecoup injury, 606
COVID-19. *See also* SARS-CoV2
   acute respiratory distress syndrome
      caused by, 407, 426
   anti-inflammatory therapy for, 421
   anti-viral therapy for, 417–418, 420
   anticoagulation for, 103, 421–422
   burn management in, 691–692
   cardiovascular system manifestations
      of, 407–408
   case fatality rate for, 422–423
   central nervous system manifestations
      of, 407
   chest computed tomography of, 413,
      414f
   chest x-rays for, 412–413, 413f, 414t
   in children, 530–531
   clinical manifestations of, 406–409
   clinical trials affected by, 313
   coagulation abnormalities in, 95, 95t
   convalescent plasma for, 108, 110,
      250t, 391–392, 420
   "corona phobia," 341
   corticosteroids for, 421
   in critically ill patients, 252, 253t
   cutaneous manifestations of, 408–409
   D-Dimer in, 95–96
   deaths caused by, 195, 245, 422–423
   delirium in, 304
   dexamethasone for, 250t
   diabetes management affected by,
      201–202, 406
   diagnosis of, 409–415, 426
   discovery of, 245
   drug repurposing for. *See*
      Repurposed drugs
   environmental infection control for,
      416
   epidemiology of, 402–403

extracorporeal membrane
   oxygenation uses in, 288–289
health care worker care during,
   334–336, 416
high-risk populations for, 403
hypercoagulability in, 115, 405
hypothalamic-pituitary axis affected
   by, 197
imaging of, 403f
immunity against, 423
incubation period for, 246
infection control for, 415–417, 418t
interleukin-6 and, 404–405
isolation for, 416–417
laboratory workup for, 412
lung-ultrasound score for, 413–414
lymphopenia in, 405
male reproductive effects of, 199
medical conditions associated with,
   252
monoclonal antibodies for, 420
mortality rates for, 422–423
myocarditis associated with, 407
neurological manifestations of, 406
noninvasive support in, 211–212
nucleic acid amplification testing with
   reverse transcriptase-polymerase
   chain reaction assay for, 409–411,
   426
pathophysiology of, 404–406
peritoneal dialysis for, 240
pneumomediastinum in, 407
pneumonia caused by, 413f
pneumothorax in, 407
post-infection syndrome, 422
prevention of, 248, 252t
prognosis for, 422–423
prone position for, 14, 25–26,
   308–309, 422
psychiatric disorders and, 321
radiologic imaging of, 412–413
recovery from, 422
reinfection, 423
remdesivir for, 53–54, 250t, 417–418,
   419t
renal involvement by, 405, 408
respiratory system features of, 407
risk factors for, 403
serology testing for, 411–412, 412t
severity of, 419t

COVID-19. *See also* SARS-CoV2
    (*Cont.*)
  signs and symptoms of, 406
  silent hypoxemia in, 407
  smoking and, 403
  summary of, 426
  symptoms of, 246
  systemic manifestations of, 407–409
  tests for, 409–410
  thyroid function affected by, 198–199
  transmembrane serine protease 2, 404
  transmission of, 245–246, 310, 402,
    415
  transplantation in, 246–248
  transthoracic echocardiogram in, 415
  treatment of, 250t–251t, 417–422
  trends in, 246, 247f
  ultrasonography for, 413–414
  vaccinations for, 423–425, 425t
  venous thromboembolism associated
    with, 94
  ventilatory support for, 253t
COVID-19 inflammatory score, 54–55
COVID-19 protocol
  anticoagulation therapy in, 103
  blood work, 9–10
  cardiopulmonary resuscitation for, 31
  CODE bags, 16
  cohort used in, 4–6
  command center in, 8
  consents, 16
  continuous screening, 18
  counseling, 18–19
  daily meetings, 4
  decontamination, 18
  discontinuation of precautions, 17–18
  endocrinologic effects of, 196t
  family communication in, 15
  goals of care in, 15–16
  high efficiency particulate air filter air
    scrubbers used in, 5
  ICU space for, 4–5
  identification of patients, 4
  imaging studies in, 9–10
  in-hospital cardiac arrest and, 31
  intravenous pumps used in, 27, 27f
  mechanical ventilation in, 13–14
  medical space used in, 6
  medications used in, 10–11
  nursing in, 11–12, 23–31

  nutrition in, 15
  overview of, 3
  patient discharge, 17–18
  personal protective equipment used
    in, 6–8, 7t, 8f, 186, 415
  pharmacy for, 10–11
  post-COVID-19 management,
    16–19
  respiratory failure management in,
    12–15
  statistics regarding, 3
  telemedicine, 8–9
  thrombosis associated with, 94
  tiered-based staffing, 11–12
  treatments, 10–11
Coxiella burnetii, 553, 568–569, 569f
CPAP. *See* Continuous positive airway
    pressure
Creatinine clearance, 312t
CRED. *See* Centre of Research on the
    Epidemiology of Disasters
CRH. *See* Corticotrophin-releasing
    hormone
Crimean-Congo hemorrhagic fever
  blood transfusions for, 109t
  causes of, 506
  in children, 538, 540
  clinical manifestations of, 507, 507f
  description of, 73t, 99
  diagnosis of, 508
  epidemiology of, 538
  outbreaks of, 506
  pathogenesis of, 506–507
  prognosis for, 508
  transmission of, 506, 538
Crisis incidents
  definition of, 357
  pediatric
    acute stress reactions caused by,
      364
    education and training for,
      357 360
    emotional considerations, 363t,
      363–365
    ethical issues in, 365–367
    full-scale exercise for, 358
    social considerations, 363t,
      363–365
    trauma management in, 360–362
  triage in, 620

Crisis standards of care
  definition of, 352
  description of, 15
  for pediatric patients, 352–355
Critical illness
  diabetes management, 200–201
  fluid overload in, 232
  glycemic control in, 200
  hyperglycemia in, 201
  thyroid disorders and, 197–198
CRRT. *See* Continuous renal
    replacement therapy
Crush injuries, 704–708
Cryptosporidiosis, 569, 570f
Cryptosporidium parvum, 569, 570f
Crystalloid fluids
  balanced, 129–130
  classification of, 129–130
  isotonic, 129
  shock treated with, 128–130, 130t, 148
CsA. *See* Cyclosporine
CSOC. *See* Crisis standards of care
Curreri formula, 683
Cutaneous anthrax, 560
cVEEG. *See* Continuous video
    electroencephalography
CXCL9, 38t
CXCL10, 38t
CXCL13, 38t
Cyanide inhalation injury, 699–701
Cyclones, 124
Cyclophilin A, 47
Cyclosarin, 580
Cyclosporine, 47
CYD-TDV vaccine, 499
Cyproheptadine, 590
Cytokine storm
  cytokines in, 35–36, 36t
  pathogenesis of, 36–38
  thrombosis and, 306
Cytokines
  anti-inflammatory, 36t
  in cytokine storm, 35–36, 36t
  pro-inflammatory, 37t, 91
  in septic shock, 139
  types of, 36t–38t

D
D-Dimer, 95–96
Dabigatran, 100

Damage-associated molecular patterns,
    91
Damage control resuscitation, 107
DAMPs. *See* Damage-associated
    molecular patterns
Decompressive craniectomy, 610
Decompressive hemicraniectomy, 614
Deconditioning, in older adults, 310
Decontamination
  COVID-19, 18
  health care workers, 86
  moist heat, 81t, 82
  nerve gas exposure, 581
  surgical instruments, 601
Decubitus ulcers, 30
Deep venous thrombosis
  in critically ill patients, 99–100
  prophylaxis for, in burn patients, 683
Deliriogenics, 585, 586t–587t, 588, 591
Delirium
  agitation associated with, 327–333
  antipsychotics for, 174–175
  in COVID-19, 304
  drug-induced, 589
  hyperactive, 328
  hypoactive, 328–329, 330t
  in older adults, 304–306, 305t
Delirium Rating Scale, 304
Dengue fever, 73t, 97, 539
Dengue hemorrhagic fever, 97–98
Dengue shock syndrome, 97–98
Dengue virus
  in children, 538–540
  clinical manifestations of, 496–497
  complications of, 497
  description of, 97–98
  diagnosis of, 497–498
  epidemiology of, 539
  high-risk populations for, 496
  imaging of, 497f
  laboratory testing for, 498
  management of, 499
  pathogenesis of, 495–496
  prognosis for, 499
  serologic testing of, 498
  serotypes of, 496
  Tourniquet test for, 498, 498f
  vaccine for, 499
  vectors of, 495, 496f
Dexamethasone, 250t, 419t

Dexmedetomidine, 165t, 172–173, 329 332
DF. *See* Dengue fever
DHF. *See* Dengue hemorrhagic fever
Diabetes mellitus
 COVID-19 effects on, 201–202, 406
 critical illness effects on, 200–201
Diabetic ketoacidosis, 11, 201–202
Diagnostic peritoneal lavage, 646–647
Diarrhea, Ebola virus as cause of, 480–482, 481t, 484
Differential multi-ventilation, 177–179
Dimercaprol, 584
Dipeptidyl peptidase 4, 384
Direct oral anticoagulants
 reversal of, 102–103
 venous thromboembolism treated with, 100–103
Disasters. *See* Natural disasters
Disease modifying anti-rheumatic drugs, 501
Disposable gowns, 83–84
Disseminated intravascular coagulation, 481
Distributive shock
 definition of, 139
 treatment of, 139, 148, 150
DKA. *See* Diabetic ketoacidosis
DMV. *See* Differential multi-ventilation
DNAR. *See* Do not attempt resuscitation
DNR. *See* Do not resuscitate
Do not attempt resuscitation, 15
Do not resuscitate, 15
DOACs. *See* Direct oral anticoagulants
Dobutamine, 133t, 136
Documentation, 28–29
Docusate sodium, 167t
Dopamine, 133t, 136–137
Dopamine receptors, 135
Doxycycline
 plague treated with, 467t–468t, 468–469
 tularemia treated with, 476
DPL. *See* Diagnostic peritoneal lavage
Drains, 640
Driving pressure, 183, 213–214
Droplet precautions, 72
Drowning

cardiopulmonary resuscitation for, 708
prognosis for, 708
venovenous extracorporeal membrane oxygenation for, 287
DSS. *See* Dengue shock syndrome
Duodenal trauma, 655
Dynamic left ventricular outflow obstruction, 143–144

E
E. coli 0175:H7, 564, 564f
Early goal directed therapy, for shock, 128
Early thoracotomy, 641–642
Earthquakes, 124, 704
Ebola hemorrhagic fever, 481
Ebola Treatment Centers, 488
Ebola virus
 atoltivimab, maftivimab, and odesivimab-ebgn cocktail for, 485, 486t
 case fatality rate for, 490
 CDC precautions for, 487
 in children, 537–538
 clinical manifestations of, 481t, 481–482
 clinical presentation of, 537
 coagulopathy caused by, 481, 485
 coinfection, 485
 complications of, 488
 description of, 73t, 98
 diagnosis of, 482–483
 diarrhea caused by, 480–482, 481t, 484
 discovery of, 478
 disseminated intravascular coagulation caused by, 480
 epidemiology of, 478–479, 537
 fluid resuscitation for, 483–484
 funeral practices for, 488
 healthcare setting practices for, 486–488
 infection control in, 485–489
 laboratory findings in, 482
 long-term functional limitations caused by, 489
 metabolic derangements caused by, 484
 mortality rates for, 490

Ebola virus (*Cont.*)
  outbreaks of, 478, 485–486
  pandemic caused by
    blood transfusions in, 109t
    nurse safety in, 24
  pathogenesis of, 480–481
  personal protective equipment for
    control of, 483, 486–487
  prognosis for, 489
  public health measures for, 488
  renal failure caused by, 484
  respiratory failure caused by, 484
  risk factors for, 478–479
  signs and symptoms of, 480–482,
    481t, 537
  superinfection, 485
  therapies specifically for, 485, 486t
  transmission of, 479, 486
  treatment of, 483–485, 537–538
  vaccine for, 486t, 488–489
  zoonotic nature of, 479
Ebolavirus, 478, 479f
Echocardiography
  shock findings, 140, 143f
  transthoracic, 415
ECMO. *See* Extracorporeal membrane
    oxygenation
EDT. *See* Emergency department
    thoracotomy
EEG. *See* Electroencephalography
Eicosanoids, 39
Elastase, 92
Elder Life Program, The, 304
Electrical burns, 679
Electroencephalography, 615
ELSO. *See* Extracorporeal Life Support
    Organization
Embolism. *See* Pulmonary embolism
Emergency department thoracotomy,
    641
Emotion-focused coping, 370
Empyema, 642
Encephalitis, 73t
Encephalopathy, post-influenza, 455
Endocrine system
  description of, 195
  hypothalamic pituitary adrenal axis,
    196–197
  hypothalamic pituitary reproductive
    axis, 199–200

  hypothalamic pituitary thyroid axis,
    197–199
Endothelial cell dysregulation, 91
Endothelium, 40
Endotracheal tubes, in prone-positioned
    patients, 30
Enteral nutrition
  for burn patients, 683
  in extracorporeal membrane
    oxygenation, 271
  in mechanical ventilation, 29
Epidemic typhus, 570
Epidural hemorrhage, 610
Epinephrine, 133t, 135
Epoprostenol, 222
Epsilon toxin, 562–563
Ervebo, 486t, 488
Erythropoiesis-stimulating agents, 113
ESAs. *See* Erythropoiesis-stimulating
    agents
Esophageal trauma, 635
Etesevimab, 420
Ethical considerations
  in extracorporeal membrane
    oxygenation, 289–292
  in pediatric mass critical care,
    365–367
Euthyroid sick syndrome, 197–199
EVs. *See* Extracellular vesicles
Expiratory positive airway pressure,
    for acute respiratory distress
    syndrome, 211
External fixators, for open fractures,
    663–664, 664f
Extracellular vesicles, 91
Extracorporeal Life Support
    Organization, 259, 281
Extracorporeal membrane oxygenation
  acute respiratory distress syndrome
    managed with, 219–220
  "chatter" during, 271
  circuit components, 259–261, 260f
  clinical uses of, 257
  complications of
    acute kidney injury, 282
    circuit-specific, 283–284
    coagulopathy, 281–282
    hemorrhagic, 281–282
    infectious, 283
    intracranial hemorrhage, 283

Extracorporeal membrane oxygenation
      (*Cont.*)
   mechanical failure, 281
   neurological, 283
   renal, 282–283
   contraindications for, 269t–270t, 271
   COVID-19 uses of, 288–289
   definition of, 257
   ECPR treated with, 284–286
   enteral nutrition in, 271
   ethical considerations in, 289–292
   evolution of, 258–259
   history of, 258
   in-hospital cardiac arrests treated
      with, 285–286
   management of, 271, 273–278, 277t
   out-of-hospital cardiac arrests treated
      with, 286
   patient selection for, 267, 270–271
   resource considerations in, 289–292
   respiratory failure treated with, 261,
      268f
   survival prediction scores for, 270,
      272t–275t
   team preparation for, 289, 290t–291t
   technological advancements in,
      258–259
   thrombosis associated with, 276f,
      281–282
   venoarterial
      acute respiratory distress syndrome
         treated with, 219
      cannulation configurations for,
         263f
      cardiac strain caused by, 263
      cardiac support goal of, 276, 278
      cardiogenic shock treated with, 261
      cerebral oxygenation in, 277
      description of, 257
      hybrid configurations, 264, 265f
      indications for, 261, 264–265, 266t
      management of, 276–278
      patient selection for, 270–271
      survival prediction score, 272t–273t
      Swan-Ganz catheter with, 276
      weaning from, 278, 279f
   venovenous
      acute respiratory distress syndrome
         treated with, 219–220
      algorithm for, 267, 268f

      in burn patients, 287
      cannulation configurations for,
         262f
      description of, 257–258
      in drowning victims, 287
      H1N1 influenza pandemic treated
         with, 287–288
      indications for, 261, 265, 267
      lung recovery signs in, 279
      lung-rest as goal of, 278
      management of, 278
      patient selection for, 270
      respiratory failure treated with,
         261, 268f
      survival prediction score, 274t–275t
      thrombosis associated with, 276f
      in trauma patients, 287
      ventilatory settings in, 278
      weaning from, 278, 280
   weaning from, 278–280, 279f
   withdrawal of care, 289, 292
Extreme temperatures, 123–124
Extubation failure, 185–186

F
Face masks, 6
Face shields, 8, 78, 78f
Facepiece respirators, 72
Factor X, 92
Falls, 307–308
Family communication, 15
Famotidine, 49
Fasciotomy, 668
FAST examination, 600, 646
Fat embolism, 670
Favipiravir, 49, 522
FDPs. *See* Fibrin degradation products
Febrile transfusion reactions, 111
Fentanyl, 164t, 168, 170
Fibrin degradation products, 95
Field hospitals, 598, 599t–600t
Filoviruses
   description of, 96
   Ebola virus. *See* Ebola virus
   Marburg virus, 490–491, 491f–492f
FiO_2, 14
First-degree burn, 676, 676t
Flail chest, 630
Flaviviruses, 97
Floods, 124, 597

Fluid overload
in acute kidney injury, 232–233
diuretic therapy for, 233
in shock, 137–138
Fluid resuscitation
for acute respiratory distress
syndrome, 222–223
for burns, 679–680, 688–689
for Ebola virus, 483–484
for sepsis, 128
for shock. *See* Shock
Flumazenil, 171
Flying foxes, 512–513, 516, 541
Foley catheters, 640, 649
Fondaparinux, 100
4-factor prothrombin complex
concentrate, 114
FOUR score, 605
Fractures
closed, 671–672
flail chest secondary to, 630
open, 661–666, 662f, 664f–665f
rib, 629–630
Francisella tularensis, 473–476, 536, 553
Fresh whole blood transfusion, 600–601
Freshwater aspiration, 705

G
G-series nerve agents, 580
GAD. *See* Generalized anxiety disorder
Gangrene, 466f, 571f
GCS. *See* Glasgow Coma Scale
Generalized anxiety disorder, 341
Gentamicin
plague treated with, 467t, 467–468
tularemia treated with, 476
GFR. *See* Glomerular filtration rate
Glandular syndrome, 474
Glasgow Coma Scale, 605, 612, 707
Glomerular filtration rate, 229
Gloves, 84–85
Glucocorticoids, 223
Glycemic control
in critical illness, 200
in older adults, 315
GM-CSF. *See* Granulocyte
macrophage-colony stimulating
factor
Gowns, 83–84
Graham, Thomas, 129

Granulocyte macrophage-colony
stimulating factor, 37t
Great vessels, 653–654
Guillain-Barré syndrome, 406–407, 455
Gustilo and Anderson classification, of
open fractures, 662

H
Haemophilus influenzae, 437
Hallucinations, 348
Hallucinogens, 585, 586t–587t, 588–591
Haloperidol, 166t, 174–175, 331
Hand sanitizers, 85–86
Hand washing, 7
Harlequin syndrome, 278
Harris-Benedict equation, 683
HBOCs. *See* Hemoglobin-based oxygen
carriers
HCQ. *See* Hydrochloroquine
Health care associated pneumonia, 149t
Health care workers
in COVID-19, 334–336, 416
decontamination of, 86
protection of, during burn
management, 692
Health crisis, 3
Heart
blunt injury to, 633–634
penetrating injury to, 637–638
Heat, for mask recycling, 81t, 81–82
Heatwaves, 123–124
Heimlich valve, 640
Heliox, 182
Helper T cells, 36
Hemagglutinin, 426, 442, 532
Hemodynamic monitoring, of shock,
138, 141
Hemoglobin-based oxygen carriers, for
hemorrhagic shock, 147
Hemophagocytic lymphohistiocytosis,
540
Hemorrhagic fever viruses
Crimean-Congo, 99
dengue virus, 97–98
Ebola virus, 98
Lassa virus, 99
overview of, 96–97
yellow fever, 98
Hemorrhagic fevers, 73t
Hemorrhagic shock, 145, 147–148

Hendra virus, 73t, 516–518
HEPA filter air scrubbers. *See* High efficiency particulate air filter air scrubbers
Heparin, 50, 182, 421
Hepatitis A, 125
Hepatitis E, 125
HES. *See* Hydroxyethyl starch
HeV. *See* Hendra virus
HFNC. *See* High flow nasal cannula
High efficiency particulate air filter air scrubbers, 4, 5f, 77
High flow nasal cannula, 12, 210–212
High-mobility group box 1 protein, 91–92
HLH. *See* Hemophagocytic lymphohistiocytosis
HMGB-1. *See* High-mobility group box 1 protein
H1N1 virus
  imaging of, 438f
  mortality caused by, 442–443
  pandemic caused by, 436t, 437–438, 454, 532
  thrombosis associated with, 93
  venovenous extracorporeal membrane oxygenation for, 287–288
H2N2 virus, 437
H3N2 virus, 437
H5N1 virus, 440, 443, 447
H7N9 virus, 440, 443, 447, 454
H9N2 virus, 440
H$_2$O$_2$. *See* Hydrogen peroxide
"Hong Kong flu," 436t, 532
Hospital
  cardiac arrests in, 31
  COVID-19 protocol, 31
  evacuation of, during natural disaster, 598
  field, 598, 599t–600t
  older adult care in, 302t, 303–311
Hospital Elder Life Program, 304
HPA axis. *See* Hypothalamic-pituitary-adrenal axis
HPV. *See* Hydrogen peroxide vapor
Humor, 374
Hurricanes, 597
Hydrochloroquine, 47
Hydrogen cyanide, 578, 699

Hydrogen peroxide, 39
Hydrogen peroxide vapor, 80, 81t, 83
Hydromorphone, 164t, 169–170
Hydroxocobalamin, 701
Hydroxyethyl starch, 131t, 132
Hydroxyl radicals, 39
Hyperactive delirium, 328
Hypercoagulability, 405
Hyperglycemia, 315, 317
Hyperkalemia, 232
Hyperlactemia, 138
Hyperlipidemia, 55
Hyperosmolar therapy, in traumatic brain injury, 613
Hyperthermia
  malignant, 328t
  neurogenic, 612
  psychotomimetic agents as cause of, 591
  after traumatic brain injury, 612–613
  treatment of, 613
Hypertonic saline, 182
Hypertriglyceridemia, 172
Hypertrophic cardiomyopathy, 141
Hypoactive delirium, 328–329, 330t
Hypoglycemia, 315, 317
Hypomania, 347
Hypothalamic pituitary adrenal axis, 140, 196–197
Hypothalamic pituitary reproductive axis, 199–200
Hypothalamic pituitary thyroid axis, 197–199
Hypothermia, 137
Hypothyroidism, 150
Hypovolemia, 361, 361f
Hypovolemic shock
  causes of, 145–147
  description of, 127, 140
  pediatric, 361
Hypoxemia
  acute respiratory distress syndrome as cause of, 206–207, 207f, 216
  in COVID-19 patients, 407
  definition of, 206
  refractory, 216–218
  silent, 407
  thrombosis and, 94–95

I

IAA. *See* Isoamyl acetate
IABP. *See* Intra-aortic balloon pump
IAH. *See* Intra-abdominal
    hypertension
ICP. *See* Intracranial pressure
ICU. *See* Intensive care unit
Idarucizumab, 102
IHCA. *See* In-hospital cardiac arrest
IHD. *See* Intermittent hemodialysis
Immersion injuries, 704–708
Immunoglobulin Manual muscle
    testing, 97
Immunothrombosis, 94
In-hospital cardiac arrest, 31
Incontinence, 310
Infection control
    for Ebola virus, 485–489
    for Hendra virus, 518
    for influenza virus, 453–454
    for Nipah virus, 515–516
    in older adults, 310
    for plague, 469–471
    for Rift Valley fever virus, 522–523
Inferior vena cava
    compressibility of, 146f
    traumatic injuries to, 654
Influenza Hospitalization Surveillance
    Network, 532
Influenza Risk Assessment Tool, 438,
    449
Influenza virus
    A, 434, 532
    antivirals for, 446–449, 448t
    B, 434
    bacterial pneumonia caused by, 444
    C, 434
    cardiac sequelae of, 455
    in children, 531–533
    clinical manifestations of, 444–445
    clinical presentation of, 533
    complications of, 454–456, 533
    conjunctivitis associated with,
        455–456
    D, 434
    deaths caused by, 532
    description of, 73t
    diagnosis of, 445–446
    encephalopathy after, 455
    epidemiology of, 435–441, 531–532

Haemophilus influenzae as cause of,
    437
    hepatic involvement by, 455
    H1N1, 93
    hospitalizations for, 532
    incubation period of, 444
    infection control in, 453–454
    masks for, 453
    myositis associated with, 456
    neurological complications of, 455
    non-pharmaceutical interventions
        for, 451–453
    novel types of, 440–441, 445
    oseltamivir for, 447–449, 448t, 533
    pandemics caused by
        "Asian flu," 436t, 437, 532
        description of, 435–438, 436f, 436t,
            532
        "Hong Kong flu," 436t, 532
        lessons learned from, 456–458
        1918, 109t, 435, 436f, 436t,
            441–442, 445, 449, 451, 532
        2009, 445
    pathophysiology of, 442–444
    personal hygiene measures for,
        453
    polymerase chain reaction detection
        of, 446
    post-exposure prophylaxis for, 451
    prevention of, 449–453
    prognosis for, 456
    pulmonary complications of, 444
    rhabdomyolysis associated with,
        456
    risk factors for, 441–442
    schizophrenia and, 456
    seasonal, 441
    signs and symptoms of, 445–446,
        533
    social distancing for, 451
    strains of, 93, 434
    surveillance of, 438, 440f
    swine strains of, 440–441
    tests for, 446, 446t
    transmission of, 441–442
    travel restrictions for, 451
    treatment of, 446–449, 448t
    vaccinations for, 450–451, 452f
    variants, 440–441
    viral shedding, 442

Inhalation injury
  burns as cause of, 680–681
  carbon monoxide, 699
  classification of, 695, 696t
  cyanide, 699–701
  definition of, 695
  radiologist's score for, 698t
  smoke inhalation, 696–698
Inhaled vasodilators, 221–222
Inmazeb, 486t, 488
Insomnia, 314–315
Institute of Medicine, 26
Intensive care unit
  analgesia in. See Analgesia
  in austere conditions, 598,
    600–601
  blood products in, 105
  burn management in, 691
  COVID-19 management, 4–5
  decubitus ulcers in, 30
  neuropsychiatric sequelae after
    leaving, 333–334
  nursing adjustments in, 11–12
  nutrition in, 29–30
  older adults in, 301, 303
  patient monitoring in, 31
  sedation in, 170–174, 329–330
  tiered-based staffing, 11–12
Interferon(s), 35, 52, 391, 393
Interferon-τ, 37t
Interferon stimulating genes, 52
Interleukin(s), 35
Interleukin-1, 37t
Interleukin-2, 37t
Interleukin-4, 36t
Interleukin-6
  antagonists of, 50–52
  COVID-19 and, 50, 404–405
  inhibitors of, 419t, 421
  thrombin stimulation of, 93
Interleukin-8, 50
Interleukin-9, 37t
Interleukin-10, 36t
Interleukin-12, 37t
Interleukin-13, 36t
Interleukin-17, 37t
Interleukin-18, 37t
Interleukin-33, 36t
Interleukin-35, 36t
Interleukin-37, 36t

Intermittent hemodialysis, 233, 234,
    237, 238t
International Society for Peritoneal
    Dialysis, 235
Intestinal trauma, 654–655
Intra-abdominal hypertension, 231
Intra-aortic balloon pump, 152
Intraabdominal pressure, 649
Intracranial hemorrhage, 283
Intracranial pressure
  monitoring of, 611–615
  rising of, 607
Intraoperative autologous transfusions,
    113
Intraosseous infusion, 126
Intravenous pumps, 27, 27f
Intubation, 12–13
IOM. See Institute of Medicine
IRI. See Ischemic reperfusion injury
Ischemia, 38–39
Ischemic reperfusion injury, 38–40
ISGs. See Interferon stimulating genes
Isoamyl acetate, 78
Isolation precautions, 71–72
Isotonic crystalloid fluids, 129
ISPD. See International Society for
    Peritoneal Dialysis
Ivermectin, 52–53

J
Janssen vaccine, 425t
Janus kinase inhibitor, 45
Jet nebulizers, 180–181
The Joint Commission, 26
Jugular bulb catheters, 616–617
"Jump START," 353

K
KDIGO. See Kidney Disease
    Improving Global Outcome
Ketamine, 10, 164t, 165t, 173–174
Kidney(s). See also Renal system
  acute injury of. See Acute kidney injury
  COVID-19 involvement of, 405, 408
  trauma to, 652–653
Kidney Disease Improving Global
    Outcome, 228, 230

L
Laceration
  renal, 653
  splenic, 650

Lactated Ringer's solution, 130t
Lactic acidosis, 138
Lactulose, 167t
Landslides, 123, 597
Large-bore straight fenestrated tubes, 640
Lassa fever, 73t, 99, 505–506, 538, 540
Lassa virus, 99, 505–506
Late thoracotomy, 642
Latex gloves, 84
Laughter, 374
LC-NE. *See* Locus coeruleus-norepinephrine
Left ventricular assist devices, 141
Left ventricular outflow obstruction, dynamic, 143–144
Leukotrienes, 39
Levofloxacin, for plague, 467t, 469
Lewisite, 579t, 584
Leydig cells, 199
Limb salvage therapy, 668
Liver trauma, 651–652
Locus coeruleus-norepinephrine, 196
Lopinavir, 52
Lorazepam, 165t, 171
Low molecular weight heparin, 96, 100, 103, 421–422
Lower extremity compartment syndrome, 669
Lung sliding, 144, 145f
Lung-ultrasound score, 413–414
LUS. *See* Lung-ultrasound score
LVADs. *See* Left ventricular assist devices
Lymphopenia, 405

M
Macrophages, 35
Maculopapular vesicles, 556f, 558f
Magnesium citrate, 167t
Major depressive disorder
  in children, 345–347, 346t
  suicidal ideation associated with, 345–346
Malaria, 125
MALDI-TOF. *See* Matrix-assisted laser desorption/ionization-time of flight mass spectrometry
Malignant hyperthermia, 328t
Mannitol, 613, 621

Mannose-binding lectin, 40
Mannose-binding lectin-associated serine protease pathways, 40
MAP. *See* Mean arterial pressure
MAP-ICP. *See* Mean arterial pressure-intracranial pressure
MAPK. *See* Mitogen-activated protein kinase
Marburg virus, 490–491, 491f–492f
Masks
  fit testing of, 78–79
  influenza virus, 453
  N95, 6–8, 9f, 76, 77f, 79
  for 1918 influenza pandemic, 78–79
  re-using, 79–83
  recycling of
    description of, 79–80
    heat, 81t, 81–82
    hydrogen peroxide for, 83
    hydrogen peroxide vapor for, 80, 81t
    ultraviolet germicidal irritation for, 80–81
  surgical, 72, 73t, 76, 76f, 79
Mass casualty events
  biological threats and, 672
  COVID-19 as. *See* COVID-19
  definition of, 162
  pediatric patients in, 351–352
Mass casualty incidents
  burn management in, 686
  pediatric trauma management in, 360–362
Massive hemothorax, 641
Massive transfusion protocol, 107
Mastomys natalensis, 505
Matrix-assisted laser desorption/ionization-time of flight mass spectrometry, 466
McConnell sign, 142, 143f, 144
MCI. *See* Mass casualty incidents
MDIs. *See* Metered dose inhalers
MDMA, 590
Mean arterial pressure, 121, 126, 139
Mean arterial pressure-intracranial pressure, 607
Meaning-focused coping, 370
Mechanical circulatory support device, 257, 267

Mechanical ventilation
  acute respiratory distress syndrome
    treated with. *See* Acute respiratory
    distress syndrome, mechanical
    ventilation for
  alternatives to, 177–183
  constipation management in, 166,
    167t–168t
  COVID-19-related respiratory failure
    managed with, 13–14
  decubitus ulcers in patients receiving,
    29
  differential multi-ventilation, 177–179
  enteral support for, 29
  extubation, 185–186, 215–216
  goals of, 180
  indications for, 177
  pressure meter dosing inhaler use in,
    180, 181t
  readiness testing, 216
  spontaneous breathing trials, 185
  synchronized intermittent, 177
  tracheostomy, 186–187
  troubleshooting, 183–187, 184t
  ventilator induced lung injury,
    183–185, 185f
Mediastinitis, 635–636
Mediastinum, 627
Medication(s). *See also* Repurposed
    drugs; *specific medication*
  administration of, by nurses, 26–28
  aerosolized delivery of, 180–182
  errors involving, 26–27
  off-label prescribing of, 313–314
  for older adults, 311–314, 312t
  pharmacokinetics of, 311, 312t
Meditation, 376
Memorial Delirium Assessment, 304
Meningeal plague, 466
Meningitis, 149t
Meningoencephalitis, 521–522
Mental health issues, 338–348. *See also*
    Psychiatric disorders
MERS. *See* Middle East Respiratory
    Syndrome
MERS-CoV. *See* Middle East
    Respiratory Syndrome-CoV
Metabolic acidosis, 232
Metered dose inhalers, 12
Methadone, 164t, 169–170

Methylene blue, 53
Methylnaltrexone, 166, 168t
Microwaves, for mask recycling, 81–82
Midazolam, 10, 165t, 171
Middle East Respiratory Syndrome
  blood transfusions in, 109t
  description of, 53, 73t
  endocrinologic effects of, 195
  extracorporeal membrane
    oxygenation in, 288
  thrombocytopenia associated with, 94
Middle East Respiratory Syndrome-CoV
  in children, 529–530
  clinical manifestations of, 387–388
  computed tomography findings in,
    388
  cytopathic effect of, 385
  description of, 93
  diagnosis of, 389–390
  epidemiology of, 382, 529
  history of, 381
  mortality rates for, 388
  pathophysiology of, 384–385, 385f
  risk factors for, 382–383
  signs and symptoms of, 529
  treatment of, 392–394
  vaccine for, 393–394
Military
  medical facility classification of,
    618–619
  traumatic brain injury in, 606
Milrinone, 134t
Mindfulness, 374
MIS. *See* Multisystem inflammatory
    syndrome
Mitogen-activated protein kinase, 45
Moist heat decontamination, 81t, 82
Monkeypox
  bioterrorism uses of, 557f–558f,
    557–558
  in children, 543–546
  clinical manifestations of, 557–558
Monoclonal antibodies, 420
Monro-Kellie doctrine, 606
Moral injury, 335
Morphine, 164t, 169
Mosquito-borne diseases
  Chikungunya virus, 499–501, 500f
  Dengue virus. *See* Dengue virus
  Rift Valley fever virus, 519

Motor vehicle accidents
  abdominal trauma caused by, 645
  blunt aortic injury caused by, 632
  thoracic trauma caused by, 626
mRNA-1273 vaccine, 425t
MTMC. *See* Multi-threat medical
  countermeasure
MTP. *See* Massive transfusion protocol
Multi-threat medical countermeasure,
  578
Multisystem inflammatory syndrome
  in adults, 408–409
  in children, 406, 408, 531
Multisystem organ failure, 138
Murine typhus, 570
Murray score for acute lung injury, 631
Mustard gases, 582–583
Mvabea, 486t, 488
Myocardial contusion, 633
Myocarditis, 407
Myositis, 456
Myxedema coma, 150
Myxedema crisis, 150

N
N-acetylcysteine, 698
N95-FFRs, 77f, 78–79, 82
N95 masks, 6–8, 9f, 76, 77f, 79, 454
N-methyl-D-aspartate receptors, 169
Naloxone, 166, 591
National Center for Immunization and
  Respiratory Disease, 72
National Institute of Occupational
  Safety and Health, 7
Natural disasters
  acute respiratory infections after, 125
  blood transfusions in, 600–601
  diarrheal diseases after, 125
  earthquakes, 124, 597
  extreme temperatures, 123–124, 597
  field hospitals for, 598, 599t–600t
  floods, 124, 597
  hospital evacuation during, 598
  infectious sequelae of, 125
  injuries caused by, 597
  landslides, 123, 597
  outbreaks after, 125
  pediatric patients in, 351–352,
    355–357
  renal replacement therapy in, 601

  shock caused by, 122–125
  Small Portable Expeditionary
    Aeromedical Rapid Response team
    for, 598, 599t–600t
  storms, 124–125, 597
  sudden-onset, 122
  tornadoes, 122–123, 597
  tsunami, 597
  ultrasound uses in, 600
  volcanic eruptions, 123, 597
  wildfires, 123, 597
Natural killer cells, 35
NCIRD. *See* National Center for
    Immunization and Respiratory
    Disease
Near-infrared spectroscopy, 617
Nebulizers, 180–181
Necrotizing fasciitis, 149t
Negative pressure vacuum assisted
    closure, 184
Neisseria meningitides, 553
Nerve agents, 578–582, 579t
NETs. *See* Neutrophil extracellular
    traps
Neuraminidase, 426, 532
Neuraminidase inhibitors, 447
"Neuro-storming," 591
Neurogenic hyperthermia, 612
Neuroleptic malignant syndrome, 327,
    328t
Neurological system
  COVID-19 manifestations of, 406
  influenza virus complications of, 455
Neuromuscular blocking agents
  acute respiratory distress syndrome
    treated with, 220–221
  description of, 175–177, 176t
Neutrophil extracellular traps, 92
Neutrophils, 35
1918 influenza pandemic, 109t, 435,
    436f, 436t, 441–442, 445, 449, 451,
    532
NIOSH. *See* National Institute of
    Occupational Safety and Health
Nipah virus
  blood transfusions for, 110t
  in children, 541–542
  clinical manifestations of, 514
  complications of, 516
  description of, 73t, 91

Nipah virus (*Cont.*)
  diagnosis of, 514–515
  epidemiology of, 512–514, 541
  infection control for, 515–516
  outbreaks of, 512–513
  pathogenesis of, 514
  prevention of, 515–516
  prognosis for, 516
  risk factors for, 512–514
  treatment of, 515
  vectors of, 512–513
Nitric oxide
  description of, 39
  inhaled, for acute respiratory distress
    syndrome, 221–222
Nitrile gloves, 84–85
Nitrogen mustards, 579t, 584
NiV. *See* Nipah virus
NMBAs. *See* Neuromuscular blocking
  agents
NMS. *See* Neuroleptic malignant
  syndrome
NO. *See* Nitric oxide
Non-invasive ventilation, 12
Nonsteroidal anti-inflammatory drugs,
  316t
Norepinephrine, 133t, 135
Nucleic acid amplification testing with
    reverse transcriptase-polymerase
    chain reaction assay, 409–411, 426
Nurse(s)
  documentation, 28–29
  medication administration by, 26–28
  medication errors, 26–27
  "prone position" team, 25–26
  safety of, 24–25
  staffing of, 23–24
Nursing
  in COVID-19, 11–12, 23–31
  in intensive care unit, 11–12
Nutrition
  for burn patients, 683, 690
  in COVID-19 protocol, 15
  immunity and, 375–376
  in intensive care unit, 29–30
  in older adults, 309

O
O_2. *See* Superoxide
Obstructive shock

acute right heart syndrome as cause
    of, 142
  cardiac tamponade as cause of,
    142–143, 143f, 151
  causes of, 142–144
  dynamic left ventricular outflow
    obstruction as cause of, 143–144
  pulmonary embolus as cause of, 142,
    144, 151
  tension pneumothorax as cause of, 144
Oculoglandular syndrome, 474
Off-label prescribing, 313–314
OH-. *See* Hydroxyl radicals
Oklahoma City bombing, 360
Olanzapine, 166t
Older adults
  age thresholds for, 300–301
  care transitions in, 317–318
  constipation in, 315
  deconditioning in, 310
  delirium in, 304–306, 305t
  demographics of, 300
  "deprescribing" in, 311
  disability in, 310
  in disasters, 301, 302t
  falls in, 307–308
  glycemic control in, 315
  goals of care for, 303
  health care resource allocation for,
    301, 302t
  hospital care for, 302t, 303–311
  hospital prescribing for, 302t
  hyperglycemia in, 315, 317
  hypoglycemia in, 315, 317
  in ICUs, 301, 303
  incontinence in, 310
  infection control in, 310
  insomnia in, 314–315
  medication management for,
    311–314, 312t
  nutrition for, 309
  pain in, 314, 316t–317t
  physical therapy for, 310–311
  polypharmacy in, 311
  pressure injuries in, 308–309
  protein-calorie undernutrition in, 309
  restraints in, 307–308
  sedatives in, 314–315
  thrombosis prevention in, 306–307
  urinary incontinence in, 310

Oleoresin capsicum, 592–594
OLV. *See* Open lung ventilation
One Health approach, 457
Open fractures, 661–666, 662f, 664f–665f
Open lung ventilation, 217–218
Open pneumothorax, 638
Opioids
  advantages of, 163, 166
  analgesic uses of, 163, 166
  constipation caused by, 166, 167t–168t
  dosing of, 170
  fentanyl, 164t, 168
  flumazenil reversal of, 171
  hydromorphone, 164t, 169–170
  hyperalgesia caused by, 166
  methadone, 164t, 169–170
  morphine, 164t, 169
  pain management using, 317t
  remifentanil, 164t, 169
  respiratory depression caused by, 166, 170
  side effects of, 166, 170
  sufentanil, 164t, 169
Organ transplantation. *See* Transplantation
Organic psychosis, 588
Orphans, 528
Ortho-chlorbenzylidene malononitrile, 592–594
Orthopedic trauma
  closed fractures, 671–672
  in combat settings, 672
  compartment syndrome, 666–671
  initial assessment of, 660–661
  open fractures, 661–666, 662f, 664f–665f
  thromboembolism in, 670–671
  triage for, 671
  wartime occurrences of, 672
Oseltamivir, 447–449, 448t, 533
Osmotic laxatives, 167t
Osteomyelitis, 149t, 309
Oxygen generators, 258, 601
Oxygen supplementation, 419t

P
P-selectin, 92
Packed red blood cells, 647

PAI-1. *See* Plasminogen activator inhibitor-1
Pain
  background, 681
  breakthrough, 681–682
  burn-related, 681–682, 690
  in older adults, 314, 316t–317t
  procedural, 681
PAMP. *See* Pathogen-associated molecular patterns
Pandemic(s), 72
  "Asian flu," 436t, 437
  blood transfusions in, 108, 109t–110t
  COVID-19. *See* COVID-19
  extracorporeal membrane oxygenation uses in, 287–289
  H1N1 virus, 436t, 437–438, 438f, 454
  "Hong Kong flu," 436t, 437
  influenza virus, 435–438, 436f, 436t
  phases of, 439f
  psychiatric disorders caused by, 334
  "Spanish flu," 435–437, 436t
  transplantations in, 254
  World Health Organization phases, 439f
Pandemic Intervals Framework, 439f, 451
Pandemic respiratory viruses, 93–96
Panic disorder, 340–342
PAOP. *See* Pulmonary artery occlusion pressure
PAPRs. *See* Powered air-purifying respirators
PAR-1. *See* Protease-activated receptor-1
Parkinsonism, 455
Parkland formula, 679
Paroxysmal sympathetic hyperactivity, 330–331
Passive leg raising, 146
Pathogen-associated molecular patterns, 36, 46, 91
Patient monitoring, in intensive care unit, 31
Pattern recognition receptors, 91
PCC. *See* Prothrombin complex concentrate
PCI. *See* Penetrating cardiac injury; Percutaneous coronary intervention

PCV. *See* Pressure control ventilation
PE. *See* Pulmonary embolism
Pediatric Index of Mortality, 354
Pediatric intensive care unit, 356–357
Pediatric patients
  adjustment disorder in, 347–348
  adults and, differences between,
    350–351
  agoraphobia in, 342
  anxiety disorders in, 339t, 339–343
  bipolar disorder in, 346–347
  Chikungunya virus in, 539
  COVID-19 in, 530–531
  Crimean-Congo hemorrhagic fever
    in, 538, 540
  crisis incidents involving
    acute stress reactions caused by,
      364
    education and training for,
      357–360
    emotional considerations, 363t,
      363–365
    ethical issues in, 365–367
    full-scale exercise for, 358
    social considerations, 363t,
      363–365
    trauma management in, 360–362
  crisis standards of care for, 352–355
  Dengue virus in, 538–540
  in disasters, 351–352, 355–357
  Ebola virus in, 537–538
  education, 528
  equipment for, 527
  extraction of, 528
  generalized anxiety disorder in, 341
  Hendra virus in, 541–542
  illness severity scoring systems for,
    352–355
  influenza virus in, 531–533
  Lassa fever, 538, 540
  major depressive disorder in,
    345–347
  in mass casualty events, 351–352
  medications for, 527
  mental health issues in, 338–348
  Middle East Respiratory Syndrome-
    CoV in, 529–530
  monkeypox in, 543–546
  multisystem inflammatory syndrome
    in, 406, 408, 531
  Nipah virus in, 541–542
  orphaning of, 528
  oxygen delivery devices for, 529
  pandemics in
    general considerations for,
      526–528
    illnesses, 529–546
  panic disorder in, 340–342
  phobias in, 341
  plague in, 533–536
  post-traumatic stress disorder in, 338,
    343–345
  providers for, 527–528
  psychotic disorders in, 348
  Rift Valley fever in, 541–542
  SARS-CoV in, 529–531
  SARS-CoV2 in, 530–531
  selective mutism in, 342
  separation anxiety disorder in,
    340
  smallpox in, 542–543
  social anxiety disorder in, 342
  surge capacity planning for,
    355–357
  traumatic brain injuries in, 362
  treatment of, 350–351
  triage of, 352–355
  tularemia in, 536–537
  yellow fever in, 539–540
Pediatric Risk of Mortality, 354
PEEP. *See* Positive end-expiratory
    pressure
Pelvic trauma, blunt, 654
Penetrating cardiac injury, 637–638
Penetrating trauma
  abdominal, 645–646
  thoracic, 626, 636–637
Pepper spray, 592
Peramivir, 447, 448t
Percutaneous coronary intervention,
    152
Perfluorocarbons, 147
Pericardial effusion, 151–152, 634
Pericardial space, 142
Pericardial window, 151
Pericardiocentesis, 151–152
Peripheral cannulation, 261
Peritoneal dialysis, 235–236,
    238t–239t
Permissive hypotension, 138–139

Personal protective equipment
  biosafety of, 71, 72t
  bioterrorism agents, 74t–75t
  bleach solution, 85
  conservation, 72, 75–76
  in COVID-19 protocol, 6–8, 7t, 8f,
    186, 415
  decontamination of, 7–8
  for Ebola virus control, 483, 486–487
  gloves, 84–85
  gowns, 83–84
  hand sanitizers, 85–86
  health care worker decontamination,
    86
  isolation precautions, 71–72
  levels of, 7t
  masks. See Masks
  minimizing patient contact with,
    75–76
  for plague, 469
  purpose of, 71
PESI. See Pulmonary embolism
    severity index
Pestis minor, 465
pFra/pMT1, 464
Phenobarbital, 165t, 174
Phenylephrine, 134t, 135
Philips Respironics V60 BiPAP, 177
Phobias, 341
Phosgene oxime, 579t, 584–585
Phosphodiesterase 3 inhibitor, 132
"Phrenitis," 589
Physical therapy, 310–311
Pigtail tubes, 640
PIRRT. See Prolonged intermittent
    renal replacement therapies
Plague
  bioterrorism uses of, 534, 536
  bubonic, 464–465, 465f, 533–535
  in children, 533–536
  chloramphenicol for, 467t, 468
  ciprofloxacin for, 468t
  clinical manifestations of, 464–466,
    465f
  clinical presentation of, 534–535
  description of, 73t
  diagnosis of, 466
  doxycycline for, 467t–468t, 468–469
  epidemiology of, 462–463, 533–534
  gangrenous fingers caused by, 466f

gentamicin for, 467t, 467–468
geographic distribution of, 462,
    534–535
infection control in, 469–471
levofloxacin for, 467t, 469
meningeal, 466
outbreak control, 469–470
pandemics caused by, 534
pathophysiology of, 463–465
personal protective equipment for,
    469
pneumonic, 464–465, 535
post-exposure prophylaxis for, 468t
preventive measures in, 469–471
public health measures in, 469–471
septicemic, 465, 535
streptomycin for, 467, 467t
tetracycline for, 467t–468t,
    468–469
treatment of, 467t–468t, 467–469
vaccine for, 470–471, 535
vectors of, 462, 470, 533
World Health Organization
    management, 470t
Yersinia pestis as cause of, 462–471,
    463f, 533, 535
Plasma
  convalescent
    for COVID-19, 108, 110, 250t,
      391–392, 420
    for MERS-CoV, 393
    for 1918 influenza pandemic,
      449
  transfusion of, 105–106
PlasmaLyte, 130t
Plasminogen activator inhibitor-1, 93,
    95
Platelet(s)
  activation of, 92
  transfusion of, 105–106
Platelet plug, 92
Pleural effusion, 142
Pleural space, 627
PLR. See Passive leg raising
pMDI. See Pressure meter dosing
    inhaler
Pneumo-hemothorax, 629
Pneumomediastinum, 183–184, 185f,
    407, 627–629
Pneumonic plague, 464–465, 535

Pneumothorax
in COVID-19, 407
definition of, 627
open, 638
spontaneous, 627–628
tension, 144, 184–185, 627
Point-of-care ultrasound, 147
Poiseuille's law, 126
Polyethylene glycol, 167t
Polymerase chain reaction
Nipah virus diagnosis using, 514–515
nucleic acid amplification testing with
reverse transcriptase-polymerase
chain reaction assay, 409–411, 426
plague diagnosis using, 466
Polypharmacy, 311
Porcine reproductive and respiratory
syndrome virus, 53
Positive end-expiratory pressure
acute respiratory distress syndrome
managed with, 209
description of, 179–180
Post-traumatic stress disorder
in children, 338, 343–345
description of, 322, 336
Powered air-purifying respirators, 7, 77
PPE. See Personal protective equipment
Pralidoxime, 582
Prayer, 376
Pressure control ventilation, 177–178
Pressure injuries, 308–309
Pressure meter dosing inhaler, 180, 181t
Pressure regulated volume cycled
ventilation, 177
Primary traumatic brain injury, 606–607
PRIS. See Propofol-related infusion
syndrome
Pro-inflammatory cytokines, 37t, 91
Problem-focused coping, 370
Procedural pain, 681
Prolonged intermittent renal
replacement therapies, 234–235
Prone position
acute respiratory distress syndrome
managed with, 218–219
advantages of, 25
complications of, 26
COVID-19-related respiratory failure
managed with, 14, 25–26, 308–309,
422
endotracheal tubes in, 30
mucosal pressure injuries in patients
in, 30
nurse's responsibilities, 25–26
Propofol, 165t, 171–172
Propofol-related infusion syndrome,
172
Protease-activated receptor-1, 92
Protease inhibitors, 391
Protein-calorie undernutrition, 309
Prothrombin complex concentrate
description of, 102
4-factor, 114
PRR. See Pattern recognition
receptors
PRRSV. See Porcine reproductive and
respiratory syndrome virus
PRVC. See Pressure regulated volume
cycled ventilation
Pseudomonas pseudomallei, 553
PSH. See Paroxysmal sympathetic
hyperactivity
Psittacosis, 567–568, 568f
Psychedelics, 588
Psychiatric disorders
in children, 338–348
COVID-19 and, 321
evaluation of, 322–323
in health care workers, 334–336
psychotropic medication for,
324–334
types of, 322
Psychotic disorders, 348
Psychotomimetic agents
clinical manifestations of, 588–589
complications of, 591
definition of, 585
deliriogenics, 585, 586t–587t, 588, 591
hallucinogens, 585, 586t–587t,
588–591
hyperthermia caused by, 591
stimulants, 585, 586t–587t, 588
treatment for exposure to, 590–591
types of, 586t–587t
Psychotropic medication, 324–334
PTSD. See Post-traumatic stress
disorder
Pulmonary artery occlusion pressure,
222
Pulmonary contusions, 629–632

Pulmonary embolism
  anticoagulation for, 100
  in critically ill patients, 99–100
  intermediate-risk, 101
  obstructive shock caused by, 142,
    144, 151
  treatment of, 151
Pulmonary embolism severity index,
  151
Push dose vasopressors, 132

Q
Q fever, 568–569, 569f
QT prolongation, 170, 175
Quetiapine, 166t, 331, 348

R
RAAS. *See* Renin-aldosterone-
    angiotensin system
Rapid response team, 30–31
Rapid sequence intubation, 12–13
Raxibacumab, 560
RDRP inhibitor. *See* RNA-dependent
    RNA polymerase inhibitor
RDRTF. *See* Renal Disaster Relief
    Task Force
Reactive oxygen species, 39–40
REBOA. *See* Resuscitative
    endovascular balloon occlusion of
    the aorta
Recombinant activated factor VII, 114
Recombinant factor VIIa, 182–183
Recombinant factor Xa, 102
Recombinant tissue type plasminogen
    activator, 101
Red blood cell transfusion, 105–107
Refractory hypoxemia, 216–218
Rehabilitation, for burns, 682–683, 690
Reintubation, 185–186
Remdesivir, 53–54, 250t, 417–418, 419t
Remifentanil, 164t, 169
Renal Disaster Relief Task Force, 237
Renal functional reserve, 229
Renal replacement therapy
  continuous, 233–234, 238t, 239
  in COVID-1P patients, 253
  in crisis, 237–240
  description of, 230–231
  extracorporeal, 234–235
  indications for, 233
  intermittent hemodialysis, 234, 237,
    238t
  modalities for, 233, 237–240,
    238t–239t
  in natural disaster situations, 601
  peritoneal dialysis, 235–236,
    238t–239t
  prolonged intermittent, 234–235
  summary of, 240
Renal system. *See also* Kidney(s)
  COVID-19 involvement of, 405, 408
  trauma to, 652–653
Renin-aldosterone-angiotensin system,
  136, 195
Reperfusion, 39–40
Repurposed drugs
  acalabrutinib, 43
  angiotensin-converting enzyme
    inhibitors, 44
  angiotensin receptor blocker, 44
  arbidol, 44–45
  azithromycin, 45
  bacillus Calmette Guerin, 46
  baricitinib, 45–46
  challenges of, 43
  chloroquine and hydrochloroquine,
    47
  corticosteroids, 47–48
  cyclosporine, 47
  eculizumab, 48
  famotidine, 49
  favipiravir, 49, 522
  heparin, 50
  interferons, 52
  interleukin-6 antagonists, 50–52
  ivermectin, 52–53
  lopinavir, 52
  methods to identify, 42–43
  methylene blue, 53
  remdesivir, 53–54, 250t, 417–418,
    419t
  ribavirin, 54
  ruxolitinib, 54–55
  sofosbuvir, 55
  statins, 55
  vitamin C, 56
  vitamin D, 56
  zinc, 56
Respiratory depression, opioid-induced,
  166, 170

Respiratory ECMP Survival Prediction score, 270, 272t

Respiratory failure
bronchodilators for, 12
continuous blood pressure monitoring in, 14–15
COVID-19-related, 12–15
Ebola virus as cause of, 484
high flow nasal cannula for, 12
intravenous access for, 14–15
intubation in, 12–13
mechanical ventilation for, 13–14, 29
prone position for, 14, 25–26, 308–309

Restraints, 307–308

Resuscitative endovascular balloon occlusion of the aorta, 653–654

Reverse transcriptase-polymerase chain reaction, 388–389, 412t

RFR. *See* Renal functional reserve

Rhabdomyolysis, 231, 456

Rib fractures, 629–630

Ribavirin
description of, 54
Hendra virus treated with, 517
Lassa fever treated with, 506
Middle East Respiratory Syndrome treated with, 393
Nipah virus treated with, 515
Rift Valley fever virus treated with, 522
SARS-CoV1 treated with, 390
yellow fever treated with, 503

Ricin toxin, 563

Ricinus communis, 563

Rickettsia typhi, 570, 571f

RIFLE, 228, 230

Rift Valley fever virus
in children, 541–542
clinical manifestations of, 520–521
complications of, 523
description of, 73t
diagnosis of, 522
epidemiology of, 518–519, 541
hemorrhagic disease caused by, 521
hepatitis associated with, 521
imaging of, 519f

infection control for, 522–523
jaundice caused by, 521
meningoencephalitis caused by, 521–522
ocular disease caused by, 521
outbreaks of, 518–519
pathogenesis of, 520
precautions for, 522–523
prevention of, 522
prognosis for, 523
transmission of, 519–520
treatment of, 522
vaccines for, 522
vectors of, 519–520

Right ventricle dilation, 145f

Riot controlling agents, 592–595

Rivaroxaban, 100–101

RNA-dependent RNA polymerase inhibitor, 53

Rocky Mountain spotted fever, 91

Rocuronium, 175, 176t

ROS. *See* Reactive oxygen species

Rotational thromboelastometry, 114–115

ROTEM. *See* Rotational thromboelastometry

RotoProne, 25

RRT. *See* Rapid response team

RSI. *See* Rapid sequence intubation

rtPA. *see* Recombinant tissue type plasminogen activator

Ruxolitinib, 54–55

RVFV. *See* Rift Valley fever virus

rVSV-ZEBOV vaccine, 486t, 488

S

SAC. *See* Sepsis-associated coagulopathy

Saccharin solution aerosol, 79

SAD. *See* Separation anxiety disorder; Social anxiety disorder

Salmonella, 566f, 566–567

Saltwater aspiration, 705

Sarilumab, 50–51, 421

Sarin, 554, 578, 580

SARS
blood transfusions for, 109t
description of, 73t
endocrinologic effects of, 195

SARS-CoV1
  blood transfusions for, 109t
  in children, 529–530
  clinical manifestations of, 385–387
  clinical presentation of, 529
  coagulation abnormalities associated
    with, 93–94
  computed tomography findings in,
    386–387
  diagnosis of, 388–389
  epidemiology of, 382, 529
  hematologic abnormalities associated
    with, 93–94
  history of, 381
  pathophysiology of, 383–385
  risk factors for, 382–383
  signs and symptoms of, 529
  treatment of, 390–392
SARS-CoV2. See also COVID-19
  anti-viral therapy for, 417–418, 420
  antigen testing for, 411, 426
  blood transfusions for, 109t
  in children, 530–531
  clinical manifestations of, 406–409
  clinical presentation of, 530–531
  coagulopathy caused by, 95
  description of, 73t, 82
  endothelial cell damage caused by,
    405
  epidemiology of, 402–404, 530
  extracorporeal membrane
    oxygenation uses in, 288–289
  gastrointestinal infection caused by,
    405
  heat decontamination of, 86
  in hepatocytes, 405
  hydrogen peroxide vapor for
    inactivation of, 83
  immune response dysregulation
    associated with, 94
  isolation for, 416–417
  laboratory workup for, 412
  monoclonal antibodies for, 420
  nucleic acid amplification testing with
    reverse transcriptase-polymerase
    chain reaction assay for, 409, 410t
  pathophysiology of, 404–406
  radiologic imaging of, 412–413
  reinfection of, 423
  sanitizers for, 85

  serology testing for, 411–412, 412t
  signs and symptoms of, 530
  systemic manifestations of, 407–409
  transmission of, 415
  treatment of, 417–418, 420
  vaccinations for, 423–425, 425t
  variants of, 409, 410t
SBT. See Spontaneous breathing trials
SCCM. See Society of Critical Care
    Medicine
Schizophrenia, 348, 456
Scrub typhus, 569–570
SE. See Surgical embolectomy
Seashore sign, 144, 144f
Second-degree burn, 676, 676t
Secondary traumatic brain injury,
    607–609, 611
Sedation
  benzodiazepines for, 170–171
  continuous, 171
  in intensive care unit, 170–174,
    329–330
  management of, 329–330
Sedatives
  clonidine, 173
  dexmedetomidine, 172–173
  ketamine, 173–174
  in older adults, 314–315
  phenobarbital, 174
  propofol, 171–172
  shortage of, 162–163
Seldinger technique, 601
Selective mutism, 342
Selective norepinephrine reuptake
    inhibitors, 344t, 346t
Selective serotonin reuptake inhibitors,
    343, 344t
Senna, 167t
Separation anxiety disorder, 340
Sepsis
  fluid resuscitation for, 128
  treatment of, 149t–150t
Sepsis-associated coagulopathy, 103
Septic shock
  cytokines in, 139
  multisystem organ failure in, 138
Septicemic plague, 465, 535
Sequential organ failure assessment,
    14, 353
Serial lactic acid, 138

Serotonin syndrome, 327, 328t, 590
Serratia marcescens, 553
Sertoli cells, 199
Shiga toxin, 564
Shigella, 553, 564, 565f
Shock
  adrenal insufficiency as cause of, 139–140, 148, 150
  anaphylactic, 139
  cardiogenic
    intra-aortic balloon pump for, 152
    pathogenesis of, 140–142
    treatment of, 152
    venoarterial extracorporeal membrane oxygenation for, 261
  definition of, 121, 129
  diagnosis of, 125–126
  distributive
    definition of, 139
    treatment of, 139, 148, 150
  early goal directed therapy for, 128
  echocardiography of, 140, 143f
  fluid resuscitation for
    access for, 126–127, 127t
    colloid fluids, 128, 131t, 148
    crystalloid fluids, 128–130, 130t, 148
    fluid overload caused by, 137–138
    intraosseous access for, 126–127, 127t
    large volume, 121
    permissive hypotension, 138–139
    responsiveness assessments, 128, 137–138, 146
    vascular access for, 126–127, 127t
  hemodynamic monitoring of, 138, 141
  hemorrhagic, 145, 147–148
  hypovolemic
    causes of, 145–147
    description of, 127, 140
    pediatric, 361
  monitoring in
    hemodynamic, 138, 141
    serial lactic acid, 138
  neurogenic, 139
  obstructive
    acute right heart syndrome as cause of, 142
    cardiac tamponade as cause of, 142–143, 143f, 151
    causes of, 142–144
    dynamic left ventricular outflow obstruction as cause of, 143–144
    pulmonary embolus as cause of, 142, 144, 151
    tension pneumothorax as cause of, 144
  pathogenesis of, 139–147
  prevalence of
    in natural disasters, 122–125
    in pandemics, 122
    in war, 121
  septic
    cytokines in, 139
    multisystem organ failure in, 138
    treatment of, 148, 149t–150t
  in thoracic trauma, 633
  treatment of, 147–152
  vasopressors and inotropes for
    acidosis, 137
    catecholamines, 133t–134t
    hypothermia, 137
    overview of, 132, 135
    push dose, 132
    route of administration, 137
    types of, 133t–134t
Shock index, 126
SI. *See* Shock index
Signal transduction, downstream, 37–38
Silent hypoxemia, 407
SIMV. *See* Synchronized intermittent mechanical ventilation
SIRS. *See* Systemic inflammatory response
Skeletal traction, 666
Skin grafts, for burn reconstruction, 684, 685t
Skull base fractures, 614
SLED. *See* Sustained low-efficiency dialysis
Small Portable Expeditionary Aeromedical Rapid Response team, 598, 599t–600t
Smallpox, 542–543, 555–557, 556f–557f
Smoke inhalation, 696–698
Social anxiety disorder, 342
Social coping, 371

Society of Critical Care Medicine
  description of, 3
  team-based care recommendations,
    23
SODs. *See* Sudden-onset disasters
SOFA. *See* Sequential organ failure
    assessment
Sofosbuvir, 55
Solid organ transplantation
  COVID-19 and, 249
  description of, 245
Soman, 580
SOT. *See* Solid organ transplantation
"Spanish flu," 435–437, 436t, 532
SPEARR team. *See* Small Portable
    Expeditionary Aeromedical Rapid
    Response team
Spike protein, 394, 404
Splenic trauma, 650–651
Spontaneous breathing trials, 185
Spontaneous pneumothorax, 627–628
SSC. *See* Surviving Sepsis Campaign
SSRIs. *See* Selective serotonin reuptake
    inhibitors
Stab wounds, 636
Standard precautions, 71–72
Staphylococcal enterotoxin B, 563–564
Staphylococcus aureus, 444–445, 563
Statins, 55
Sterofundin, 130t
Stimulant laxatives, 167t
Stool softeners, 166, 167t
Storms, 124–125
Streptococcus pneumoniae, 444
Streptomyces avermitilis, 52
Streptomycin
  plague treated with, 467, 467t
  tularemia treated with, 476
Stress hyperglycemia, 200–201
Stroke volume, 146–147
Stroke volume variation, 147
Subcapsular hematoma, 650–651
Subcutaneous emphysema, 183–184,
    185f
Subdural hemorrhage, 610
Submersion injuries, 704–708
Substance P, 593
Sudden-onset disasters, 122
Sufentanil, 164t, 169
Suicidal ideation, 345–346

Sulfur mustards, 579t, 582–583
Superior mesenteric artery, 653
Superoxide, 39
Surge capacity planning, for pediatric
    patients, 355–357
Surgical embolectomy, 151
Surgical instrument sterilization, 601
Surgical masks, 72, 73t, 76, 76f, 79
Surgical tracheostomy, 186–187
Surviving Sepsis Campaign, 128–129,
    135, 177, 252
Sustained low-efficiency dialysis,
    234–235, 238t
Swan-Ganz catheter, 264, 276
Swollen baby syndrome, 540
Synchronized intermittent mechanical
    ventilation, 177
Synesthesia, 591
Systemic inflammatory response, 677

T
T3. *See* Triiodothyronine
T4. *See* Thyroxine
t-PA. *See* Tissue plasminogen
    activator
Tabun, 580
TACO. *See* Transfusion associated
    circulatory overload
TBI. *See* Traumatic brain injury
TCD. *See* Transcranial Doppler
TEG. *See* Thromboelastography
Telemedicine, 8–9, 248, 252t
Tension pneumothorax, 144, 184–185,
    627
Tertiary traumatic brain injury, 609
Tetracycline, for plague, 467t–468t,
    468–469
Third-degree burn, 676t, 676–677
Thoracic trauma
  anatomy of, 627
  blunt
    aortic injury, 632–633
    cardiac injury, 633–634
    description of, 626, 630
    survival rate for, 641
  chest tubes for, 639–640
  description of, 626
  esophageal trauma, 635
  flail chest, 630
  mediastinitis, 635–636

Thoracic trauma (*Cont.*)
  motor vehicle accidents as cause of, 626
  open pneumothorax, 638
  penetrating, 626, 636–637
  pericardial effusion, 634
  pneumomediastinum, 627–629
  pneumothorax, 627–629
  pulmonary contusions, 629–632
  rib fractures, 629–630
  shock in, 633
  stab wounds, 636
  thoracotomy for, 640–642
  tube thoracostomy for, 638–639
Thoracotomy
  definition of, 640
  early, 641–642
  emergency department, 641
  late, 642
  thoracic trauma treated with, 640–642
  urgent, 641
Thorax, 627
Thrombin, 93
Thrombocytopenia
  in dengue hemorrhagic fever, 97
  Middle East Respiratory Syndrome and, 94
Thromboelastography, 114–115
Thromboembolism
  mechanisms of, 94
  venous. *See* Venous thromboembolism
Thrombosis
  in COVID-19 patients, 94
  hypoxemia stimulation of, 94–95
  in older adults, 306–307
  pandemic respiratory viruses and, 93–96
  pathophysiology of, 90–93
  platelet activation in, 92
  prevention of, 306–307
Thromboxane A2, 103
Thyroid disorders
  COVID-19 and, 198
  critical illness and, 197–198
Thyroid releasing hormone, 198
Thyroid stimulating hormone, 198
Thyroxine, 198
Tiered-based staffing, 11–12
Tissue plasminogen activator, 151

TMPRSS2. *See* Transmembrane serine protease 2
Tocilizumab, 50–51, 419t, 421
Tornadoes, 122–123, 597
Total body surface area, 677–678
Tourniquet test, 498, 498f
Toxic shock syndrome, 445
TP. *See* Trendelenburg position
Tracheostomy, 186–187
TRALI. *See* Transfusion-related acute lung injury
Tranexamic acid, 113, 183, 648
Transcranial Doppler, 617
Transforming growth factor-ß, 36t
Transfusion(s)
  acute hemolytic transfusion reaction, 111
  blood alternatives, 112–113
  blood products, 104–105
  in burn-injury patients, 108
  complications of, 110–112
  febrile reactions, 111
  fresh whole blood, 600–601
  human error in, 110–111
  intraoperative autologous, 113
  massive transfusion protocol, 107
  in pandemics, 108, 109t–110t
  plasma, 105–106
  platelets, 105–106
  red blood cells, 105–107
  restrictive strategy, 105
  in trauma, 106–107
Transfusion associated circulatory overload, 110–111
Transfusion-related acute lung injury, 110–111
Transfusion-related immunomodulation, 112
Transmembrane serine protease 2, 404
Transplantation
  candidates for, 246–248
  challenges associated with, 246
  in COVID-19 patients, 246–248, 254
  epidemiology of, 245–246
  ICU admittance after, 252
  immunosuppression for, 249
  overview of, 245
  in pandemics, 254
  recipients of, 249–252
  solid organ, 245

Transthoracic echocardiogram, 415
Trauma
  abdominal. *See* Abdominal trauma
  blood transfusions in, 106–107
  intestinal, 654–655
  liver, 651–652
  orthopedic. *See* Orthopedic trauma
  pelvic, 654
  shock caused by, 121
  splenic, 650–651
  thoracic. *See* Thoracic trauma
  war-related, 121
Trauma-focused cognitive behavioral
    therapy, 345
Trauma-induced coagulopathy, 104, 114
Traumatic brain injury
  blood-brain barrier disruption caused
    by, 608
  brain swelling caused by, 608
  burr hole craniotomy for, 619–620
  cerebral perfusion pressure in, 607,
    611
  cerebrospinal fluid leaks after,
    614–615
  closed, 614
  in combat environments, 618
  computed tomography of, 610
  in crisis environments, 618–620
  in crisis situations, 620
  decompressive hemicraniectomy
    after, 614
  definition of, 604–605
  diagnosis of, 609
  early resuscitation for, 620–621
  emergency department transport for,
    621
  epidemiology of, 605–606
  epidural hemorrhage caused by, 610
  EVD for, 611
  extra-axial hematoma in, 619
  FOUR score for, 605
  Glasgow Coma Scale, 605, 612
  herniation syndrome secondary to,
    619
  hyperosmolar therapy for, 613
  hyperthermia after, 612–613
  incidence of, 605–606
  intracranial pressure
    monitoring of, 611–615
    rising of, 607

  level of consciousness affected by, 610
  mild, 605, 618
  in military personnel, 606
  monitoring in
    ancillary techniques, 615–617
    automated pupillometry, 616
    carbon dioxide, 612
    cerebral venous thrombosis, 613
    continuous video
      electroencephalography, 615
    electroencephalography, 615
    intracranial oxygenation, 616
    intracranial pressure, 611–615
    invasive devices for, 617
    jugular bulb catheters, 616–617
    near-infrared spectroscopy, 617
    transcranial devices for, 616
    transcranial Doppler, 617
  neurogenic hyperthermia caused by,
    612
  outcome predictors, 621
  in pediatric patients, 362
  penetrating injuries, 606
  primary, 606–607
  secondary, 607–609, 611
  severity classifications for, 604–605,
    618
  skull base fractures, 614
  subdural hemorrhage caused by, 610
  tertiary, 609
  treatment of, 609–617
  venous thrombosis risks, 613–614
Trendelenburg position, 128
TRH. *See* Thyroid releasing hormone
Triage
  of abdominal trauma, 646–647
  for burns, 687
  in crisis incidents, 620
  for orthopedic trauma, 671
  of pediatric patients, 352–355
Tricyclic antidepressants, 344t
Triiodothyronine, 198
TRIM. *See* Transfusion-related
    immunomodulation
TSH. *See* Thyroid stimulating hormone
Tsunami, 597
Tube thoracostomy, for thoracic
    trauma, 628–629, 638–639
Tularemia, 73t, 473–476, 536–537
Tumor necrosis factor, 37t

TXA. *See* Tranexamic acid
Type III secretion system, 463
Typhoidal syndrome, 474
Typhus fever, 569–570, 571f

U
UFH. *See* Unfractionated heparin
Ulceroglandular syndrome, 474
Ultraviolet germicidal irritation, 80–81
Unfractionated heparin, 101, 103, 182, 421
United Organ Network for Organ Sharing, 246
UNOS. *See* United Organ Network for Organ Sharing
Urgent thoracotomy, 641
Urinary incontinence, 310
Urinary tract infection, 149t
UVGI. *See* Ultraviolet germicidal irritation

V
V-series nerve agents, 580
Vaccines
    anthrax, 560
    COVID-19, 423–425, 425t
    dengue virus, 499
    Ebola virus, 486t, 488–489
    influenza virus, 450–451, 452f
    MERS-CoV, 393–394
    plague, 470–471, 535
    Rift Valley fever virus, 522
    smallpox, 542–543, 546
    yellow fever, 503–505
VAD. *See* Ventricular assist device
Variola major, 542
Variola minor, 542
Vascular endothelial growth factor, 37t
Vasodilators, 221–222
Vasopressin, 134t, 136
Vasopressors
    catecholamines, 133t–134t
    hypothermia, 137
    hypothermia and, 137
    overview of, 132, 135
    push dose, 132
    route of administration, 137
    types of, 133t–134t
VATS. *See* Video-assisted thoracoscopy
VC. *See* Volume cycle ventilation

Vecuronium, 175, 176t
VEGF. *See* Vascular endothelial growth factor
Vena cava filters, for venous thromboembolism, 101
Venoarterial extracorporeal membrane oxygenation
    acute respiratory distress syndrome treated with, 219
    cannulation configurations for, 263f
    cardiac strain caused by, 263
    cardiac support goal of, 276, 278
    cardiogenic shock treated with, 261
    cerebral oxygenation in, 277
    description of, 257
    hybrid configurations, 264, 265f
    indications for, 261, 264–265, 266t
    management of, 276–278
    patient selection for, 270–271
    survival prediction score, 272t–273t
    Swan-Ganz catheter with, 276
    weaning from, 278, 279f
Venous filters, 307
Venous thromboembolism. *See also* Pulmonary embolism
    anticoagulation therapy for, 103
    antiplatelet therapy for, 103–104
    in COVID-19 patients, 94
    direct oral anticoagulants for, 100–103
    management of, 99–104
    in orthopedic trauma, 670–671
    pandemic respiratory viruses associated with, 93
    pathogenesis of, 670
    prophylactic therapy of, 419t
    traumatic brain injury as cause of, 613–614
    vena cava filters for, 101
    vitamin K antagonists for, 100–101
Venovenous extracorporeal membrane oxygenation
    acute respiratory distress syndrome treated with, 219–220
    algorithm for, 267, 268f
    in burn patients, 287
    cannulation configurations for, 262f
    description of, 257–258
    in drowning victims, 287

Venovenous extracorporeal membrane
    oxygenation (*Cont.*)
  H1N1 influenza pandemic treated
      with, 287–288
  indications for, 261, 265, 267
  lung recovery signs in, 279
  lung-rest as goal of, 278
  management of, 278
  patient selection for, 270
  respiratory failure treated with, 261,
      268f
  survival prediction score, 274t–275t
  thrombosis associated with, 276f
  in trauma patients, 287
  ventilatory settings in, 278
  weaning from, 278, 280
Ventilator induced lung injury, 183–185,
    185f
Ventricular assist device, 141
Vesicants, 582–585
Vibrio cholerae, 553, 565f, 565–566
Video-assisted thoracoscopy, 628m642
Vinyl gloves, 84–85
Viral hemorrhagic fevers, 96–97, 538–540
Virchow's triad, 306, 670
Visceral pleura, 627
Vitamin A, 375
Vitamin B9, 375
Vitamin B12, 375
Vitamin C, 56, 375
Vitamin D, 56, 375
Vitamin E, 376
Vitamin K antagonists
  international normalized ratio
      affected by, 106
  venous thromboembolism treated
      with, 100–101
Volcanic eruptions, 123, 597
Volume cycle ventilation, 177
von Willebrand factor, 91
VWF. *See* von Willebrand factor

W

Wang-Zwische, 261
Warm immersion injuries, 707
Weibel–Palade bodies, 92
Whole blood, 104–105
Wildfires, 123, 597
World Society of Emergency Surgery, 650

Wound care, for burns, 681, 682t,
    689–690
WSES. *See* World Society of
    Emergency Surgery

X
Xanthine oxidase, 39

Y

YEL-AND. *See* Yellow fever associated
    neurological disease
Yellow fever
  in children, 539–540
  clinical manifestations of, 502–503
  cytoarchitectural changes caused by,
      504f
  description of, 73t, 98
  diagnosis of, 503, 504f
  outbreaks of, 502
  pathogenesis of, 502
  prognosis for, 505
  treatment of, 503–505
  vaccine, 503–505
  vectors of, 501
  virions of, 502, 502f
Yellow fever associated neurological
    disease, 504
Yersinia outer membrane proteins, 463
Yersinia pestis, 462–471, 463f, 533, 535,
    553
Yersinia pseudotuberculosis, 471
YOPS. *See* Yersinia outer membrane
    proteins

Z
Z-plasties, 684
Zabdeno, 486t, 488
Zanamivir, 447, 448t
Zika virus, 109t
Zinc, 56
Zone of coagulation, 677
Zone of hyperemia, 677
Zone of stasis, 677
Zoonotic infections
  Ebola virus, 479
  Hendra virus, 516–518
  Nipah virus, 512–516
  Rift Valley fever virus, 518–523